Managed Care Pharmacy Practice

Second Edition

ROBERT P. NAVARRO, PharmD
Navarro Pharma, LLC

JONES AND BARTLETT PUBLISHERS

Sudbury, Massachusetts

BOSTON   TORONTO   LONDON   SINGAPORE

World Headquarters

Jones and Bartlett Publishers
40 Tall Pine Drive
Sudbury, MA 01776
978-443-5000
info@jbpub.com
www.jbpub.com

Jones and Bartlett Publishers
Canada
6339 Ormindale Way
Mississauga, Ontario L5V 1J2
Canada

Jones and Bartlett Publishers
International
Barb House, Barb Mews
London W6 7PA
United Kingdom

Jones and Bartlett's books and products are available through most bookstores and online booksellers. To contact Jones and Bartlett Publishers directly, call 800-832-0034, fax 978-443-8000, or visit our website www.jbpub.com.

Substantial discounts on bulk quantities of Jones and Bartlett's publications are available to corporations, professional associations, and other qualified organizations. For details and specific discount information, contact the special sales department at Jones and Bartlett via the above contact information or send an email to specialsales@jbpub.com.

The authors, editor, and publisher have made every effort to provide accurate information. However, they are not responsible for errors, omissions, or for any outcomes related to the use of the contents of this book and take no responsibility for the use of the products and procedures described. Treatments and side effects described in this book may not be applicable to all people; likewise, some people may require a dose or experience a side effect that is not described herein. Drugs and medical devices are discussed that may have limited availability controlled by the Food and Drug Administration (FDA) for use only in a research study or clinical trial. Research, clinical practice, and government regulations often change the accepted standard in this field. When consideration is being given to use of any drug in the clinical setting, the health care provider or reader is responsible for determining FDA status of the drug, reading the package insert, and reviewing prescribing information for the most up-to-date recommendations on dose, precautions, and contraindications, and determining the appropriate usage for the product. This is especially important in the case of drugs that are new or seldom used.

Production Credits

Publisher: David Cella
Editorial Assistant: Maro Asadoorian
Production Director: Amy Rose
Production Assistant: Julia Waugaman
Associate Marketing Manager: Lisa Gordon
Manufacturing and Inventory Control Supervisor: Amy Bacus

Composition: Arlene Apone
Cover Design: Brian Moore
Cover Image: © Aura Castro/ShutterStock, Inc.
Printing and Binding: Malloy Incorporated
Cover Printing: Malloy Incorporated

Library of Congress Cataloging-in-Publication Data
Managed care pharmacy practice / [edited] by Robert P. Navarro. — 2nd ed.
    p. ; cm.
Includes bibliographical references and index.
ISBN-13: 978-0-7637-3240-0
ISBN-10: 0-7637-3240-0
1. Pharmacy—Practice—United States. 2. Managed care plans (Medical care)—United States. 3. Insurance, Pharmaceutical services—United States. I. Navarro, Robert.
[DNLM: 1. Pharmaceutical Services—organization & administration. 2. Insurance, Pharmaceutical Services. 3. Managed Care Programs—organization & administration. QV 737 M2648 2009]
RS100.3.M356 2009
615'.1068—dc22
                                        2008035267
6048

Printed in the United States of America
12 11 10 09 08   10 9 8 7 6 5 4 3 2 1

DEDICATION

This book is dedicated to pharmacists everywhere who have developed and executed cost-effective managed prescription drug benefit programs. I include pharmacists within the pharmaceutical industry and government who support managed care programs.

This book is also dedicated to pharmacists and other healthcare professionals to whom we pass the challenge and responsibility to continue the evolution of future prescription drug benefits. Your patients, your profession, and indeed our country, depend upon your creativity and success.

Personally, my dedication includes Polly, who provided encouragement to complete this revision, and to Auggie, who faithfully stood watch, to make sure I did my job up until the end.

CONTENTS

v

FOREWORD

The evolution of the pharmacy profession has at its heart a migration to managed care principles. The spotlight now focused on our practice was spurred by the creation of the Medicare Part D program, which created unparalleled access to pharmaceuticals for millions by expanding medication coverage to the age 65-plus and disabled American population. The practice of pharmacy is truly coming of age with this incorporation of managed care elements that have produced quality, cost effective, and appropriate care for legions of patients.

The tools that managed care pharmacy uses to deliver on its promise of affordable access to appropriate medication therapy are intrinsic to a coordinated population-based approach to healthcare services. Forged in the crucible of providing medication coverage to more than 200 million Americans, formulary system management, drug utilization review, prior authorization programs, and the appropriate use of generics have all contributed to taming the escalation of prescription expenditures. These factors, combined with the transition of pharmacists from dispensers of pharmaceuticals to system design experts, to practitioners engaged in the hands-on delivery of medication therapy management services will establish a new level of excellence for the profession. Add in managed care's emphasis on external validation of quality of care and the stage is set for the profession to advance smartly.

What, you may ask, are the factors that will allow a pharmacist to succeed in this dynamic developing environment? The answer lies in the words of the experts in the field who have shared their knowledge and expertise in this volume. To do well in this emerging scenario demands an understanding and use of the concepts integral to the practice of managed care pharmacy. You have at your fingertips the know-how of those who have met the challenges of the insatiable demand for cost effective delivery of quality medication therapy.

Read, learn, embrace, and succeed.

Judith A. Cahill
Executive Director
Academy of Managed Care Pharmacy

INTRODUCTION

Healthy citizens are the greatest asset any country can have.
Winston Churchill

Many of us have witnessed, and indeed orchestrated, the evolution in the financing and delivery of managed pharmacy benefits over the past 30 years. Without rules or the crushing regulations that encumber us today, we created managed prescription drug benefits with the simple but arduous goal of optimizing pharmacy benefit quality while managing cost and utilization.

We came to early HMOs often with hospital or community pharmacy experience. While the principles of sound drug formulary development and management were congruent, the administration and execution of an outpatient managed pharmacy benefit was an art we learned on the job during our uncharted journey. We launched the Academy of Managed Care Pharmacy to provide a forum for others engaged in managed care pharmacy to share and learn from our successes and failures. At that time, we had no textbook to follow and no rulebook to chart our progress.

The *First Edition* of this textbook, published almost a decade ago, was an attempt to capture the best practices from some of the pharmacists who were responsible for developing managed prescription drug benefits. This *Second Edition* is the response to requests for an updated, contemporary text.

All chapters are updated to reflect recent changes in pharmacy benefit design, most notably the Medicare Modernization Act, the growth of specialty pharmacy, and the increasing use of health and economic outcomes data. The Medicare Part D benefit is perhaps the most dynamic benefit design change thus far this decade. Part D continues to evolve almost monthly, and the reader is advised to consult the Centers for Medicare and

Medicaid Services for the latest guidance on the Medicare drug benefit to supplement information provided in this textbook.

The passage of time and leadership are unrelenting and inevitable. What we have begun, others will build upon, although the process will never fully be complete. My desire is that future leaders will continuously pursue the adoption of new technologies and apply the science of pharmacy in ways that promote the individualized and appropriate use of the most cost-effective pharmaceuticals, and to be able to communicate the value of managed prescription drug benefits to healthcare policymakers.

I wish to acknowledge the significant contributions of Albert I. Wertheimer. Albert coauthored chapters, obtained the involvement of other authors, and provided valuable guidance during the long course of completing this revision.

On behalf of the chapter authors, we hope this textbook will be a valuable source of information and will help readers develop the next generation of managed prescription drug benefits.

Robert P. Navarro
S/V CIEL BLEU

CONTRIBUTORS

Mila Ann Aroskar, EdD, DSc(hon)
Emeritus Faculty Associate
Center for Bioethics
University of Minnesota
Minneapolis, MN

Allen W. Becker, BS Pharm, RPh
Director, Clinical Account Services
CVS/Caremark
Palatine, IL

Joseph E. Biskupiak, PhD, MBA
Research Associate Professor
University of Utah College of Pharmacy
Salt Lake City, UT

Garth E. Black, MBA
Vice President of Analytics and Insights
SXC Health Solutions, Inc.
Lisle, IL

Diana I. Brixner, RPh, PhD
Professor and Chair
Department of Pharmacotherapy
Executive Director Outcomes
    Research Center

President, International Society of
    Pharmacoeconomics and Outcomes
    Research (ISPOR)
Salt Lake City, UT

Judith A. Cahill, CEBS
Executive Director
Academy of Managed Care Pharmacy
Alexandria, VA

Kim A. Caldwell, RPh
Director, Competitive Health Analytics
Humana Pharmacy Solutions
McKinney, TX

Vicky Chan, PharmD, BCPS, CDE
Sr. Medical Scientific Liaison—
    Managed Care
Medical and Scientific Affairs, Diabetes
Novo Nordisk Inc.
Princeton, NJ

Michael J. Dillon, MS, RPh, FAMCP
Scientific Affairs Liaison
Santarus, Inc.
Cliffton Park, NY

William Francis, MBA, RPh
Director Business Development
MedImpact Healthcare Systems
Tucson, AZ

Raulo S. Frear, PharmD
Director, Pharmacy Services
The Regence Group
Plymouth, MN

Richard N. Fry, BS Pharm
Director of Programs
Foundation for Managed Care Pharmacy
Alexandria, VA

James E. Grzegorczyk, RPh, MS
Director of Pharmacy
Blue Care Network
Blue Cross Blue Shield of Michigan
Southfield, MI

**Rusty Hailey, PharmD, DPh,
   MBA, FAMCP**
Chief Pharmacy Officer and
Senior Vice President, Pharmacy Services
Coventry Health Care, Inc.
Franklin, TN

Elizabeth Taylor Holland, BS, MS
Regional Account Manager
Biogen Idec MA, Inc.
Atlanta, GA

**Kjel A. Johnson, PharmD, BCPS,
   FCCP, FAMCP**
Vice President, Strategic Operations
ICORE Healthcare
Orlando, FL

Vijay N. Joish, PhD
Director, Evidence Based Medicine–
   Health Outcomes
Internal Medicine and Oncology
Sanofi-Aventis
Bridgewater, NJ

John D. Jones, RPh, JD, FAMCP
Senior Vice President, Professional Practice
   & Pharmacy Policy,
Prescription Solutions
A UnitedHealth Group Company
Irvine, CA

Denise Kehoe, MBA, PhC, RPh, FAPhA
Vice President of Business Development
PharmMD
Deerfield, IL

James T. Kenney, BS, RPh, MBA
Pharmacy Operations Manager
Harvard Pilgrim Health Care
Wellesley, MA

Dale Kramer, RPh
Remark Associates LLC
Danville, CA

Alan Lyles, ScD, MPH, RPh
Henry A. Rosenberg Professor of Public,
   Private and Nonprofit Partnerships,
   University of Baltimore
Docent of Pharmaceutical Policy and
   Pharmacoeconomics, University
   of Helsinki
Senior Fellow, Center on Drugs and Public
   Policy, University of Maryland School of
   Pharmacy
Baltimore, MD

Daniel C. Malone, RPh, PhD
Professor
College of Pharmacy
University of Arizona
Tucson, AZ

Elaine Manieri, BS Pharm, RPh
Vice President, Strategic Product
   Management
CVS/Caremark
Hunt Valley, MD

Kevin J. McDermott, BA, BS
Vice President, Managed Markets
Daiichi Sankyo, Inc.
Parsippany, NJ

**Darlene M. Mednick, RPh, MBA,
  PhD, FAMCP**
Senior Vice President, Strategic
  Business Development
CareMed Pharmaceutical Services
Lake Success, NY

Mary Kay Owens, RPh, CPh
Clinical Associate Professor
Department of Pharmacy Health
  Care Administration
College of Pharmacy
University of Florida
President
Southeastern Consultants, Inc.
Tallahassee, FL

Andrew M. Peterson, PharmD
Associate Professor of Clinical Pharmacy
  and Chair
Department of Pharmacy Practice/
  Pharmacy Administration
Philadelphia College of Pharmacy
University of the Sciences
  in Philadelphia
Philadelphia, PA

Claiborne E. Reeder, RPh, PhD, FAMCP
Director
Xcenda
Distinguished Professor Emeritus
University of South Carolina
Columbia, SC

Timothy S. Regan, BPharm, RPh, CPh
Executive Director, Customer Insights
Xcenda
Palm Harbor, FL

Debi Reissman, PharmD
President
Rxperts, Inc.
Irvine, CA

John H. Romza, MS
Executive Vice President Research and
  Development / CTO
SXC Health Solutions, Inc.
Lisle, IL

Thomas M. Santella, BS, MLA
Assistant to the CEO & President
Lannett Company, Inc.
Philadelphia, PA

Kenneth W. Schafermeyer, PhD
Professor and Director of Graduate Studies
Director, Department of Liberal Arts and
  Administrative Sciences
St. Louis College of Pharmacy
St. Louis, MO

Hemal Shah, PharmD
Executive Director, Health Economics
  & Outcomes Research
Boehringer Ingelheim
  Pharmaceuticals, Inc.
Ridgefield, CT

Joan M. Siegel, MA
Consultant
JSB Healthcare Services
Longwood, FL

Douglas Stephens, RPh
Pharmacy Benefit Consultant
Stephens Pharmacy Benefit Consulting, LLC
Scottsdale, AZ

Lowell T. Sterler, RPh, MBA, FAMCP
Vice President, Pharmacy Services
Blue Cross Blue Shield of Florida
Jacksonville, FL

**Craig S. Stern, RPh, PharmD, MBA,
FASCP, FASHP, FICA, FLMI, FAMCP**
President
Pro Pharma Pharmaceutical Consultants, Inc
Northridge, CA

Norrie Thomas, PhD, MS, RPh
The Center for Leading Healthcare Change
University of Minnesota
Minneapolis, MN

Celynda Tadlock, PharmD, MBA
Regional Vice President
WellPoint NextRx
Roswell, GA

Paul N. Urick, RPh
Senior Vice President, Pharmacy Services
FutureScripts, LLC
FutureScripts Secure, LLC
Philadelphia, PA

Albert I. Wertheimer, BS, MBA, PhD
Director, Center for Pharmaceutical Health
Services Research
Temple University School of Pharmacy
Philadelphia, PA

T. Jeffrey White, PharmD, MS
Director, Clinical Analytics and
Health Outcomes
WellPoint NextRx
West Hills, CA

James M. Wilson, BS, MBA
President
Wilson Health Information, LLC
New Hope, PA

Marcus D. Wilson, PharmD
President
HealthCore
Wilmington, DE

Allan Zimmerman, RPh, MBA
Principal
RxDirections, LLC
Lincoln, NE

ROLE OF MANAGED CARE IN THE U.S. HEALTHCARE SYSTEM

ROBERT P. NAVARRO

JUDITH A. CAHILL

INTRODUCTION

Managed care is an approach to the delivery of healthcare services in a way that puts scarce resources to best use in optimizing patient care. Managed care principles are the basis for effective administration of pharmacy benefits. While it is true that a small portion of prescription drugs, less than 15%, is purchased through unreimbursed cash transactions, this amount is negligible and dwindling. The tenets of managed care, described below, have transformed the U.S. healthcare delivery system. The healthcare delivery revolution grew rapidly, especially in densely populated geographic regions following the passage of the Health Maintenance Organization (HMO) Act of 1973. However, rudimentary yet impressive managed care initiatives could be found in the United States almost 100 years ago. Managed care developed in response to unmet economic and social needs. Managed care is neither a singular process nor a static event. Rather, managed care is chimeric and dynamic, and is a highly regionalized—even local—phenomenon that is molded by territorial demands. The impact of managed care is both historic and immutable, yet even today, with the early growth of consumer-driven healthcare, managed care continues to morph, embracing vestigial elements of fee-for-service pharmacy. Managed care struggles to balance quality of care with cost efficiency, and it continues to evolve in an attempt to meet the needs of private and government plan sponsors as well as patient-members.

This chapter briefly explains the genesis, evolution, and fundamental features of managed care within the U.S. healthcare delivery system. By understanding the nature and purpose of managed care delivery and its financial principles, the reader will be able to identify, and perhaps forecast, future evolutionary states of managed healthcare pharmacy benefits.

While *managed* care implies a certain genetic structure, fundamental traits may be expressed or repressed to accommodate current and near-term market needs. Recognizing this element, the reader should bear in mind that although this chapter defines managed care from a classical, genealogical perspective, various types of organizations are, by definition, managed, yet may appear and function quite differently.

MARKET EVENTS SUPPORTING THE DEVELOPMENT OF MANAGED CARE IN THE UNITED STATES

At the beginning of the 20th century, health insurance was virtually nonexistent in the United States. Very early managed care plans developed in isolated pockets in the early and mid-twentieth century, often provided by an employer as an employee benefit (e.g., Western Clinic, Tacoma, WA, in 1910; Blue Cross and Blue Shield organizations during the 1930s; Kaiser Foundation Health Plans in 1937; Health Insurance Plan of Greater New York in 1944).[1] Broad medical insurance coverage is generally assumed to have begun with indemnity insurance post-World War II. Pilot HMO projects began in some progressive cities in the late 1960s and more broadly after the HMO Act of 1973 signed by President Richard Nixon, which provided funding for federally qualified HMOs. It is alleged that Paul Ellwood, MD, a Minnesota physician who found himself in Washington as a healthcare policy consultant, created the term *health maintenance organization (HMO)* as an egalitarian membership health promotion and delivery system that encouraged wellness and health prevention in addition to comprehensive acute and chronic care.

Throughout the second half of the twentieth century, Americans began to consider health insurance as a necessity rather than a luxury. Although many consider access to appropriate health care a right of citizenship, the United States is the only developed industrialized nation that does not provide universal health insurance coverage on a federal level to all of its citizens. The federal government does offer coverage to those over the age of 65 and the disabled through the Medicare Program and to the needy through a partnership arrangement with states through the Medicaid programs. The Medicare Modernization Act of 2003 added outpatient prescription drug coverage for Medicare beneficiaries through the establishment of Part D. As a result, the vast majority of Americans have some type of medical and pharmacy benefits. Tragically, there remain 46.6 million Americans, or 15.9% of the population, who had no healthcare coverage in 2005.[2] Health insurance coverage has become a highly coveted employee benefit as well as an emotionally-charged political issue. Often the ability to obtain health insurance is a reason people seek employment until they qualify for Medicare benefits or can self-insure.

FUNDAMENTAL CONCEPTS OF GROUP INSURANCE

Individuals who self-insure pay cash from their personal funds for all healthcare needs and services. Most individuals cannot afford to personally pay for surgery, chemotherapy, and expensive imaging studies. The group health insurance concept is built on a large group of individuals pooling a fixed amount of money (premiums) to pay for defined healthcare services needed by members of the group. Actuaries statistically forecast the anticipated healthcare needs of the group and the costs associated with their provision. The actuarial projections become the basis for determining the premium that must be collected in order to fund reimbursement for the covered services. The group may purchase reinsurance from an insurance carrier to protect themselves from extraordinary catastrophic claims. The group insurance concept allows covered healthcare costs and financial risk to be spread over an entire membership group, such that the *per capita* costs are reasonable and manageable.

In addition to paying a monthly premium, individuals who use covered healthcare services usually pay an out-of-pocket user fee in the form of a fixed copayment, a percent coinsurance, and/or a deductible amount. Copayments, coinsurance, and deductibles call for a portion of the actual costs for healthcare services to be paid by the individual using the services as a method of sharing the financial risk. Copayments, coinsurance, and deductibles also may be used as a tool to encourage individuals to use only necessary medical resources. Copayments and coinsurance are further discussed in Chapters 2 and 4. Healthcare services that are not a covered benefit are either payable in full by the individual receiving the service or end up being written off as a bad debt by the providing institution.

From the 1960s through the 1980s, the predominant type of group health insurance was indemnity insurance. The benefit design of indemnity insurance typically required covered individuals to pay 20% of billed charges after satisfaction of an annual deductible. The indemnity insurance company paid the 80% balance. This 80% balance was paid out of the pooled insurance premiums collected on behalf of the eligible group insurance members. The 20% coinsurance paid by the individual spread the financial risk between the group member and the insurer. It also discouraged the use of unnecessary medical resources. Often there was a cap or out-of-pocket maximum on the amount individuals had to pay in the event of an expensive healthcare catastrophe.

As a result of the 1973 HMO Act, managed care insurance became an option in many cities by the mid to late 1980s. Managed care was an evolutionary step beyond indemnity insurance that expanded the financial risk-sharing beyond member individuals and their insurance plans. For the first time it required healthcare providers—physicians, hospitals, pharmacies, and others—to also accept and share financial risk. In addition to expanding risk-sharing, managed care developed programs for greater integration of administrative claims, communication among healthcare providers, and the introduction of wellness and prevention programs. Finally, managed care became much more explicit in defining the benefits that were covered and those that were not as well as the rules patients had to access covered benefits.

GROWTH OF MANAGED CARE

Healthcare is a competitively market-driven industry in the United States. Similar to other markets, health insurance changed in response to current or anticipated customer desires and unmet needs. Both health insurers and HMOs (especially the federally qualified plans) became subject to state and/or federal regulations and oversight. The primary forces that continue to influence the evolution of healthcare delivery and insurance in the United States are local and national competitive market and healthcare policy issues.

In the 1980s and 1990s, the cost of covering the increasing number of both private commercial members, state Medicaid eligibles, and federal Medicare beneficiaries continued to climb without restraint. The 1990s saw most traditional healthcare insurers develop *de novo* managed care plans or modify existing indemnity products by introducing managed care tools such as utilization review and quality measurement.

Additionally, in the spirit of the original HMO concept of comprehensive services and preventive medicine, healthcare policy leaders believed that a managed healthcare plan could better coordinate healthcare delivery, manage resource utilization, and implement preventive care and disease management systems superior to fragmented indemnity insurance.

Managed care offered to solve two fundamental societal health issues: rising healthcare costs, and fragmented healthcare delivery.

1. Managed care promised cost savings for healthcare purchasers compared to traditional indemnity insurance. Under traditional indemnity insurance, healthcare resource utilization was uncontrolled, and resources were prescribed and consumed at the caprice of physicians and patients. Physicians were not at financial risk, and often did not consider the cost of the resources they ordered. Conversely, managed care had a defined, inclusive list of covered benefits and services, and used financial incentives to influence physicians and patients to follow health plan policies and procedures and use resources in a cost-effective manner. Whereas traditional indemnity insurance accepted and paid fee-for-service claims from any provider, managed care only paid claims submitted by contracted healthcare providers willing to accept discounted reimbursement. Managed care plans monitored and controlled health resource utilization, and prevented over- or unnecessary utilization by requiring prior authorization for non-emergency surgeries and expensive drugs or procedures.

2. Managed care offered an integrated financing and delivery system that included preventive care and coordinated chronic care for members. By processing all covered health encounter claims, health plans were able to monitor an individual's total healthcare experience, and coordinate care when appropriate. The comprehensive claims database also allowed health services researchers to measure clinical and economic outcomes, and recommend improvements in the delivery of quality care.

Thus, it was concern over rising costs and the desire to better manage both healthcare delivery and health outcomes that drove the growth and acceptance of managed care by private and public purchasers and by healthcare policymakers. In general, managed care was successful in accomplishing these two objectives when compared with traditional fee-for-service medicine and indemnity insurance. In the 1990s, a managed prescription drug benefit could reduce pharmacy costs by 10% to 40% compared with an unmanaged pharmacy program, depending upon the aggressiveness of the pharmacy benefit management. Managed care systems incorporated tools that coordinated care in a cost-efficient manner through:

- Implementation of population-based healthcare screening programs
- Use of disease and case management
- Development of an integrated database that allowed the measurement of and reduction in practice variation
- Use of health outcomes research to identify the most cost-beneficial expenditure of healthcare resources

Today, a dizzying array of managed care organizations and benefit designs are managing the cost and care of almost 85% of the U.S. population, notwithstanding the 46 million uninsured. **Figure 1-1** illustrates the rise in U.S. healthcare expenditures (in millions of dollars) from 1975 to 2005.[3] From the mid-1980s onward, managed care began to replace indemnity insurance. The graph shows the cost of healthcare has continued to spiral upwards, seemingly undaunted by the growing presence of managed care. However, what is not known is what the expenditures would have been if managed care had not been introduced.

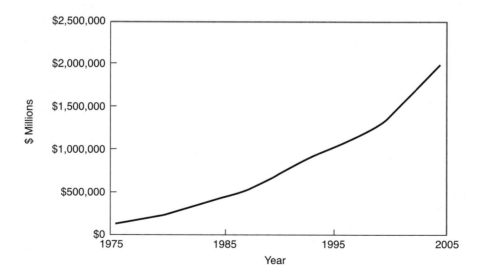

FIGURE 1-1   U.S. Healthcare Expenditures 1975–2005 (Millions of Dollars).
Source: Data are from the CMS U.S. Health Expenditures 1960–2005. Available at http://www.cms.hhs.gov/NationalHealthExpendData/ 02_NationalHealthAccountsHistorical.asp#TopOfPage. Accessed 26 May 2008.

MANAGED CARE TERMINOLOGY

A new lexicon of terms accompanied the growth of managed care, some of which are not universally accepted and require further definition. We have already introduced the term *health maintenance organization (HMO)* to refer, in general, to a managed care health plan. Two decades ago, we more easily categorized HMOs as one of four discrete types, or models, using classical definitions[4]:

1. *Staff model:* The staff model HMO owns healthcare facilities (e.g., physician offices with pharmacies, hospitals), and healthcare professionals are salaried employees. Staff model HMOs have high control and lower costs, but offer fewer choices of providers for members. Although several staff model plans flourished in the 1980s and 1990s, most are no longer in existence.
2. *Group model:* Pure group model HMOs contract with a large multispecialty physician group. Physicians are employed by the group practice but not the HMO. Kaiser Permanente and Geisinger Health Plan are examples of group model HMOs.
3. *Network model:* In a network model HMO, the HMO contracts with more than one multispecialty group practice. Health Insurance Plan (HIP) of New York was an example of a network HMO.
4. *Independent practice association (IPA) model:* This popular HMO model contracted with many independent community-based physicians (individual physicians as well as group practices) to provide care.

The greater level of control of staff in group model plans often resulted in lower costs but with reduced freedom of choice of providers and benefit levels for members. In contrast, the network, and especially the IPA model HMOs, offered more choice but because they were able to exert a lower level of control over providers and members, often had higher costs. Therefore, plan purchasers had to choose between lower costs and greater freedom of choice. In this book, staff and group models are often combined together as similar "closed" models that use a limited number of defined, and owned or affiliated, medical groups, often with employee providers and owned facilities. Similarly, network and IPA models are often combined together as "open" models that generally contracted with a broad array of independent community-based providers or large medical groups and rarely owned facilities. The general relationship between level of control, benefit richness, and cost is shown in **Figure 1-2**.

By the late 1980s, many HMOs began offering plans with more options with broad provider networks, often at a slightly higher cost. An example of such a plan is a Preferred Provider Organization (PPO). Some HMOs combined a higher benefit/higher cost option with a lower benefit/lower cost plan, called a Point-of-Service (POS) plan. A POS gave the member the choice within a single plan to access more HMO benefits (at a lower copayment) or PPO benefits (at a higher copayment). Plans with similar names often have very different levels of benefits covered within a broad cost structure. Plan sponsors desired more choice of benefits and larger community-based providers, and favored open

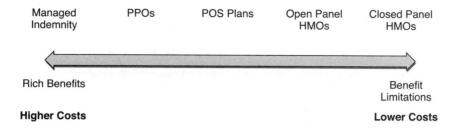

FIGURE 1-2 Continuum of Cost and Control Among Managed Care Organizations.

model plans (network and IPA HMOs) more than closed model plans (staff and group HMOs). Today, it is rare to find a pure HMO model plan, as most are hybrids that offer a broad array of health benefit programs (often called "products") under one company. Additionally, another type of specialized organization exists that exclusively manages pharmacy benefits called *pharmacy benefit managers* (*PBMs*). They are discussed in depth in Chapter 3. This range of control, costs, and level of benefits of HMOs and other insurance products are illustrated in Figure 1-1.

We use the terms *managed care organizations (MCOs)* and *health plans* interchangeably to refer to a managed care delivery system that is not a pure PBM. We will use the term *PBM* when we wish to address only pharmacy benefit management organizations.

In addition to the health benefit programs offered to employer groups and corporations, often termed *commercial plans*, many managed care organizations developed an array of product offerings:

- Managed Medicaid and Medicare programs
- Individual products offered to an individual or family
- Department of Defense TRICARE programs

Entities that purchase healthcare benefit products are often termed *plan sponsors*, as they may design, select, and purchase a program on behalf of their employees (for commercial purchasers) or beneficiaries (for state Medicaid programs, or the Centers for Medicare and Medicaid Services, [CMS], for Medicare programs). The terms *payer* or *payor* or *third party payor* is often confusing, and may refer to the MCO or health plan, or the plan sponsor (employers, Medicaid, or CMS [for Medicare]). We will use the term *payor* to refer to plan sponsors.

Individual patients who enroll in a commercial plan are termed *subscribers*. Often dependent family members are also covered under the policy. Together, subscribers and covered dependents are collectively termed *members, covered lives,* or *enrollees* of a health plan. Patients and dependents that are enrolled in Medicare programs are termed *beneficiaries*. Patients who are covered by state Medicaid programs are termed *eligibles*. Managed behavioral or mental health organizations call their members *clients*. Healthcare professionals, including physicians, pharmacists, and nurses, are generally referred to as *providers*, and pharmacies are often called *pharmacy providers*.

COMPONENTS AND ATTRIBUTES OF MANAGED HEALTH CARE

While all managed care organizations are slightly different in their version of managed care, three seminal tenets embody the philosophy of all healthcare that is "managed."

1. First, managed care is a subscription, partially pre-funded healthcare delivery system with explicitly defined contributions and covered benefits. Through a contract filed with state regulatory agencies, the health plan or PBM defines what benefits are and are not covered, the premium cost to the plan sponsor and members as well as individual member deductibles, benefit caps (maximums), copayments, or coinsurance amounts to be paid whenever a specifically covered healthcare service (e.g., prescription, physician visit, surgery) is accessed.
2. Second, all stakeholders and participants of the managed care system (healthcare providers as well as health plans, plan sponsors, and individuals) are financially and contractually linked so that each participant shares in the financial risk, and has the ability to have some level of control or influence over the use and cost of covered services.
3. Managed care controls overall costs by controlling the supply and demand of all healthcare resources. The supply of all resources is controlled through defined benefit limitations, and contracts with all providers of products and services, including all hospitals, physicians, pharmacies, venders, and other providers. The demand of all healthcare resources is influenced by requiring a member to pay a copayment or coinsurance amount whenever a resource is accessed.

In-patient hospital benefits, outpatient medical benefits, and pharmacy benefits are the three largest cost centers for health plans. Hospital and outpatient medical services (including physician, dental, diagnostic, and other services) are generally managed under the medical benefit, whereas the pharmacy benefit is generally managed separately. Infused drugs are often managed by the pharmacy department but may be a financial component of the medical benefit. Specialty pharmacy benefits are discussed in Chapter 22. Pharmacy benefits can be managed internally by a health plan pharmacy department, externally by a separate PBM, or the pharmacy benefits can be jointly managed by the internal health plan pharmacy department with assistance by an external PBM (discussed in Chapter 3). The reader is also referred the glossary of managed care terms on the Academy of Managed Care Pharmacy Web site (http://www.amcp.org).

The legal contract between a health plan, MCO, or PBM, and the purchasing plan sponsor is often called the *Certificate of Coverage (CoC)*. *Evidence of Coverage (EoC)* is another similar term. The CoC explicitly defines what benefits are included in the contract, what benefits are excluded by the contract, and the manner in which the member must access covered benefits (e.g., by using only a participating provider with payment of a defined copayment). This is called the *benefit design*. One MCO may offer numerous benefit designs to accommodate the needs of various plan sponsors. Indemnity insurance coverage of the past had few coverage limitations, which produced higher and less predictable costs. By contrast, managed care covers selective, appropriate healthcare services to meet member needs. These services focus on the fundamental healthcare needs of members. Not all healthcare services may be covered, particularly those that are highly discretionary. Some services may be covered with a high copayment or coinsurance.

The CoC is a legal document and is filed with the regulatory authority that would be a state agency for a state chartered plan or CMS for a Medicare program. As the CoC may be a cumbersome legal document, health plans often provide members with both the CoC and a simplified summary of benefits and instructions on how to access covered services. Chapter 4 addresses the contractual relationship between the health plans and plan sponsors.

HOW MANAGED CARE ORGANIZATIONS MANAGE FINANCIAL RISK

A fundamental cost management strategy of managed care is to use financial risk-sharing to influence the behavior of all stakeholders in the healthcare delivery system to make cost-effective decisions. All providers of care (physicians, hospitals, pharmacies, etc.) must accept discounted reimbursement rates and often have financial incentives to influence cost-effective decisions. Physicians may receive incentives for achieving performance standards (Pay for Performance), and members pay lower copayments to access lower cost drugs or those known to produce valuable outcomes for patients with chronic conditions. Equipment vendors offer competitive bids to acquire contracts. Drug companies offer discounts and rebates in exchange for preferred formulary coverage (discussed in Chapter 15). Plan sponsors pay a premium for defined benefits, and member must pay a copayment whenever care is accessed. The financial risk-sharing mechanisms are summarized in **Table 1-1**, and the relationship among the stakeholders is illustrated in **Figure 1-3**.

TABLE 1-1   Examples of Managed Care Financial Risk-Sharing Mechanisms

Managed Care Stakeholder	Financial Risk-Sharing Mechanisms
Physicians	Discounted reimbursement (capitation, discounted fee-for-service); performance incentives
Hospitals	Discounted reimbursement (contract and case rates; per diem rates)
Pharmacies	Discounted reimbursement; generic dispensing incentives; drug formulary; quality, step, and other edits; prior authorization of certain drugs
Plan Sponsors	Premium increases for excessive costs
Members	Premium share payments; copayments and coinsurance

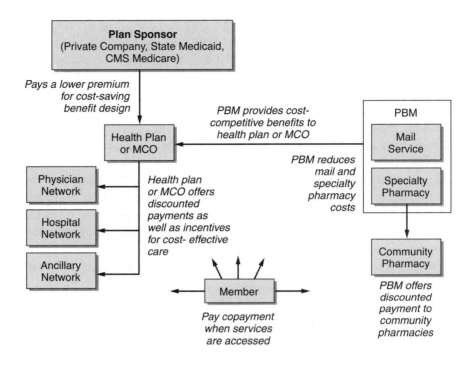

FIGURE 1-3   Managed Care Flow of Money and Financial Risk-Sharing Relationships.

UNDERWRITING TO FORECAST PLAN SPONSOR FINANCIAL RISK

Managed care organizations statistically examine the defined population they are expected to provide with health benefits coverage in order to forecast how much it will cost to provide the expected level of resource utilization. Through this analysis, called *underwriting*, the health plan or insurer can forecast the financial cost (risk) the health plan may incur to provide the medical and pharmacy benefits that are defined in the benefit product the plan sponsor decides to purchase. Based upon the projected financial risk, the health plan or insurer can determine the monthly fee (premium) the plan sponsor and members will pay as well as the copayment or coinsurance the members will pay to access covered health services. The group members covered by the plan are referred to as the *risk pool*. The value of a large population risk pool is that the costs generated by healthcare claims (e.g., high cost, high prevalence diseases, health wellness programs, rare diseases, transplants, catastrophic claims) may be spread over the entire risk pool for a lower *per capita*, or per-member cost, although costs depend upon the benefit design. The benefit design is developed to share the financial risk with the plan sponsor through premiums as well as members through copayments, coinsurance, and deductibles, and to encourage the cost-effective use of healthcare resources.

Health plans assess the financial performance (profitability or loss) of each plan sponsor contract. Health plans divide the total healthcare expenditures by the total premium income for a specific plan sponsor to determine the *medical loss ratio (MLR)*. For example, if $100 is taken in as premium, and $90 is spent on medical services, the MLR is 90% (and the health plan saved 10%, part of which is kept as profit or retained earnings for non-profit organizations). An MLR of 90 or better is generally acceptable. If the premium taken in is $90 but the cost of healthcare services provided is $100, the MLR is 111%, and the health plan lost money. For the subsequent year, the health plan will increase the plan sponsor's premium, or insist that the sponsor's benefit design include more strident limitations (e.g., higher copayment) to help reduce inappropriate utilization or increase member cost-sharing. If the plan sponsor refuses, the health plan may not offer the plan sponsor a contract for the subsequent year. Through this mechanism, plan sponsors are encouraged to develop an effective benefit design, and copayment structure to encourage member responsibility in accessing healthcare services.

PHYSICIAN CONTRACTING AND REIMBURSEMENT MECHANISMS

Physician reimbursement depends upon the organizational structure of the managed care organization. Physicians employed by a staff model HMO are usually salaried, and often receive a bonus or incentive linked to plan performance. Physicians not salaried are often reimbursed through either capitation, or a discounted fee-for-service (FFS) contract. They may also qualify for a bonus linked to plan or individual performance (termed *pay for performance*, or abbreviated *P4P*). Physician capitation or discounted FFS reimbursement are the two reimbursement mechanisms most commonly used by MCOs, which are predominantly not staff or group model plans.

Capitation Reimbursement Under capitation arrangements, a physician (or medical group) receives a fixed monthly fee for providing covered services based upon the number of enrolled members that are assigned to the physician or medical group for a given month. The physician or medical group receives the same monthly fee per capita (per assigned member) regardless of how many times the members may see the physician or how many covered services the physician provides for members. Through capitation, the HMO transfers a portion of the financial risk to the physician. Theoretically, this will serve as an incentive to the physician to cost-effectively provide only needed care. While covered services will vary by contract, they often include all outpatient visits, preventive care, common laboratory, and other office-based services. Prescriptions may or may not be included. If the capitation includes pharmacy costs, the medical group will often develop its own drug formulary to encourage the use of the most cost-effective drugs. Physicians often share the financial risk for patients who are hospitalized, as an incentive to provide appropriate outpatient care and to prevent unnecessary admissions.

Discounted FFS Reimbursement Under discounted FFS reimbursement mechanisms, physicians receive a payment whenever they provide covered services to a health plan patient. However, their reimbursement is discounted from usual and customary (U & C) reimbursement rates, and may be based upon the Resource Based Relative Value Scale (RBRVS) reimbursement rates developed by the California Medical Society. This provides a mechanism to reduce costs per service, and the reimbursement is often adjusted geographically as well as by demographic underwriting of the covered population. Also, physicians generally receive only a portion of the reimbursement at the time services are rendered (often 80%). The remaining 20% is withheld and maintained in a reserve to be paid out at the end of the year if certain plan and physician performance objectives are met. At the end of the year, the utilization of services and financial performance of physicians within a specialty group are reviewed and compared. High-risk outlier members that may unfairly skew the financial performance are eliminated. Physicians that do not perform efficiently (i.e., are most costly) forfeit their 20% reserve payment. Physicians that consistently are poor performers may be terminated from participating with the MCO. Physicians who are "average" performers receive their 20% reserve payment. Physicians who are the most efficient and least costly will receive a bonus, that is essentially the 20% withhold from the least efficient physicians. Through this mechanism, physicians within each specialty group compete among themselves, and physicians receive periodic "report cards" to help them monitor their performance and reduce inefficient practice variation.

Primary Care Physicians as Gatekeepers The "gatekeeper" concept, less common today, required members to obtain permission from their primary care physician (PCP) in order to consult a physician specialist. The dual purpose for gatekeeping was to allow the PCP to coordinate care and to minimize the use of more expensive specialists. Most MCOs found this to be inefficient and realized that specialists may be more cost-effective for many medical conditions. Most MCOs have eliminated the gatekeeper concept and allow members to "self-refer" to specialists, although there may be a higher copayment charged for specialist services.

Pay For Performance A logical extension of financial risk-sharing with physicians is to pay physicians a financial incentive when they achieve pre-defined clinical and or financial performance benchmarks that are structured to encourage the achievement of preferred clinical outcomes at the lowest net cost (cost-efficiency). Examples of managed care pay for performance programs include:

1. CMS P4P programs for cost-efficient care in Medicare.[5]
2. Employers and MCOs that embrace the Bridges to Excellence (Diabetes Care Link, Cardiac Care Link, and Spine Link) programs.[6]
3. MCOs pay incentives to physicians for improving HEDIS[7] measure scores.
4. State Medicaid physician Pay for Performance programs.[8]

Ancillary Service "Carve Outs" Managed care is an extremely competitive business and is evolving to meet the expanding expectations of payers and members. Many MCOs offer a variety of optional "ancillary" benefits (beyond traditional hospital, physician, and pharmacy benefits), including dental, chiropractic, podiatry, vision, wellness, massage therapy, expanded durable medical equipment, mental health, acupuncture, and other alternative healthcare options. MCOs can customize a benefit design and premium and member cost sharing schedules to meet specific plan sponsor needs.

The term *carve-out* means that the plan sponsor removes (or carves out) a specific benefit from the internal health plan delivery system and offers the benefit through an external company that specializes in providing a particular ancillary benefit in a cost-efficient manner. Carve-out benefits often include benefit maximums (e.g., a maximum number of covered visits), and may include a higher copayment or coinsurance.

PURSUIT OF QUALITY

Managed care has created unprecedented competition among U.S. healthcare delivery systems. As a result of comprehensive claims databases, health plans could measure their costs as well as their clinical and economic outcomes, and identify the most cost-effective physicians, hospitals, and drugs. If these outcomes can be measured, they can be managed to minimize variation, and optimize use of resources. MCOs have identified the top medical conditions by cost, prevalence, incidence, and other parameters, and have implemented disease and care management programs to deal with these top diseases. The Disease Management Association of America[9] provides educational resources and is a clearinghouse for disease management activities focused on high cost and high prevalence medical conditions, including obesity, hypertension, dyslipidemia and coronary heart disease, asthma, congestive heart failure, and several others.

National organizations, such as National Committee for Quality Assurance[10], The Leapfrog Group[11], The Joint Commission (JCAHO)[12], URAC[13], and various local organizations began measuring, accrediting, and publicly publishing health plan, physician, and hospital performance report cards to prospective purchasers as an incentive for plans to provide the most cost-effective healthcare. As a result of the market competition, plans must provide the benefits, cost, and outcomes demanded by plan sponsors in order to remain in business.

Health care, and especially commercial managed care, is a highly competitive, market driven business. Plan sponsors and members have access to an increasing amount of information to select the health plan that best satisfies specific cost management and benefit design demands. Managed care organizations are constantly evolving to meet and anticipate market demands. The market is also consolidating, with health plans acquiring others, PBMs merging, chain pharmacies buying PBMs through various horizontal and vertical integrations.

The plan sponsors and consumers should benefit from the market competition; however, with costs continuing to increase, plan sponsors and health plans are requiring members to pay higher and higher copayments and coinsurance percentages, and are subjecting members to higher deductible amounts and lower benefit caps. The future consumer of health care must be better informed, must practice self care for disease prevention, and must make wise choices when accessing more restrictive healthcare benefits.

FUTURE TRENDS AND CONSUMER-DRIVEN HEALTH CARE

Despite the pervasiveness of managed care, healthcare costs continue to escalate. However, the U.S. market has been dynamic, and significant changes have occurred over the past two decades, most of which have contributed to an increase in utilization of healthcare resources.

- The population grew by 20% to 300 million.[15]
- A greater percent of the U.S. population (85%) has healthcare insurance and pharmacy benefit coverage, including expensive subgroups (e.g., Medicaid, Medicare).
- The average life expectancy grew by almost 5 years to 77 years, increasing the percent of the population over 65 years, the highest utilizers of healthcare services.[16]
- The cardiovascular, cerebrovascular, cancer, homicide death rates declined, while the death rate from diabetes has increased.
- New drugs, including biotechnology agents, have improved outcomes for many life-threatening illnesses (see previous bullet), but the pharmacy benefit cost of managed care organizations has quadrupled.

Despite the improvements in quantity and quality of care, the U.S. population and plan sponsors are unable to maintain the same level of medical and pharmacy benefit coverage without greater cost-sharing with members. In response to plan sponsor requests, MCOs and PBMs are making significant changes in benefit design and healthcare delivery:

- Many new drugs are high cost, often injectable, bioengineered drug products. Managed care is depending upon specialty pharmacies (see Chapter 22) to optimize cost and utilization.
- Benefit designs include more formulary limitations and edits to better manage utilization of high costs drugs. The use of generic drugs before branded agents is often required, or heavily incentivized.
- Benefit coverage maximums are often capped at lower amounts, thus limiting the total dollar amount of benefits covered.
- Up-front member deductibles are more common and higher, and the member must pay $2,500 out-of-pocket before health insurance covers any benefits.
- Member copayments and coinsurance levels are increasing. Twenty years ago, the average brand copayment represented 25% of the total prescription cost. Today it is often 40% or more.

In summary, there will be increased financial authority and responsibility given to the member through deductibles, copayments, and coinsurance amounts. Rather than have "first dollar" coverage with no deductible, the member will have to "spend down" his or her deductible with out-of-pocket dollars before covered benefits are accessible. This benefit change is termed *consumer-driven healthcare (CDH)*, and indicates the member will be given the authority and responsibility to make healthcare decisions and spend his or her healthcare resources with benefit design limitations.

CDH is a general concept that takes on many different forms among health plans and insurers. One of the popular CHF insurance products is called a *Health Savings Account (HSA)*, which is essentially a personal healthcare savings account that can follow a member for life, through many different insurers. HSAs typically have a relatively lower premium cost, but also has much higher front-end deductibles (often $2,500 per individual or $5,000 per family) that must be paid out-of-pocket before benefits are accessed. After the deductible is satisfied, covered benefits are accessed. HSAs often waive a deductible payment for certain preventive care services, such as an annual physician exam.

CDH-type plans present cost-sharing opportunities for MCOs, but must be accompanied with member education so that members spend their money wisely to make the best long-term healthcare decisions. An uneducated member may refuse to spend his or her own money for necessary preventive or wellness care, and may not avoid a preventable illness. This may result in an avoidable and expensive hospitalization that will be a covered benefit, thus shifting the costs back to the insurance company. As a result of these potentially perverse and misaligned incentives, MCOs are spending enormous resources on health and wellness education, health risk assessment and screening, and often paying members to access such services.

CONCLUSION

Managed care is the current primary economic and social choice in the United States for delivering quality health care in a cost-efficient manner. Managed care has specific policies and procedures all stakeholders must follow for the system to function properly. A basic tenet of managed care is to involve all stakeholders in the financial risk of the healthcare delivery process. Managed care is no longer an alternative form of healthcare delivery. It is now considered the main financing and delivery mechanism for healthcare within the United States. CDH changes in health care coverage promise to contain rising costs for plan sponsors, but can only do so if members are educated and become a partner in achieving clinical, economic, and quality of life outcomes.

REFERENCES

1. Fox P.D. and Kongstvedt P.R, "The Origins of Managed Care," in Kongstvedt P.R. (ed.): *Essentials of Managed Health Care*, 5th Ed., Sudbury, MA: Jones and Bartlett Publishers; 2007, p. 3–18.
2. Center on Budget and Policy Priorities, "The Number of Uninsured Americans Is at All-Time High," 29 August 2006. Available at http://www.cbpp.org/8-29-06health.htm. Accessed 26 May 2008.
3. Department of Health and Human Services, Centers for Medicare & Medicaid Services, National Health Expenditures by Type of Service and Source of Funds: Calendar Years 1960–2006. Available at http://www.cms.hhs.gov/NationalHealthExpendData/02_NationalHealthAccountsHistorical.asp. Accessed on 26 May 2008.
4. Wagner E.R. and Kongstvedt P.R., "Types of Managed Care Organizations and Integrated Health Care Delivery Systems," in Kongstvedt P.R. (ed.): *Essentials of Managed Health Care*, 5th Ed., Sudbury, MA: Jones and Bartlett Publishers; 2007, p. 19–40.
5. Department of Health and Human Services, CMS Office of Public Affairs, "Medicare Pay For Performance (P4P) Initiatives," 31 January 2005. Available at http://www.cms.hhs.gov/apps/media/press/release.asp?Counter=1343. Accessed 26 May 2008.
6. Bridges to Excellence homepage. Available at http://www.bridgestoexcellence.org/. Accessed 26 May 2008.
7. National Committee for Quality Assurance. 2006 NCQA HEDIS measures. Available at http://www.ncqa.org/tabid/366/Default.aspx. Accessed 26 May 2008.
8. The Commonwealth Fund homepage. Pay-for-Performance in State Medicaid Programs: A Survey of State Medicaid Directors and Programs. 12 April 2007. Available at http://www.cmwf.org/publications/publications_show.htm?doc_id=472891. Accessed 26 May 2008.
9. The Disease Management Association of America (DMAA) homepage. Available at http://www.dmaa.org/dm_definition.asp. Accessed 26 May 2008.
10. National Committee for Quality Assurance, The NCQA homepage. Available at http://web.ncqa.org/. Accessed 26 May 2008.
11. The Leapfrog Group homepage. Available at http://www.leapfroggroup.org/. Accessed 7 May 2007.
13. Utilization Review Accreditation Commission, The URAC homepage. Available at http://www.urac.org/. Accessed 26 May 2008.
14. Consumer Driven Health Care homepage. Available at http://www.consumerdrivenhealthcare.us/. Accessed 26 May 2008.
15. Infoplease homepage. Available at http://www.infoplease.com/year/1985.html. Accessed 26 May 2008.
16. Center for Disease Control and Prevention, National Center for Health Statistics, *Fast Stats A to Z: Life Expectancy.* Available at http://www.cdc.gov/nchs/fastats/lifexpec.htm. Accessed 8 May 2007.

Chapter 2

OVERVIEW OF PRESCRIPTION DRUG BENEFITS IN MANAGED CARE

ROBERT P. NAVARRO
RUSTY HAILEY

INTRODUCTION

A prescription drug program is a vital component of comprehensive healthcare benefits offered by managed care organizations. Virtually all managed care organizations offer pharmacy benefits, and over 92% of commercial managed care customers purchase pharmacy benefits for their employees. In addition to commercial health plans, Medicaid programs include a pharmacy benefit, and as of 2006, Medicare Part D offers an outpatient prescription drug benefit to the 41 million Medicare beneficiaries. Therefore, other than the 46 million uninsured, the vast majority—approximately 85%—of the U.S. population may obtain prescription coverage through a private or public third-party managed pharmacy benefit program. Correspondingly, as a result of the Medicare Part D drug benefit, the Centers for Medicare and Medicare Services (CMS) projects that by 2008, 80% of prescription drug expenditures will be paid by a public or private third-party prescription program.[1] The 2004 to 2008 change in prescription drug expenditures by payer source is illustrated in **Figure 2-1**.

Prescription drug benefits are a highly coveted and a highly utilized benefit by plan sponsors as well as members. Plan sponsors should understand that offering all health plan members comprehensive pharmacy benefits makes clinical as well as economic sense. Clearly, prescription drugs are a management linchpin of many high-cost and high-prevalence medical conditions, including hypertension, outpatient infections, hyperlipidemia, congestive heart failure, diabetes, cancer, seizure disorders, migraine headache, asthma, allergic rhinitis, depression, psychosis, gastroesophageal reflux disease (GERD), seizure disorders, and many others. Effective outpatient treatment with a pharmaceutical may obviate the need for more expensive and less benign medical resources, such as hospitalization and surgery.

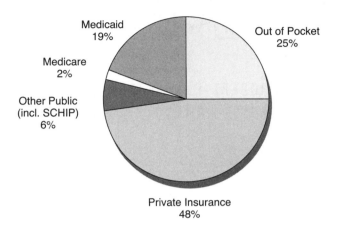

2004 Prescription Drug Expenditures by Payer ($188.5B)

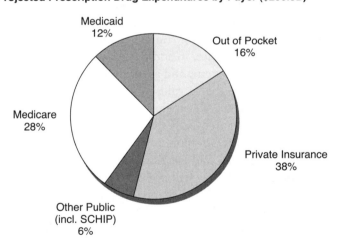

Projected Prescription Drug Expenditures by Payer ($255.8B)

FIGURE 2-1   Change in Payer Source of Prescription Drug Expenditures (2004 and 2008).
Source: Data obtained from National Healthcare Expenditure Projections: 2005–2015. Prescription Drug Expenditures (Table 11). Available at http://www.cms.hhs.gov/NationalHealthExpendData/03_NationalHealthAccountsProjected.asp. Accessed 30 May 2008.

GOALS OF PHARMACY BENEFIT MANAGEMENT

Health care in the United States is a highly competitive market-driven business. Public (Medicaid and Medicare) and private (employer groups) plan sponsors have many competitive alternative sources for prescription drug benefits. As a result, providers of pharmacy benefits must understand and anticipate the varied expectations and demands of purchasers, who are quite willing to switch to another pharmacy benefit provider on an annual basis if they are dissatisfied with their current provider. Generally, payers are interested in pharmacy benefit providers who are able to manage program costs, provide reasonable access to necessary medications, and provide excellent customer support programs. However, payers are different in their demands, and whereas one plan sponsor may place greater importance on cost containment and accept very limited benefits, another group, such as a union trust, may desire a broad range of drug coverage with very low copayments, and still another employer may be more interested in providing greater drug coverage supported by disease management programs. Pharmacy program providers counsel their clients on how they may achieve their desired outcomes by crafting their own customized pharmacy benefit management program.

Pharmacy directors attempt to manage the *supply cost* as well as the *utilization demand* of pharmaceuticals. This is accomplished by influencing the behavior of all individuals and entities that can control the supply and demand of pharmaceuticals by sharing with them the program financial risk. From a pharmacy benefit perspective, managed care implements supply side contracts with pharmaceutical manufacturers and dispensing pharmacies that essentially extract discounts on the drug ingredient cost (through manufacturer rebates and pharmacy reimbursement discounts) and a discounted pharmacy dispensing fee. Demand-side controls involve member prescription copayments or coinsurances paid by patient-members when they access and obtain pharmacy services. Member cost sharing is designed to encourage use of the most cost-effective products. Some managed care organizations (MCOs) also share a portion of the pharmacy benefit financial risk with prescribing physicians. The theory behind this strategy is that physicians will prescribe more cost-efficiently if they share in the cost of the drugs they prescribe. Despite the fact that this practice has been criticized for appearing to pay physicians for prescribing certain drugs, physicians with shared financial risk generally prefer generic or less expensive brand products, which also benefit patients through a lower copayment. In summary, pharmacy program managers attempt to obtain discounts on the drug ingredient cost as well as encourage the use of the least expensive yet therapeutically effective products to optimize pharmacy budget expenditures, which benefits plan sponsors as well as members.

As a result, pharmacy benefit managers (PBMs) must offer a broad range of program benefit design options to meet varied plan sponsor desires, while involving all stakeholders financially to achieve program objectives for each unique customer. The relationships and the flow of money among various stakeholders involved in medical and pharmacy benefits are shown in **Figure 2-2**. A general rule in identifying entities that may influence supply and demand is to "follow the money" trail. This model includes an MCO that contracts with a PBM for certain pharmacy benefit services (e.g., pharmacy distribution network and to contract with pharmaceutical manufacturers). However, large MCOs can provide complete pharmacy benefits directly without using a PBM. The relationships

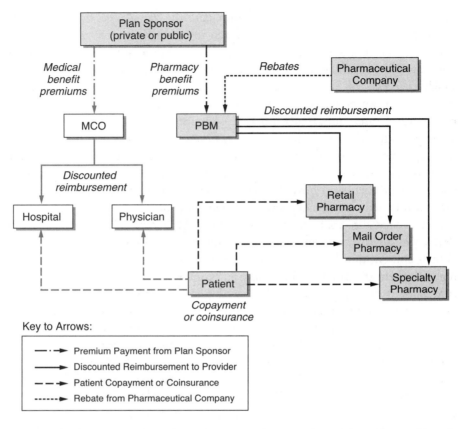

FIGURE 2-2   Relationships Among Stakeholders in Managed Prescription Drug Benefits (PBM model; medical benefit delivery de-emphasized).

involved in medical benefit delivery in Figure 2-2 are de-emphasized to highlight the pharmacy benefit delivery.

Both public and private MCOs continue to aggressively manage pharmacy benefits in an attempt to promote the appropriate level of prescription utilization rate as well as optimize the drug expenditure spend. This focus on pharmacy benefit management may seem antithetical to the cost-effectiveness value of pharmaceuticals. However, health care in the United States is a market-driven business. Since the inception of managed healthcare concepts in the early part of the 20th century, purchasers of care have demanded cost-containment as well as a broad spectrum of healthcare benefits. Although managed care has aggressively managed all healthcare products and services, pharmaceutical benefits continue to be aggressively managed for three primary reasons:

1. Although pharmacy benefits are the third largest healthcare benefit expenditure of managed care plans (after hospital and outpatient medical benefits), the annual trend

rate of prescription drug benefits had been rising faster than the other two major benefits for the past several years. Today, pharmacy benefits consume approximately 20% of total managed care healthcare costs, compared with approximately 5% two decades ago. This trend seems to be slowing a bit since 2005, and may be reduced more by the loss of patent protection of a number of important high cost and high utilization drugs over the next three years.

2. Pharmacy benefits are highly visible to government and private plan sponsors and accessed more than hospital or outpatient medical benefits. The average commercial MCO members uses approximately 8 to 11 prescriptions per year, and the average Medicare Part D member uses approximately 17 to 23 prescriptions per year, whereas the average commercial member consults a physician 5 to 6 times per year, and many of these encounters are pediatric visits.

3. Pharmacy benefits *can* be easily managed. The recipe for managing prescription drug costs and utilization is well known and can be implemented within months with adequate resources, and if payers and members are willing to accept benefit limitations. The management strategies used today were initiated almost 25 years ago, and used by every pharmacy benefit manager to manage pharmacy benefits. However, while the strategies are well known, successful implementation is challenging.

Rather than severely restrict or eliminate pharmacy benefits, MCOs and PBMs attempt to counsel their customers to purchase a cost-effective benefit. That is, an intelligently managed pharmacy benefit will provide easy access to necessary drugs, even encourage the appropriate use of cost-effective pharmaceuticals, and guard against inappropriate use of unnecessary, ineffective, or overly expensive drugs.

Pharmacy benefit management has been successful in reducing pharmacy benefit costs by 25% to 45%, compared to unmanaged drug costs, depending upon the aggressiveness of the managed program. As pharmacy benefits evolve, and outcomes data demonstrate the comparative value of competitive pharmaceuticals, PBMs and purchasers of health care will be in a better position to develop and implement an intelligent pharmacy benefit that optimizes the appropriate use of the most cost-effective pharmaceuticals to achieve the best clinical, economic, and humanistic outcomes.

Pharmacists managing prescription drug benefits must provide high quality pharmacy benefits while managing program costs. The quest to *manage* costs, rather than merely *minimize* costs, remains the challenge. As pharmacy program costs continue to escalate at an annual trend rate of approximately 10% to 15%, it is tempting to merely restrict expensive drugs, require the use of only generic drugs, and to significantly increase the patent co-patient tier amounts. However, simply focusing on cost-minimization may be myopic and ultimately cost-ineffective in several therapeutic categories. High cost drugs *may* produce superior clinical and economic outcomes compared with less expensive alternatives. Also, very high member copayments may be a barrier to drug utilization and adherence, and may result in drug failure, which may require more expensive medical treatment. Thus, pharmacy directors must consider the cost as well as outcomes associated with competing drug products when developing and managing their pharmacy benefit.

Health plan administrators as well as commercial and government payers often consider pharmacy benefits only as a cost center, and do not appreciate the value that a well-managed pharmacy benefit can bring to clinical, economic, and humanistic outcomes. In fact, a successfully managed pharmacy benefit should be considered an *investment* in cost-effective health care, rather than only a necessary expense. Health outcomes research in health plans, addressed below, provides the linkage between appropriate use of cost-effective drugs and positive outcomes, and helps administrators and payers migrate from cost-minimization to optimizing value. To achieve this goal, pharmacy benefit managers attempt to select the most cost-effective drugs for formulary inclusion, implement programs to promote the appropriate use and adherence, and document value by measuring outcomes. These goals are no different than those of hospital pharmacists, but are more difficult to control as the MCO pharmacy director is often managing prescription benefits for hundreds of thousands, or even millions of patients, from pediatric patients to Medicare beneficiaries, with literally every known disease for a prolonged period of time.

NOVEL CHALLENGES AND EFFECTIVE MANAGEMENT STRATEGIES

Pharmacy benefit management has evolved over the past 25 years to meet and—if possible—anticipate the clinical and financial market challenges threatening effective prescription drug benefit management. The events of the years leading up to 2010 and beyond provide some unique market trends not seen in the past two decades. The three most important concerns and challenges managed care pharmacy directors face include:

- Successful implementation of the Medicare Modernization Act Part D Medicare pharmacy benefit. Although some health plans have had experience in Medicare health benefits, very few have offered a comprehensive pharmacy benefit. Medicare Advantage plans (formerly Medicare + Choice) will hold financial risk for medical as well as pharmacy benefits in this population subgroup with 40 million elderly beneficiaries, which typically have more diseases, comorbidities, and consume more medications.
- Management of injectable biological medications, which are generally extremely expensive and often used in severe or life-threatening medical conditions (e.g., rheumatoid arthritis and other autoimmune disorders, HIV-AIDS, Crohn's disease, end-stage renal disease, and a variety of cancers). Many health plans and PBMs are using specialty pharmacies to provide and manage injectable biologicals, as these products require specialized distribution systems and patient management strategies. Injectable products may not be a component of the pharmacy budget, and are often part of the medical budget. However, even if injectables are not a financial responsibility of the pharmacy budget, often the pharmacy department is involved in managing injectable drug selection and utilization.

- Successfully implementing consumer-driven healthcare (CDH) initiatives that include health spending accounts (HSAs), and higher and more complicated copayments and coinsurance schemes. CDH initiatives should motivate and reward the consumer for self-management and include financial incentives and cost-sharing, without the unintended consequence of inadvertently building in financial disincentives to delay preventive care.

In addition to these novel challenges, health plans and PBMs continue to face the daily challenge of developing and implementing cost-effective pharmacy benefit programs customized for each of their customers. To meet the long-term and unique pharmacy benefit management challenges, pharmacy and medical directors routinely consider the following strategies as most effective (these strategies are discussed in depth later in this chapter)[2]:

1. Increasing the use of generic drugs. Health plans and PBMs frequently report that 50% to 60% of the prescriptions they reimburse are dispensed with lower priced generic alternatives. Some closed-model plans estimate they may be able to increase this rate to 70% or even 80%, especially in upcoming years when some important high-cost and highly utilized drugs lose patent protection (e.g., statins, calcium channel blockers, antidepressants, inhaled and nasal corticosteroids).

2. Raising patient prescriptions copayments and coinsurance amounts. Health plans and PBMs continue to increase copayments and coinsurance levels to encourage the use of lower cost preferred formulary products and to share the cost of medications with members who use them. The impact of copayments will be discussed below in the Drug Formulary Development and Management section.

3. Health plans and PBMs will more aggressively limit open access to the use of certain expensive drugs, or drugs with a misuse or abuse potential, through the use of prior authorization (physician and/or pharmacist must obtain approval to prescribe or dispense certain drugs), step-care edits (a lower priced drug must be used before a similar expensive drug is reimbursed), and other limits (e.g., quantity of units dispensed at one time, and the duration of use).

4. Health plans and PBMs may again promote more closed drug formularies. Closed formularies (a limited of drugs are reimbursed) were more common in the late 1980s and early 1990s, but formularies became more open (increased number of drugs reimbursed using expanded tiered copayments) by the late 1990s. However, with increasing drug program costs, and demands from plan sponsors for greater cost containment, pharmacy directors may again encourage the use of closed formularies. This reoccurring trend may be reinforced by the recent implementation of Medicare Part D formularies, which were generally more restrictive or closed.

Pharmacy directors will continue to use these and other strategies in the future, but will use them more aggressively and with more therapeutic categories. The following sections discuss important information systems, and commonly used prescription drug program management strategies in greater depth and detail.

PHARMACY INFORMATION SYSTEMS AND HEALTH INFORMATICS

Similar to other healthcare delivery components, pharmacy benefit administration is critically dependent on efficient data and information systems. The basic information systems involved in pharmacy benefit management include the following:

- Internal health plan administrative data systems that include member eligibility files, group benefit claims adjudication files, provider files, and drug files that are used for accurate claims adjudication.
- In-pharmacy, point-of-service (POS) third party claims adjudication systems that dispensing pharmacists use to verify member, provider, and drug eligibility, and obtain copayment and reimbursement information in an online, real-time environment.
- Health plan or PBM pharmacy administrative claims file, used for drug utilization review, pharmacy program performance analysis, research, patient and physician intervention programs, and financial report generation. Drug files are often merged with medical files to generate an integrated claims database suitable for research.

The presence of a universally accepted electronic data interchange standard for pharmacy claims transmission and adjudication has accelerated the adoption of pharmacy e-commerce. This standard, maintained by the National Council for Prescription Drug Programs (NCPDP), "creates and promotes standards for the transfer of data to and from the pharmacy services sector of the healthcare industry."[3] This universal standard has allowed the pharmacy claims systems to be suitable for electronic commerce.

PHARMACY CLAIMS ADJUDICATION

Observation of the NCPDP data standards allows 99% percent of all managed care prescription claims to be processed electronically online and usually in real-time. Pharmacists rely on the third-party prescription drug program benefit design and coverage information provided to them through the in-pharmacy POS system. Pharmacy benefits programs, even within a single MCO or PBM, may be highly variable, may change frequently, and may have complex benefit design elements, so dispensing pharmacists simply must rely on electronic messaging to efficiently process prescriptions. When a pharmacist fills a managed care prescription, the required patient, drug, and prescriber data are input into the pharmacy POS system. Within seconds, the pharmacist is informed if the patient and drug are eligible for coverage, is informed of the copayment to be collected, and is provided any pertinent clinical information (e.g., drug interactions or clinical edits). If correct, the pharmacist completes the transaction and within seconds the claim is adjudicated online, informing the pharmacist of the reimbursement amount. The online pharmacy management systems provide patient-specific information at the point-of-dispensing that will identify adherence problems, drug interactions, dispensing errors, and print a patient information document. Pharmacy claims data are also used to identify members that may benefit from disease or case management, such as patients who appear to be misusing or abusing redundant prescriptions from multiple providers, or displaying other inappropriate or excessive drug use patterns.

PHARMACY AND MEDICAL CLAIMS INTEGRATION AND CLINICAL PROGRAM SUPPORT

Over the past decade, healthcare information system standards have allowed easier integration of medical, administrative, and pharmacy claims datasets. Merging of these databases is accomplished through linking the common shared dimensions, such as identifiers for member, physician, and employer group benefit level. Health plans and PBMs compete on price as well as quality of care and services. Thus, health plans in particular are interested in measuring clinical and economic outcomes, and use comparative health plan data for marketing to potential customers. For example, a population of case-mix–adjusted patients with a specific medical condition can be stratified according to severity, age, comorbidities, and other characteristics, to compare the clinical and economic outcomes of each cohort. Similarly, physician drug prescribing patterns also may be evaluated and compared. A well-constructed merged database may be used to identify clinical "best practices" that are associated with the most cost-effective outcomes.

Most health plans participate in the National Committee for Quality Assurance (NCQA) accreditation process, and allow their performance metrics to be compared against competitive plans using the NCQA Health Plan Report Card.[4] The NCQA has also established many "effectiveness of care" indicators through its Health Plan Employer Data and Information Set (HEDIS®) program. The NCQA HEDIS are a list of almost 70 measures designed to collect data about the quality of care and services provided by the health plans.[5] Approximately one-half of these measures relate to appropriate pharmaceutical or immunization use, and can be used to measure pharmacy benefit contributions at a high level. Health plan quality initiatives are addressed elsewhere in this book.

ELECTRONIC PRESCRIBING

The rapid expansion of information technology applications in health care presents novel opportunities and challenges for pharmacists. Although electronic prescribing is not universal, many MCOs are experimenting with real-time electronic data transfer of prescription-related information among trading partners: the health plan, physician, and pharmacy. Electronic prescribing refers to the use of computing devices to enter, modify, review, and output or communicate drug prescriptions. For inpatient care, electronic medication ordering increases prescribing accuracy, dispensing efficiency, and reduces the number of adverse drug events and redundant medications. A number of outpatient pilot projects and initiatives in electronic prescribing are proliferating within managed care organizations to achieve the same goals, and also providing medication history, drug formulary options, drug hypersensitivities, and other clinically relevant data to the prescriber at the point of prescribing.

Electronic prescribing is an electronic data interchange application that provides electronic connectivity among all trading partners involved in prescription generation, adjudication, and analysis.[6] E-prescribing links the health plan or PBM, with the physician and pharmacy. E-prescribing allows the physician, using a desktop or handheld device to access a patient's medication history, drug allergies, pharmacy benefits, and drug formulary drugs covered, and transmits a "clean" prescription to the patient's preferred pharmacy: all online and in real-time. **Figure 2-3** illustrates the electronic connectivity among trading partners.

There are several potential financial and patient care advantages to the physician, health plan, pharmacy, and patient. Point-of-prescribing medication information helps enforce drug formulary conformance, informs the physician of the member copayment impact of selected drugs, and prevents rejected prescriptions at the pharmacy. Prior authorization or step-care protocols may be enforced through e-prescribing, and the system can alert physicians of any drug interactions, history of adverse events, redundant prescriptions from other physicians, and incorrect dosages before the patient leaves the physician's office. The potential cost savings from e-prescribing result from reduced administrative costs and less physician and pharmacist time involved in the prescription process, reduction in drug interactions and adverse effects, improved safety and reduced medication errors, and improved medication compliance.

In the ambulatory environment, recent research shows that adverse events are common and can be serious. The Center for Information Technology Leadership reports that more than 8.8 million adverse drug events occur each year in ambulatory care, of which over 3 million are preventable, many resulting in deaths. In addition to reducing adverse

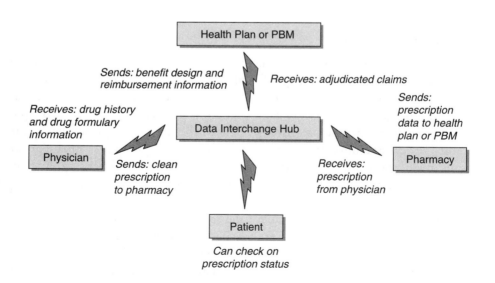

FIGURE 2-3 E-Prescribing Connectivity Among Managed Care Trading Partners.

drug effects, electronic prescribing can improve quality, efficiency, and reduce costs through other benefits, including[7]:

- Actively promoting appropriate prescription use and adherence.
- Providing information about formulary options and copay information.
- Improving dispensing efficiency and accuracy by providing instant electronic connectivity between the physician, pharmacy, health plans and PBMs.

More than 3 billion prescriptions are written annually.[6] Given this volume, even a small improvement in quality attributable to electronic prescribing would translate into significant healthcare cost and safety benefits if electronic prescribing is broadly adopted. Studies suggest that the national savings from universal adoption of electronic prescribing systems could be as high as $27 billion, including $4 per-member-per-year (PMPY) savings from reducing preventable adverse drug events, and $35 to $70 PMPY savings from more appropriate use of medications, for a total savings of $39 to $74 PMPY.[6] Electronic prescribing has significant benefits for pharmacists as well. The Institute for Safe Medication Practices estimates that pharmacists spend a significant amount of their time each day on clarifying prescription orders, and make 150 million phone calls to physicians annually on prescription accuracy related issues.[8]

RxHub® provides a universal portal that supports prescription electronic data interchange among trading partners.[9] Originally formed in 2001 by three PBMs, the enterprise now enjoys participation of PBMs, health plans, and numerous e-prescribing solution venders, for the purpose of:

> ". . . creating a single point of communication for all participants in the prescription creation and delivery process the founders formed a neutral organization, whose primary mission is to accelerate the adoption of electronic prescribing resulting in better medicine and lower administrative costs."[9]

All advantages of e-prescribing can lead to improved clinical, economic, and quality of life outcomes. E-prescribing will unquestionably increase, especially as it is an eventual requirement in the Medicare Modernization Act.

COMPONENTS OF A MANAGED PRESCRIPTION DRUG BENEFIT

Prescription drug benefits are provided through an internal pharmacy department within an MCO* or by a stand-alone pharmacy benefit manager (PBM; the role of PBMs will be addressed below and in Chapter 4). Regardless of the source (e.g., MCO or PBM), there is great consistency in the management strategies used to develop and manage a prescription drug program. Pharmacists operating health plan pharmacy benefits have borrowed many management strategies from hospital pharmacy programs, including the Pharmacy

---

* In this context, the term *managed care organization* refers to HMO, PPO, POS, and other health plans; Medicaid programs; Medicare Part D plans.

& Therapeutics (P & T) Committee, the drug formulary, pharmaceutical company contracting, physician academic counter detailing, utilization review, and health outcomes research. However, MCOs have had to include additional capabilities, such as development of a pharmacy distribution network, innovative pharmacy benefit design, member copayment schemes, member communication and education, and massive computer systems to process millions of claims in a real-time environment. This section will list and illustrate the components of a successful managed care prescription drug benefit program.

LEGAL BASIS FOR PHARMACY BENEFIT PROGRAMS

All states have regulatory bodies that control health-related benefit plans as well as licensing boards that control the practice of specific healthcare providers. The Employee Retirement Income Security Act of 1974 (ERISA) is a federal law that sets minimum standards for most voluntarily established pension and health plans in private industry to provide protection for individuals. The ERISA act has been supplemented by two important amendments. The Consolidated Omnibus Budget Reconciliation Act (COBRA) provides workers and their families the ability to continue their health coverage after loss of employment, and the Health Insurance Portability and Accountability Act (HIPAA) provides protection for patients from discrimination related to pre-existing medical conditions as well as enhanced confidentiality of medical information.[10]

MCOs and PBMs, as corporate entities, do not practice medicine or pharmacy, and do not claim to provide any and all desired pharmacy products and services. Rather, they arrange for defined medical and pharmacy benefits to be provided by licensed healthcare professionals within a defined structure and process. Healthcare professionals participating with an MCO or PBM provide pharmacy benefits that are specified and defined in a state regulated contract (e.g., Certificate of Coverage or other similar legal document) between the MCO or PBM and the purchaser of pharmacy benefits. Physicians and pharmacists agree to participate according to policies outlined in their respective provider manuals and contracts, which are generally filed with a state regulatory agency. The contract defines included and excluded benefits as well as the access rules through which members must obtain benefits. Drugs eligible for reimbursement are normally those included in the drug formulary (a list of reimbursed drugs) that is reviewed and updated from time to time. Drugs typically excluded from reimbursement include the following:

- Experimental or investigational drugs (drugs not approved by the U.S. Food and Drug Administration for commercial sale in the United States).
- FDA approved drugs when prescribed for unapproved indications ("off-label" indications). This is generally unenforceable through community pharmacies, as pharmacists are generally unaware of the prescribed indication or medical diagnosis for most prescriptions dispensed. The approved indication may be enforced if the pharmacist must obtain a prior authorization from the MCO or PBM prior to receiving reimbursement for the drug product.

- Drugs used for cosmetic purposes (e.g., Botox® for wrinkles) or possibly life enhancement drugs (e.g., PDE-5 inhibitors).
- A brand name drug for which there is an identical generic equivalent that is subject to mandatory generic substitution (e.g., drugs subject to a maximum allowable cost [MAC] reimbursement).
- Drug available without a prescription (or over-the-counter [OTC] drugs), including brand name drugs for which there is an identical OTC equivalent. Insulin is an exception, as it is a non-prescription drug in most states but remains covered by health plan pharmacy benefits.

It is important to note that all health plans and PBMs allow for medical exceptions to defined benefits. That is, a physician may appeal to a health plan or PBM for coverage and reimbursement for a non-covered benefit based upon an individual patient's medical needs. Additionally, patients have the ability to directly purchase any non-covered benefit outside of the pharmacy benefit, on a cash basis, with a physician's prescription. Pharmacy benefit design does not limit what a physician may prescribe; benefit design only limits what an MCO or PBM will reimburse.

CHANGES IN PHARMACY BENEFIT DESIGN

There are two principal changes occurring in benefit design. The first is greater use of formulary prescription copayment and coinsurance tiers as well as higher copayment tier dollar and coinsurance percent amounts, especially for non-preferred and injectable medications. The second major benefit design change is the growth of CDH and HSAs, which are encouraged by state and federal regulatory agencies as well as employer groups and health plans.[2,11] HSAs usually have lower monthly premiums and higher annual deductibles (often $2,500 for individuals and $5,000 for families), and give members more latitude and freedom in using HSA funds for health-related expenditures. A potential downside is that HSA members, used to near first-dollar coverage for medical and pharmacy benefits, will now have to spend $2,500 or more in out-of-pocket deductible expenses before benefits are covered 100% by the health plan. Early experiences of a few employer groups have found some members are reluctant to spend their own out-of-pocket money, and may delay preventive care, thus resulting in a need for delayed and more expensive acute medical treatment.[12] HSAs are most effectively used by informed members who are educated and motivated to optimize their health care, and are given appropriate information to make intelligent healthcare access decisions. HSA members are important targets for pharmaceutical companies with direct-to-consumer advertising for both prescription and over-the-counter medications.

DISTRIBUTION CHANNELS FOR OUTPATIENT PHARMACEUTICALS

Managed care organizations and PBMs must develop a pharmaceutical distribution system that meets member needs for easy access to prescription services as well as controlling drug ingredient and dispensing costs. Closed model health plans (e.g., staff or group model MCOs) or large employer groups may have in-house, owned pharmacies for member convenience, supplemented with community pharmacies, often with mail service. Open model plans (e.g., independent practice associations [IPA] and network MCOs) will use a community-based pharmacy network including chain pharmacies, independent pharmacies, and often mail service pharmacy. Today, a pure MCO rarely exists, and most staff and group model plans now offer a hybrid distribution network consistent of in-house pharmacists supplemented by community and mail service pharmacies.

Generally 80% to 90% of third party outpatient prescriptions are dispensed through community pharmacies (pharmacy chains, independent pharmacies, supermarkets, or mass merchandise stores such as WalMart and Target). Most of the remaining prescriptions are dispensing through mail services pharmacies, often owned or associated with PBMs or chain pharmacies. A small percent of prescriptions, mostly generic drugs and often in rural areas, are dispensed in physician offices, which may not be reimbursed by MCOs or health plans. Of the $221 billion spent on outpatient prescription drugs in 2004, the National Association of Chain Drug Stores (NACDS) reports that 42.2% were dispensed through chain pharmacies, 18.7% through community independent pharmacies, 18.3% through mail service pharmacies, 12.2% through supermarkets, and 9.6% were dispensed through mass merchandise stores.[13] As a result, the basis of a managed care outpatient prescription network is often chain pharmacies, supplemented by other types of pharmacies. However, the NACDS reports that the largest annual growth in prescription sales from 2002 to 2003 occurred in mail service pharmacies, which grew by almost 18%, in contrast with all other pharmacy types, which grew between 5% and 8%.

Pharmacies participating in the pharmacy provider network agree, by contract, to dispense drugs prescribed by participating physicians to eligible members according to the drug formulary and other benefit design requirements. Open-access of POS plans may reimburse prescriptions from any licensed physician. Pharmacists participate in many different managed pharmacy programs, and by contract must use an online, real-time POS computer system to verify coverage information (eligible drug, member, and physician), learn any dispensing limitations or requirements (e.g., quantity limits, step-care protocols), obtain copayment information, and know the level of reimbursement from the health plan or PBM. Busy pharmacists dispensing 200 prescriptions per day simply must rely on an accurate and efficient online system to verify and adjudicate claims.

All participating pharmacies are bound by a provider agreement that stipulates they will provide approved prescriptions dispensed to their members in accordance with drug benefit and coverage policies, and for a specified discounted reimbursement. These policies are usually detailed in a Participating Pharmacy Policy and Procedure Manual that is updated from time to time by the MCO or PBM. Participating pharmacies agree to follow the drug formulary and dispensing requirements, use the POS system to adjudicate claims online and in real-time whenever possible, promote the use of generics, discourage the use of "dispense as written" prescriptions that encourage the use of brand drugs, and agree to participate in on-site audits of third party prescription records.

Pharmacists receive a discounted ingredient cost reimbursement based upon a discount off the drug average wholesale price (AWP) plus a discounted dispensing fee. The elements and calculations involved in determining pharmacy reimbursement of a brand drug in formulary copayment Tier II (brand preferred) is illustrated in **Table 2-1**. Wholesale acquisition cost (WAC) is the published drug list price, but is not used in determining pharmacy reimbursement from health plans or PBMs (WAC is de-emphasized in Table 2-1).

As shown in the example, the drug AWP is generally used to determine drug ingredient reimbursement. In Table 2-1, the AWP is discounted by 15%. This level of discount is used to approximate the actual acquisition price (AAC) by the pharmacy. It is actually quite difficult to positively identify the AAC for a particular prescription, as the pharmacy inventory is based upon volume discounts, special offers, and early payment discounts. Thus, rather than burden pharmacies with the requirement to identify the exact AAC of a prescription, MCOs and PBMs approximate this amount using a discounted AWP. Brand drug AWP discounts may be 15% to 18%, and generic drug discounts are often in the AWP less 40% to 60% range. Other payments may exist, such as for special incentives for generic substitution or member clinical consultation, and medication therapy management (MTM) program activities, as mandated by the Medicare Part D regulations.

SPECIALTY PHARMACY DISTRIBUTION

The increasing use of high-cost injectable biological products is identified as the greatest threat to pharmacy benefit management. However, despite the challenge in managing cost and utilization of expensive products, injectable biologicals present unique, advanced therapy for many severely debilitating and life-threatening illnesses. Thus, as much as health plans welcome the launch of life-saving drugs, they are faced with the reality that uncontrolled

TABLE 2-1 Calculations Involved in Determining Pharmacy Reimbursement from a Managed Care Plan

	Preferred Brand Drug Tier II
Wholesale Acquisition Cost (WAC)*	$80.00
Average Wholesale Price (AWP)	$100.00
Drug Reimbursement (AWP—15% Discount)	$85.00
Dispensing Fee (+)	$2.50
Subtotal	$87.50
Member Tier II Copayment (–)	$25.00
MCO Reimbursement to Pharmacy	$62.50

*WAC is not used in pharmacy reimbursement.

utilization may place a plan in financial peril. Health plans support the use of evidence-based treatment guidelines and protocols, and usually implement prior authorization edits on expensive biological injectables to encourage appropriate use for Food and Drug Administration (FDA)-approved indications. A large Blue Cross and Blue Shield plan found that 37% of injectable expenses were for oncology and related products, 11% were for inflammatory diseases of the colon, 9% of injectables were for leucocyte stimulants, and 2% was spent on anti-inflammatory and anti-arthritis injectable products.[14]

The unique distribution, storage, and utilization consideration of injectables has caused the development of carve-out specialty pharmacy distributors (SPDs). Specialty pharmacy services may also be offered internally through PBMs and health plans. Specialty pharmacies manage the distribution and use of self- and physician-administered injectable products. SPDs may send injectables directly to a physician's office or infusion center specifically for a patient appointment, or self-injectable drugs may be mailed directly to a member's home. Volume purchasing by SPDs introduces cost efficiencies into the system that are passed on to payers and members. SPDs also use rebates, formulary-style product steerage, copayments and coinsurance, and provider discounts as other methods of controlling injectable drug costs. Chapter 6 contains further discussions about specialty pharmacy distribution.

Health plans also may use SPDs to buy and store inventory on behalf of physicians, which prevents physicians from stocking and storing expensive mediations, and removes them from the flow of dollars. In this scheme, the SPD bills the health plan and/or member directly, and the physician is paid an infusion and/or administration fee by the health plan. The growing availability to biotechnology pharmaceuticals will likely increase the role and importance of SPDs in the future. Traditional discounted reimbursement of injectable products as a Part B Medicare Benefit will be altered through the use of a CMS average selling price (ASP) plus 6% method. Many plans are adopting this Medicare-style cost-plus reimbursement for injectables in their commercial plans as well. The implementation of the CMS competitive acquisition program (CAP) for injectable has been delayed, and the impact of the CAP is unknown at this time.

INTERNET PHARMACY ACCESS

Internet pharmacies developed in the late 1900s, and were thought to be a future threat to community and mail service pharmacies. However, this has not occurred, and although some Internet pharmacies remain in existence (e.g., http://www.drugstore.com), others have ceased business. In reality, Internet pharmacies were simply an online method to access traditional pharmacy services with mail delivery. Internet pharmacy access allows patients to refill prescriptions and purchase non-prescription drugs, vitamins, and other health products online. However, rather than Internet pharmacies threatening mail service pharmacies, we have seen chain and mail service pharmacies develop patient-friendly Internet portals, and have developed their own Internet pharmacy capabilities. Managed care supports Internet access to pharmacy services of U.S. licensed participating pharmacies because Internet access increases the use of the mail service pharmacy component, which is considered a growing source of pharmacy budget savings.

While Internet access to licensed U.S. chain and mail service pharmacies is a patient convenience, there remains a safety concern about unregulated Internet pharmacies outside of the United States. Counterfeit and inert drugs from international sources have been distributed through Internet pharmacies, and international commerce through the Internet is impossible to control.

In response, the National Association of Boards of Pharmacy® (NABP) developed the Verified Internet Pharmacy Practice Sites(tm) (VIPPS) program in 1999.[15] To be VIPPS certified, a pharmacy must comply with the licensing and inspection requirements of each state to which they dispense pharmaceuticals. In addition, pharmacies displaying the VIPPS seal have demonstrated to NABP compliance with VIPPS criteria. According to the NABP Web site, twelve Internet pharmacies have satisfied VIPPS criteria,[15] including the mails service pharmacies of PBMs (e.g., Caremark, Medco Health Solutions, Prescription Solutions), health plans (e.g., CIGNA, Coventry), pharmacy chains (e.g., CVS, Walgreens), and Internet pharmacies (e.g., http://www.Familymeds.com, http://www.Drugstore.com).

PHYSICIAN DISPENSING

Some health plans may reimburse physicians for dispensing drugs directly from their office, but this is an uncommon practice and most often occurs only in rural areas without adequate coverage of community pharmacies. Health plans will often not reimburse physicians for dispensing drugs unless the physician's office agrees to accept the same level of reimbursement as is paid to pharmacies and if the physician's office submits pharmacy claims through a POS terminal. Physician dispensing units often contain a limited amount of acute care drugs and generally promote the use of generics. Some applications link in-office physician dispensing units for acute care drugs with mail order for chronic care medications. The American Academy of Family Practice supports the right of physicians to dispense,[16] but thus far most medical groups have not focused on developing in-house dispensing activities, other than through a co-located and usually independent community pharmacy (state law may allow the medical group to own the pharmacy space, and obtain rent, but may prevent the medical group from owning the licensed pharmacy practice itself).

PHARMACY AND THERAPEUTICS COMMITTEE MANAGEMENT

Managed care has borrowed the P & T Committee concept from hospitals as a source for formulary development and drug coverage decisions. In addition to the clinical drug review, the Committee must make recommendations on drug formulary coverage and copayment tier, and other dispensing limitations or restrictions. A managed care P & T Committee typically consist of 10 to 15 physicians and pharmacists who meet quarterly.

Clinical pharmacists with the health plan or PBM conduct a review of available data and information, and prepare a drug monograph for distribution to members of the P & T Committee that contains a recommendation for formulary inclusion or exclusion. Chapter 13 provides an in-depth discussion on P & T Committees.

The data and information reviewed by clinical pharmacists includes the following:

- Peer-reviewed published clinical efficacy and effectiveness studies
- Safety and toxicity data
- Published health outcomes and economic data
- Data on file and economic models submitted by the pharmaceutical manufacturer that is usually organized according to the Academy of Managed Care Pharmacy *Format for Formulary Submissions*[17] (see also Chapter 11)
- Plan-specific expected utilization patterns
- The positioning and impact on other formulary drugs
- Manufacturer contracts

Due to concerns about drug safety and utilization patterns, a new drug is usually not formally reviewed for formulary consideration for at least three to six months after its launch. During that time, the drug may be available for reimbursement as a non-formulary or non-preferred drug, usually on the copayment Tier III. The Medicare Part D regulations require that a drug be reviewed within 90 days, and a formulary decision must be made within 180 days. Medicare Part D regulations also require a separate Medicare P & T Committee and members appropriate to evaluate drugs for the elderly. Many health plans share members between commercial and Part D P & T Committees, and often hold their meetings sequentially.

Clinical data (efficacy, effectiveness, and safety) are the two primary formulary decision criteria, but net cost ranks quite high as a decision consideration as well. Increasingly, credible health outcomes and economic data are available and considered by managed care P & T Committees, and formulary decisions are becoming more based upon clinical, and economic outcomes, rather than solely on pharmacy budget cost minimization. Humanistic or quality of life outcomes remain less important for most drugs, but quality of life data are used subjectively when appropriate and convincing. The Academy of Managed Care Pharmacy *Format for Formulary Submissions*[17] has made a significant and positive impact on improving the quality and quantity of data available for reviews, as well as the ability of clinical pharmacists to review the body of existing data.

DRUG FORMULARY DEVELOPMENT AND MANAGEMENT

Health plans and PBMs have used drug formularies for the same reasons they are used in hospitals: to identify and promote the most cost-effective pharmaceuticals in the most appropriate manner. A drug formulary is a preferred list of medications developed by the health plan or PBM P & T Committee to guide physician prescribing and pharmacy dispensing. Formularies are not novel but have been used for decades by hospitals, health plans, and other healthcare institutions as a method of inventory control and to promote the use of the most cost-effective products.[19] Early formularies in the United States were primarily compilations of formulas and recipes used to prepare medicines. The first hospital formulary, the Lititz Pharmacopoeia (1778), attempted to standardize compounding and dispensing of medicines in military hospitals that were set up during the Revolutionary War.[19] A formulary system is the method and process used that continually updates the formulary's content of prescription medications. The formulary system is a uniquely dynamic system that represents the current body of pharmaceutical knowledge and medical community practice standards resident in the healthcare setting it serves (see also Chapter 9).

The benefit design is enforced through the formulary, which is the basis for the drug and reimbursement information used by the pharmacist to process eligible claims using the POS system. Formulary booklets are mailed to participating physicians and often abridged formulary documents are provided to members. However, paper documents are often discarded, and many plans and PBMs provide pharmacy benefit and formulary information for physicians and members online. This allows for more frequent changes, and efficiency in communicating formulary matters to providers and members.

Some formularies are "open," signifying that most drugs are eligible for reimbursement although the level of member copayment varies with formulary position. Some drugs are "on formulary" but available only if the patient satisfies certain prior authorization (PA) criteria. Drugs may be subject to a PA based upon cost or safety issues, to attempt to control use for labeled indications only, or to limit use for certain types of patients.

Other formularies may be "closed," indicating a select number of drugs are eligible for reimbursement, while others are not. Closed formularies do not allow for reimbursement of non-formulary products, and if one is prescribed, the pharmacist must contact the prescribing physician to request a change to a formulary product, or the patient must pay cash for a non-formulary product. The open and closed nature of formularies is cyclical. Since the mid-1990s, formularies were often more open and inclusive, with non-preferred or even non-formulary products covered on Tier III. However, due to rising costs and the recent development of Medicare formularies, many MCOs are returning to more restrictive, closed formularies as well as including higher and tiered copayments.

Physician and member formulary conformance may be enforced using different mechanisms depending upon if the formulary is inclusive or exclusive. Closed and open formularies both use a tiered copayment structure, described below, to encourage physician prescribing and member use of generic or preferred formulary products. Some health plans and PBMs use pharmacists to "academically detail" directly to physicians who continuously disregard the formulary. Many health plans and PBMs provide physicians "formulary conformance report cards" and indicate opportunities for prescribing changes that favor formulary products. Some plans and PBMs offer financial incentives to physicians for high levels of formulary conformance.

FORMULARY COPAYMENT TIERS

MCOs and PBMs often use tiered formulary copayments as an integral component of their pharmacy benefit design. Two copayment tier plans have been in existence for over 20 years, but in the last decade more plans are adopting three or more copayment tier benefit plans. The purposes of tiered copayments are to:

1. Share some of the prescription costs with the utilizing member, and help reduce some of the pharmacy program costs to the plan sponsor, and,
2. Encourage physicians to prescribe, and patients to accept, lower cost drugs, which usually have a lower patient copayment.

Through a copayment system, members pay a flat dollar payment per prescription (i.e., $12.00, or $30.00), while with a coinsurance, a patient pays a percent of the total prescription cost (e.g., 50%), sometimes up to a maximum cap amount.

Drugs are placed into copayment tiers generally based upon their value to the plan and payer. A drug's value is based upon its clinical benefits as well as the net cost. Generic drugs are generally less expensive than brand name alternatives, and as a result, generic drugs are found on the lowest copayment tier, Tier I. Preferred formulary brand drugs are placed into copayment Tier II, and non-preferred or non-formulary drugs are found in Tier III. Three-tier formularies are the most common tiered formulary structure, although some programs, notably union trust groups, may still have two tier formulary copayments (generics in Tier I and all brands in Tier II).

We are seeing some large MCOs and PBMs offer greater copayment tier options for their customers, and may include four and five tiered formularies. Tier IV may include unessential, lifestyle, or cosmetic drugs, and Tier V may contain self-injectable drugs. Copayments are more common today, but coinsurance payments are becoming more popular with self-injectable biologicals and expensive non-essential drugs in higher copayments tiers. An example of a common three tier open formulary copayment structure is found in **Table 2-2**.

Copayments continue to increase in dollar amount, especially for Tier III non-preferred products. Many large health plans and PBMs have announced options for Tier III copayments over $60.00 for clients who desire such cost containment measures. A summary of average copayment amounts from a number of large health plans over the past five years is shown in **Figure 2-4**.

TABLE 2-2   Example of Three-Tier Drug Formulary Copayment Structure
Three Tier Formulary Example

Tier I Generic Drugs	Tier II Preferred Formulary Brand Drugs	Tier III Non-Preferred or Non-Formulary Brand Drugs
Copayment $13.00	Copayment $31.00	Copayment $53.00

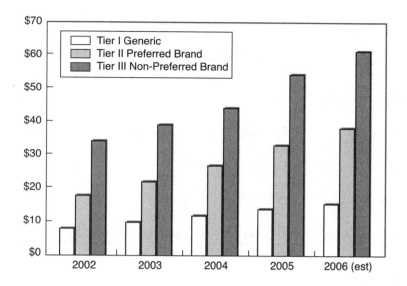

FIGURE 2-4 Examples of Average Copayment Amounts for Various Tiers 2002–2006.

Source: Average health plan copayments were compiled from a variety of research projects and personal communications with pharmacy and medical directors, 2002–2006.

Examples of formularies and copayment tiers used to encourage the use of lower priced medications are found in **Table 2-3.** This table shows possible entries for the hydroxymethylglutaryl-coenzyme A (HMG Co-A) reductase inhibitor therapeutic category (e.g., statins), a high cost and high utilization category, for 2006 and for 2008 (before and after simvastatin and pravastatin lose patent protection). The number of dollar signs ($) is a graphic indication of the relative price of the products within the therapeutic category.

The 2006 statin formulary category includes one generic statin in Tier I, two preferred formulary brand drugs in Tier II, and two non-preferred brand drugs in Tier III. The 2008 formulary includes three generic statins in Tier I, one high potency statin in Tier II, and the two remaining non-preferred brand statins in Tier III. This copayment structure will encourage physicians to prescribe, and members to prefer, generic statins first, and, if necessary, Lipitor® on Tier II, before the non-preferred Tier III statins.

The formulary position of a drug, and the resulting prescription copayment, can have a significant impact on the cost of the drug to a health plan and the member. **Table 2-4** illustrates the impact of a Tier II and Tier III copayment on the health plan payment to a pharmacy as well as to the member. The WAC is a realistic price that approximates the actual acquisition cost of a drug. The AWP is an artificial calculated number, somewhat archaic, which often remains used in pharmacy reimbursement calculations.

TABLE 2-3 Examples of potential HMG Co-A Reductase Inhibitor Therapeutic Category Drugs (Statins) in a Commercial Formulary in 2006 and 2008

HMG Co-Reductase Inhibitor Formulary (single entity statins)—2006

	Tier I	Tier II	Tier III
Type of Drugs	Generic	Preferred Formulary Brand	Non-Preferred or Non-Formulary Brand
Drugs Included	$ lovastatin	$$$ Pravachol (pravastatin) $$$ Lipitor (atorvastaton)	$$$$$ Crestor (resuvastaton) $$$$$ Zocor (simvastatin)
Copayment Amount	$12.00	$25.00	$45.00

HMG Co-Reductase Inhibitor Formulary (single entity statins)—2008

	Tier I	Tier II	Tier III
Type of Drugs	Generic	Preferred Formulary Brand	Non-Preferred Non-Formulary Brand
Drugs Included	$ lovastatin $ simvastatin $ pravastatin	$$$ Lipitor (atorvastaton)	$$$$$ Crestor (resuvastaton)
Copayment Amount	$18.00	$35.00	$65.00

Non-reimbursed drugs: Pravachol (brand of pravastatin) and Zocor (brand of simvastatin)

TABLE 2-4 Impact of a Tier II and Tier III Copayments on the Cost of a Drug to a Health Plan and Member

	Preferred Brand Tier II	Non-Preferred Brand Tier III
Wholesale Acquisition Cost (WAC)	$80.00	$80.00
Average Wholesale Price (AWP)	$100.00	$100.00
Drug Reimbursement (AWP—15%)	$85.00	$85.00
Dispensing Fee (+)	$2.50	$2.50
Subtotal	$87.50	$87.50
Member Tier II Copayment (–)	$25.00	$45.00
MCO Reimbursement to Pharmacy	$62.50	$42.50

In this example, drugs with identical AWPs ($100.00) are put in Tier II and Tier III. In Tier II, the patient pays a $25.00 prescription copayment, and the MCO payment to the pharmacy is $62.50. In the Tier III example, the patient pays a greater portion of the drug cost ($45.00 copayment), and as a result, the payment from the MCO to the pharmacy is less ($42.50). This illustrates how a health plan or PBM can reduce costs, which are passed on to the plan sponsor, by increasing the member copayment cost. When on Tier II, the MCO pays approximately 60% of the AWP to the pharmacy, whereas when on Tier III, the MCO pays approximately 40% of the AWP to the pharmacy, over a 30% savings, although the patient must pay a copayment that is 180% of the Tier II copayment.

Generic drugs are one of the most important cost containment components of an effective drug formulary. Members are well accepting of generics, and most often ask for a generic drug. Generic drugs generally cost a fraction of the brand costs, and AB-rated products (considered to be bioequivalent and generically substitutable), are increasing in importance, as several high cost and high utilization drugs will soon lose their patent protection. In addition to encouraging the use of generics through lower copayments, health plans and PBMs also have a mandatory generic reimbursement program, often referred to as a MAC program.

Through a mandatory generic program, the generic form of drug is assigned a MAC, which is the upper level of pharmacy reimbursement by the MCO or PBM. This means that if a pharmacist dispenses a brand name equivalent to a drug with a MAC, the pharmacist will only be reimbursed at the MAC level, which approximates the acquisition cost of the generic. This almost guarantees a generic drug will be dispensed if the drug is subject to a MAC, unless the patient is willing to pay cash for the brand drug, or the physician demands the brand drug through a "dispense as written" order. Pharmacists are advised of drugs subject to a MAC as well as the MAC level of reimbursement through the POS pharmacy claims adjudication system.

Health plans and PBMs often develop their own proprietary MAC programs and list of drugs subject to a MAC, and the mechanism they use to establish a MAC level may vary. However, in general, a product is assigned a MAC if there are three or more generic products available from reputable generic manufacturers, and the AAC is significantly lower than the AAC or WAC of brand drugs. The level of significance varies with different health plans and PBMs, but generally if the AAC of a generic product if more than 50% less than the AAC or WAC of a brand drug, and the generic AAC has stabilized, a MAC will be assigned.

The use and impact of high tiered copayments on pharmacy program costs and prescription adherence are controversial topics. Certainly copayments can reduce the cost of drugs by 20% to 40% or more, depending upon the copayment amount. However, critics of high dollar copayments claim the high copayment amounts are financial deterrents to members obtaining, and remaining on, prescribed drugs, and high copayments results in poor adherence and failed outcomes. Such negative outcomes may occur, but critics must also realize that lack of adherence is caused by a number of other factors, such as lack of member understanding, forgetfulness, belief that mediations are unnecessary, adverse effects or fear of adverse effects, and cultural barriers to medication use.[20–23] Some employer groups have adopted novel copayment structures, and have reduced the copayment for chronic medications for several high cost and high prevalence medical conditions, such as diabetes, asthma, hypercholesterolemia.[24,25]

PHARMACEUTICAL MANUFACTURERS' REBATE CONTRACTS

Borrowed from hospitals and other industries, health plans sought—and received—a financial incentive (rebate) to more favorably position contracted drug products. It is important to note that the price or rebate are not the most important drivers in formulary positioning; clinical efficacy and safety appropriately remain the most important decision criteria. However, in the absence of statistically and clinically significant differentiation among similar drugs, the net cost (which may be reduced by a rebate) can have an important impact on ultimate formulary positioning. This is especially true in crowded, relatively undifferentiated therapeutic categories, such as angiotensin converting enzyme (ACE) inhibitors, angiotensin II receptor blockers (ARBs), and proton pump inhibitors as well as expensive, competitive categories with clinical product differentiation, such as antidepressants, statins, and inhaled corticosteroids. Rebates are also discussed in Chapter 15.

However, a rebate may make a drug more attractive by making it less expensive than competitors, and a rebate may result in a preferred formulary position *if* the clinical features and benefits of the rebated drug are somewhat similar to non-rebated, more expensive alternatives. The rebate savings obtained reduce the net price of contracted drugs, which in turn reduces the overall prescription drug program expenses. A reduced net price will result in a more favorable cost-effectiveness ratio, and may result in more positive economic outcomes. These savings are passed on to plan sponsors through lower premiums (or, lower than would be without rebates) and to patients through a lower prescription copayment (rebated products are usually in Tier II, which has a lower prescription copayment than Tier III).

The effect of rebates is similar to discounts. Health plans and PBMs that contract with community pharmacies, and do not take possession of drug products, are usually offered rebates. In contrast, health plans with in-house, owned pharmacies that take possession of drug products may qualify for a discount (often a wholesale chargeback). The net result is similar, although the administration and flow of money of rebates and discounts are dissimilar.

Rebates' contract terms are varied and somewhat complex. However, in simplest terms, rebates provide health plans with incentives to position contracted products in a favorable position because rebates reduce the net cost of the product. The favorable formulary position helps pharmaceutical manufacturers, because physicians and members generally prefer drugs with lower copayments, such as those found in Tier II. Rebate contracts often contain two components, an access rebate and a performance component. The flat, access rebate (the smaller of the two contract components) is offered for a Tier II preferred formulary status. The value of the access rebate may vary based upon the number of competitive products sharing Tier II. For example, if a product has an exclusive Tier II position, the access rebate may be higher, but if the product shares Tier II with one or more other products, the access rebate may be lower. Traditionally with three-tier open formularies, rebates were not offered for Tier III positioning. However, with closed formularies, commonly seen in Medicare Part D, rebates are offered for Tier III status, because if a product is not covered on Tier I, II, or III, it is not reimbursed in a closed formulary. Thus, manufacturers pay for access to Tier III, which is preferable than their product not being reimbursed at all.

The performance rebate component, greater than the access component, may be based upon market share (in plan or national), volume growth, or other similar metric. Although a rebate contract may allow a health plan or PBM to include more than one product on a formulary tier, there is a better chance of achieving performance tiers if there are a limited number of products in a tier. There is a trend away from two component contracts (access and performance) to only a flat access rebate.

Rebates are additive, and highly variable based on the therapeutic category, number of similar products, competitive nature of the category, and the clinical and safety differentiation among products. Frequently, the ceiling on total rebate income for a specific drug will be capped at 15.1%, the "best price" limit required in Medicaid statutes (discussed below). If this amount is exceeded in commercial plans, the pharmaceutical companies must provide the same amount to all Medicaid plans under contract. Products in crowded and undifferentiated therapeutic categories may be associated with total rebate potential of 20% to 30% or more. Conversely, unique, highly differentiated products may have no rebate offered or a very low rebate (e.g., 5% total rebate). Products and categories associated with no, or very low rebates include many unique injectable biological products, HIV/AIDS drugs, and atypical antipsychotics.

Health plans and PBMs are relatively transparent regarding sharing rebates with their clients, although the exact terms of rebate contracts remains confidential. However, rebates are generally passed on to clients, or used to reduce pharmacy program cost. An example of how a rebate may reduce the net cost of a contracted drug is shown in **Table 2-5**. In the illustration, the drugs of the same WAC have significantly different net costs based upon formulary tier, member copayment, and rebate (paid for Tier II positioning). As stated above, WAC is a realistic price that approximates the actual acquisition cost of a drug. AWP is an artificial, calculated number that is often approximately 20% higher than the WAC, is somewhat archaic, but often remains used in pharmacy reimbursement calculations. Rebate calculations are usually based on the WAC.

In this example, the net cost of two drugs with identical WACs is shown. The drug on the preferred Tier II position is associated with a 20% rebate off the WAC. The rebate value is $32.00, which results in a net cost $12.00 less than the Tier III product, despite

TABLE 2-5   Impact of Copayment and Rebate on Drug Net Cost to an MCO or PBM

	Preferred Brand Tier II	Non-Preferred Brand Tier III
WAC	$128.00	$128.00
AWP	$160.00	$160.00
Drug Reimbursement (AWP – 15%)	$108.80	$108.80
Dispensing Fee (+)	$2.50	$2.50
Subtotal	$111.30	$111.30
Member Copayment (–)	$25.00	$45.00
MCO Reimbursement to Pharmacy	$86.30	$66.30
Rebate (15% of WAC)	20%	0%
Rebate Amount (–)	$32.00	$ 0.00
Net MCO Cost	$54.30	$66.30

the higher member copayment associated with the Tier III drug. Rebates will remain an important cost containment strategy to manage the net cost of brand drugs.

Although the regulation is somewhat more complex, the primary impact of the Omnibus Budget Reconciliation Act of 1990 (OBRA '90) required pharmaceutical man-ufacturers to extend commercial drug rebates 15.1% or greater to State Medicaid pro-grams. As a result, the rebate on many drugs would not exceed this percentage, although in competitive therapeutic categories, rebates could reach the 20% to 45% range, which is extended to Medicaid programs. Additionally, some state Medicaid programs mandate payment of a "supplementary rebate" to assist in reducing program costs. Other novel rebate contracts, including outcomes-based rebates, adherence-based rebates, and drug expense guarantees are interesting, but often difficult to administer.

CLINICAL PHARMACY AND DISEASE MANAGEMENT SERVICES

Health plans and PBMs offer an array of clinical pharmacy services, many of which are online and real-time edits provided to the dispensing pharmacist. Others include prospec-tive or retrospective utilization monitoring, adherence intervention, and disease manage-ment program support.

Online, real-time point-of-dispensing edits provide commonly used guidance regarding drug interactions, early refill prevention, duplicate medications, age and gender edits, and step-care edits. Health plans and PBMs also provide computerized drug utilization review (DUR), screening for drug misuse and abuse, polypharmacy, and non-adherence, and other dangerous or inappropriate drug use patterns. Interventions may include patient and or physician communications requesting clarification of the potential dangerous pattern.

Health plans may offer disease-specific management programs to augment healthcare services provided by plan physicians that may include general disease education, diagnostic screening events, and case management. Most common diseases included in clinical programs include diabetes, asthma, cardiovascular disease (hypertension and lipid disorders), chronic obstructive pulmonary disease (COPD), congestive heart failure (CHF), and behavioral health. Disease management programs in managed care are addressed elsewhere in this book.

MCO pharmacy departments and PBMs often play a supportive role in health plan and employer disease management programs. Pharmacy program drug utilization data are often used to identify patients with poorly controlled medical conditions (identified by the number and type of medications used) or have drug adherence problems (through inconsistent prescription refills records). Pharmacy departments may obtain resource support from pharmaceutical manufacturers that often provide unbranded disease management resources (e.g., physician or patient education materials or educational grants) to supplement health plan efforts. Disease management offering from pharmaceutical manufacturers will not influence formulary decisions, and in fact the reverse influence exists. That is, health plans and MCOs may seek clinical program support from manufacturers whose drugs have been previously selected for preferred formulary positions.

Clinical pharmacy programs are important in supporting health plan quality of care initiatives, such as NCQA accreditation and improvement of NCQA HEDIS measures. This was previously discussed in the Pharmacy and Medical Claims Integration and Clinical Program Support section.

PHARMACY BENEFIT MANAGERS

Pharmacy benefit managers, such as Medco Health Solutions, CVS Caremark, Express Scripts, Inc., Prime Therapeutics, MedImpact, WellPoint Pharmacy Management, and many others, are stand-alone companies that specialize in all aspects of pharmacy benefit management. They sell their services to private or public purchasers, including MCOs, self-insured employers, Medicaid programs, and Medicare Advantage Part D plans, as well as directly to Medicare members, and other purchasers of pharmacy benefits. **Table 2-6** provides a list of the largest PBMs.

Pharmacy benefit managers have evolved as specialized experts in pharmacy benefit management. Many large health plans, such as Aetna, Humana, CIGNA, and Coventry, manage their pharmacy benefit programs through an internal "captive" PBM. Although many large MCOs manage their pharmacy benefit through an internal pharmacy department, they may use a PBM for claims processing, pharmaceutical manufacturer contracting, and other "back end" commodity services. Other small MCOs, large self-insured employers, and state Medicaid agencies may use a PBM for full-service, turn-key prescription drug benefits.

Although PBMs do not offer any services a health plan could not develop through an internal pharmacy department, they manage many millions of lives, and offer economies

TABLE 2-6 Membership of Largest U.S. PBMs

Approximate Membership of the Largest U.S. PBMs	
CVS Caremark	82 million
Medco Health Solutions	71
Express Scripts, Inc.	51
WellPoint Pharmacy Management	36
MedImpact	21
Prime Therapeutics	13

Source: Compiled by RP Navarro from PBM Web sites and marketing material, 2006–2007.

of scale to MCOs regarding computer services, patient call centers, contracting with pharmacies and with pharmaceutical manufacturers, and other services. The PBM may offer such services less expensively than could be developed by an MCO.

The amount of PBM services purchased by MCOs, Medicaid plans, and self-insured employers depends entirely on the needs of the PBMs' customer. Some of the offered services include the following:

- Pharmacy distribution network (community, mail, and possibly specialty products)
- Drug formulary development and management
- P & T Committee support services
- Pharmaceutical manufacturer contracting
- Physician and member communications
- Member service help line support
- Health plan pharmacy benefit Web site development and maintenance
- Clinical pharmacy services (utilization review, adherence monitoring, clinical edit development) and disease management program support
- Claims processing and report generation

The PBM market is very competitive, and most large PBMs offer similar services. Decisions on PBM selection usually come down to aligned interests (e.g., cost containment, member services, and clinical programs), transparency, quality of service, and cost.

MEASURING PHARMACY BENEFIT MANAGEMENT PROGRAM PERFORMANCE

The competitive managed care environment requires that health plan and PBM pharmacy programs are effectively managed to achieve desired clinical, economic, and quality of life objectives. Health plans have been criticized for managing pharmacy costs separate from medical costs, when the use of resources—and outcomes—of both may be inextricably linked for many medical conditions. As discussed earlier, appropriate use of cost-effective pharmaceuticals may result in higher pharmacy program costs, but may prevent use of more expensive medical resources, such as hospitalizations and emergency department visits.

However, despite the awareness that the pharmacy program must be managed to optimize the drug spend, the pharmacy director must focus on pharmacy program performance metrics as well. The pharmacy program director will monitor specific performance metrics on a monthly basis and attempt to modify controllable factors if performance measures suggest costs are rising more than forecast, member satisfaction is declining, drug-related clinical outcomes are being achieved, or other markers of poor pharmacy program performance are indicated.

Some of the basic performance benchmarks monitored (monthly, quarterly, or annually) will include the following financial and quality of care metrics:

- Total prescription program costs as well as costs and trends of selected therapeutic categories and specific high cost and/or highly utilized drugs
- Monthly per-member-per-month (PMPM) and annual per-member-per-year (PMPY) program costs, PMPM and PMPY or high cost therapeutic categories, and cost trends
- Prescription utilization (PMPM and PMPY) overall and for selected highly utilized therapeutic categories
- Administrative and claims processing fees (overall and per prescription)
- Prescription discount or rebate (total amount, per prescription, PMPM, and PMPY)
- Generic dispensing rate (overall, by pharmacy, by group, by therapeutic class, and by physician), and missed generic substitution opportunities
- Drug formulary conformance rate (overall, by physician, and by pharmacy)
- Patient satisfaction and member complaints related to the pharmacy program
- Number of drug formulary prior authorization exception requests and approvals, and review of authorization trend
- NCQA HEDIS measure scores related to pharmacy (e.g., percent of post-myocardial infarction patients receiving a beta blocker)
- Trend of all the preceding performance measurements measured monthly, quarterly, or annually.

There are many more performance measurements that pharmacy directors routinely monitor, especially with more sophisticated programs that may include drug formulary conversion, compliance, and persistence activities. However, with the preceding basic performance measurements, a pharmacy director can evaluate the effectiveness of his or her prescription drug management program.

CONCLUSION

Pharmacy benefits are an important component in comprehensive healthcare benefits and, when optimized, can contribute to clinical, economic, and quality-of-life outcomes of benefit to plan sponsors as well as members. Purchasers of pharmacy benefits have many options for obtaining a customized pharmacy program, and must identify their objectives clearly to their pharmacy benefit provider to make certain the benefit is appropriately designed. Primary future challenges will be control of expensive biologicals, and implementing a successful consumer-driver healthcare benefit, such as through a health savings account.

Pharmacy directors see increased use of generics and higher member copayments as two important methods to help contain costs. However, the pharmacy benefit must be integrated in the broad medical benefit to demonstrate the contribution of appropriately used, cost-effective pharmaceuticals.

REFERENCES

1. National Health Care Expenditure Projections: 2005–2015. Prescription Drug Expenditures (Table 11). Available at http://www.cms.hhs.gov/NationalHealthExpendData/downloads/proj2005.pdf. Accessed 30 May 2008.

2. Navarro R.P., personal communication with pharmacy and medical directors, 2005–2006.

3. National Council for Prescription Drug Programs (NCPDP) homepage. Available at http://www.ncpdp.com. Accessed 30 May 2008.

4. NCQA homepage. Available at http://hprc.ncqa.org/. Accessed 30 May 2008.

5. NCQA HEDIS® homepage. Available at http://www.ncqa.org/tabid/59/Default.aspx. Accessed 30 May 2008.

6. eHealth Initiative: Electronic prescribing: toward maximum value and rapid adoption. Recommendations for optimal design and implementation to improve care, increase efficiency and reduce costs in ambulatory care. Available at http://ccbh.ehealthinitiative.org/communities/community.aspx?Section=97&Category=250&Document=269. 2004: 11, 32 Accessed 30 May 2008.

7. *Medical Expenditure Panel Survey (MEPS).* From: Justification for Budget Estimates for Appropriations Committees, Fiscal Year 2003. February 2002. Agency for Healthcare Research and Quality, Rockville, MD. Available at http://www.ahrq.gov/about/cj2003/meps03.htm. Accessed 9 July 2008.

8. Institute for Safe Medication Practices. A Call to Action: Eliminate Hand-Written Prescriptions Within 3 Years. Available at http://www.ismp.org/msaarticles/whitepaper.html, 2000. Accessed 30 May 2008.

9. RxHub homepage. Available at http://www.rxhub.net. Accessed 30 May 2008.

10. U.S. Department of Labor in the 21st century. Health Plans & Benefits. Employee Retirement Income Security Act—ERISA. Available at http://www.dol.gov/dol/topic/health-plans/erisa.htm. Accessed 30 May 2008.

11. "States Consider Encouraging Increased Use of HSAs," *California Healthline*, 13 February 2006. Available at http://www.californiahealthline.org/articles/2006/2/13/States-Consider-Encouraging-Increased-Use-of-HSAs.aspx?topicID=37. Accessed 30 May 2008.

12. The Consumer Driven Health Care Institute homepage. Available at http://www.cdhci.org/. Accessed 30 May 2008.

13. National Association of Chain Drug Stores. Available at http://www.nacds.org/user-assets/PDF_files/2004results.PDF. Accessed 2 June 2006.

14. "Minnesota Blues Injectable Drug Cost July 2003–June 2004," *Specialty Pharmacy News*, January 2006, 3(1): p. 11.

15. National Association of Boards of Pharmacy. Verified Information and Verification Pharmacy Practice Sites™ (VIPPS®). Available at http://www.nabp.net/. Accessed 30 May 2008.

16. American Academy of Family Physicians (AAFP). Available at http://www.aafp.org/online/en/home/publications/news/news-now/practice-management/20080306getconnected.html. Accessed 30 May 2008.

17. Academy of Managed Care Pharmacy (AMCP). Professional Resources. AMCP Format for Formulary Submissions, Version 2.1. Available at http://www.amcp.org/amcp.ark?c=pr&sc=link. Accessed 30 May 2008.

18. Goldberg R.B., Managing the pharmacy benefit: the formulary system, *J Managed Care Pharmacy.* 1997; 3(5): 565–573.

19. King N.M., *Pharmacopoeias and Formularies: A Selection of Primary Sources for the History of Pharmacy in the United States.* Madison, WI: American Institute of the History of Pharmacy; 1985, p. 9–11.

20. Rector T.S., Finch M.D., Danzon P.M., et al., Effect of tiered prescription copayments on the use of preferred brand medications. *Medical Care.* 2003; 41(3): 398–406.

21. Sokol M.C., McGuigan K.A., Verbrugge R.R., Epstein R.S., Impact of medication adherence on hospitalization risk and healthcare cost. *Medical Care.* 2005; 43(6): 521–530.

22. Landsman P.B., Yu W., Liu X., Teutsch S.M., Berger M.L., Impact of 3-tier pharmacy benefit design and increased consumer cost-sharing on drug utilization. *Am J Manag Care.* 2005; 11(10): 621–628.

23. Gibson T.B., Ozminkowsk R.J., Goetzel R.Z. The effects of prescription drug cost sharing: a review of the evidence. *Am J Manag Care.* 2005; 11(11): 730–740.

24. The Rand Corporation news releases. Cutting drug copayments for sicker patients can cut hospitalizations and save money. 11 January 2006. Available at http://www.rand.org/news/press.06/01.11.html. Accessed 30 May 2008.

25. "Total Value/Total Return(TM) Tells the Pitney Bowes Experience: Healthier Employees Translate into a Healthier Bottom Line," *PRNewswire*, 17 April 2006. Available at http://media.prnewswire.com/en/jsp/tradeshows/events.jsp?option=tradeshow&beat=BEAT_ALL&eventid=1001951&view=LATEST&resourceid=3187226. Accessed 30 May 2008.

ACRONYMS

AAC	actual acquisition price
ACE	angiotensin converting enzyme
ARB	angiotensin receptor blocker
ASP	average selling price
AWP	average wholesale price (drug)
CAP	competitive acquisition program
CDH	consumer-driver healthcare
CHF	congestive heart failure
CMS	Centers for Medicare and Medicare Services
COBRA	Consolidated Omnibus Budget Reconciliation Act
COPD	chronic obstructive pulmonary disease
DUR	drug utilization review
ERISA	Employee Retirement Income Security Act of 1974
FDA	Food and Drug Administration
GERD	gastroesophageal disease
HEDIS	Health Plan Employer Data and Information Set
HIPAA	Health Insurance Portability and Accountability Act
HSAs	health spending accounts
MAC	maximum allowable cost
MCOs	managed care organizations

MTM	medication therapy management
NACDS	National Association of Chain Drug Stores
NABP	National Association of Boards of Pharmacy
NCPDP	National Council for Prescription Drug Programs
NCQA	National Committee for Quality Assurance
OBRA '90	Omnibus Budget Reconciliation Act of 1990
OTC	over-the-counter (drugs)
PA	prior authorization
PBMs	pharmacy benefit managers
PMPM	per-member-per-month
PMPY	per-member-per-year
POS	point-of-service (pharmacy)
P & T	Pharmacy & Therapeutics (Committee)
SPD	specialty pharmacy distributor
VIPPS	Verified Internet Pharmacy Practice Sites™
WAC	wholesale acquisition cost

PHARMACY BENEFIT DESIGN, MARKETING, AND CUSTOMER CONTRACTING

JOHN D. JONES

BUSINESS BASIS OF PHARMACY BENEFIT MANAGEMENT

Pharmacy benefit management is a business that developed during the late 1980s and early 1990s to address concerns regarding double-digit pharmacy inflation.

Early pharmacy benefit management involved simple contracting for discounts with a network of pharmacies and the development of information systems to adjudicate claims electronically. Such basic efficiencies in claims handling and contracting for network discounts were quickly recognized by payers of pharmacy benefits as necessities of modern pharmacy benefit management. The growing need for expertise in pharmacy benefit management spawned the development of specialized company, pharmacy benefit managers (PBMs), which brought management skill and efficiency to health plans, employer groups, and Medicaid agencies. PBMs also delivered lower drug costs, higher quality drug therapy programs, and expanded access for beneficiaries whom previously could not afford prescription medications. PBMs are discussed in depth in Chapter 4.

While a commitment to lower costs and higher quality has remained, as a business, the PBM industry has changed considerably over the past two decades. Today, the business basis of pharmacy benefits management has developed with advances in technology, increasing utilization, and the rising cost of health care. Total U.S. drug expenditure is now more than $230 billion annually. More than 95% of all Americans with drug coverage receive their benefit through a PBM. As discussed in Chapter 2, many large health plans manage their pharmacy benefits through an internal pharmacy department, or "captive" PBM, and many comments included in this chapter apply to these pharmacy programs as well.

Finding ways to manage costs and ensure appropriate access to drug therapies will remain a key objective for American business. Due to the introduction of promising yet costly drug therapies, expansion of drug coverage through Medicare Part D as well as an overall aging population, the growth of the empowered consumer, and more aggressive direct-to-consumer marketing (DTC), drug utilization will only increase over the next several years.

Although the use of pharmaceuticals as an integral component of quality health care is not disputed, the appropriate use of drugs to deliver the most value to members and plan sponsors is of great concern. In today's media driven environment, what consumers want, and what they need in terms of clinically appropriate care, are not always in alignment. Many plan sponsors view prescription drugs as a component cost of health care and will not tolerate unabated inflation of those costs without a quantifiable benefit to the overall cost or quality of health care. Balancing these two demands is one of the more important and challenging tasks for PBMs today.

As a result of market demand for strong management of the pharmacy benefit, the PBM industry has grown and has become highly competitive. There have been considerable acquisitions, mergers, and closings over the past decade. While there are more than 60 PBMs today, for the past five years, the industry has been dominated by three to five major PBMs that manage more than 70% of the market.

Many analysts believe this control may be waning, as a growing number of companies are turning to smaller niche players that have more innovative approaches to pharmacy benefit-cost containment and outcomes-focused programs. These plan sponsors also are looking for the more tailored, non-standard approaches to PBM management that smaller PBMs are willing to provide. Large companies with member populations in excess of 50,000 will be able to design and implement innovative strategies, as PBMs are always willing to look for creative ways to help their largest clients accomplish their objectives. However, mid-size and smaller companies will need to consider alternatives to the major PBMs as non-standard programs will be viewed as too costly for any but the largest of organizations.

The opportunities for PBMs willing to take the time to identify and define their areas of expertise, and to match their strengths to an organization's specific needs, are significant. In short, the business is there; however, it will take considerable work and effort to secure *and retain* that business.

Services offered by pharmacy benefit management companies include:

- Claims processing
- Network development
- Formulary management
- Medication therapy management
- Mail service
- Specialty pharmacy

This chapter explores some of the issues affecting pharmacy benefit design, management, and marketing today, and how PBMs can better meet the challenges of an increasingly complex and dynamic marketplace.

CORPORATE AND GOVERNMENT IMPETUS FOR PHARMACY BENEFIT MANAGEMENT

GROWTH OF PHARMACY BENEFITS

Corporate America has long recognized the need for effective pharmacy benefit management. Although early efforts in managing these benefits were relegated to obtaining network discounts and processing claims electronically, the increasing costs of providing pharmaceuticals to their employees has created a focus on pharmacy benefits and the way they are provided. The need for corporate competitiveness in the global market is constantly weighed against the value of providing a rich, yet costly healthcare benefit to employees.

Ongoing efforts at corporate competitiveness continue to pressure organizations to find ways to better manage pharmaceutical benefit costs. In the late 1990s and early 2000s, companies began to move away from managed benefit programs, to programs that purported to offer greater choice and flexibility. It should be noted that cost remained a key concern; however, due to intense government and consumer demand, corporate America realized that a seemingly overly restrictive approach to healthcare benefits simply would not be tolerated.

In addition, corporations and plan sponsors began to recognize the importance of quality, as witnessed by the growth in influence of organizations such as the regional and national Business Groups on Health. While continuing to value choice and cost, these organizations stressed that lower costs—at the expense of quality of care—should not be tolerated. To ensure quality, many corporations also adopted quality measurement criteria that were used to differentiate managed care programs. In addition, organizations dedicated to identifying, developing, and benchmarking quality measurements began to proliferate. Corporations looked to these organizations and their standards for determining quality of health care. Pharmacy benefits and their administration soon entered the mainstream delivery of health care and are now also subject to quality measurements.

In the early 2000s, there began to be a greater exploration of consumer driven health plans (CDHP), which provided more information regarding the actual cost for benefits and gave greater choice, flexibility, and responsibility to the plan member. In addition, many companies turned to cost sharing—specifically, higher copays or coinsurance—as a strategy to manage pharmacy costs.

MEDICARE

The complexity of today's Medicare marketplace, along with rising costs, has challenged many plan sponsors in both commercial and public programs. Guidance appeared from Congress in 2003 with the Medicare Modernization Act of 2004. The new Medicare Act relies heavily on the principles of managed care to help control pharmaceutical costs. In a 2001 report from the Federal Trade Commission and Department of Justice, the government stated that when PBMs are allowed to operate in a competitive marketplace, and to use managed care tools such as formularies, drug utilization review, tiered cost share and mail service, they could play a significant role in helping Medicare Part D plan sponsors to manage costs.[1]

In past decades, employers and plan sponsors paid little attention to Medicare when considering prescription drugs. Other than with some Medicare + Choice programs, prescription drugs weren't part of the covered benefit. Medicare supplemental programs covering drugs were relatively expensive and not embraced by the majority of Medicare beneficiaries. However, consultants and industry analysts note that now many employers and plan sponsors appear to be closely studying the benefit design options available under Part D, and that many may adopt similar benefit design strategies for their retirees and active employees. Therefore, the industry can expect to see much more emphasis on promotion of generics, tiered cost share, drug use management, outcome studies, and other traditionally managed care approaches to pharmacy benefits for retirees.

STATE MEDICAID PROGRAMS

While Medicare will clearly be the dominant factor influencing pharmacy benefit design over the next decade, actions taken at the state level should interest all employers and plan sponsors also. One of the most significant changes of the past five years has been the aggressive, and some would say bold actions of state governments to rein in rising pharmaceutical costs. The move is surprising to many as just a few years ago, many states were demanding full coverage of all drugs for their Medicaid members and paying top dollar to pharmacies that supplied the drugs. Over the past few years, some states and municipalities launched programs to purchase drugs from foreign markets. Even more have actively adopted managed care plans for state employees and the Medicaid population.

In addition, many states have developed healthcare insurance purchasing cooperatives that allow individuals and small employers to combine to purchase in the same manner as large groups. This structure allows for managed care purchasing at large purchaser discounts for smaller employers. Pharmacy benefit management is a part of the services offered to such organizations.

Large groups of state workers also have had an effect on the development of pharmacy benefit management. The public employee retirement systems are among the largest purchasers of pharmacy services and insist on high quality at a low cost for their members. The size of the groups and their interest in the delivery of health care has resulted in tremendous influence exerted on the quality and pricing of pharmacy services.

LEGAL CONSIDERATIONS IN PHARMACY BENEFIT MANAGEMENT

Pharmacy benefit management relies on a number of factors allowing the organization to exercise controls on utilization.

- Pharmacy practice is regulated by boards of pharmacy in each state, individual state agencies regulating controlled substances, and federal agencies such as the United States Food and Drug Administration and the United States Drug Enforcement Administration

- Many states have established regulations governing the operation and administration of health insurance companies and health maintenance organizations (HMOs). Most involve enforcement by regulatory agencies such as the state Departments of Insurance, Departments of Corporations, or Health Services.
- A number of states have initiated legislation to directly regulate PBM organizations. While such laws have been introduced in many states, to date, only a few have direct requirements that license or regulate PBMs. Perhaps one reason is that most states are still not sure about how to classify PBMs. They do fall under direct regulatory oversight by state boards of pharmacy if the PBM owns and operates one or more mail service pharmacies, but PBM activities outside of mail service have not been directly regulated. A key challenge to regulation by state Departments of Insurance is that PBMs do not generally take risk on the provision of prescription drugs. To provide oversight, some states have required that PBMs become licensed as third party administrators (TPAs).
- A body of federal law governing the provision of health benefits is the Employee Retirement Income Security Act of 1974 and the rules and regulations promulgated subsequently. Collectively, they are known as the *ERISA laws*. Employer groups, PBM companies, and HMOs are generally protected by federal ERISA laws from state liability for their administration of pharmacy benefits designed or selected by the plan sponsors for their covered beneficiaries (although some states are challenging this liability exemption with state legislation).
- ERISA laws protect PBMs, in part, because these organizations were not considered to fit the definition of ERISA fiduciaries. PBMs do not prescribe or practice medicine; they administer prescription drug benefits and determine coverage according to parameters established by the employer or health plan (which more clearly fall under the definition of an ERISA fiduciary). To the degree the PBMs act as fiduciaries, however, they may be treated as such. Factual analysis of the PBM's activities will determine their fiduciary status. Performing functions such as initial benefit determination or performing fair and impartial first level appeals may establish a fiduciary responsibility if the PBM is exercising discretion in those acts.
- Formularies are lists of drugs selected by a pharmacy and therapeutics (P & T) committee via a deliberative process. Formularies are administered by the PBM according to the client approved benefit design. Plan members are not prohibited from receiving prescriptions for non-formulary drugs, but under state and federal statutes, the plan is not generally bound to pay for non-formulary drugs unless the laws require the plan to cover all medically necessary drugs. Medical necessity is generally determined based upon the prescription drug treatment guidelines spelled out in the plan and supported by specific criteria established by the P & T committee. Medical necessity also may be established by a pharmacist or physician review of the facts during the prior authorization process or upon an appeal. Denials of prior authorization requests may be done by pharmacists in most states but denials of appeals usually require a physician. Reasons for

denials are explained in communication with the prescribing physician and the member. Beneficiaries are notified that their prescription drug benefits are limited. This notification is generally done through an explanation of benefits (EOB) document that beneficiaries receive from their health plan or employer. (An example of an EOB is found in Appendix 3-1.) In a number of states, laws specify that the EOB must clearly state which drugs are covered and which are excluded from the formulary, either naming the drugs individually or by treatment category.

- Some states, the Federal Employees Healthcare Benefit Plan (FEHBP), and a number of federal government plans, have established mandatory coverage of certain drug treatment categories. An example of a state mandate is an insured plan that is required to offer oral contraceptives, unless they are a recognized faith-based organization.
- PBMs contract with pharmacies to provide services to members. The contractual obligations must satisfy state and federal licensure, record-keeping, access, and consumer protection requirements.
- Many states have regulatory agencies that enforce laws created to govern the activities of health plans and to protect consumers. Generally, the health plans must provide medically necessary treatment within the guidelines of the health plan benefit policy for its members. Health plans and their contracted vendors, including PBMs must comply with the laws of those states (e.g., observing prompt pay laws or regulatory restrictions on marketing to plan members) in order to properly serve their clients' needs.
- Pharmacy network contracting may be subject to any-willing-provider laws that are present in some states. Others may have laws prohibiting prescription drug copays that provide incentive to prefer one provider (i.e., mail service) over other contracted providers.

PRESCRIPTION DRUG BENEFIT DESIGN; INFLUENCES AND EVOLUTION

FACTORS INFLUENCING BENEFIT DESIGN

A number of factors influence pharmacy benefit design and these range from federal and state requirements, plan sponsor and member needs and expectations, and more. To determine the specific elements of benefit design to be recommended to clients, PBMs rely on a wide range of strategies. PBMs conduct formulary management, including a review of the product monograph, dossier (see Chapter 11), primary literature, pharmacoeconomic data, and statistical research on populations as well as industry and society trends.

EXPLANATION OF COVERAGE LANGUAGE

Pharmacy benefit management companies, health insurance companies, and health plans must provide documents to their members that explain the prescription drug benefit in detail. Although the wording of the explanation of coverage (EOC) may incorporate by reference other healthcare coverage documents, it is generally comprehensive in content. An example of this document is listed in Appendix 3-1.

EOC INCLUSIONS, EXCEPTIONS, FORMULARY, COPAYMENT AND COINSURANCE

The EOC will include a statement of the pharmacy benefit including any specific riders that the plan sponsor has selected (contraceptives, smoking cessation, weight management, sexual dysfunction, infertility, etc.). Benefit exceptions or specific exclusions must be clearly stated in easy-to-read text. If a formulary is a feature of the benefit, the EOC should state what a formulary is, how it affects the use of the benefit, and how to obtain a copy of the formulary. An important benefit component to explain is that of direct member reimbursement. If a member has an emergency situation or is traveling out of the coverage area and does not have access to a network pharmacy, many plans allow for the member to pay for the prescription, submit a claim to the PBM, and receive direct reimbursement. It is also important for the EOC to provide a method of obtaining a complete listing of approved pharmacies within the network and to fully explain the cost and penalties for securing prescriptions outside the network.

PLAN SPONSOR EXPECTATIONS

Plan sponsors expect benefits language to be clear and unambiguous. If the language is confusing to the members of an employer group or health plan, the uncertainty is generally viewed in favor of the member. Many years of experience have gone into the development of EOB language that represent most PBMs' and health plans' pharmacy products. The plan sponsors generally view the EOB as the total terms of the benefit. Any reference to other limitations of the benefit that relate to other documents must be clearly stated to allow the member to quickly and easily access the language that may limit their benefit.

BENEFIT COST

The cost of the benefit to members is carefully described in the EOC. The member's copay amounts for generic, branded formulary, preferred drugs, and branded or generic non-formulary drugs should be spelled out. Any benefit caps, deductible amounts, or coinsurance percentages are also listed to allow the member to fully understand their financial obligation when exercising each benefit coverage option.

PATIENT SATISFACTION

Evidence of coverage language often includes information regarding customer service telephone numbers, Web site addresses, and the availability of non-formulary drugs or exceptions to drug therapy exclusion via the formulary exceptions or prior authorization process. It also provides the terms of the appeals process, and states the addresses and telephone numbers to allow the member an opportunity to redress complaints with their benefit. The member services function also may include consumer ombudsman services and in some instances a nonaffiliated third party review of grievances.

PRINCIPLES OF MARKETING PHARMACY BENEFITS

FACTORS INFLUENCING PBM PRODUCTS AND SERVICES

In the late 1980s and into the early 90s, the pharmacy benefits industry was ripe for expansion and growth. At that time, only about 60% of pharmacy benefit programs were managed by a PBM or MCO. Today, more than 90% of all pharmacy programs are managed by businesses that provide claims processing or other pharmacy services. In addition to market saturation, there has been a reduction in the number of businesses providing services due to mergers and acquisitions.

Consolidations in the marketplace do not necessarily mean that new business opportunities have vanished, however. Organizations needing specialized services as well as businesses unhappy with current providers offer opportunities for expansion. In addition, with the growth of Medicare plans, many PBMs have developed or expanded programs for the burgeoning senior market. While there are a number of restrictions and requirements for PBMs serving Medicare clients, this business remains a significant growth opportunity for PBMs with the experience and capabilities to meet the compliance requirements of public programs.

While the growth of Medicare plans will clearly influence the market, PBMs will continue to face traditional challenges with regard to product offerings and costs as well as significant new challenges from the federal government and an increasingly empowered and knowledgeable base of consumers. In particular, PBMs will need to take note that their approach to issues such as pricing and rebate contracting may no longer be confidential due to a growing interest from customers and regulators in transparency and full disclosure.

Detailed information describing revenues derived by the PBM from the plan sponsors business is expected, as is the ability to assure that the financial agreement between the parties is being honored. Contract language detailing the financial arrangement and spelling out the rights of the client to audit the PBM's transactions on behalf of the plan are becoming common. Simply offering the lowest cost benefit will no longer be enough to retain or win business. To ensure they are getting the best price possible, plan sponsors will demand greater openness and disclosure of business practices.

DRUG PRICE

As noted, due to intense scrutiny of PBM business practices, pricing of PBM services has become one of the most complex and potentially troublesome issues facing the industry. In the past, pharmacy benefit managers would provide pricing based on average wholesale price (AWP) or the government's maximum allowable cost (MAC). However, due to variable therapies and lack of standards and guidelines in the numbers and pricing as well as undefined terms, knowledgeable employers no longer rely solely on those pricing mechanisms. Today's plan sponsors want to know specifically how prices are developed. What percentage of generics receives the lowest publicized MAC rate? How is AWP calculated? What benchmarks are used and who establishes and maintains them? What other sources of revenue does the PBM have? As a result, PBMs have responded to market demands to be more flexible, and more open when it comes to pricing as purchasers have clearly become more knowledgeable and sophisticated.

Pricing a product will depend on the level of competition and the services provided. Challenging an entrenched competitor that gives good service and offers a reasonably priced product is very challenging in today's market. The PBM entering a market will need to determine whether the product intended to compete in the market can be offered at a price competitive enough to be attractive and still give an adequate profit margin. PBMs may at times need to offer their products at a price below their profit goals in order to make an entrance into a particular market. Once a market presence is established, the product prices can be adjusted to retain business but satisfy the financial goals of the PBM.

Pricing also should reflect the amount and type of services demanded by the plan sponsor and provided by the PBM. Processing prescription drug claims using an open formulary and maintaining an open access pharmacy network involves minimal effort on the part of a PBM. There are many PBMs that provide this service, making it suitable for commodity pricing.

PBM programs that provide clinically focused programs, sophisticated services, and intensive program management command higher prices, but offer more in return. Disease-specific case management, prior authorization, client specific ad hoc reporting, auditing tailored to the client, and specialized utilization analysis and consultation are the type of services that provide a value that will increase the price of services offered.

However, plan sponsors will not simply pay more for such services. PBMs will need to perform extensive pharmacoeconomic and market research and develop strong models for return on investment (ROI) for disease and care management programs. Plan sponsors are not averse to such programs, but they will demand proof that they will secure value for their increasingly scarce benefit dollars.

MARKETING CHANNELS

Advertising   Marketing a PBM is more complex than ever before. To adequately address key issues and effectively communicate points of differentiation and value, PBMs will need to consider a comprehensive and broad sales, marketing, and public relations program. The good news is there are a wide range of marketing opportunities available to PBMs today. Trade magazines—whether focused on the MCO or employer marketplace—which specialize in healthcare benefit articles are a natural focus for PBM advertising. However, developing effective programs can be costly.

There are options emerging within the advertising industry. Some of the nation's largest healthcare trade publications have experienced significant drops in advertising over the past few years. To attract and retain advertisers, many are offering lower rates and enhancements to existing ad purchasing programs. PBMs interested in traditional advertising should work closely with publishers and advertising representatives to ensure that they are aware of discounts and special programs. For example, the publication may be interested in co-sponsoring events at trade shows or may offer use of mailing lists to advertisers or advetorials. The point is to look beyond simply the placement of ads to work with publishers of trade journals in a more strategic and cooperative program. The result will provide considerably more value than simply purchasing space in a trade magazine.

Meetings and Conventions   National managed care meetings are also popular targets for marketing efforts. Presentation of new programs, reports on outcomes, a review of emerging trends, and how to use the latest technologies are all topics for presentations. There are a number of national associations offering annual conventions, including:

- The Academy of Managed Care Pharmacy
- The Pharmaceutical Care Management Association
- National Managed Health Care Congress
- National Council on Prescription Drug Programs
- America's Health Insurance Plans
- Annual events from Blue Cross and Blue Shield associations
- National Business Groups on Health

There are also a number of employer-focused meetings and conferences that are key targets for PBMs seeking to expand their business. While securing speaking invitations is not easy and is often highly competitive, interesting, and engaging presentations that focus on innovative real world approaches to the problems of pharmacy benefits today, and that provide insights into how to improve the benefit, are popular and remain of interest. Spending time and effort developing effective speaking and presentation proposals can provide significant dividends in the end.

Some PBMs also sponsor exhibits and displays at leading conferences. However, if organizations opt to invest in the expense of creating an exhibit and sending key staff out of town, they need to ensure that they develop a comprehensive plan and strategy for securing optimal value from the exhibit. Simply staffing an exhibit will likely be a waste of funds. Consider creating a special event that will attract the "right" attendees to the exhibit, train the staff to engage potential prospects, conduct follow-up. Exhibiting can be an important marketing tool. However, it must be supported with a clear plan and specific goals to ensure that time and money are not wasted.

Consultant Outreach   As the healthcare benefits marketplace becomes more complex, many employers are turning toward healthcare consulting firms to help them develop requests for proposals (RFPs) and to identify those organizations that can best meet their needs. Recognizing the important role consultants play, PBMs aggressively court their business through relationship-building with key consultants, advertising, trade shows, and other marketing and sales tactics.

PBMs also strive to gain information on when large employer groups or purchasing coalitions are planning changes to pharmacy benefit programs. Direct marketing to these groups is common. The goal of such efforts should be to secure an opportunity to submit an RFP when new business opportunities become available.

PROMOTION

A variety of other factors are influencing the PBM marketing today. Due to the intensity of competition, all forms of promotion—not just advertising and marketing—are utilized by companies seeking ways to grow and retain business. To be viable, a PBM cannot rely on word-of-mouth marketing of its services alone. More importantly, PBMs today are subject to intense scrutiny from state and federal legislators, consumer advocate groups, employers, special interest groups, and others. Many of the nation's largest PBMs have experienced significant negative publicity due to questionable pricing tactics and general business practices. Negative coverage tends to position PBMs as nothing more than middlemen that add cost and no value to the healthcare system.

As a result, not only must PBMs find ways to market in a highly competitive market, they must fight a strong battle to educate and communicate to a diverse audience the value they provide in today's healthcare environment.

To address these challenges, many PBMs turn to strategic public relations campaigns. These campaigns may include news releases on new products and services, articles written by company experts that highlight innovative disease management programs or new technologies, public affairs programs aimed at communicating the PBM value proposition and a wide range of other strategies designed to help educate and inform key audiences on the nature and goal of PBM programs today.

While in the past, many PBM marketing programs were aimed at employers or health plans, with the advent of CDHPs and Medicare PBMs, many companies will now need to consider advertising and marketing that more directly reaches consumers.

This will involve a new mindset for many PBMs, as factors motivating consumers vary greatly from those that influence employers or MCOs. PBMs will need to better understand the knowledge level of consumers, and other factors contributing to purchasing decisions.

THE INTERNET

While a number of factors have influenced PBM marketing over the past five years, one of the most significant is the growth of the Internet as a communication channel with a wide range of audiences. PBMs can use the Internet to directly communicate news releases and other communication materials, and as a distribution channel for direct marketing. In addition, company Web sites are now a crucial source of information and insights into a company's expertise, products, and service. Current and potential customers as well as members will use the Internet or a PBM's Web site to gather pertinent information. The good news about the growth of the Internet is that it enables an organization to more fully communicate the messages they believe best portray the organization. Therefore, a strong Web site, with information of interest to key audiences including employers, MCOs, consumers, and other audiences, is critical to an effective marketing campaign.

In addition to a strong company Web site, leading industry associations and publications now offer the opportunity to post articles and white papers onto their Web sites. These Web sites also offer advertising opportunities at prices much lower than print advertising. PBMs should research those online opportunities that provide a good fit to their messages and budget, and fully explore the marketing opportunities provided by the Internet.

Another emerging feature offered by the Internet is the use of audio conferences tailored to meet the needs of specific audiences. Recognizing the value of this new communication method, leading trade publications are seeking to collaborate with customers to develop programs targeted to directly reach key audiences. While typically reaching a smaller number of prospects, such vehicles enable the creation of much more direct and meaningful programs that often go beyond marketing, to providing important and highly sought-after "how-to" insights. Such programs are generally viewed much more favorably by current and prospective customers and enable PBMs to better position themselves as knowledgeable leaders and resources.

While providing tremendous value as a marketing tool, the Internet also allows for negative information to be more quickly communicated. PBMs today must be proactive and not reactive. If a PBM is aware of a negative industry story or a drug recall, it should be prepared to immediately respond to all key audiences; gone are the days when a company could spend several days developing and refining messages. The Internet spreads news quickly and delays in response put an organization at risk of seeming ill-prepared, lacking knowledge, or being uncaring. These responses do not necessarily need to be targeted toward the media. However, information correcting significant errors or clarifying misinterpretations should be communicated to current and prospective customers quickly if management deems it a critical issue.

THE GROWTH OF BLOGS

While the Internet is a communications tool, it is also used as a forum for those with similar interests. The use of "blogs" or online journals has grown from an informal means for people to communicate personal experiences, preferences, etc., to sophisticated experts' forums to marketing vehicles for large corporations or politicians. While many blogs are offered today by well-known and respected PBM consultants, some are simply mediums for disgruntled former or current employees, members, general gossip, and individual rants. It is important for organizations to be aware of these sites and to ensure that inaccurate or inflammatory information is not posted. Informed bloggers guard their freedom to write the truth as they see it. (They most definitely do not want to receive news releases or promotional materials.) PBMs should make note of reputable industry experts that have blogs and ensure there is an ongoing dialogue with them so that they are aware of successful programs and of issues the organization believes are appropriate for industry discussion.

Member Retention   While companies spend considerable time and effort developing programs to attract new business, few spend time retaining existing business. Business retention is not typically thought of as a marketing tactic. However, in the competitive world of pharmacy benefit marketing today, it should be.

Companies that invest in marketing should also consider how their programs could be tailored to reach existing customers. For example, presentations at key conferences can be designed that include existing customers so that they can secure exposure and acknowledgment for successful and innovative programs. The key is for the PBM to consider existing client's need for information and outreach as much as that of prospects. Customer service, which is discussed later in this chapter, also must become a critical component of retention efforts. A satisfied client, one who will share their positive experiences with other prospects, is among the best marketing tools a PBM can have.

PLAN SPONSOR AND PATIENT EXPECTATIONS AND DECISION POINTS

Virtually every member category within a PBM's business has undergone considerable change over the past five years. Due to high-profile coverage of the PBM industry, there is not only greater knowledge as to what PBMs are, but there are more questions and concerns about the impact of industry practices on organizations and individuals. Therefore, PBMs need to ensure they thoroughly understand plan sponsor, patient and member expectations, needs, and factors influencing purchasing decisions.

SELF-INSURED PLAN SPONSORS

Self-insured businesses expect PBMs to perform benefit administration smoothly and deal with member concerns and complaints quickly and with positive outcomes. They expect a level of autonomy but with intelligent guidance in determining benefit design. As government regulations change through new rulings and court cases, self-insured companies also will look to their PBM to help them navigate the often-changing legal landscape to maintain their compliance and to avoid regulatory liability.

MANAGED CARE ORGANIZATIONS AND HEALTH PLANS

MCOs, HMOs, and health plans frequently demand a high level of pharmacy benefit management services because they are more likely to employ the use of formularies, limited networks, and incentive-based benefits for providers and members. With traditional HMO membership shrinking, organizations want their PBMs to help them move beyond simply the image of "cost-cutter" to that of an organization that can improve quality, outcomes, and member satisfaction. MCOs will want their PBM to provide insights into innovative programs that can help them better retain and attract new business.

PLAN MEMBERS

Plan members today are becoming much more knowledgeable about their healthcare and prescription benefit. The good news is that many are much more willing to accept generics and to participate in disease management programs. However, due to cost-shifting, rising copays, and the growth of CDHP, plan members are demanding more value, better service and more information with which to better manage their benefit. PBMs that do not provide strong customer service run the risk that members will become unhappy and complain to their plan sponsors or regulators. As noted, as the new Medicare plan takes effect in 2006, PBMs will also have to find ways to manage the distinct needs of a new member population: seniors.

TAFT-HARTLEY TRUSTS

Not long ago, most Taft-Hartley Trusts (unions) simply wanted uncomplicated, problem-free, and low-cost administration of their members' benefit and the highest possible level of rebates. However, as pharmacy costs have risen, unions have been challenged to ensure the value of the benefit while protecting the trust's assets. The health benefit is perceived as part of the total compensation package under the union contract. Union members continue to view benefits as a crucial attribute of membership, yet they also recognize that with costs rising, some concessions will need to be made. Union members and retirees are also reflective of the population, and the fact that they are aging increases utilization and the need for more targeted disease management programs. While traditionally shunning managed care techniques such as formulary and prior authorization, many unions are now willing to consider such strategies if they are tied to higher quality, value, stronger service, and preservation of their benefit. Therefore, union trusts will be motivated by PBMs that can prove they can provide low cost, attractive benefits, and strong customer service.

MEDICAID

Medicaid programs are put out to bid by the Medicaid administration in each individual state. The RFPs are usually comprehensive in nature, requesting information on all aspects of pharmacy benefits management activities.

Medicaid plan sponsor expectations include:

- The operational capacity to handle the volume of Medicaid enrollees.
- The ability to work within federal and state regulations and to quickly address changes in legislation and regulatory rulings.
- The capability to implement new business with little member impact and to administer the benefit seamlessly.
- Program offerings that can be tailored to meet the distinct needs of the Medicaid population.

It is also important for PBMs interested in bidding for Medicaid programs to understand the often significant political nuances involved in any public program. The administration and design of the benefit is often less influenced by what the PBM recommends, but more by political negotiation and budgetary considerations.

One of the most challenging components for Medicaid programs is that the PBM must have the ability to contract with a wide range of network pharmacies at a rate dictated by the Medicaid contract. Because pharmacies pay state and federal taxes, the right to participate at the rate established is often guaranteed to pharmacies traditionally serving the Medicaid population. Providing benefits to Medicaid populations within those restrictions can be challenging. However, many states have focused on development of high quality, outcomes-focused, and low-cost programs. Therefore, while the political nature of Medicaid should be acknowledged, it should not preclude a PBM from seeking such business. Thorough research can help to identify those programs that will welcome a PBM's approach to pharmacy benefits. Another approach the states have taken involves transferring risk to health plans that are allowed to manage the Medicaid medical and pharmacy benefits similarly to private health plans. The plans bid for the business and manage the benefits to meet financial and regulatory requirements.

MEDICARE

Attention has been given in this chapter to the significant influence Medicare will have on all aspects of pharmacy programs over the next several years. Even after a few years, these programs are so complex, that there continue to be questions and uncertainties. It will be difficult for organizations with no experience in developing prescription benefits to seniors to manage and implement successful programs. PBMs that wish to market prescription drug programs (PDPs; stand alone Medicare Part D prescription drug benefits) or Medicare Advantage Prescription Drug Programs (MAP; Part D programs with integrated medical and prescription drug benefits) to Medicare enrollees need to recognize the needs of the plan sponsors, which include employers, MCOs, and health plans, and of individual Medicare enrollees. The marketing needs are special in that these plans are highly regulated by the federal government and need to follow strict guidelines. They are subject to regulatory oversight and must generally be approved by both the plan and the regulator prior to use. A PBM that is experienced with Centers for Medicaid and Medicare Services (CMS) oversight requirements concerning marketing materials has an advantage in successfully serving its clients.

Plan sponsors will be motivated not just by cost, but by the PBM's level of experience in developing and implementing programs for Medicare eligibles. They will want assurances that their PBM is fully aware of all requirements and regulations and that it has the capabilities and depth to meet demands. Medicare remains complex and—as it has become a program highly influenced by politics—is viewed as a somewhat less predictable segment of the marketplace. Extensive expertise in legislative initiatives and knowledge of the marketplace will be crucial for plan sponsors. Those PBMs that elect to enter this volatile market will still need to understand the factors motivating plan sponsors and members. For example, employers—as they will be at risk for pharmacy programs—will rely heavily on their PBM to guide their choices toward programs that meet the needs of members, manage costs, and help to control overall pharmacy and medical expenses. Members selecting a PDP or MAP will continue to be motivated by factors ranging from cost and trust in the organization to disease management programs and customer service. This is among the most demanding market segments and PBMs will need to ensure their programs are designed to meet expectations.

Marketing a PDP or MAP may be costly. Competition will be intense and to break through the clutter of marketing "noise" will take considerable presence. There are questions as to profitability in the near term, especially if the laws and regulations surrounding Part D are subject to change by Congress and/or CMS. Indeed, some plans are holding off on entering the market until some of the competition has thinned out. However, those that enter now, and that have experience in the market, will gain considerable knowledge. They will refine their products and their marketing. As they do so, those organizations will continue to grow.

ROLES OF THE MEMBER IN PHARMACY BENEFIT PROVIDER SELECTION

While Medicare members will have high expectations from their new PDP or MAPD programs, commercial members are expected to become more demanding as well. As a cost-cutting tool, small- to mid-sized companies will likely continue to mandate a single health plan and PBM provider. However, larger employers will likely continue to offer one or more choice of benefit plans. Today, member acceptance of the benefit and the PBM is integral to the success of the programs instituted to improve quality or control costs. There are several scenarios that occur which influence the member selection of the PBM provider.

Employer Competitiveness   Members who are unhappy with their pharmacy benefit management perceive their benefit as substandard and tend to vote with their feet. An employer in a job market where there is low unemployment needs to offer current and prospective employees a benefit that is perceived to be of high quality and strong value. Health benefits are considered by many employees as a critical part of their compensation. PBMs that perform poorly in benefit management, create inconvenient access to network pharmacies, provide poor customer service, or otherwise produce a high level of dissatisfaction, are a liability for an employer.

Employee Interaction with Employer Health Benefits Managers   It is common for employees to comment on the employer's current choice of PBM if they are dissatisfied with service. Employees also are quick to suggest those PBMs and benefit designs that they would like their employer to consider. Employee complaints are a significant reason for decisions made by employers on health care issues. Therefore, strong customer service is essential to an effective PBM program. Investing in technology such as high quality automated voice response (AVR) systems and focusing on training of customer service staff will be well-worth the time and money.

Customer Satisfaction Surveys   Routine customer satisfaction surveys take individual member views of the PBM services into account. Although the surveys are done using a representative sample, most include individual member input. This information should become a key source of insight and provide the foundation for program improvements and enhancements. Improvements in satisfaction should be communicated to employers and employees. Lack of improvement should be carefully studied and new plans developed to ensure appropriate changes are made.

Consumer Focus Groups   Many health plans conduct focus groups using representative consumers from their markets. While most consumers are not familiar with a specific PBM company, they are well aware of the features offered that they would like. For example, computer savvy consumers may prefer online access to information such as formularies, copays, generic alternatives, mail service ordering or a record of the prescriptions they have filled.

Taft-Hartley Plan Members   Members of union group benefit plans are able to influence their union benefit management representatives to choose PBMs and network pharmacies based on union affiliation and relationship with organized labor. A pharmacy network design rejecting non-union pharmacy participation is a common differentiation with standard benefit models.

Influence of Customer Satisfaction   Assertions that the individual has no ability to influence selection of PBMs or benefit designs ignore the facts of the competitive marketplace. Customer satisfaction with the PBM is measured by the plan sponsors through their individual members. Because most PBMs have a common method of doing business, benefit administration practices that negatively impact individuals are quickly recognized and corrected before they result in a substantial member backlash and termination of the PBM services. No benefit provider can afford to develop the reputation that they ignore the needs of their covered members.

PHARMACY PERFORMANCE MEASUREMENTS IMPORTANT IN MARKETING

As the PBM industry becomes more complex and competitive, performance measurements will become increasingly more important to plan sponsors and members. Some pharmacy functions are measurable as performance criteria and become standards for comparing the quality of the PBM against its competitors. In categories where performance is exemplary, a PBM will use such information for promotional marketing. Examples of measurable performance categories include:

- Per member per month drug expense
- Average rebated discount per prescription
- Customer service wait time and call abandonment rate
- Customer satisfaction surveys
- Average turnaround time for mail service prescriptions
- Standard and ad hoc reporting turnaround times
- Complaint reporting (formulary, network, benefit design, customer service, prescription errors, etc.)
- Accreditation programs such as URAC[2] (formerly Uniform Standards of Utilization Review) or the National Association of Boards of Pharmacy's Verifiable Internet Pharmacy Practice Site (VIPPS)[3] accreditation and other industry standards and guidelines
- Fraud and error detection and reporting

Competencies that are less easily measured but are also important in marketing the PBM are:

- Ability to forecast and communicate drug trends
- Legal and regulatory compliance expertise
- Presence of quality improvement programs and ability to assist in preparation for health plan URAC or Nation Commission for Quality Assurance (NCQA)[4] accreditation
- Medicare/Medicaid management expertise
- Benefit design and plan management expertise
- Successful implementation experience

Competitive PBMs continually receive RFPs. Many of these are extremely detailed in the nature of their questions. The RFPs are often written by benefit consultants who are experienced in pharmacy benefit management and pose in-depth and detailed questions about the ability of the PBM to support pharmacy benefit designs that are envisioned by the entity submitting the RFP or its consultant. The process of responding to RFPs helps the PBM define areas on which the market will focus when judging their success or failure. By developing measurement tools to gauge the PBM's performance successes, the PBM is also able to determine which areas of their performance will be suitable for inclusion into their marketing programs. This information also allows the PBM to understand the areas of its performance where it may later contract for risk or performance incentives.

A new performance category that PBMs are recognizing is communication of revenue stream, pricing, and transparency. This is an area of great interest to the purchasers of pharmacy benefit management services and is reflected in the RFP questions of both private and public plan sponsors. PBMs that are perceived as open, honest, and forthcoming will be better able to position themselves as trusted and reliable resources for current and prospective customers. Likewise, companies that are not forthcoming with requested information will have challenges in securing business and will face greater scrutiny. PBMs should carefully examine current transparency policies and revise as necessary. Such efforts not only help the company with its competitive positioning, but will also reduce the likelihood of state and federal regulatory oversight.

PBM MARKETING CAMPAIGN

Examples of trade advertising materials for a PBM are shown in **Figures 3-1 through 3-3**. Other marketing materials will include direct mail, sponsorships, teleconferences or other strategies as identified by the marketing team.

MARKETING PROCESS: ROLE OF PHARMACISTS IN MARKETING

Pharmacists may undertake many roles in the marketing of their organization's pharmacy benefit. In recent years, many pharmacists have expanded their post-professional education to obtain advanced degrees or certificates in business administration. This specialization has been especially attractive to pharmaceutical manufacturers and managed care companies. Marketing is one business activity where these dual-disciplined pharmacists can add value for their employer.

With the increasing issues of prescription drug inflationary trends, the marketing of a managed care pharmacy benefit requires the involvement of PBM or health plan staff that can easily reduce the concepts to the level of the lay purchaser of services. More importantly, these pharmacists possess insights that can help marketing executives better understand the clinical issues that impact benefit design and to identify program outcomes that will have meaning to purchasers in terms of quality, productivity, and ability to manage costs. These people become subject matter experts to the sales and marketing staff.

The managed care pharmacist involvement in marketing may include:

- Providing strategic analysis of the market
- Acting as an issue spokesperson with the media
- Developing market-competitive pharmacy programs
- Pricing of the marketed services
- Developing marketing materials
- Participating in or conducting events where the PBM/health plan has marketing presentations or displays
- Joining the marketing team on sales calls to potential or existing clients
- Responding to requests for proposals
- Obtaining positive references from existing clients
- Participating in the contract negotiation process with new and renewing clients
- Responding to concerns of potential clients regarding pharmacy network adequacy or benefit design

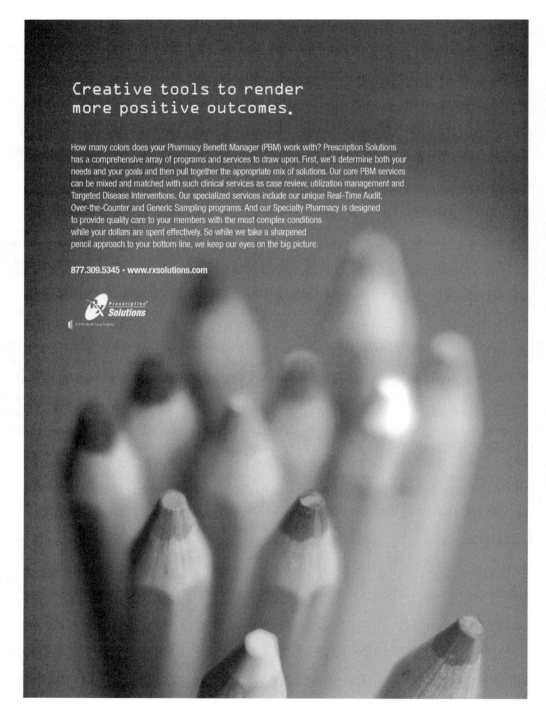

FIGURE 3-1   Example 1 of trade advertising materials for a PBM.
Source: Prescription Solutions. www.rxsolutions.com.

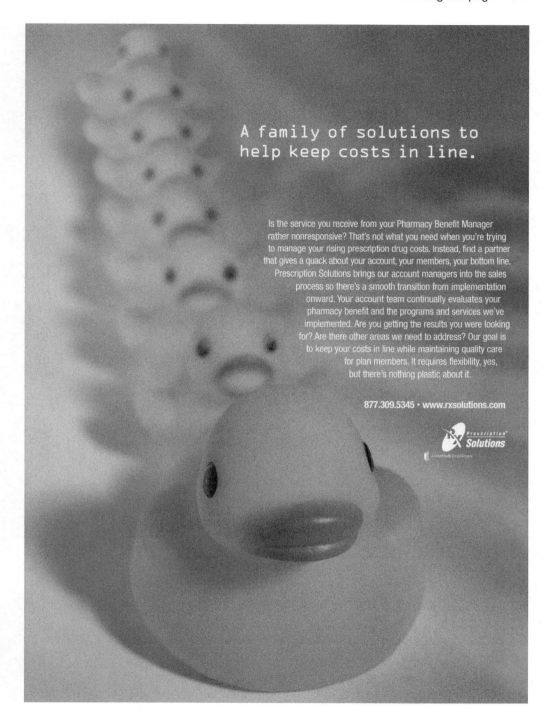

FIGURE 3-2   Example 2 of trade advertising materials for a PBM.
Source: Prescription Solutions. www.rxsolutions.com.

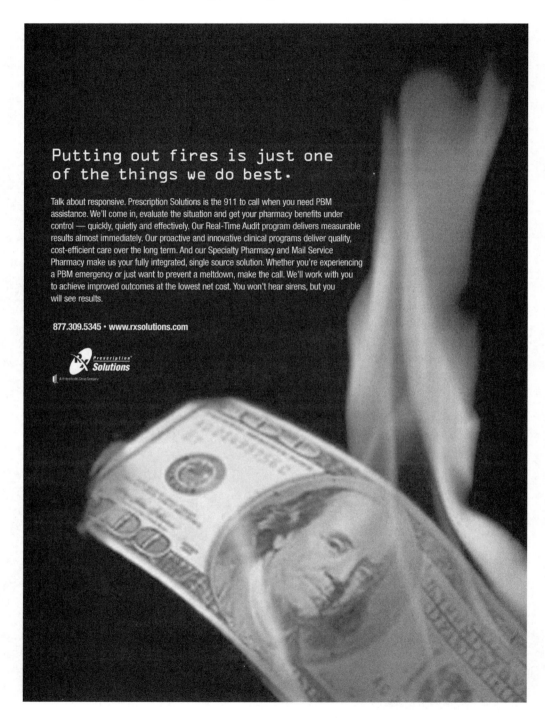

FIGURE 3-3 **Example 3 of trade advertising materials for a PBM.**
Source: Prescription Solutions. www.rxsolutions.com.

Pharmacists in a managed care marketing capacity need to develop a set of skills that are generally not emphasized during their pharmacy education. Sales and marketing skills are often required. Strong speaking and writing skills are essential, as professional presentations to a discriminating purchaser of pharmacy benefits are expected in this competitive environment.

Analytical skills are important as clients will discuss their benefit options and the obvious and hidden advantages and disadvantages of each. Pharmacists can discuss therapeutics and the relative value of making benefit changes on the overall cost of the healthcare program. A pharmacist can bring balance to the marketing discussion when the only consideration is the price of the services to be contracted and not the savings brought by the quality of a well designed and managed benefit. Many of the activities that make the management of the pharmacy benefit successful and please the individual program members are not obvious to the buyer of services, so their importance must be carefully explained. A marketing advantage stemming from superior program administration or innovative methods of management has to be sold by marketing staff with the ability to convey its importance and value.

Pharmacists will have a growing involvement in the marketing of pharmacy benefit management services as the costs of pharmaceuticals continue to escalate. Explaining the methods used by PBMs, their relative value to the buyer, the therapeutic soundness of the benefit design, and the ways in which appropriate management will increase enrollee outcomes and satisfaction will become more important than ever in fielding a successful benefit management marketing effort.

CONTRACTING, INTERNAL HEALTH PLAN AND CARVE-OUT PBM SERVICES, SELF-FUNDED PROGRAMS, AND INTERNAL HEALTH PLAN CONTRACTING ISSUES

Health plans with pharmacy departments will be required to establish a variety of contracts for efficient pharmacy benefit management. Depending on the level of operational independence, the health plan will need to either develop an information system competency for claims processing or contract this function to an information technology vendor that specializes in development and maintenance of that function. The health plan can contract for licensed software and customize the program to suit its needs. It can purchase or contract to lease the hardware to support claims processing or contract the whole claims processing function to a third party with the pharmacy department performing clinical and utilization management functions.

The internal pharmacy department will need to contract with network pharmacies, clinical consultants, auditing companies, and potentially a mail service pharmacy if that capability is desirable as part of the benefit being offered. Finally, rebate contracting with pharmaceutical manufacturers may be performed internally or subcontracted to an outside vendor of these services. Formulary management, while kept separate from rebate contracting, must communicate its decisions to the contracting team to allow efficient negotiation of pharmaceutical contracts and maximum price concessions. This creates a challenge if the formulary is managed by the pharmacy department and the rebate contracting is done outside of the health plan.

CARVING OUT PHARMACY BENEFIT MANAGEMENT TO PBMs

Many health plans, large employers and self-funded programs choose to carve out the management of their pharmacy benefits to a PBM. The PBM generally contracts to provide all management functions including claims processing, formulary management, rebate contracting, pharmacy network contracting, network support, and customer service. The PBM contract has many features. Primary among them is the articulation of rights and responsibilities of the parties, including all of the contracted functions of the PBM. The responsibilities state in detail the functions the PBM will be performing in the course of benefit administration for their client. It is important to describe each activity of the PBM and disclose all standard and exceptional costs for the services performed.

Contracts generally include performance standards that list the expectations of the health plan or self-funded program regarding the services performed by the PBM. Common performance standards include accuracy of prescriptions filled, member wait time on the telephone for customer service calls, mail service turnaround time, member satisfaction with the PBM, timeliness of utilization report generation, and minimum rebate amounts. The contracts also may include liquidated damage clauses and termination clauses if performance does not meet minimum standards stated in the contract.

There is a current trend toward including disclosure of PBM revenue sources in the PBM client services agreement. Administrative fees paid to the PBM by drug manufacturers, data sales fees and additional revenues received from contracted network pharmacies are examples of areas of disclosure specified in the contract.

PRODUCT OFFERINGS AND TARGET MARKET

PBMs design their products to reflect their areas of strength and the customers' wants and needs. A PBM that processes claims with a high level of efficiency and maintains a broad access pharmacy network with strong brand recognition by network pharmacies will appeal to purchasers that are interested in providing a benefit with few customer service problems. Other PBMs develop programs to meet the needs of more demanding customers. Their programs may include:

- Strong management of the pharmacy benefit
- Administering closed formularies
- Performing prior authorization of non-formulary drugs
- Conducting therapeutic interchange and disease management programs
- Contracting with pharmaceutical companies for rebates as well as for restricted access network discounts

These services appeal to plan sponsors interested in obtaining the highest quality for the best value.

Each market is different. A mail service PBM that tailors its services to transplant or AIDS patients can narrowly define its target markets and appeal to those health plans or physician groups that serve large numbers of those patients. States where managed care is the prevalent method for delivering pharmacy benefits require PBM products that are capable of providing aggressive and effective management. Medicaid and Medicare programs form markets that also may require aggressive contracting for pharmacy network discounts and strong management of member utilization.

PRODUCT OFFERINGS FOR VARIOUS MARKETS (WHO BUYS WHAT?)

PBMs will improve their sales opportunities by developing products that differentiate them from competitors and by advertising those products to the appropriate markets. Markets that emphasize tight drug utilization management will be likely to choose PBM products such as analytical reports and sophisticated formulary management.

Some health plans focus on providing access to all FDA approved drugs and depend on tiered pricing using a preferred drug list to influence member utilization. Such a plan will need clinical support to determine which drugs to prefer and a flexible system of electronic edits and customer service support to provide members with information as to which drugs provide the best value under the program.

Yet another market, Taft-Hartley union trusts, historically have been more likely to look for an open formulary and a pharmacy network that is price competitive but with broad access for its members. Both labor and management have come to realize, however, that the pharmacy benefit is erosive of their overall wage and benefit package if left unmanaged. Many unions are allowing significantly more aggressive management of their pharmacy benefits to preserve their overall compensation. A PBM that is able to work with the labor client's needs in balancing access with effective cost controls will be able to appeal to this market.

CONTRACTING TRENDS

Electronic Medical Records and PBM Database Contracting Contracting for pharmacy benefit management services has moved to providing a more integrated approach with the goal of integrating medical and pharmacy claims and tracking overall outcomes. Although the ability of PBMs and HMOs to integrate the medical claim has been very slow in coming, there is a continuing effort to standardize the medical database and automate the capture of its information from medical groups and clinical laboratories. As companies are able to successfully implement systems including an electronic medical record and an electronic prescribing system, managed care organizations will either develop or contract for the information systems to support these programs and provide access to the resulting data.

E-prescribing, whether as a stand-alone capability or as an integrated program with other physician practice management programs will aid the PBM in reducing negative member interactions at the pharmacy while improving formulary compliance by prescribers. The initiatives for developing an electronic medical record and establishing e-prescribing programs has been given new momentum by the CMS to complement the new Medicare Part D prescription drug benefit. Contracting for e-prescribing capabilities will become more important as new standards come to the market and the technology is adopted by, and integrated into, the business practices of prescribers, pharmacies, and PBMs.

GROWING ROLE AND IMPORTANCE OF MEDICARE AND MEDICAID TO PBMs

BRIEF OVERVIEW OF IMPACT OF THE MEDICARE MODERNIZATION ACT

Late in 2003, Congress passed a historic Medicare reform bill. This bill includes the most sweeping legislative reforms in the Medicare program's then 38-year history, including the first funded Medicare Prescription Drug Benefit.

The new Medicare legislation was created to provide financial relief to Medicare beneficiaries and to make prescription drugs more affordable for all those eligible for Medicare benefits. As of January 1, 2006, coverage for prescription drugs is being provided through a funded Prescription Drug Benefit Program (PDP) provided under Medicare Part D. Additionally, the Medicare + Choice program is now the Medicare Advantage Prescription Drug (MAPD) program. Both programs can only be offered by plan sponsors approved by the CMS.

This legislation was developed by congressional policymakers who carefully examined an exhaustive array of issues. They determined that private companies (i.e., health plans, insurers, and PBMs), through their ability to provide quality and affordable drug coverage, were a critical component of a strong Medicare Prescription Drug Benefit (PDP) program. Specifically, the legislation validates the model exemplified by pharmacy benefit managers with a managed care heritage by preserving proven tools and techniques that such organizations rely upon—medication therapy management and quality assurance programs, specialty pharmacy services, drug utilization review, and compliance programs—to make prescriptions safer, more effective, and more affordable for Americans.

UNIQUE BENEFITS DESIGN AND CONTRACTING REQUIREMENTS

Plan components vary by region and plan. However, Part D standard prescription drug coverage includes a $250 deductible, 25% coinsurance up to the initial coverage limit of $2,250, and catastrophic coverage after an individual incurs $3,600 in out-of-pocket expenses. Low-income individuals earning below 135% of poverty, and less than $6,000 in assets for individuals and $9,000 for couples, will receive premium subsidies of 100% of the average premium in their area.

Within certain guidelines outlined in the legislation, approved Medicare Advantage (MA) and Employer-Sponsored programs have the freedom to design the coverage that they believe is best for their members, provided the drug coverage has an actuarial value equal to or greater than the actuarial value of Part D standard prescription drug coverage.

The new legislation includes numerous incentives that encourage employers to continue to offer retiree benefits. Retiree plans offering actuarially equivalent coverage receive 28%

payment for drug costs between $250 and $5,000. These subsidies are not counted as taxable income providing further savings to seniors. It should be noted also that many employers are turning to private companies that have experience in providing benefits to seniors to help them manage their programs. This creates significant opportunities for companies that have relationships with employers and that possess an ability to manage pharmacy costs.

MEDICAID

It is estimated that Medicaid programs will see the most significant increase in prescription drug expenditures over the next decade. CMS projects that, by 2011, Medicaid will be paying for almost 20% of all U.S. prescriptions. To help manage these costs, many states are turning to private sector pharmacy benefit managers.

The percentage of Medicaid beneficiaries receiving pharmacy benefits through managed care and the level of PBM or health plan involvement in the Medicaid program varies by state and at times by county. Benefits generally are required to be at the level of the state fee-for-service programs although some states do not require the health plans or PBMs to use the same preferred drug list.

The advantages of transferring the state Medicaid pharmacy programs to managed care entities are to increase the efficiency of providing services, achieve significant cost reductions through network and rebate contracting, provide strong clinical programs and formulary management, and decrease the size and complexity of government.

Pharmacy benefits may extend to items beyond prescription drugs. Many benefits include adult diapers, durable medical equipment, prosthetic devices, over-the-counter (OTC) drugs, and diabetic supplies. Contracting for Medicaid risk or administration will generally require inclusion of all aspects of the previous Medicaid drug benefit in order to successfully gain a contract award.

Working with Medicaid programs opens up the health plan or PBM to oversight from CMS and the Office of Inspector General (OIG) at the Department of Health and Human Services. In particular, there will be considerable scrutiny of PBMs that manage drug therapy by moving patients from one drug to another: a key component of programs designed to improve outcomes and manage costs. The OIG will also carefully monitor health plan formulary development procedures, and PBM contracting programs.

The federal government is also focused on drug pricing mechanisms and understanding how pricing is developed. CMS has become more involved with Part B pricing benchmark standards and will pay under the average sales price standard that it maintains. Some analysts believe that the industry is moving closer to adopting government established benchmark pricing mechanisms as opposed to traditional AWP or MAC methodologies.

Other requirements for some Medicaid programs include setting a limit on maximum copays and eligibility that does not extend beyond 30 days. This means that the PBM is constantly working to identify whether or not a patient is eligible for benefits. This particular requirement makes the use of automated systems, such as those used in many mail service programs, particularly difficult.

PLAN SPONSOR EXPECTATIONS

Purchasers of pharmacy benefits expect a number of outcomes in dealing with a PBM or MCO. Plan sponsors want the greatest value possible for their benefit dollar. They want to please their members or employees with the benefit they have offered. They want few if any surprises from their pharmacy benefit manager. Plan sponsors do not want to hear a litany of complaints from their covered members regarding their pharmacy benefits. To those ends, the following twelve issues are important.

Customer Service   The benefits manager must have a customer service program that is responsive to beneficiary concerns before they become critical and result in complaints. The customer service hours must be adequate to cover the normal needs of members in filling prescriptions in the time zones covered. Many large pharmacy benefit managers have added 24-hour, 7-day-a-week coverage in order to accommodate members' after-hours needs and issues. Average wait times must be at or below industry standards (generally under two minutes), as should the percentages of call abandonment (generally under 5%). The customer service function should handle most member issues routinely while elevating only unusual member issues to the attention of the employer.

Efficient Claims Handling   Plan sponsors expect seamless processing of claims. Member complaints due to poor eligibility handling benefit administration, or network systems issues will not be well received. PBMs must plan for adequate capacity and have sufficient infrastructure to handle the volume and complexity of claims for all of their clients. System redundancy and emergency planning are essential also in providing the claims administration expected by plan sponsors.

Access to Information   With the advent of the empowered consumer and Consumer Directed Health Plans (CDHP), including Health Savings Accounts (HSAs) and Flexible Spending Accounts (FSAs), plan sponsors expect their pharmacy benefit manager to provide comprehensive, accurate, and easily accessible information about the benefit. Information on how members or employees can secure optimal value from the benefit is also important. Plan sponsors will want their PBM to provide Internet access so that their employees or members can access information on cost and efficacy of drug options, particularly generics; copay or coinsurance amounts. If the plan sponsor offers a CDH plan, or one that provides a specific dollar limit for pharmacy, beneficiaries will want to be able to readily access account status.

Access to Pharmacies   An important emerging benchmark for care is the TRICARE Standard, which was developed for the Department of Defense health plans such as CHAMPUS. This standard sets a number of guidelines PBMs must meet, including access to pharmacies for members. TRICARE states that within urban areas, at least 90% of beneficiaries, on average, must live within two miles of a network pharmacy. In a rural area, at least 70% of members must live within 15 miles of a pharmacy.[5] Similar standards are used by CMS for Medicare Part D. Many commercial plans are using these standards as guidelines for access when contracting their pharmacy networks.

Plan sponsors expect adequate network access, although the exact definition of *adequate* will vary by plan sponsor. Some plan sponsors require nearly open networks with a very high level of access to enable their members to fill prescriptions in almost every pharmacy location. This level of access generally involves a greater cost due to the need to satisfy the margin requirements of an expanded number of pharmacies. Other plan sponsors are willing to accept significant restrictions on the number of pharmacies available to their members if there is a corresponding level of quality, savings or other value offered that meet specific needs. For example, union trusts may want to eliminate non-union pharmacies from their network. Other plans may be willing to reduce network pharmacies in exchange for greater control in the management of medication therapy or other quality-based programs performed by a selected group. The important message for pharmacy benefit managers is that many plan sponsors today want flexibility in their pharmacy benefit programs, not a standardized cookie-cutter approach.

Formulary Management   Most plan sponsors today expect strong clinical management of their pharmacy benefit. After years of drug benefit inflation, even the plan sponsors offering the most generous benefits are interested in adopting moderate to aggressive formulary management for their members. Formularies are expected to serve the therapeutic needs of the plans' members, and provide the best chance for positive outcomes while also offering the greatest value to the plan sponsor. Other plan sponsors are eager to have nearly all drugs available on their formulary and then vary the member cost share according to status of the drug on their preferred drug list. Beneficiaries have an incentive through a lower share of cost to use the drugs featured on the preferred drug list of the formulary.

Contracting for Rebates and Discounts   Many plan sponsors have developed a high level of sophistication in negotiating contracts with PBMs and have taken into account the rebates that may result from utilization of the formulary products by their members. The amounts of the rebates vary considerably depending on the contracting abilities of the pharmacy benefit manager, the number of covered lives, pharmacy benefit design, and utilization patterns of the group. The allocation of rebates and discounts resulting from the plan sponsor's utilization is often aggressively negotiated between the pharmacy benefit manager and his/her client. Sophisticated plan sponsors also will demand information on any revenue that a PBM might secure as a result of doing business with them as well as audit rights to confirm that they are receiving the value of their bargain. Thus, well disclosed, auditable rebate contracting and management has become an expectation of many plan sponsors.

Mail Service   Most plan sponsors and their members have come to expect that PBMs or affiliated organizations will provide a mail service benefit. Many members find value in receiving their refill prescriptions via the mail and request this convenience. Most importantly for plan sponsors, mail service offers a more cost-effective, highly efficient, and accurate method of delivering prescription drugs. While the benefit design does not work for every member or employee, it is particularly valuable for long-term employees or members on chronic medications. Mail service also should provide other services to members, including education (particularly on the importance of compliance) and drug therapy management. Customer service is of vital importance to a mail service program. Members will want to be able to call and immediately secure answers to questions. In particular, customer service at the mail service pharmacy should provide prompt access to pharmacists if patients or physicians have specific questions.

Pharmacy Benefit Design Expertise   Pharmacy benefit managers have moved well beyond simply administering programs and processing claims. Modern pharmacy benefit managers employ not only clinical pharmacists, statisticians, and pharmacoeconomic experts, they also provide actuaries and professionals experienced in benefit design and pricing. Predictive modeling and other capabilities provided by pharmacy benefit managers allow plan sponsors to analyze various benefit options and discover the impact of a particular design on their population in terms of costs and outcomes.

Reporting   Within the confines of patient confidentiality, plan sponsors expect strong reporting capabilities for drug utilization by their members. The PBM should be able to produce comprehensive utilization reports, trend reports, and narrowly focused ad hoc reports to the plan sponsor. Some PBMs also offer extensive online reporting capabilities, meaning that plan sponsors can instantaneously access information on utilization, outcomes, and cost. This access allows the plan sponsor to recognize potential problems more quickly as well as the ability to judge how well programs are working.

Auditing   Fraud remains a significant issue in health care today. It is estimated that plan sponsors lose millions of dollars to either fraud or simple errors annually. Plan sponsors today demand that the pharmacy network management offer a vigorous network auditing program to reduce the likelihood of fraud and inappropriate submission of claims. The best pharmacy benefit programs will provide "real time" auditing capabilities to quickly identify fraud and prevent payment of fraudulent claims while having strong retrospective on-site audit capabilities for fraud recovery.

Medication Error Detection   As the number of people on multiple medications from multiple prescribers increases (known as *polypharmacy*), so do opportunities for medication errors. Often these errors involve drugs that are potentially harmful if used together or drugs that are inappropriate for a patient due to age, weight, or other factors. Technology, specifically online edits and review can help to eliminate many such errors. In addition, as the use of electronic prescribing grows, medication errors will be further reduced as electronic decision paths will guide and aid prescribers in avoiding errors.

Medication Therapy Management   Medication therapy management has become a widely used term in health care. However, the value it provides is often difficult to clearly define. The ability to provide effective and targeted management programs—particularly those that have data to highlight cost, productivity, morbidity, or other measurements—can become an important differentiator for PBMs. As noted, the key will be to identify the needs of the plan sponsor and to ensure that medication therapy management programs specifically address those needs. Plan sponsors will be much more likely to select a pharmacy benefit manager that can prove that their medication therapy management program improves outcomes while managing costs.

As the services offered by pharmacy benefits managers and health plans evolve, plan sponsors' expectations will follow. Best practice standards will gradually move the bar higher and as quality standards organizations such as URAC move to define the quality differences in managing pharmacy benefits. This effort will further help plan sponsors to articulate what they expect from their pharmacy benefit manager.

PERFORMANCE MEASUREMENT

Pharmacy is unique in its development as a data-driven profession. Today, nearly all claims are adjudicated online and captured electronically. The use of pharmacy benefit manager databases has been of great value to health plans, insurers, research organizations, and pharmaceutical manufacturers. Pharmacy benefit performance can be measured using a variety of datasets. In addition to reviewing pharmacy claims within an integrated healthcare system, additional analysis can be obtained by reviewing medical and lab data.

NATIONAL AND INDUSTRY PERFORMANCE MEASURES

The key national performance standards of interest to the pharmacy benefit manager marketplace are: URAC,[2] the nation's largest healthcare accreditation organization with its forthcoming pharmacy benefit manager specific accreditation standards; the Verified Internet Pharmacy Practice Sites (VIPPS)[3] mail service accreditation by the National Association of Boards of Pharmacy; and the National Committee for Quality Assurance (NCQA),[4] which benchmarks healthcare quality for health plans and uses the Health Plan Employer Data and Information Set (HEDIS®),[6] a set of metrics for health plan performance. These organizations represent professionals and companies involved in pharmacy benefits and can help organizations better compare performance indicators. The URAC pharmacy benefit manager Accreditation Standards, released in July 2007, specifically address plan compliance with best practices in the pharmacy benefit manager industry. The PQA (a pharmacy quality alliance)[7] is another example of a disparate group of private and public parties that have come together to create quality metrics for the provision and management of prescription drugs. In addition, pharmacy benefit associations, including the Academy of Managed Care Pharmacy (AMCP) and Pharmaceutical Care Management Association (PCMA) are involved in developing quality assessment standards in collaboration with CMS for Medicare PDPs. Six key PBM performance standards to measure are described below.

Quality Initiatives   Programs intended by PBMs and plan sponsors to improve the quality of the pharmacy benefit must be studied to determine whether or not they ultimately provided value. Quality initiatives should specifically target high impact, high-cost disease states including depression, diabetes, congestive heart failure, and migraines. Programs must be able to quantify either very specific outcomes such as improved adherence to industry guidelines, or improvements in compliance and quality of life. For example, a program designed to improve compliance among diabetic patients should show a corresponding improvement in monitored hemoglobin A1c levels.

Long-Term Measurements   One of the more difficult clinical factors to measure within pharmacy benefit managers is long-term outcomes for chronic disease states. Typically, health outcomes are measured over time; for example, morbidity rates occurring within cardiovascular or diabetes management programs. However, a limitation in managed care performance measurements is the fact that many members change plans (and therefore medication therapy management programs) and long-term performance measurement is often impractical. Pharmacy benefit managers should be able to provide analysis of long-term outcomes for members and organizations that have been with the company for an extended period (multiple years). Other data, including compliance with therapy and member satisfaction can help provide insights into overall performance.

Financial Performance   Fiscal performance can be measured in a variety of ways. However, plan sponsors should look beyond performance measurements that compare net drug spend and level of rebates. A better way to determine financial performance is to look at pharmacy benefit managers that can show how pharmacy benefits help to lower costs on the medical side of the benefit through reduced hospitalizations, fewer hospital visits, and reduction in overall prescription drug utilization.

Mail Service   Mail service is one of the most commonly measured services offered by a pharmacy benefit manager. Plan sponsors can determine mail service performance by looking at a range of factors, including:

- The prescription filling rate accuracy
- Time between order and receipt of prescriptions

- Customer service features, including average time on hold
- Call abandonment
- Overall member satisfaction with care provided

Contractual Performance Criteria   Managed care plan sponsors often include performance standards in their contracts with health plans and pharmacy benefit managers. Types of performance measurement reports provided may include:

- Customer service call handling
- Prior authorization call statistics
- Claims handling efficiency, including loading of member eligibility
- Mail service turnaround times
- Member complaints
- Member retention

Customer Satisfaction Studies   The ability of the PBM to administer the benefit in a manner that affects the members positively is reflected in customer satisfaction surveys conducted by the plan sponsor, a contracted firm, or the PBM. The customer survey must be designed in such a way that measurable criteria are easily recognized and understood by system users and ensure a high likelihood that the survey will be completed and returned. Self-serving satisfaction studies are easily recognized by their design and are of little value. A good customer satisfaction study should show strong and weak points and allow a pharmacy benefit manager to identify areas for improvement.

Performance measurement will improve with advances in technology and individual measurement acceptance by the healthcare community. Most physicians have not yet embraced the technology necessary to integrate their data with the health plans they serve. Thus, it is very difficult to obtain patient encounter data, accurate diagnosis codes, and medical information formatted in a standard manner and submitted in a timely way. Acceptance of this new technology will come sooner if it becomes obvious that there is a financial benefit that outweighs the expense in time and attention. There is strong, nationwide attention focused on technological solutions to improve quality and safety in medicine. Under the new Medicare laws and regulations, there have been efforts to standardize the transaction data necessary for development of electronic medical records and e-prescribing, which promise to bring broader availability and adoption before the end of the decade.

FUTURE TRENDS IN BENEFIT DESIGN AND CONTRACTING

Prescription drug benefits will continue to be an integral part of health care. As newer, more sophisticated and expensive drugs are developed and brought to market, pharmacy benefit designs will need to evolve to ensure appropriate utilization and reasonable costs. Over the next decade, plan sponsors will become less concerned with marketing materials that highlight low administrative costs, and more concerned with finding pharmacy benefit managers that have the ability to meet the dramatic changes that will continue to shape the healthcare marketplace.

SPECIALTY PHARMACY

Specialty pharmaceuticals, also known as *injectables* or *biotech drug therapies*, have become one of the most talked about segments within pharmacy benefits over the last several years. While expensive, many biotech agents are also highly promising in terms of their ability to improve the quality of life for patients with devastating diseases such as multiple sclerosis or rheumatoid arthritis, and also their ability to control drug spending and overall medical services. The ability to offer comprehensive, integrated specialty pharmacy programs, or to collaborate with organizations that have that expertise, will become an important feature for PBMs to publicize and market. However, because of the cost of biotech agents, PBMs will need to ensure they work with pharmacists, clinicians, and other experts within the industry to develop data that can highlight to plan sponsors the return on investment (ROI) such programs can provide.

PHARMACOGENOMICS

The next evolution in specialty pharmaceuticals promises to be pharmacogenomics, which use an individual's genetic inheritance to determine the body's response to prescription drugs. Scientists and clinicians believe that through pharmacogenomics, drugs might one day be tailor-made for individuals and adapted to each person's own genetic makeup. Their promise is impressive; but the cost and implications for the pharmacy benefit potentially troublesome on a number of levels. Plan sponsors are already being exposed to the fact that pharmacogenomics will likely be a reality in the next decade. To ready themselves for this future, plan sponsors will want to align themselves with PBMs that have expertise in the area and have the ability to help the plan sponsor determine medically, legally, and ethically how to best design a pharmacy benefit to include these new therapies.

DRUG RECALLS

The voluntary recall of popular prescription drugs can cause considerable apprehension among plan sponsors and consumers. Of primary concern is how quickly the PBM can get information from the manufacturer and FDA to patients and providers. Next, plan sponsors will want to ensure the PBM has a plan to facilitate changing patient medications to appropriate alternatives; and finally, they will want to ensure that cost and risk to the plan is minimized. Of equal importance, plan sponsors will want assurances that organizations providing pharmacy benefits have the capabilities or programs to help recognize drug therapies with potential problems well before there is a recall or a black box warning (special labeling on drugs that have potential serious side effects in some instances and that require providers to take special note of clinical concerns before prescribing the drug). Plans should consider marketing programs that help to highlight their firm's ability to incorporate stringent, clinically focused review and utilization control programs with tools such as prior authorization that may help to anticipate and more rapidly and effectively respond to recalls.

IMPROVED DISCLOSURE OF DRUG STUDIES

Due in large part to the extraordinary impact of drugs taken off the market, or that have faced serious questions as to their safety, legislators, consumer advocates, and some clinicians are heavily pushing reforms with regard to how information on new drugs is communicated. One of the most important changes is that manufacturers are now required to publish *all* findings and not just to publish positive articles in journals. The result will likely provide a more thorough discussion of the pros and cons of new and existing drugs; but it will also create much more data to sift through and therefore many more questions for plan sponsors and members. Today's PBMs must have the clinical staff to help their clients understand the pros and cons of therapies discussed in new studies. For example, if there is a potential danger with a cholesterol medication, should all patients be immediately taken off the drug? What dangers will that pose? What is the best response? PBMs have a critical role to play in terms of helping their customers understand drug studies and more importantly, in helping them design and implement effective programs based on study information.

UTILIZATION MANAGEMENT

Utilization management (UM) has been associated with managed care plans for decades. While once considered a strategy that limited access to care or drug therapies, plan sponsors now recognize that effective UM programs must be integrated into the pharmacy benefit to ensure access to appropriate therapies and promote consistent, therapeutically sound use of those drugs. The aging population, aggressive direct-to-consumer marketing, and other factors will have a significant impact on UM programs. Pharmacy benefit managers that can develop and communicate the value of programs that promote access to the right drugs, to the right people, and for the right length of time will find both plan sponsors and plan members are much more open to such programs. The key will be to highlight value and quality and not simply control of costs.

PLAN DESIGN

Over the past five years, PBMs and plan sponsors have experimented with a number of enhancements to basic plan design elements. Most significant has been the growth of tiered benefits as a strategy to involve members and employees in sharing the resulting costs of their prescription decisions. In addition, there has been strong interest in CDHP, and in coverage options for lifestyle drugs. Plan sponsors should expect ongoing innovations in plan design strategies. However, PBMs and MCOs will need to take aggressive steps to help educate their clients on the dangers of overly restrictive or unmanaged pharmacy benefit programs. For example, the ability to simply provide employees or members with $1,000 to cover prescription drug expenditures may seem tempting to some plan sponsors. However, how can the plan ensure that their money is being spent wisely? What happens if those benefit dollars are spent on the wrong medications that end up increasing costs on the medical side? Providing education and insight into the optimal plan design for an organization will become an increasingly important task for all pharmacy benefit managers. Patient education also will become increasingly important, as patient choices will have a significant impact on their health outcomes.

TECHNOLOGY

Technology is not necessarily a future trend. Many technological innovations have already been introduced, from Internet access to benefit information to electronic prescribing to formularies online. What will change over the next few years are innovations within existing technologies, access, and utilization. Today, only a handful of health plans require electronic prescribing; within the next decade, virtually all health plans will require it and many will integrate that information with electronic medical records (EMRs). The rapidity of change will be impressive and plan sponsors will expect their PBMs to support and keep pace with these changes. The ability to highlight technological capabilities will become a critical marketing and competitive differentiator over the next several years.

AGGREGATE PURCHASING

From employer groups to large government purchasers, a growing number of organizations want the ability to directly purchase their pharmaceuticals. The goal of this approach is to improve savings by carving out drug purchasing from the PBM relationship. However, what plan sponsors may not realize is that securing the ability to purchase drugs directly may not fully address their concerns regarding cost. Moreover, many plan sponsors may not be aware of the full range of services that their PBM may be, or should be, providing. As noted throughout this chapter, from benefit design to program development to clinical services, PBMs today can play an important role in improving the health of plan members and employees while they work to manage costs. Also, discounts and rebates on prescription drugs are not solely a function of volume purchasing. Formulary placement, market share, and utilization management performance may improve rebates beyond that which may be achieved by increased volume. Clearly, there are important issues to communicate to large purchasers and coalitions as to the value provided by PBMs today. However, the pharmacy management industry should also take note of the real concerns plan sponsors have with regard to drug pricing. By discussing this issue fully, and highlighting the many services pharmacy benefit managers provide, it is likely that both sides will be better able to come up with compromises and approaches that meet the needs of plan sponsors and their members.

REFERENCES

1. Iz P. (federal project manager), HCFA Study of the Pharmaceutical Benefit Management Industry. Atlanta: PricewaterhouseCoopers LLP; 2001. Available at http://www.pcmanet.org/assets/2008-03-25_Research_hcfastudy.pdf. Accessed 1 June 2008.
2. URAC homepage. Available at http://urac.org/. Accessed 1 June 2008.
3. National Association of Boards of Pharmacy, Verified Internet Pharmacy Practice Sites™ (VIPPS®) Web site. Available at http://www.nabp.net/indexvipps.asp. Accessed 1 June 2008.
4. National Committee for Quality Assurance (NCQA) homepage. Available at http://web.ncqa.org/. Accessed 1 June 2008.
5. RUPRI Center for Rural Health Policy Analysis, North Carolina Health Research and Policy Analysis Center, Definition of Rural Health in the Context of MMA Access Standards for Prescription Drug Plans, Sept. 27, 2004. Available at http://www.unmc.edu/ruprihealth/Pubs/p2004-7.pdf. Accessed 1 June 2008.
6. National Committee for Quality Assurance, NCQA HEDIS Programs homepage. Available at http://web.ncqa.org/tabid/76/Default.aspx. Accessed 1 June 2008.
7. PQA homepage. Available at http://www.pqaalliance.org. Accessed 1 June 2008.

Appendix	PRESCRIPTION SCHEDULE OF BENEFITS
3-1	

HOW TO USE THE PROGRAM

- Present your ID card at any XXX PBM contracted pharmacy.

- Pay your copayment for up to one month supply of medication or the retail cost of the prescription, whichever is less.

WHAT IS THE FORMULARY?

The formulary is a list of outpatient prescription drugs that are covered by XXX PBM when prescribed by a licensed provider and filled at a XXX PBM contracted pharmacy. The formulary was created and is regularly updated by a pharmacy and therapeutics committee, which consists of practicing physicians and pharmacists. This committee decides which prescription drugs provide quality treatment for the best value. Your physician has a copy of the formulary and will use it as a reference when prescribing medications.

The formulary list of medications is also available on the Internet. Formulary drugs are available at different copayment levels, as shown in **Table 3-1**.

Please contact the customer service phone number on your ID card if you would like more information about the formulary.

TABLE 3-1   Prescription Schedule of Benefits

Prescription Drugs XXX PBM Formulary with Select Preauthorization	Generic Formulary	Brand Formulary	Non- Formulary
Retail Pharmacy Copayment (up to one month)	$10	$30	$60
Mail Service Pharmacy Copayment (up to three months)	$20	$60	$120

ARE MEDICATIONS NOT LISTED IN THE FORMULARY COVERED?

Medications not listed in the formulary are known as non-formulary medications. Your employer has purchased a three-tier pharmacy plan. You can obtain a non-formulary medication at the higher copay listed above.

WHAT DOES SELECT PREAUTHORIZATION MEAN?

A benefit plan may select certain medications that would require that the member go through a type of preauthorization or step therapy process. Preauthorization means that certain select medications will not be covered until one or more formulary alternatives or "first-line" drugs have been tried first.

XXX PBM reserves the right to preauthorize, institute step therapy and/or limit the quantity of any prescription to ensure that the following coverage criteria are met: (1) the prescription is for the treatment of a medical condition, (2) there is sufficient evidence to draw conclusions about the effects of the prescription on the medical condition being treated and on the health outcome of the member, (3) the expected beneficial effects of the prescription outweigh the expected harmful effects, and (4) the prescription represents the most cost-effective method to treat the medical condition.

WHAT DOES "GENERIC" MEAN?

A generic drug is a medication that has met the standards set by the Food and Drug Administration (FDA) to assure its bioequivalency to the original patented brand name medication. Once a generic drug is approved by the FDA as being bioequivalent, its level of safety, purity, strength, and effectiveness is the same as the brand name product. When new generic drugs are approved by the FDA and added to the formulary, XXX PBM will cover the generic version in place of the brand name drug. By using these equivalent medications, you can maintain quality while realizing substantial savings.

If there is no generic equivalent available for a specific brand name drug, your physician may prescribe a "therapeutic substitute" instead. Unlike a generic, which has the identical active ingredient as the brand name version, a therapeutic substitute has a chemical composition so close to its brand name counterpart that it has the same clinical—or therapeutic—effect.

HOW MUCH MEDICATION CAN I OBTAIN FOR A COPAYMENT?

Members may receive up to one month supply of covered medications for a single copayment.

A three (3) month supply of maintenance medications can be obtained through the mail service program. If you use the mail service program, you may receive up to a three (3) month supply for two (2) copayments.

Medications such as Schedule II substances (e.g., morphine, amphetamines, and methylphenidate), antibiotics, and other medications for short-term or acute illnesses, and drugs with special packaging requirements, are not available through the mail service program.

HOW MUCH MEDICATION CAN I OBTAIN AT ONE TIME?

A maximum of one-month fill of any covered medication can be obtained at one time. A three (3) month supply of maintenance medications can be obtained through the mail service program.

ADDITIONAL INFORMATION

MEDICATIONS COVERED BY YOUR BENEFIT:

- Federal Legend Drugs: Any medicinal substance that bears the legend: "Caution: Federal Law prohibits dispensing without a prescription."
- State Restricted Drugs: Any medicinal substance that may be dispensed by prescription only according to state law.
- Federal Legend oral contraceptives and prescription diaphragms.

For the purposes of determining coverage, the following items are considered prescription drug benefits: glucagons, insulin, insulin syringes, blood glucose test strips, lancets, inhaler extender devices, and anaphylaxis prevention kits.

EXCLUSIONS AND LIMITATIONS:

- Prescription medication for the treatment of sexual dysfunction, including erectile dysfunction, impotence and anorgasmy or hyporgasmy.
- Elective or voluntary enhancement procedures, services, supplies and medications, including weight loss, hair growth, sexual performance, athletic performance, cosmetic purposes, anti-aging, and mental performance.
- Procedures, services, supplies, and medications until they are reviewed for safety, efficacy, and cost effectiveness and approved by XXX PBM.

- Therapeutic devices or appliances including hypodermic needles, syringes (except insulin syringes), support garments and other non-medicinal substances.
- All nonprescription (over-the-counter) contraceptive jellies, ointments, foams, and devices.
- Medications available without a prescription (over-the-counter) or for which there is an over-the-counter equivalent, even if ordered by a physician.
- Drugs used for diagnostic purposes.
- Saline and irrigation solutions.
- Dietary supplements, including vitamins and fluoride supplements (except prenatal), health or beauty aids, herbal supplements, and/or alternative medicine.
- Dental related products.
- Smoking cessation products including, but not limited to, nicotine gum, nicotine patches, and nicotine nasal spray.
- Unit dose pre-packaged medications.
- Disposable all-in-one prefilled insulin pens, insulin cartridges, and needles for non-disposable pen devices.
- Injectable drugs are covered as part of the medical benefit.
- Medications prescribed for experimental or non-FDA approved indications unless prescribed in a manner consistent with a specific indication in Drug Information for the Health Care Professional, published by the United States Pharmacopeia Convention, or in the American Hospital Formulary Services edition of Drug Information; medications limited to investigational use by law.
- Replacement of lost, stolen, or destroyed medications.
- Drugs or medicines purchased and received prior to the member's effective date or subsequent to the member's termination.
- Medications to be taken or administered to the eligible member while a patient in a hospital, rest home, nursing home, sanitarium, etc.
- Drugs or medicines delivered or administered to the member by the prescriber or the prescriber's staff.
- Compounded medication: Any medicinal substance that has at least one ingredient that is Federal Legend or State Restricted in a therapeutic amount. All compounded medications are subject to XXX PBM's prior authorization process.
- Medication for which the cost is recoverable under any Workers' Compensation or Occupational Disease Law or any state or government agency, or medication furnished by any other drug or medical service for which no charge is made to the patient.
- Medications dispensed by a non-participating pharmacy (except for prescriptions required as a result of an urgent or emergent situation).

This summary of benefits is intended only to highlight your benefits and should not be relied upon to fully determine coverage.

ACRONYMS

AMCP	Academy of Managed Care Pharmacy
AVR	automated voice response
AWP	average wholesale price (drug)
CDHP	consumer-driven health plans
CMS	Centers for Medicare and Medicare Services
DTC	direct-to-consumer (marketing)
EMRs	electronic medical records
EOB	explanation of benefits
EOC	explanation of coverage
ERISA	Employee Retirement Income Security Act of 1974
FDA	Food and Drug Administration
FEHBP	Federal Employees Healthcare Benefit Plan
FSAs	flexible spending accounts
HEDIS	Health Plan Employer Data and Information Set
HMOs	health maintenance organizations
HSAs	health spending (or savings) accounts
MAC	maximum allowable cost
MAP	Medicare Advantage Prescription Drug Programs
MAPD	Medicare Advantage Prescription Drug
MCOs	managed care organizations

NCQA	National Committee for Quality Assurance
OIG	Office of the Inspector General (at DHHS)
OTC	over-the-counter (drugs)
PBMs	pharmacy benefit managers
PCMA	Pharmaceutical Care Management Association
PDPs	prescription drug programs
P & T	pharmacy & therapeutics (committee)
RFP	requests for proposals
ROIs	return on investment
TPAs	third party administrators
UM	utilization management
URAC	(formerly, the Uniform Standards of Utilization Review)
VIPPS	Verified Internet Pharmacy Practice Sites™

PHARMACY BENEFIT MANAGEMENT COMPANIES

ROBERT P. NAVARRO
ALLEN W. BECKER
WILLIAM FRANCIS
CELYNDA TADLOCK
ALLAN ZIMMERMAN

INTRODUCTION

Pharmacy benefits are a highly visible and highly valued health benefit as health plan members obtain prescriptions at a rate almost twice that of physician visits. Pharmacy benefits present unique management issues. Pharmaceuticals are perhaps the most cost-effective form of preventive and acute care for many high cost and high prevalence conditions. However, the cost of pharmaceuticals has increased steadily in the recent past, prompting managed care organizations to apply stringent cost-containing strategies. This apparent paradox—limiting the use of cost-effective therapies—requires judicious and specialized expertise in appropriately managing access to and utilization of prescription drugs. For the first time, the cost trend of non-specialty outpatient pharmacy benefits is moderating, largely due to the patent loss of some of the more expensive and highly utilized prescription drugs. Pharmacy benefit management companies, or pharmacy benefit managers (PBMs), have emerged and evolved over the past three decades to provide specialized services to the health care delivery system.

Managed care began to aggressively control pharmacy program costs in the late 1980s, after hospital and physician service costs were addressed. In response to dramatic managed care growth and the resulting unmet need for pharmacy benefit management, specialized companies came into existence to provide prescription drug benefit management for a broad spectrum of customers. These PBMs have taken a dominant role in the management of prescription drug benefits and currently have a role in managing more than 70% of the 3 billion prescriptions dispensed in the United States. This equates to 95% of all prescriptions of commercial and public members with a managed pharmacy benefit. This chapter describes the genesis and evolution of PBMs and their role in managed care.

GENESIS OF PBMs

Pharmacy benefit managers are specialized business enterprises established for the sole purpose of developing and managing comprehensive and cost-efficient prescription drug benefits for a broad array of diverse plan sponsors, including self-insured employer groups, health plans, and government-sponsored programs (e.g., Medicaid, Medicare Part D). Over the past thirty years, PBMs have developed as a result of a market demand and unmet prescription drug management needs, and continue to evolve today. The PBM industry is extremely competitive, so successful PBMs must not only respond to customer needs but also act as an advisor and create innovative benefit design strategies that anticipate near and long-term future market events and healthcare policy changes.

As described in Chapters 1 and 2, the 1973 Health Maintenance Organization (HMO) Act promoted the development of HMOs in many states. Initially, HMOs sought to manage the large cost center, hospital, and physician outpatient costs. In 1980, hospital costs consumed 42% of healthcare expenses, while physician outpatient services represented 18% of all healthcare costs. At that time, pharmacy program costs represented only 5% of total healthcare expenses.[1] Pharmacy costs were a lesser concern, and received attention only after hospital and physician costs were addressed. In the early 1980s, HMOs managed their pharmacy programs internally through their own pharmacy department where staff and group model HMOs distributed drugs through their own internal pharmacies. Independent practice associations (IPAs) and network HMOs contracted this function through community pharmacies. By the mid-1980s, first generation PBMs were marketing rudimentary pharmacy management services to IPA and network model HMOs.

THE EARLY PBMS: 1970S AND 1980S

The PBM industry began in the late1970s with two separate entities: Prescription Card Services (PCS) and Medco Containment Services. Each company provided very different embryonic prescription drug management programs initially to private and public plan sponsors, and by the 1980s that service extended to HMOs.

In the late 1970s and early 1980s, PCS developed a national network of contracted community retail pharmacies that agreed to accept slightly discounted prescription reimbursement rates for PCS customers, which included employer groups and eventually Medicaid programs. PCS promised to help customers contain prescription drug costs, and installed a proprietary stand-alone card reader device (named RECAP) in pharmacies to process third-party prescription claims. The PCS program provided some discounts and caps on prescription drug reimbursement, and slightly discounted the dispensing fee. PCS became a full-service PBM in the late 1980s, offering comprehensive pharmacy benefit management services. Extending the PCS lineage forward to 2007, the original entity has evolved through six changes in ownership and is now a component of CVS Caremark (**Table 4-1**), the largest PBM in the United States, serving approximately 95 million people.

TABLE 4-1 History of Major Ownership Events of the Three Largest PBMs

CVS Caremark[5,7,9-11]	Medco Health Solutions[12,13]	Express Scripts, Inc.[2-4]
PCS, Inc. (original public corporation)	Medco Containment Services (original entity)	Express Scripts created in 1986 by Sanus Corporation Health Systems.
1990—McKesson Corporation purchased 100% of PCS, Inc. stock. Company changed to PCS Health Systems.	1994 Merck Pharmaceutical Company purchases Medco Containment Services.	1989—Express Scripts was purchased by New York Life.
1994—Eli Lilly purchases PCS Health Systems.	2003—Merck spins off Medco as Medco Health Solutions to Merck shareholders.	1992—Express Scripts, Inc. (ESI) becomes a publically traded PBM.
1998—Rite Aid Pharmacy Corporation purchases PCS Health Systems.		
2000—Advance Paradigm PBM purchases PCS Health Systems to create Advance PCS.		
2003—Caremark Rx purchases Advance PCS and ceases using the PCS name.		
2007—CVS Pharmacy Corporation merges with Caremark Rx. The combined name is CVS Caremark.		

Separately, during the late 1970s and early 1980s, Medco Containment Services developed mail service pharmacy prescriptions, and began processing pharmacy claims for state Medicaid programs through its PAID Prescription unit using a contracted community pharmacy network. By the late 1980s, Medco became a full-service PBM, and was acquired by the Merck pharmaceutical company in 1994. It was spun off as a separate unit to Medco shareholders in 2003 as Medco Health Solutions. Today, Medco Health Solutions is the nation's second largest PBM with almost 80 million members (see Table 4-1).

PCS and Medco originated as *de novo* companies established for the purpose of satisfying the nascent but burgeoning need for managed prescription drug benefits. However, two other PBMs, Express Scripts and Diversified Pharmaceutical Services, had their mid-1980 genesis borne from early managed healthcare companies. Their parent organizations began by managing pharmacy benefits internally and quickly realized pharmacy benefit management was a highly specialized skill that presented external commercial opportunity. They too saw a growing need and opportunity for marketing such expertise to other non-competitive HMOs.

In 1983, United HealthCare (UHC) initiated comprehensive pharmacy benefit management, including a closed outpatient drug formulary, online claims adjudication, clinical point-of-service (POS) edits, and manufacturer rebate contracts on behalf of IPA HMOs. By 1986, the UHC pharmacy department was marketing pharmacy benefit management services for other non-UHC HMOs and public employee groups. In 1987, UHC formalized the pharmacy department as a subsidiary PBM named Diversified Pharmaceutical Services (DPS). DPS was later sold by UHC to the SmithKline Beecham pharmaceutical company in 1995.

In 1986, the Sanus Corporation Health Systems established Express Scripts initially as a mail service pharmacy company to service Sanus members. New York Life purchased Express Scripts in 1989, and eventually developed a complete suite of PBM services.[2,3] Express Scripts, Inc. (ESI) became a publicly traded company in 1992 and remains so today. In 1998, ESI acquired PBM ValueRx, and in 1999, ESI purchased rival PBM DPS from SmithKline Beecham (see below).[4] By 2007, ESI was the third largest PBM, with approximately 55 million members (Table 4-1).

PHARMACEUTICAL INDUSTRY OWNERSHIP OF PBMs

In 1993, Merck shocked the managed care and pharmaceutical industries by purchasing Medco Containment Services for $6.6 billion, which was $182 per covered person. Immediately, other pharmaceutical manufacturers began courting PBMs for purchase. In May 1994, SmithKline Beecham (SKB) purchased the DPS unit of United HealthCare for $2.3 billion, or $177 per covered person. Later the same year, Eli Lilly purchased PCS for $4.1 billion, or $80 per covered person.[5,6] By the end of 1994, three of the largest PBMs, with the potential to influence over 80% of the entire covered pharmacy benefit market, were owned by the pharmaceutical industry: Merck owned Medco; Eli Lilly owned PCS, and Smith Kline Beecham (SKB) owned DPS.

The U.S. Federal Trade Commission (FTC) expressed strong concern about Eli Lilly's acquisition of PCS Health Systems and the drug formulary options used by PCS. The FTC stated that the PBM could in fact become a direct distribution channel for Eli Lilly. The concern of the FTC was that PCS would prefer Lilly products on its closed drug formulary and perhaps "force" patients to use an inappropriate or costly Lilly drug in place of a more appropriate drug from a different manufacturer. The FTC required Eli Lilly to operate its PBM subsidiary as a separate and functionally independent unit and to implement a firewall to prevent inappropriate communication and information flow between the PBM and the parent pharmaceutical company. The FTC also required PCS to maintain and offer open formularies to its customers. In a joint statement, Janet D. Steiger, then FTC chairman, and Commissioner Christine A. Varney stated, "We remain concerned about the overall competitive impact of vertical integration by drug companies into the pharmacy benefits-management market."[7] These FTC requirements for the Lilly PCS acquisition cascaded to the two other vertically integrated PBMs (Merck–Medco and SKB–DPS), which voluntarily complied with offering an open formulary in addition to a restricted formulary to their customers. In addition, these companies implemented a corporate firewall like the one between PCS and Eli Lilly.

The vertical integration of pharmaceutical manufacturers with PBMs heightened the general concern about factors influencing all PBM formulary decisions. The concern focused on whether a PBM, through ownership or through contractual relationship, would make formulary decisions based upon manufacturer price concessions. In fact, in a survey of 263 HMOs using PBMs, 55% reported moderate or great concern about the potential for bias in the PBMs' drug product selection process as a result of their alliance (by contract or ownership) with pharmaceutical manufacturers.[8]

Today, none of the three PBMs that were purchased by pharmaceutical manufacturers in 1993 and 1994 remain owned by a drug company. In 1999, Eli Lilly sold PCS Health Systems to Rite Aid chain pharmacy for $1.5 billion.[9] PCS was subsequently purchased by Advance Paradigm to become Advance PCS, and that company was purchased by and incorporated into the Caremark PBM.[10] CVS and Caremark merged in March of 2007.[11] In 1999, SKB sold DPS to Express Scripts, an independent PBM, for $700 million.[7] PCS and DPS were each sold in 1999 for approximately one-third of their sales price in 1994, despite the fact that the respective memberships were substantially unchanged over the previous five years. Medco was spun off by Merck as Medco Health Solutions in 2003, and today is the second largest PBM.[12,13]

GROWTH OF THE PBM INDUSTRY: 1990S TO PRESENT

The growth for expertise in managed pharmacy benefits continued, and this spawned the development of an entire PBM industry in the 1990s. Some PBMs were started *de novo* (e.g., MedImpact, National Prescription Administrators), some as part of pharmacy chain organizations (e.g., Walgreens Health Initiatives, CVS PharmaCare) while others grew out of health plan organizations (e.g., WellPoint Pharmacy Management, Prescription Solutions). As PBMs developed, mergers and acquisitions occurred resulting in a more consolidated PBM industry. Although more than 100 PBMs have been developed, today there are about 50 PBMs, and 90% of the membership is covered by the top ten PBMs. The membership of some of the largest PBMs is found in **Table 4-2**.

TABLE 4-2 Approximate Membership of the Largest PBMs

Pharmacy Benefit Manager	Millions of Members
CVS Caremark	82
Medco Health Solutions	71
Express Scripts, Inc.	51
WellPoint Pharmacy Management	36
MedImpact	21
Prime Therapeutics	13

Source: Compiled from PBM Web sites and marketing material, 2006 to 2007.

RATIONALE FOR USING PBM SERVICES

The growth of MCOs and the diversity of new product offerings (e.g., PPO, POS, managed indemnity, Medicaid) tested the resources of internal HMO infrastructure. There are generally considered to be six primary resource-consuming operational components of a typical managed care prescription drug benefits program:

1. *Human resources.* Skilled pharmacists trained in business administration, pharmaceutical contracting, clinical evaluation, health outcomes research, and other areas are required to develop and successfully operate a managed care pharmacy department.

2. *Technological resources.* Prescription drug benefits are highly transactional and 99.5+% of pharmacy claims are adjudicated on-line and in real time. Enormous capital expenditures are necessary to maintain and upgrade leading edge data processing systems to support an efficient pharmacy program (see Chapter 7).

3. *Drug distribution network and systems.* Health plans must establish and manage a network of independent and chain retail pharmacies and specialty pharmacies. Larger PBMs invest millions of dollars to develop internal mail services pharmacies as an optional distribution and revenue channel (see Chapter 5).

4. *Drug evaluation and formulary management processes.* Maintaining a clinically responsible drug formulary requires the pharmacy department to have skilled clinical pharmacists collect and critically review drug information and drug product dossiers, analyze utilization reports, prepare Pharmacy & Therapeutics (P & T) Committee monographs, and respond to provider and member concerns.

5. *Pharmaceutical contracting.* An experienced pharmacy staff is required to negotiate, monitor, and manage rebate contracts with pharmaceutical companies (see Chapter 15).

6. *Clinical pharmacy programs management.* Clinical pharmacy staff is required to develop and monitor utilization reports, perform drug utilization review (DUR), monitor adherence, and administer disease management and medication therapy management (MTM) programs.

Certainly, a large MCO can develop all of the capabilities to successfully operate a comprehensive pharmacy department, and many do so without the need of an external PBM (e.g., Blue Shield of California, Kaiser Permanente, Aetna, and many others). However, as discussed below, there may be long-term cost and quality of care reasons for using an external PBM rather than expending capital on internal pharmacy benefit program capabilities for certain undifferentiated, commodity processes. Pharmacy management strategies that can be internally implemented by an MCO or outsourced to a PBM are generally similar in concept, but the resources and operational efficiencies offered by a PBM may make the outsourcing route more cost-efficient. This is an important concept: If the internally-developed pharmacy benefit management program, or specific components, do not offer differentiating or competitive cost or quality advantages, it may be a wise business decision for the MCO to "buy" services from a PBM. The *raison d'être* for

PBMs is that they are highly cost-efficient and flexible in managing pharmacy services due to a singular focus on pharmacy benefit management and economies of scale. The PBM industry is highly competitive and as a result, PBMs are generally quite eager to satisfy—or exceed—customer cost and quality expectations.

Claims processing was outsourced to PBMs because computer system maintenance and upgrades are expensive capital investments that require continuous maintenance and updating. PBMs often had massive and scalable computer processing capability, and all but the largest MCOs could buy claims processing for less than they could build it internally. Also, because all MCOs, PBMs, and pharmacies observed the National Council for Prescription Drug Programs (NCPDP) data processing and transmission standards, prescription claims processing was an undifferentiated, commodity expense, and PBMs could often provide claims adjudication for a lower per transaction cost. The cost of claims processing is volume-dependent, and the more claims processed reduced the per claim processing fee.

Retail pharmacy network development and management was often outsourced to PBMs as this function was time-consuming and, as most pharmacies participated with most MCOs and PBMs, pharmacy networks were often not exclusive and considered a commodity component. Because all participating pharmacies are required to adjudicate prescription claims online and in real-time, and all use the NCPDP standard protocol, it often made sense for PBMs to maintain the pharmacy network that was also electronically sending the claims to PBMs for processing. PBMs often develop and support several different retail pharmacy networks to meet various plan sponsor needs. A vast, national network of 50,000 or more pharmacies may include a higher pharmacy reimbursement rate (and cost to the plan sponsor) compared to a smaller, limited network with a smaller number of pharmacies that has been customized to the needs of a specific plan sponsor. The pharmacies in the limited network may accept a lower fee in exchange for having exclusive access to a defined, captive population. Networks with a smaller number of pharmacies may be inconvenient to members, but often are less expensive to the member and plan sponsor.

Although drug formulary decisions and management remained the providence of health plans, the pharmaceutical rebate contracting function was often outsourced to PBMs. Leverage in rebate contracting came from the number of covered lives that were subject to an enforceable drug formulary. While the health plan retained formulary enforcement authority, PBMs demonstrated that if they pooled the covered lives of many health plans with enforceable formularies, the PBM was able to negotiate greater rebate amounts than possible by each individual MCO. Rebate contract management requires significant claims analyses utilization reports, and a system for invoicing drug manufacturers to collect rebates on the contracted drugs. This is often all provided by the PBM that is doing the MCO's claims adjudication. Efficiencies are often realized by allowing the PBM processing prescription claims and providing management utilization reports to also provide the rebate management function. In summary, PBMs supported MCO rebate contracting by negotiating high value contracts, and by processing all required rebate management reports.

Health plans maintained control of non-commodity, differentiated services, including benefit design, clinical programs, formulary management, and P & T Committee operations, as these were the components that contributed unique and competitive pharmacy benefit advantages. Today, many health plans purchase a broad array of services from PBMs. Some plans purchase comprehensive, turnkey pharmacy benefits while others only use PBMs for claims processing, rebate contracting, and reporting. PBM services shall be discussed in greater depth below.

PBM SERVICES AND BUSINESS RELATIONSHIPS

Pharmacy benefit managers may market comprehensive or component pharmacy benefit management services to health plans, self-insured employer groups, union health and welfare trusts, state Medicaid programs, state and federal employee groups, Medicare Part D beneficiaries, and other plan sponsors. A typical PBM has 35% of customers as health plans, 33% as self-funded employer groups, 21% as other insurance companies, and 11% as other customers.[14] Some PBMs service a broad array of customers, while others may specialize and exclusively serve commercial populations or public sector programs such as Medicaid or Medicare Part D programs. Health plans that do not manage pharmacy benefits internally use a PBM for some or most pharmacy benefit services (**Figure 4-1**). Health

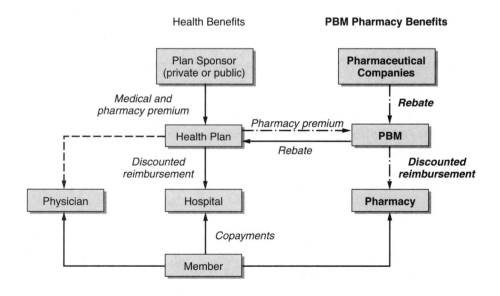

FIGURE 4-1 Plan Sponsor Obtains Pharmacy Benefits Indirectly from a PBM Through a Contract with a Health Plan.

plans generally maintain local control over pharmacy benefits, often have their own P & T Committee, and make their own local drug formulary decisions.

Non-health plan customers (e.g., self-funded employer groups and union trust funds) typically have no internal medical and pharmacy benefit management resources or expertise, and contract with a health plan for medical benefits. The health plan may provide the PBM service directly or may subcontract these to an external PBM. The non-health plan customer also may contract directly with a PBM to provide and manage pharmacy benefits (**Figure 4-2**).

In summary, PBMs offer pharmacy programs directly to plan sponsors and employer purchasing coalitions, or indirectly to a plan sponsor through a health plan.

PBMs match their service offerings and capabilities to the services needed by their plan sponsor customers. **Table 4-3** illustrates managed pharmacy benefit program components (discussed more fully in Chapter 2), and associated services. PBMs must be able to support a broad array of plan sponsors with very different needs. Some self-funded employers or union trust funds may desire to offer rich benefits with low copayments. Other smaller employers may offer limited pharmacy benefits with high copayments. Many Medicaid programs are required by state legislation to offer a broad formulary, covering certain OTC drugs, with no or low copayments. Medicare Part D programs may have closed formularies with multiple tiers and may or may not fill the coverage gap. Health plans may have the most complex needs, as each may also serve hundreds of employer groups, many with very different benefit designs.

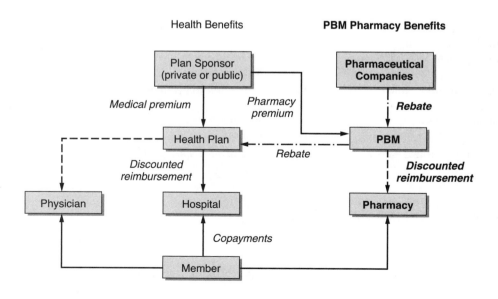

FIGURE 4-2 Plan Sponsor Contracts Directly with PBM for Pharmacy Benefits.

TABLE 4-3   PBM Services Matched to Pharmacy Benefit Management Components

Pharmacy Benefit Management Components	PBM Service(s)
Pharmacy benefit plan design	Recommend plan benefit design to meeting plan sponsors' business objectives (i.e., rich benefits vs. cost containment).
Pharmacy distribution network	Develop a retail and mail prescription distribution network customized to meet plan sponsors' needs.
New drug data review	PBM clinical pharmacy departments and National P & T Committees review new drug clinical and economic data, and provide analyses and monographs to plan sponsor customers.
Drug formulary management	Develop a National Drug Formulary that may be used by plan sponsors, or may be modified to meet unique plan sponsor needs. Health plan customers often develop their own formulary independently through their own P & T Committee.
Patient prescription cost-sharing (e.g., copayment or coinsurance)	Recommend formulary tier and copayment structures customized for each plan sponsor as part of the benefit design (see above).
Mandatory generic drug program (e.g., maximum allowable cost [MAC] list)	Develop their own proprietary MAC list that is applied as needed to meet individual plan sponsor needs.
Pharmaceutical manufacturer rebate contracts	Consolidate all plan sponsor membership, aggregated by level of formulary control, and negotiate aggressive rebate contracts on behalf of their plan sponsor customers.
Online, real-time point-of-sale pharmacy claims adjudication system	Implement and maintain administrative, claims processing, and reporting computer capabilities to meet plan sponsor needs.
Clinical pharmacy and medication therapy management (MTM) services	Develop and operate administrative systems to support various plan sponsor clinical pharmacy services (e.g., reports to identify risk-stratify members, or screen members for clinical pharmacy and MTM services).
Physician and member communications and member services support	Develop communications to members and/or physicians as requested by plan sponsors. PBMs also develop and operate prior authorization and member service departments on behalf of plan sponsors.
Specialty pharmacy services	Develop and manage specialty pharmacy services for plan sponsors consistent with their benefit design.

CONTRACTING FOR PBM SERVICES

Plan sponsors may contract for PBM services in a variety of manners. Typically, PBMs prefer not to accept financial risk for the pharmacy benefits they offer or support, although they will accept program performance risk. Those PBMs that are CMS approved as Medicare Part D PDPs are expected to accept program financial risk.

In no-risk business relationships, prescription drug claim costs are funded by the plan sponsor and paid to providers by the PBM on behalf of the plan sponsor. PBMs may be paid an administrative fee based upon the services they provide, such as a per-transaction fee for claims processing, or a per-capita administrative fee for broader program development and management. PBMs may be paid an administrative fee based upon the services they provide, such as a per-transaction fee for claims processing, or a per-capita administrative fee for broader program development and management. PBMs pass on rebate income according to the contract with their plan sponsors, and may be paid a separate fee (paid by the pharmaceutical company or the plan sponsor) for administering the rebate program. PBMs frequently include cost and quality benchmarks in their contracts with plan sponsors, and failure to meet performance benchmarks may result in PBMs paying a penalty to the plan sponsor.

BASIS OF THE PBM: PLAN SPONSOR RELATIONSHIP

The plan sponsor selects a PBM that is best able to deliver the program objectives, which generally include supporting a specific benefit design, specific member services expectations, clinical programs, and cost containment requirements. The contract between the PBM and the plan sponsor will include specific cost and performance expectations. Examples of some of the typical contract terms of a PBM contract with a health plan are noted below.

Basic Administrative Fee   The health plan may pay a fee on a per claim basis, based upon total claims volume, which is based upon the individual plan sponsor's contract. This fee includes maintaining administrative files and databases, member identification cards, claims processing, basic point-of-service adjudication edits, basic member communications, maintaining a drug file history, basic reports, basic member service support, and other standard services. Alternative fee arrangements based upon a per-member-per-month (PMPM) also may be available from some PBMs.

Additional Administrative Fees   The PBM will charge additional fees based upon specific requests of the health plan, such as identification card replacement, special reports, paying paper claims, disease management support, and special clinical pharmacy programs, such as utilization management, drug utilization review, and adherence programs.

Prescription Claim Reimbursement   Prescription drug claim costs are paid by the health plan to the PBM within a specified time period, often two days, via electronic funds transfer.

Performance Guarantees   PBM contacts often include performance benchmarks and guarantees based upon cost savings, claims adjudication system availability and accuracy, program PMPM costs, generic dispensing rate, member services telephone abandonment, member complaints, rebate income, or other metrics. The PBM may be paid a performance incentive, or may pay the health plan a penalty if performance guarantees are met or missed.

Rebate Program Fees   Health plans may pay an administrative fee to the PBM based upon a percent of rebate income (e.g., 5%–10%).

PBMs' ROLE IN REBATE CONTRACTING

As discussed above, PBMs aggregate their covered lives, sorted by level of formulary control (e.g., open, closed) and product (e.g., commercial, Medicaid, Medicare), and negotiate rebates with pharmaceutical companies on behalf of their plan sponsor customers. Rebates, extensively discussed in Chapter 15, are paid by pharmaceutical companies in exchange for a specific drug formulary reimbursement position. Rebate money received by the PBM on behalf of their plan sponsors' members is then dispersed to plan sponsors in accordance with their contract with the PBM. The 2001 HCFA report states that rebates typically result in a 5% to 15% reduction of a contracted drug's cost, although rebates may be lower or higher, depending upon the drug and contract terms.[14] The relationship with and provision of rebates, samples, and other services of pharmaceutical companies to managed care organizations, and especially Medicaid and Medicare programs has created questions regarding fraud, abuse, and undue influence by the U.S. Office of Inspector General.[15–17] As a result, PBMs, MCOs, and pharmaceutical companies have established their own compliance departments to assure observance with Federal anti-fraud guidelines. Although specifically focused on Federal programs, commercial MCOs and PBMs are vigilant to carefully collect and account for rebate dollars as well as other sources of income, grants, and resources offered by pharmaceutical companies that may be considered to be of monetary value. Some PBMs are reluctant to accept program resources from pharmaceutical companies except rebate payments as specified by contract that are passed through to plan sponsors according to the terms of their contract with the PBM. Other PBMs may accept non-rebate financial support, or non-financial resources, but monetize their value and consider them as rebate income.

IMPACT OF PBMs ON PHARMACY BENEFIT MANAGEMENT

Since the mid-1980s, PBMs have focused exclusively on developing the most efficient systems and processes to provide the pharmacy benefits that yield the high quality outcomes at the lowest possible cost. The diverse array of public and private plan sponsors and the various types of products they offer requires enormously flexible information systems and management expertise to meet highly variable and dynamic customer and member expectations.

PBMs and large health plans that internally manage pharmacy benefits have been effective in leading the development of cost-effective pharmacy benefit management in the United States. A 2004 PricewaterhouseCoopers report found that effective pharmacy benefit management reduced prescription costs by 15% to 40% depending upon the level of program aggressiveness, compared with an unmanaged program, reduced commercial per-member-per-year (PMPY) costs by $268 in 2005, and reduced Medicare pharmacy PMPY costs by $937.[18]

In addition to aggressive cost containment, PBMs are well equipped to support clinical edits through the POS claims adjudication system, perform DUR to monitor for drug abuse and misuse, monitor and improve adherence, conduct pharmacoeconomic research, and provide plan sponsors with member risk stratification reports. Clinical edits are commonly used to control the quantity of drugs dispensed, ensuring compliance with labeled dosing guidelines and preventing misuse and overuse of costly and potentially harmful drugs. Claim system edits also can be used to enforce step therapy programs in which the use of first-line and often less expensive therapies must be found in a patient's drug claim history before a prescription for a more advanced and often more costly therapy is allowed. PBMs can use their database of pharmacy claims to run retrospective drug use queries and identify patients at risk due to patterns of controlled substance drug use that appear to be abusive. Similarly, compliance with drug regimens can be evaluated by examining refill histories over time. Patients can be notified with refill reminders and prescribing physicians can be informed when patients are not refilling critical medications in a timely fashion. Some PBMs also have the capability to combine medical claims data with prescription drug data to draw even more specific conclusions such as the impact of drug therapy on medical costs.

The complexion of some of these programs is varied and dependent on the ability of the PBM Client or Health Plan to implement more rigorous programs that will ensure member safety, appropriate, and cost-effective utilization of the drug benefit. Example of some of these programs are: Concurrent DUR, Retrospective DUR, Controlled Substance DUR, Prior Authorization, Quantity Limitations, Step Therapy, Medical Exception, and other programs that are more specific in nature and proprietary to the respective PBM. In the past, some clients have chosen not to implement programs that may be construed to be "invasive in nature." As healthcare dollars continues to escalate, clients are now more receptive than ever to apply tools that will ensure both the member and plan of becoming a good steward of the drug benefit.

COMPETITION AMONG PBMs BENEFITS PLANS SPONSORS AND MEMBERS

PBMs must continuously strive to be more cost effective and exceed customer service performance expectations because the PBM industry is extremely competitive. The U.S. General Accounting Office (GAO) has also confirmed the financial benefit using PBMs for federal employees and Medicare recipients.[19,20] The June 2001 *HCFA Study of the Pharmaceutical Benefit Management Industry*[14] reports that due to the highly competitive industry, PBMs operate on thin profit margins of approximately 5%, and are subject to competitive bids when awarded business from plan sponsors. A 2004 PricewaterhouseCoopers report on the PBM industry supports this conclusion.[18] However, PBM margins are the subject of some scrutiny because of their mode of computation. A case can be made that the 5% margin referenced is artificially low by the common practice of most PBMs of classifying plan sponsor prescription claim costs as revenue, offset by a not always equivalent cost of goods sold (CGS) expense. Without the inclusion of prescription claim dollars as a revenue and expense line item on the profit and loss, PBM margins may be viewed by some in a considerably different light.

Competition has benefited pharmacy benefit corporate sponsors as well as individual members and beneficiaries, and has reduced the administrative costs of pharmacy benefit management. Large employer groups use health benefit consultants to advise them about PBM selection. The large consultancies review and compare the services, quality programs, and prices of all major PBMs. To become a finalist, PBMs must satisfy the expectations and requirements of benefit consultants as well as the employer plan sponsors.

Most established PBMs perform administration tasks well but fall short of providing consistent innovative management. One health plan executive in Arizona, described his PBM as, "good at the Pharmacy and Benefit part of their relationship but lacking in terms of any real Management." PBMs must seek to develop new ways to differentiate themselves from their competitors. This is critical in an industry that views administration as a commodity.

As the competition grows within the PBM industry, we are seeing consolidation of some of the major forces, but also some niche players have surfaced. These niche players will contact various vendors for claims processing, DUR, Specialty Prescriptions, and offer packages to clients based on deals for services these intermediaries can negotiate. The depth and breadth of the services provided may vary widely.

FUTURE PBMs

PBMs will continue to evolve to anticipate and meet the quality and cost desires of their private and public plan sponsors. Some of the market events likely to occur in the future that will influence the PBM market include the following:

- Specialty pharmacy services that focus on distribution and management of high-cost oral and injectable drug therapies will become as much a commodity as mail order pharmacy is currently.
- Increased use of electronic prescribing technology will allow for drug therapy based on diagnosis and development of more specific utilization management programs.
- The growing trend toward high deductible health plans and healthcare savings accounts (HSAs) will drive consumers towards use of less expensive drug therapies (e.g., generics) and remove the impact that formularies will have on drug choice. As a result, PBMs will be driven to become less reliant on pharmaceutical manufacturer rebates and more reliant on clinical and customer services. Programs that assist a member in maximizing the use of their HSAs will have appeal to health plan sponsors.

PBMs have pursued a variety of activities to improve drug adherence, including the following:

- Educate the patient about their chronic illness on a level they understand.
- Provide opportunity for patient with chronic illnesses to afford medications, such as a preventative drug list that either lowers or negates copay for drugs to treat their condition.
- Engage the patient to become a prudent purchaser of the health benefit with consumer-driven/high-deductible health plans.
- Provide incentives toward becoming a "good" patient.
- Clients or payors will engage in member health via PBM tools and outreach.
- Offer the opportunity to have the patient to contact a "health advocate" to walk the member through their medication questions, issues, concerns, and use.
- Work in an integrated approach with the member and physician to close the gaps in therapy.

Ultimately, the payor and consumer market will drive the near future changes. PBMs will have to adapt to these pressures with different business models as well as improve their internal organizational structure to support that change. These changes focus on four broad market needs that payors want from their PBM relationship:

1. Objectivity/Innovation
2. Accountability
3. Transparency
4. Management

PBMs must align goals with their business partners to help payors achieve low net cost for their prescription benefit while ensuring high clinical quality and high member satisfaction. Organizations, such as the Center for Health Transformation, have evolved to foster innovation that will deliver quality health services in the future. URAC is among a number of organizations working towards standards of accountability for the PBM industry and the means to validate performance of those standards.

PBMs also must be able to respond to an increasing demand for transparency. This transparency includes both financial and operational disclosure and openness with the plan sponsor and their members. The plan sponsors' perception that many PBMs do not fully disclose revenue streams, pharmaceutical company relationships, and general business practices that may have a detrimental influence on the plan sponsors' overall program costs, has driven many purchasers to demand a higher degree of transparency. As a result, niche PBM players have emerged in the marketplace to respond to this demand over the past few years.

The Center for Medicare and Medicaid Services (CMS) Medication Therapy Management requirement for Medicare Part D plans may in some way act as a platform for driving the quality improvement of prescription drug therapy in all prescription programs. Clinical management will become more focused as PBMs are able to analyze claims data to finer levels of granularity. Interventions can then move from the traditional "shot gun" approach to those tailored to individual patients and specific health conditions (**Table 4-4.**)

TABLE 4-4 Categories of Clinical and Disease Management Programs

Type of Program	Example(s)	Program Goal or Objective
Benefit Design	Diabetes Management Program	Copay reduction/forgiveness for medication refill when member has been compliant to treatment.
Drug/Drug Class	Multisource Brand to Generic (MSB) Single Source Brand to Generic (SSB)	Promote generic medication use. Reach a balance between low net cost and maximizing rebates.
Retail Pharmacy	Asthma Management	Enlist retail pharmacy in promoting patient education about proper use of inhalers.
Disease Specific	High-Risk Diabetic Program Asthma Care Management Program	Promote adherence to treatment protocols and guidelines. • Asthma: Appropriate use of controller medications. • Diabetes: Identify patients at risk for heart disease.
Quality of Care	Appropriate use of Atypical Antipsychotic Medication Migraine Treatment Program	Improve clinical outcomes. Improve standard of clinical practice.
Member Compliance	Depression Management Program	Improve member compliance; adherence and persistence to treatment.
Medicare Part D	Polypharmacy in the Elderly	Identify elderly members who are at risk of adverse events due to number of medications taken.
Population Management	Chronic Renal Disease	Identify patients at high risk for developing chronic renal disease. Promote early identification and treatment of causes for renal damage.
Behavioral Modification	Chronic Disease Management	Assess member's willingness and capability to take positive steps toward self-management and appropriate care. Risk stratify identified members and match resources, interventions, and goals to level of member's willingness and capability for management.

CONCLUSION

Prescription benefit managers have a place in our healthcare system and have provided a tremendous paradigm shift in how we administer health care in the last twenty years. The "3 P's" are now engaged—physician, patient, and payors—and now partnering to offer a higher quality of both the drug benefit and medical benefit, which will ultimately lower overall healthcare costs. In the future, you will see a more integrated approach to look at individualized therapy for chronic illness and specialization or targeting for specialty bio-pharmaceuticals based on patient genetic testing.

REFERENCES

1. Health Care Financing Administration, Office of the Actuary, National Health Statistics. Washington, DC; 1998.

2. Express Scripts Incorporated. Wikipedia Web page. Available at http://en.wikipedia.org/wiki/Express_Scripts. Accessed 2 June 2008.

3. Express Scripts Web page. Available at http://www.express-scripts.com/aboutus/. Accessed 2 June 2008.

4. Express Scripts to Acquire Diversified Pharmaceutical Services, press release, February 9, 1999. Available at http://phx.corporate-ir.net/phoenix.zhtml?c=69641&p=irol-newsArticle&ID=36148&highlight=. Accessed 2 June 2008.

5. PCS buy-back looms; future not sure. *Chain Drug Review*, January 1990. Available at http://findarticles.com/p/articles/mi_hb3007/is_199001/ai_n7867747. Accessed 2 June 2008.

6. FTC OKs Lilly's PCS buy, but not without restrictions, *Drug Store News*, November 21, 1994. Available at http://findarticles.com/p/articles/mi_m3374/is_n20_v16/ai_15893262. Accessed 2 June 2008.

7. Burton T.M., "Eli Lilly Accepts FTC Curbs, Clearing Way for Its $4 Billion Purchase of PCS," *The Wall Street Journal*, 4 November, 1994.

8. Office of Inspector General, Department of Health and Human Services. Experiences of Health Maintenance Organizations with Pharmacy Benefit Management Companies. Washington, DC: DHHS; 1997: p. 10.

9. "Rite Aid in $1.5 Billion Deal for Lilly Unit." *The New York Times*, November 18, 1989. Available at http://query.nytimes.com/gst/fullpage.html?sec=health&res=9405E5DA1630F93BA25752C1A96E958260. Accessed 2 June 2008.

10. Caremark, Advance PCS deal would join two major PBMs. *Business Insurance*, September 22, 2003. Available at http://www.princeton.com/pbm/pdfs/BusinessInsurance-Caremark.pdf. Accessed 2 June 2008.

11. "CVS Corporation and Caremark Rx Provide Update on Closing of Merger." CVS Corporation press release, March 20, 2007. Available at http://phx.corporate-ir.net/phoenix.zhtml?c=99533&p=irol-newsArticle&ID=975828&highlight=. Accessed 2 June 2008.

12. Assessing the Merck-Medco deal. (Merck and Company Inc.; Medco Containment Services Inc.). *Chain Drug Review*, April 2004. Available at http://findarticles.com/p/articles/mi_hb3007/is_199404/ai_n7964733. Accessed 2 June 2008.

13. "Medco Spin-Off," press release, Merck & Co., Inc. Available at http://www.merck.com/finance/shareholder_letter.html. Accessed 2 June 2008.

14. HCFA Study of the Pharmaceutical Benefit Management Industry. PricewaterhouseCoopers, June 2001. Available at http://www.pcmanet.org/assets/2008-03-25_Research_hcfastudy.pdf. Accessed 2 June 2008.

15. Compliance Program Guidance for Pharmaceutical Manufacturers, U.S. Office of Inspector General, April 2003. Available at http://oig.hhs.gov/fraud/docs/complianceguidance/042803pharmacymfgnonfr.pdf. Accessed 2 June 2008.

16. Fraud, Waste and Abuse Oversight in Medicare Part D Program. *Federal Register,* Vol. 66, No. 112, Monday, June 11, 2001; Notices 31245. Available at http://www.npdb-hipdb.hrsa.gov/

legislation/fedreg/Federal_Register_2001-06-11. pdf. Accessed 2 June 2008.

17. Pharmaceutical Commerce. CMS' Office of Inspector General is preparing to enforce new guidelines on billing and incentive practices, April 30, 2006. Available at http://www.pharmaceuticalcommerce. com/frontEnd/main.php?idSeccion=295. Accessed 2 June 2008.

18. The Value of Pharmacy Benefit Management and the National Cost Impact of Proposed PBM Legisla-tion, PricewaterhouseCoopers, July, 2004. Available at http://www.pwc.com/Extweb/pwcpublications. nsf/docid/D5E8B5900A6E17C880256EFB0037 73AA. Accessed 2 June 2008.

19. United States General Accounting Office. Federal Employees' Health Benefits: Effects of Using Pharmacy Benefit Managers on Health Plans, Enrollees, and Pharmacies. Available at http:// www.gao.gov/new.items/d03196.pdf. Accessed 2 July 2008.

ACRONYMS

CMS	Centers for Medicare and Medicare Services
DPS	Diversified Pharmaceutical Services
DUR	drug utilization review
ESI	Express Scripts, Inc.
FTC	U.S. Federal Trade Commission
HCFA	Health Care Financing Administration
HMOs	health maintenance organizations
HSAs	health spending (or savings) accounts
IPA	independent practice associations
MCOs	managed care organizations
MTM	medication therapy management
NCPDP	National Council for Prescription Drug Programs
OTC	over-the-counter (drugs)
PBMs	pharmacy benefit managers, pharmacy benefit management (companies)
PCS	Prescription Card Services
PDPs	prescription drug programs
PMPM	per-member-per-month
PMPY	per-member-per-year
POS	point-of-service (pharmacy)

PPO	preferred provider organization
P & T	Pharmacy & Therapeutics (Committee)
SKB	Smith Kline Beecham
UHC	United HealthCare
URAC	originally Utilization Review Accreditation Commission, now accredits other types of organizations as well

Chapter 5

PHARMACY DISTRIBUTION SYSTEMS AND NETWORK MANAGEMENT

LOWELL T. STERLER
DOUGLAS STEPHENS

A comprehensive pharmacy distribution system is a critical component of any pharmacy benefit management program. A successful distribution system must provide patients with convenient access to the most clinically appropriate and cost-effective medications. Several cost and patient satisfaction goals must be considered when designing a distribution system. In the patient's mind, convenient access to a participating pharmacy provider is foremost. Managed care uses in-house pharmacies, community independent and chain pharmacies, mail-order, and specialty pharmacies to construct a comprehensive distribution system. Patients expect a trustworthy and informed pharmacist to be available to answer medication questions. Patients are assuming more responsibility for their own health and wellness, and members of the media are increasingly focusing on healthcare issues. Thus, a better-educated, inquisitive consumer enters the pharmacy with enhanced expectations, including the expectation that prescriptions will be dispensed in a reasonable time because of improved technology and greater use of technicians in the dispensing function.

Increasingly, patients are turning to pharmacists to provide economic counsel as well. The growth of managed care has resulted in empowered patients who are acutely aware of broad price differences for similar therapeutic drugs. The patient, payer, provider, and pharmacy benefit manager in a managed care organization (MCO) or pharmacy benefit management company (PBM) all have a common goal: to contain costs while ensuring clinical quality and broad access to pharmacy services. This chapter describes the development and operation of three of the basic prescription drug distribution systems used by managed care (PBMs are discussed in Chapter 4; specialty pharmacy is covered in Chapter 6). It also discusses pharmacist roles and responsibilities within each of these distribution alternatives.

PHARMACY PROGRAM DISTRIBUTION OPTIONS

MCOs and health plans, including health maintenance organizations (HMOs), preferred provider organizations (PPOs), state Medicaid programs, Medicare Part D programs, and PBMs will construct a pharmacy distribution system based upon the organizational structure, client needs, and distribution area of members. There are four major options for a pharmacy distribution system: retail network, in-house, mail service, and specialty.

A retail network of pharmacy providers is a group of licensed community independent, supermarket, or chain pharmacies that have contracted with a health plan or PBM to provide pharmacy services to eligible members. These networks are generally referred to as community pharmacy networks. The reimbursement requirements are established and agreed upon in advance. The pharmacies must comply with the MCO or PBM benefit design, performance standards, claims transmission standards, and quality assurance parameters, such as permission for the payer or PBM to audit the pharmacy. To receive the maximum benefit, plan members must use the contracted network. There is usually a higher member copayment, or penalty, for using a pharmacy outside the contracted network.

An in-house pharmacy is located within a staff or group model HMO, mixed model HMO, or on-site at an employer's facility. These pharmacies are usually limited to providing service only to their HMO members or employees. In-house pharmacies rarely are part of a PBM's standard national network that provides services to members of other payers or MCOs that contract with the network.

The third distribution option is mail service (also commonly referred to as home delivery). Through this option, a licensed pharmacy provides maintenance medications to members through mail delivery. Often, mail service providers will be an added option to the standard network of retail providers. As a response to mail service, many MCOs today offer an extended supply network (ESN) at retail. This network allows members to obtain a 90-day supply at participating retail pharmacies for up to three copays.

COMMUNITY PHARMACY PROVIDER NETWORKS

There are four basic types of community pharmacy networks: (1) open, pre-contracted, or shelf; (2) restricted, preferred, or customized; (3) exclusive or closed; and (4) specialized. An open, pre-contracted, or shelf network will enroll any pharmacy that agrees to the contract and reimbursement parameters, giving the benefit plan the advantage of the broadest access. Because the base reimbursement rate is inversely proportional to the size of the network, open networks usually have the highest reimbursement rate and program costs.

A restricted, preferred, or customized network is a subset of an open network. It is designed to meet the needs of an individual plan sponsor with fewer pharmacies and, therefore, lower reimbursement rates and lower costs than an open network. It is easier to ensure performance consistency through communications and education because fewer pharmacies are involved.

A closed, or exclusive, network locks out any pharmacy not enrolled in the network. It has the smallest access and, therefore, the lowest reimbursement rate and lowest costs because the lockouts channel members to only the participating pharmacies.

A specialized network is developed to accommodate a specific class or type of drug (e.g., interferon, acquired immune deficiency syndrome therapy, injectables) or services available (e.g., anticoagulation clinics or home infusion). The services may require specialized education in a particular disease state, patient monitoring, or extensive patient consulting. It may require the willingness to maintain an inventory of specialized medications or injectables. Credentialing or certification may be required to ensure quality and consistency when delivering professional services. Reimbursement can be based on both the product cost and the amount of time necessary to deliver the service.

Community pharmacy networks offer several advantages to the payer and patient. A network of community pharmacies ensures as broad an access as a payer desires; consistency or standardization of processes, procedures, and programs that ensure quality; audit controls; economies of scale; and administrative uniformity. In most cases, the community pharmacy network is used in combination with mail order, giving patients the ability to use either option when getting prescriptions filled.

All four types of community pharmacy networks normally consist of a combination of chain and independent pharmacies. Using chain pharmacies has advantages and disadvantages. It is administratively easier to communicate with several hundred or even a few thousand stores with a single mailing (or fax) to the chain headquarters. It is the chain headquarters' responsibility to see that the educational materials, policies, procedures, or other managed care pharmacy communications and other tools are distributed to each of the chain's stores. In addition, many chain stores are open 24 hours a day, are widely available in many urban areas, and may offer internal mail service.

Using independent pharmacists has advantages and disadvantages as well. Independent pharmacists are typically local businesses with a strong community commitment. Independents have the opportunity to join a variety of wholesale buying groups or Pharmacy Service Administrative Organization (PSAO) coalitions. These groups give the independent pharmacy some additional leverage to purchase at competitive prices, negotiate with managed care entities in a large block, and enhance the network access in the same manner as a chain. The ability to resemble and negotiate like a chain allows independents some of the same administrative and competitive efficiencies as chains. In addition, some independent pharmacies offer "on-call" 24-hour services.

PHARMACY PROVIDER NETWORK DEVELOPMENT

Developing a participating pharmacy provider network today is both an art and a science. Most PBMs have large national pre-contracted networks that are ready to activate once a plan sponsor decides to utilize the network. As most claims processing is completed online electronically and in real-time through in-pharmacy point-of-service (POS) computers, the

PBM only needs to input the plan sponsor's files of plan members eligible for coverage and the entire national network is capable of dispensing medications to the plan members.

However, today's sophisticated networks require another complete set of tools, including contracting, training, and reimbursement methodologies. The three fundamental goals of all provider network development are access, cost, and quality. Pharmacy directors must determine how broad the access to pharmacies is for all members, what is the cost to the plan sponsor for a specific network, and what will be the depth and quality of the network services.

The first step is to identify the plan sponsor's goal. Usually, it will be to provide the broadest access to members in the most cost-effective manner. Some plan sponsors choose greater access instead of a marginally less expensive reimbursement rate. It is necessary to obtain the member ZIP code list from the plan sponsor to determine the actual pharmacy access in an existing or customized network. Then, using sophisticated geographic information systems (GIS) software, member ZIP codes are matched with the pharmacy ZIP code locations.

Current standards usually dictate that a pharmacy provider must be within one to five miles of each plan member's home in a metropolitan area, five miles or less in a suburban area, and ten miles or less in a rural area. Sophisticated GIS programs make possible accurate comparisons between an MCO's membership and the pharmacy network locations. Many patients also are offered the option of having prescriptions mailed directly to their homes.

After this analysis is complete, it is possible to model various access scenarios involving combinations of chains and independents. The plan sponsor can obtain a close estimate of the percentage of pharmacies that may be required to participate under each scenario, along with the average drive time or distance from each member's home to the nearest participating pharmacy.

Cost containment is the second fundamental goal. This will vary by the competitiveness of the environment, restrictions of the plan design, mix of pharmacies, number of lives covered by the plan sponsor, past experience with the PBM, and other factors. Cost will usually be inversely proportional to the size of the network; in a smaller network, each of the pharmacies contracted through the network may receive more business than they would were the network large.

Most contracts stipulate reimbursement at the lowest of retail price (e.g., usual and customary price), maximum allowable cost for generics, or the contract rate. This permits accurate administration of all types of benefit designs (flat dollar copayments, percentage copayments, deductibles, maximums, and cash at the POS).

Performance characteristics of the network providers also factor heavily into the overall cost for a plan sponsor. In addition to the base product cost and dispensing fee, it is necessary to consider other economic variables, such as generic substitution rate, brand effective rate, purchasing efficiency, and preferred drug intervention programs. The brand effective rate is the average reimbursement of a single-source brand drug from all sources of payment. This concept is discussed as follows.

Quality is the third fundamental program goal. The basic claims adjudication process must minimize system downtime and ensure that the benefit design is being administered accurately. Frequency and reliability of payments to the pharmacies ensure the financial integrity of the system. There must be a consistent, easily identifiable member identification card to reduce confusion at the pharmacy. The ability to target pharmacies that should be audited is also important. Enforcement of the formulary and compliance with drug utilization review (DUR) messages must be maintained.

In recent years, an additional quality component has become more visible to patients and drug benefit payers alike. This component deals with the depth of services that are available at community pharmacies. Traditionally, the services available at a community pharmacy have focused on accurately dispensing medications and providing or having available some minimal level of patient consultation. However, evidence supporting the value of providing more in-depth consultative services at the pharmacy continues to grow. As a result, more and more community pharmacies are beginning to offer an expanded level of service. These additional services can include:

- Comprehensive medication reviews
- In-depth education and monitoring services for specific diseases (diabetes, asthma, hypertension, etc.)
- Immunization services
- Screenings
- Drug- or disease-specific clinics (blood thinners, osteoporosis, hormone therapy, etc.)

Although the cost of providing a drug benefit continues to rise, it is becoming increasingly evident that medications are often not utilized in the most effective manner. In fact, inappropriate medication use can result in increased medical costs, often in the form of increased hospital and outpatient medical facility use. As a result, pharmacy networks that offer services designed to maximize medication therapy (using programs like those mentioned above) can be utilized to help reduce overall medical costs even if the cost of providing such services results in increased drug benefit costs.

PHARMACY PROVIDER NETWORK CONTRACTING

If analysis of the plan sponsor's needs indicates the desirability of a network other than an existing pre-contracted network, it will be necessary to solicit, negotiate, and enroll a customized network. Frequently, a request-for-proposal is distributed to potential community pharmacies. Criteria for provider acceptance may include cost considerations, willingness to offer specialized services, location of stores, hours of operation, and delivery options. After a pharmacy has been selected, an agreement is executed that binds the pharmacy to the network policies and procedures.

After enrolling pharmacies in a basic or pre-contracted network, further changes or additions are accomplished through an addendum to the original agreement. Additionally, the contractor may choose either a positive or a negative solicitation. A positive solicitation requires the pharmacy to sign the actual agreement, an addendum, or a legal acknowledgment indicating acceptance of the terms. For a negative solicitation, the provider is automatically subject to the terms of the agreement as of a stated date, unless the provider specifically notifies the contractor of unwillingness to agree to the terms.

PARTICIPATING PHARMACY PROVIDER AGREEMENT

The provider agreement is a legally binding contract that ensures providers follow the rules set forth in the agreement and any related documents. **Appendix 5-1** contains an example of a provider agreement. Typical topics addressed in the provider agreement include the following:

- Amendments that specify the terms by which the contractor may terminate the agreement
- Services and standards such as licensing, certification, and continuing education
- Prior authorization policies that may require the pharmacy to contact the physician in specified circumstances
- Documentation, including the signature log, which is a record that counseling was performed and the patient or other authorized person accepted the prescription
- Record retention requirements beyond those set by state pharmacy or other laws
- Electronic communication standards requiring transmission and display of all online messages from the claims processor (i.e., drug formulary compliance, drug interactions, patient eligibility, DUR, and drug use evaluation [DUE]) and that appropriate action is taken
- Requirements for pharmacist compliance with the drug formulary
- Pharmacy provider insurance standards
- Expectations for online and real-time claim submission in the required format
- Requirements for participation in national pharmacy provider networks
- Taxes that must be collected
- Reimbursement policies and accompanying payment reports
- Enrollment fees the pharmacy must pay to participate in a network
- Audit and inspection rights of the contractor, and responsibilities of the pharmacy
- Definition of the pharmacy provider records that must be maintained
- Advertising and trademarks privileges of the contractor

PARTICIPATING PHARMACY PROVIDER MANUAL

The provider manual details the specific policies and procedures the participating pharmacies must follow to be in compliance with the provider agreement. Therefore, the manual must be consistent with the performance criteria outlined in the provider agreement. Typical topics addressed in the manual include the following:

- Systems requirements (hardware requirements of the in-pharmacy POS system as well as data transmission standards)
- DUR message definitions for messages transmitted on the electronic system
- Enhancements to electronic messages
- Incentive programs associated with dispensing performance requirements
- Contract compliance and audits
- Operational procedures (e.g., signature log and dispense-as-written [DAW] codes)
- Software requirements that include current and future upgrades
- Pharmacy Distribution Systems and Network Management
- Components of performance evaluation service requirements (beyond traditional dispensing and counseling)
- Delegation rights, authorization, and expectations

PARTICIPATING PHARMACY NETWORK MANAGEMENT ISSUES

Once the network has been contracted, the health plan members have been enrolled, and some have begun using the network, ongoing management is critical. Various methods are used to communicate with the network providers. Periodic newsletters update the providers on any procedural changes and offer clinically-oriented continuing education articles. Other news items about the claims processor or plan sponsors, or tips from colleague providers, are highlighted. A more comprehensive policies and procedures publication may be distributed as needed. This publication would summarize the various claim record fields, DAW explanations, identification card fields, and other areas of operational interest. A complete drug formulary and maximum allowable cost (MAC) list may be included.

In addition to these publications, regular notices of new plan sponsors may be distributed, inserted along with the regular payments made to pharmacies or mailed separately. With the increased use of Internet technology, most of these communication items are also distributed online. It is now common to find documents such as formularies, MAC lists, and preferred drug lists on a Web site for two reasons: the reduction in mailing costs and the possibility of instant updates.

Payments to pharmacies are usually biweekly or monthly. However, some pharmacies subscribe to a service that permits them to receive funds overnight. Along with the actual payment check, a remittance advice (R/A) details the reimbursement for each claim. The R/A may include a breakdown of performance-related payments or service charges.

Management of the network also involves maintenance of the various databases. Addresses, telephone numbers, and provider numbers for pharmacies and physicians need to be kept current. Changes are constantly taking place with drugstore mergers and store openings and closings.

Provider compliance must be monitored. The PBM, as network administrator, ensures that pharmacies submit accurate provider numbers; the numbers are needed to secure the most accurate information for DURs and other clinical evaluations. The PBM also must ensure that pharmacies submit their current usual and customary pricing, as stated in the agreement. Compliance monitoring covers the percentage of formulary drugs dispensed, observance of DUE, and patient counseling practices, too.

Maintaining good relations with professional and trade associations, state boards of pharmacy, and other healthcare-regulating entities is a key to effective network management. Pharmacies often contact association officers with concerns or issues pertaining to various third-party groups. By keeping the associations informed and maintaining regular communications, the network administrator can avoid some needless misunderstandings. Because all operations need to comply with the guidelines and regulations set by each of the 50 state boards of pharmacy, it is essential that network policies, procedures, and products meet legal standards.

ADDITIONAL NETWORK MANAGEMENT ISSUES

- Multiple MAC lists: Pharmacies may find significant differences in the MAC lists that are utilized to support a managed care contract. These differences may include the number of products on the MAC list, the unit pricing paid for individual MAC drugs, or both. Also, there are situations where the pharmacy MAC list could differ from the MAC list used by the payer.
- "Spread pricing": In some cases, pharmacy reimbursement formulas can differ from the formula used to bill a payer client. Quite often, this billing technique is used so that a payer will see consistent pricing while the pharmacy reimbursement amount will vary according to their contract (e.g., lower usual and customary [retail price; U&C] vs. average wholesale price [AWP] based discounts, etc.)
- Access fees: Commonly used for physicians and dentists, access fees are seldom used for pharmacy providers but are becoming more common. They can be considered a "surcharge" for the use of a provider that does not agree to accept the base reimbursement rate.
- Zero balance billing: Pharmacies negotiate for the right to charge a member the full copay even if the U&C or contract rate is less than the copay.
- Minimum prescription price: Pharmacies negotiate a minimum or floor reimbursement rate for any prescription.

MEASURING PERFORMANCE

Plan sponsors, in general, regard a network's overall financial performance as the primary indicator of its success. In the early days of networks, the basic indicator was the reimbursement rate for ingredient cost and dispensing fee. In today's environment, it is possible that the network with the most favorable ingredient cost and dispensing fee may be the least economically favorable from a performance or level of service standpoint.

Performance is measured by both clinical and economic factors. A common economic measure is the *generic substitution rate*, which is the number of times a pharmacy dispensed a generic product divided by the total number of opportunities to dispense generics. A normal generic substitution rate would be 80% to 90%.

The brand effective rate achieved by the pharmacy network, and the percentage below AWP at which all the brand drugs are dispensed by the pharmacy network, are two additional performance metrics. For example, the actual contract rate may be AWP – 14% plus $2.00, but the brand effective rate may be AWP – 16% plus $2.00. The difference can be attributed to the fact that the pharmacy received reimbursement for several claims at a cash (or U&C) rate, which was lower than the contract rate. Additionally, some claims may be submitted below the contract rate simply because the submitting pharmacy may be using a different pricing database or may not have updated their pricing database in a timely manner.

A third economic performance measure is purchasing: the effect of bottle size on drug costs. When a pharmacy submits a drug claim, the National Drug Code number on the claim indicates the package size, among other things. Pricing per tablet for small bottles (i.e., 50 or 100 units) can be more expensive than pricing per tablet for larger bottles (i.e., 500+ units). If pharmacies consistently use large bottle sizes, which increase purchasing efficiency, savings for the plan sponsor can be significant.

In addition to economic performance, there are many ways to measure clinical performance and service levels. The number of responses to online DUR alerts and accuracy of prescriber identification numbers are two indicators of performance. Another performance measure is the number of times that a non-preferred drug is changed to a preferred drug (generic or brand). (Chapter 24 has a broader discussion on pharmacy program performance.)

Clinical service programs that measure and reimburse pharmacists for patient care initiatives (e.g., disease management, medication compliance, and wellness counseling) are available today at many community pharmacies. Performance measures in these programs often require access to medical records or documented comparisons to similar programs that have already published measurement markers. In addition, provider surveys, patient complaint tracking, patient surveys, and service-based audits can be utilized to measure both the levels of service and satisfaction with the services that are offered.

AUDITS

The potential for fraud and abuse is always present within the network but can be curbed with a well-designed and thorough auditing system. Fraud or abuse can arise from actions of a member, pharmacy, or prescriber. Often, it is unintentional and simply due to a lack of appropriate education about a certain procedure. The first line of defense is on-line claims adjudication. Edits applied at the POS by the electronic system act as an automated management tool to monitor and ensure compliance to program parameters before the prescription is dispensed.

The second line of defense is the audit. One type of audit is the *bench* or *desk audit*, in which reports are analyzed based on utilization and cost data to identify erroneous billings and confirm that billed drugs were, in fact, provided to the plan sponsor's members. A more controversial form of desk audit uses pre-established algorithms to indicate the highest boundaries within which a pharmacy's claims may fall. For all claims that fall outside these boundaries, the pharmacy is held responsible for the dollar amount of these claims. This method is called *extrapolation*. Because the monetary impact is detected through only exception reports, as opposed to actual reviews of claims, this auditing method is more frequently challenged.

A more common type of audit is the actual *field* or *on-site audit*, where an auditor visits the pharmacy and reviews claims, signature logs, and other substantive documentation within the pharmacy. Pharmacies are targeted for a field audit if the claims analysis indicates a potential problem or if tips are received from regulatory agencies, plan members, providers, or plan sponsors. Possible actions include on-site inspection of pharmacy documentation, a contact with the prescriber-of-record for validation, or a contact with the patient for validation of receipt of the drugs.

Another form of the field audit is an *educational audit*. Auditors will answer questions about claims processing, inform pharmacists about programs and policies, and relay pharmacists' concerns back to the processor. Educational material is reviewed to help the pharmacy prevent future problems. Some common criteria used to screen pharmacies for potential problems include:

- U&C price submission
- Claim submission exceeding a specified number of claims per patient per day
- Average ingredient cost paid
- Average amount paid per prescription filled
- Percentage of compounded claims
- Percentage of controlled drugs
- Percentage of brand-name claims for multisource drugs
- Dispense-as-written (DAW) classification
- Percentage of refilled prescriptions
- Percentage of DAW prescriptions

As set forth in the provider agreement, the network contractor has the right to examine prescription information and other related records during normal business hours. If the contractor is denied admission to the pharmacy or if the provider does not present prescription records, signature logs, and supporting documentation, the contractor has the right to charge back 100% of the reimbursed claims. While the time frame for an audit may encompass all retained records, an auditor will usually review claims dispensed during the past three years. This review will be of claims paid, not necessarily filled, during the period.

A hard copy of each prescription must be readily retrievable upon request. This hard copy of a prescription, including prescription by telephone, must contain data elements required by state law and all of the prescriber's instructions that support the claims transmission. A signature log in date order is usually mandated for all claims submitted to the processor. The patient or authorized representative must sign the signature log for every prescription dispensed, even prescriptions delivered or mailed. Logs usually must be maintained for three years or longer, according to the state law for retaining prescription hard copies. The transition to electromagnetic signatures currently under way in many pharmacies will likely change this historic requirement.

Incorrect DAW codes are the most common cause of pharmacy charge backs and may lead to removal from a network. The pharmacy has a specified period of time (usually 30 days) from the receipt of the audit report to document problems identified during the audit. Collection methods for an audit liability may include but are not limited to a request for a check or offset against future claims payment, and the use of a collection agency. Terminated pharmacies, if granted reinstatement, may be required to pay a reinstatement fee, post a bond, or meet other criteria.

REPORTS

With the increased sophistication of performance-based networks comes the necessity for concise and comprehensive reports to illustrate the success of the entire network as well as each pharmacy's results. A few sample reports that are routinely used to monitor performance are presented below. These reports can be extremely useful for comparing pharmacy performance and permitting health plans to see the value of a specific network.

Missed Opportunity Report This report provides prescription level detail on generic substitution or preferred drug interchange opportunities in which no action was taken by the pharmacy. Pharmacies can review this report and analyze how to take better advantage of such opportunities in the future. Pharmacies can be compared to like pharmacies (independents, chains, etc.) within a specific geographic area. Comparing a pharmacy to its peers and identifying a benchmark or threshold provides an incentive for the pharmacy to perform more efficiently. Clients can review these reports to find the better performing pharmacies within their network.

Interchange Detail Report This report is used to determine successful interchanges within a reporting period and by therapeutic class. It provides an opportunity for identifying therapeutic classes that are problematic and therefore less profitable versus therapeutic classes that are less problematic and more profitable.

Therapeutic Class Analysis This report lists all drugs within the therapeutic drug classes in an interchange program. It also indicates the preferred and non-preferred products for all drugs dispensed.

Program Savings Report This report details overall savings from various components of a performance network.

MEMBER SATISFACTION

Member satisfaction is a key indicator of a network's success. Periodic surveys of members who have recently utilized the network can help assess this parameter. It is important to find out how the member was treated throughout the pharmacy encounter and whether a pharmacist met the member's expectations. Additionally, surveys help determine whether a pharmacy is charging members the actual usual and customary fee when that fee is lower than the contracted rate.

Under the Omnibus Budget Reconciliation Act of 1990 (OBRA '90), pharmacists were directed to counsel Medicaid patients. In most states, this standard has been expanded and is now expected for every patient. Appropriate and thorough counseling of patients with regard to their medication regimen, its impact, potential side effects, drug interactions, dietary interactions, appropriate scheduling, and other related information can greatly improve compliance and decrease overall medical costs. In recognition of this fact, many well-designed pharmacy care programs are being carefully assessed to potentially reimburse pharmacies for going beyond the basic standard covered by OBRA '90. As pharmacy care programs proliferate, the true value of retail pharmacy should become apparent (see Chapter 10 for a discussion on member satisfaction).

IMPACT OF MANAGED CARE ON THE DESIGN AND OPERATION OF A PHARMACY

CONSIDERATIONS FOR STAFF MODEL "IN-HOUSE" PHARMACIES

Although developing and operating an in-house pharmacy is normally associated with a staff model HMO, an employee benefit manager, a large employer, or any location with large numbers of health plan members may consider the option. Some employers have installed pharmacies in a convenient workplace setting. Typically, though, operating an in-house pharmacy does not result in the cost savings employers had hoped to achieve.

ADVANTAGES OF AN IN-HOUSE PHARMACY

Probably the most important advantage of a staff model HMO in-house pharmacy is significantly increased control over prescribing patterns. Generally, staff physicians and pharmacists work together to develop the most therapeutically advantageous and cost-effective drug regimens. The resulting list of drugs is the health plan's drug formulary, available in the pharmacy. When staff physicians play a role in developing an in-house formulary, compliance is often much higher and physicians are more likely to embrace the formulary concept. Also, there is more peer pressure among staff physicians and a stronger working relationship between in-house pharmacists and physicians than exist in an HMO using contracted community pharmacies.

Other advantages of an in-house pharmacy are the ability to better manage dispensing practices in the pharmacy (e.g., generic utilization), the ability to integrate pharmacy data with medical data, and the potential to improve member satisfaction because of pharmacists' familiarity with the drug benefit and plan design. In addition, in-house pharmacies improve control over the purchasing of pharmaceuticals and reduce the need to negotiate reimbursement rates with community pharmacies.

Often overlooked is the in-house pharmacy's ability to more easily develop, implement, and manage pharmaceutical care programs. These can be integrated into the health plan's programs to improve patient care and reduce patient utilization of other, more expensive types of medical treatment. For example, intensive pharmacy based educational programs for asthma patients ensure familiarity with proper inhaler use and peak flow meter techniques, resulting in improved control over the disease and reduced use of the emergency room. Other examples include intensive monitoring to ensure proper medication compliance as well as rapid detection and correction of side effects or inappropriate dosages. Through use of the proper feedback techniques, these programs can also improve the productivity and effectiveness of staff physicians.

DISADVANTAGES OF AN IN-HOUSE PHARMACY

Limited patient access is probably the greatest disadvantage of an in-house pharmacy. Many patients are willing to travel long distances to receive primary medical care but not to access pharmacy services. Because pharmacy services are often the most frequently utilized component of a health benefit plan, easy access to a conveniently located pharmacy becomes a determining factor when patients select a health plan. To address this issue, the health plan must carefully consider the locations of clinics as well as the possibility of combining in-house pharmacy services with at least a limited number of community pharmacies.

Using community pharmacies to improve access can negatively impact formulary compliance and adherence to the generic dispensing policies desired by the health plan. Also, community pharmacies are less likely to be familiar with the health plan's drug benefit policies and, as a result, may not handle benefit issues in the same responsive manner as an in-house pharmacy. Moreover, although on-line adjudication of claims submitted by community pharmacies is readily available for health plans, community pharmacy claims data cannot easily be integrated in real time with in-house pharmacy and medical data. Most often, integration is accomplished using daily, weekly, or monthly bulk transfer of claims data.

Other disadvantages of having only an in-house pharmacy include potential compliance issues due to the difficulty (limited access) of refilling prescriptions; a negative impact on member recruitment due to the limited pharmacy network; and the need for supplemental emergency, after-hours pharmacy service. Although it is not always the case, in-house pharmacies often do not produce the anticipated overall cost savings once the total costs of salaries and overhead are considered.

FINANCIAL CONSIDERATIONS FOR USING IN-HOUSE VERSUS COMMUNITY PHARMACIES

The costs of operating an in-house pharmacy can be considerable, ranging from bricks and mortar to staffing and inventory. If the in-house pharmacy is to deliver a broad range of pharmaceutical care services, the pharmacist-to-prescription ratio common to most retail pharmacies may not apply. As modern pharmacy practice moves away from routine dispensing functions toward managing patient drug therapy, more time must be available for interaction with patients and other members of the healthcare team. Thus, maximizing the use of pharmacy technicians, computers, and automated dispensing equipment is essential to success. This increases the initial investment but, theoretically, provides significant overall cost savings in the long run.

Physical Space Requirements The size and location of the pharmacy can significantly affect its success. Clearly, it is best to locate the pharmacy in a high traffic area, preferably where patients enter and exit the facility, with prominent directional signs. The waiting area should be designed to eliminate congestion. **Figure 5-1** provides an example of a pharmacy design for delivering pharmaceutical care in a professional pharmacy or staff model HMO pharmacy.

An in-house pharmacy often lacks an area with comfortable chairs that will accommodate patients waiting for prescriptions to be filled. Because in-house pharmacies are

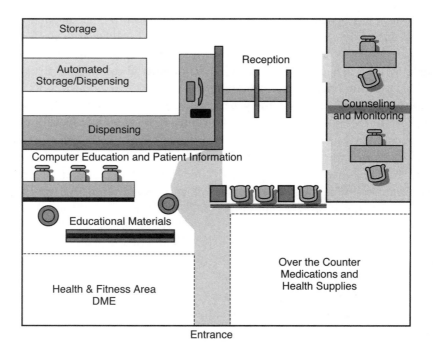

Entrance

FIGURE 5-1 Pharmacy Design for Delivering Pharmaceutical Care in a Professional Pharmacy or Staff Model HMO Pharmacy.

often located further from home than a community pharmacy might be, it is more likely that patients dropping off new prescriptions will wait for them to be filled as opposed to coming back later in the day for pick up. As a result, amenities offered in the waiting area can be critical. Wood tones, background music, and magazine stands are often used. In addition, kiosks and video terminals that offer healthcare information can improve the usefulness of the waiting area.

CONSIDERATIONS FOR ALL PHARMACIES THAT SERVICE MANAGED CARE PATIENTS

Additional Design Considerations Other important aspects of the pharmacy design are the location of patient consultation areas (private and/or semiprivate), a prescription-filling area that accommodates the appropriate use of technicians, computer screens, and prescription-filling automation. Some pharmacies may buy large quantities of drugs to capitalize on limited buying opportunities, making adequate storage space imperative. In cases where pharmacies provide clinics with injectables and sterile solutions, the use of a clean room and laminar flow hood may be required.

Staffing Issues When developing pharmacy staffing requirements, functional goals should be considered. A larger staff will be required for intensive drug therapy management aimed at improving overall drug therapy, physician productivity and reduced overall medical costs. Conversely, a smaller staffing level will be adequate if the pharmacy offers only a quick, convenient, and cost-effective way to deliver prescriptions to members. The pharmacist-to-prescription ratio can vary widely, depending on the use of technicians, the availability of automation and computerization, and the expected duties of the pharmacist.

Recruiting qualified pharmacists can be difficult. Some pharmacists pursue positions that promote expanded clinical services because they want to use a broader range of their clinical skills. The rapid expansion of managed care programs and PBMs has also resulted in a high demand for pharmacists with managed care experience.

Managed Care Impact on Pharmacy POS Computer System Selecting an appropriate POS computer system for the pharmacy can be a challenge. The first step is to determine the level of sophistication necessary. A pharmacy could use a commercially-available basic dispensing and billing system. Or it could use a customized system designed to facilitate an expanded level of services. Capabilities to consider include:

- Basic dispensing and billing requirements (including basic DUR capabilities)
- Automation of the prescription-filling process
- Integration with a phone system that allows patients to order prescriptions and access information about prescription status using touch-tone or voice-activated phone technology

- Sufficient terminal access for both the technician filling prescriptions and pharmacists engaged in clinical activities or patient counseling
- Integration with medical and other data integration with other pharmacy distribution methods (e.g., mail-order, in-clinic distribution during office visits)
- Data and performance analysis and reporting capability
- Expanded "pharmaceutical care" capabilities (e.g., expanded patient data intake to develop patient care plans, initiate follow-up activities, automate documentation and billing for services, or quantify potential cost savings)
- Ability to manage an expanded level of pharmaceutical care services (e.g., protocol-driven standards of care, capture of additional patient demographics and medical information, ability to utilize medically-based service codes, ability to provide patient educational materials, and ability to issue patient care reminders and daily "to do" logs)

Predicting Success In the past, the success of a pharmacy was almost entirely dependent on minimizing operational costs and maximizing the volume of prescriptions that could be driven into the location. Today, additional measurements can be made. Pharmacists can work with physicians to impact drug mix and reduce overall costs by maximizing the use of generic drugs and preferred brand (formulary) drugs. Advancements in technology (handheld prescribing devices, Internet formulary access, etc.) have made it possible to better manage drug therapy in both community and staff model pharmacies.

Financial/feasibility projections for an in-house pharmacy can be difficult. In most cases, the health plan's sales and marketing staff will project utilization by using membership demographics (e.g., average age of members) and other corporate or commercially available data. These sources can also be used to project the average cost of a prescription.

The projected membership multiplied by expected utilization (prescription drugs [Rxs] per-patient-per-year) will provide an estimate of the annual prescription volume that can be expected from a managed care contract. Further analysis will be required to consider the market share that will result from a managed care contract. If the pharmacy network is broad and includes most pharmacies, there will be little impact on market share. However, if the pharmacy network is restricted, the pharmacy will need to project the potential increase in market share (Rx volume).

The technique for projecting impact on operating costs are not much different from the technique for projecting costs for any other operational department: fixed costs (e.g., staffing, fixtures, and equipment) plus variable costs (cost of goods sold, etc.). Again, overall profitability may not be the sole consideration. Based on prescription data alone, the impact on overall medical costs and clinic operations could prompt the decision to operate an in-house pharmacy, even if it proved minimally profitable.

Measuring Performance Pharmacists should be encouraged to develop and implement programs to lower overall drug costs, control inappropriate drug utilization, improve productivity, or improve member drug therapy. Of primary importance would be reports that track average drug costs, generic utilization rates, drug utilization rates, physician prescribing patterns, and market share changes in high-volume and high-cost drug categories. Standard operational reports are necessary. These include daily profit and loss reports, inventory turn reports, short order reports, and others, most of which are included with a standard pharmacy management computer system.

To the extent possible, the pharmacy staff should be challenged to assign cost savings for each activity outside the normal dispensing process. For example, if the pharmacy staff chooses to implement a program in which the pharmacists spend additional time working with noncompliant patients, a mechanism should be developed to measure any increase in overall patient compliance. In addition, an attempt should be made to quantify whether improved compliance has reduced overall medical costs.

MAIL SERVICE PHARMACY

Most plan sponsors today want an integrated delivery system with both retail and mail components. In 2001, 87% of large employers offered a mail service option. A mail service provider is a licensed pharmacy that offers primarily maintenance medications to members through mail delivery. Mail service pharmacies provided 5.5% of all prescription medications in 2002, or approximately 174 million prescriptions. The costs for those medications accounted for $33.54 billion of the prescription drug market or 18.4% of total prescription sales. Mail service is distinguished mainly by price and the ability to contain costs. As with other distribution systems, there are both advantages and disadvantages.

ADVANTAGES

- *Single pharmacy provider.* Administrative costs are minimized with only one mail-order location that serves as a single pharmacy provider with one provider number.
- *Volume leverage.* By dispensing average quantities of 90 days, a mail service provider can leverage high volume to gain maximum wholesaler discounts.
- *Technology.* The high volume of mail service makes it cost-effective to acquire the most advanced and most efficient technology, such as robotics, computer chip encryption, conveyor belt, computerized graphics, and automatic high-speed counting machines. For many retail pharmacies, such advanced, efficient technology is cost-prohibitive.
- *Error minimization.* Advanced technology provides multiple automatic safeguards to help minimize errors.
- *Delivery convenience.* Prescriptions delivered to the patient's home by mail are especially convenient for members who are older or have disabilities.
- *Centralized interchange opportunities.* Most mail service providers have call centers for contacting members and physicians about interchange opportunities.
- *Deeper manufacturer discounts.* With the aggressive use of both generic and therapeutic interchange, PBMs are able to negotiate deeper manufacturer discounts.

- *Toll-free drug information line.* Most mail service providers have a 24-hour, toll-free telephone line with access to registered pharmacists.
- *Large quantities.* The average 90-day quantities minimize dispensing time for technicians and pharmacists, resulting in lower administrative costs.
- *Compliance refill reminders.* Many mail service providers contact (e.g., phone, mail, email) patients a few days before their prescriptions are due to run out, which enhances overall compliance.
- *Education material.* Patient education materials can be triggered to automatically be included with each prescription.
- *Increase community pharmacist availability.* By moving stabilized chronic therapies to a highly automated system, the community pharmacy network becomes more available to counsel patients with acute, newly diagnosed conditions.

DISADVANTAGES

- *Lack of personal contact.* There is no opportunity for face-to-face counseling or discussions with a pharmacist. As the value of pharmacy care programs is quantified more precisely, this lack of in-person contact could become an even bigger issue in the future.
- *Increased waste.* With an average of a 90-day supply, there is potential for waste if the medication is discontinued.
- *Advance request.* The member must request their refill well in advance of depletion of their current supply.

STRUCTURING A MAIL SERVICE BENEFIT

Mail service benefit programs began with fixed-dollar copayments, a method that was perceived as reasonable to both patient and health plan. However, the flat copayment has not kept pace with rising drug prices and may not yield an equitable share from the member, especially because ordering a 90-day supply through the mail (as compared with a 30-day supply at retail) essentially waives two copayments. Moreover, with mail, members are less likely to understand the true value of their drug benefit program.

Many payers have implemented a mandatory mail service benefit. This can either be limited to medications in specified therapeutic classes or can be used after an initial fill at a community pharmacy. The concept is to force the purchase of all chronic medications through mail order. Even when the program is not mandatory, the member is normally incentivized to use mail service.

Exhibit 5-1 lists the indicators for quality prescription mail services.

DEVELOPING AN INTEGRATED DISTRIBUTION SYSTEM

The drug benefit business is the only segment of the healthcare insurance industry that can operate in a totally automated environment. Virtually all pharmacies in the United States today use a computer system to submit drug claims and to receive payment.

EXHIBIT 5-1 INDICATORS FOR QUALITY PRESCRIPTION MAIL SERVICES

Cost management
- Aggressiveness of benefit management
- Physician interaction and education
- DUR and formulary capabilities
- Generic substitution rate achieved
- Size and stringency of MAC list
- Impact of MAC provisions and generic discounts on overall costs for a population and the mix of products used

Service
- Customer service and telephone support resources
- Turnaround time
- Shipping capabilities: cool packs, express delivery
- Administrative support to place (e.g., a dedicated account representative)
- Protocols for working with physicians
- Availability and expertise of pharmacists

Site visit
- Adequacy of physical plant
- Use of advanced technology such as bar coding, robotics, computerization
- Match between marketing promises and reality
- Flexibility and responsiveness to plan needs

Quality assurance
- Error rates and prevention procedures
- Classification and correction of errors
- Presence of total quality management program
- Billing accuracy

POS and reporting
- Ability to process claims on line in real time
- Integration with retail networks
- Understandable, useful management reports
- System back-up provisions

Source: Courtesy of Midwest Business Group on Health, 1994; Chicago, Illinois.

The ability to integrate data from community pharmacies, mail order pharmacies, and in-house pharmacies is an important aspect of drug benefit automation. Prescription drug claims from each entity can be submitted via an automated online environment, allowing the entire claims processing function to occur at the POS. This processing capability accumulates all claims information in a central database and establishes the foundation for an unlimited number of drug benefit products and services.

Although difficult to accomplish in some cases, data integration for drug claims has proven most beneficial for health plans with multiple distribution systems. For example, using both in-house and community pharmacies and integrating the data can improve plan member satisfaction. Members may be dissatisfied if they are forced to rely solely on an in-house pharmacy. To remedy the problem, the delivery network can be expanded to include community pharmacies and mail order pharmacy, which can submit claims data that can be integrated with in-house pharmacy data. The resulting database permits quick and efficient detection of drug utilization problems, makes possible reports drawn from drug benefit information, and provides much faster computation of drug market share information.

The integrated data can be used to compare the cost of an in-house prescription to the cost of a prescription from a contracted community pharmacy. In addition, pharmacy performance can be evaluated and performance improvement programs established. Using the physician identifier submitted by the pharmacy with each prescription, prescribing patterns can be monitored to identify physicians with high non-formulary or non-preferred drug prescribing habits. Physicians can be targeted for educational mailings that will demonstrate potential plan savings associated with the use of formulary drugs.

It is also possible to integrate mail-order pharmacy prescription activity. The mail-order pharmacy will, in some cases, submit claims online just like a community pharmacy. More commonly, the mail-order pharmacy will submit *batch* or *bulk claims data* using a computer tape or once-a-day online modem transmission. Information formatted in this way facilitates integration with prescription data submitted by the in-house or community pharmacy. Integration of claims data from all three sources provides plan members and payers with maximum safety and cost-effectiveness.

PHARMACIST'S ROLE

Pharmacists are members of perhaps one of the most stereotyped professions in the United States. The pharmacist is seen solely as a person behind the prescription counter who is responsible for dispensing medications prescribed by the physician. In a managed care environment, however, pharmacists are involved in a number of different functions, and their work varies greatly depending on the practice setting.

RETAIL/COMMUNITY PHARMACY PRACTICE

The primary role of the community pharmacist is to oversee the dispensing function. Recently, however, community pharmacists have been able to expand that role. Pharmacists involved in a chain, supermarket chain, mass-market retail chain, or independent pharmacy will dispense medications, counsel patients, and participate in store management. A limited number will become involved in corporate operations. In addition, pharmacists are often involved with basic computer functions, inventory control, record keeping, staff supervision, and overall store operations. In some cases, chains operate their own pharmacy benefit management division, coordinating pharmacy services for employer groups and insurance providers.

THIRD-PARTY INSURED PATIENTS

In most areas of the United States, patients obtain prescriptions as part of an insurance benefit sponsored by a third party. Starting in the late 1990s, third-party insured patients became the largest segment of pharmacies' patient base, outnumbering cash-paying customers. As a result, pharmacists have had to sharpen their business skills to remain profitable in an environment where payers will reimburse for prescription services delivered to insured members only if pharmacies are willing to accept reduced reimbursement levels. At the same time, complicated insurance benefit plan requirements demand additional time with each patient.

Many pharmacists have learned to meet the demands of third party customers. Of increasing importance is the ability to process prescription orders quickly and effectively, utilizing enhanced computerization, pharmacy technicians, and prescription-filling automation. By maximizing efficiency, the pharmacist can spend more time reviewing medication profiles and counseling patients. In addition, many third-party plans offer incentives for discussing generic or less costly brand alternatives with the patient and physician. By familiarizing themselves with the benefit programs offered by most payers (insurance companies or employers), pharmacists can help patients to better understand their drug benefit. Quick and efficient prescription-filling capability, combined with pharmacist-based patient counseling and drug benefit information, are sure to please managed care patients.

PHARMACY PRACTICE IN AN IN-HOUSE PHARMACY

In general, pharmacists working in an in-house pharmacy environment are less likely to be involved with operational issues and more likely to encounter opportunities for expanding their role in support of clinical programs. In-house pharmacists may handle patient counseling and drug therapy management. The lack of an extensive retail section means more opportunity for semiprivate or private patient counseling. Pharmacists are able to work with staff physicians in developing drug formularies and drug therapy protocols that will be supported as part of the overall operation of the HMO. Also, as part of the operation of an outpatient pharmacy, many staff model pharmacies become involved with extensive patient care clinical programs.

In a staff model HMO, pharmacists are likely to be salaried, as are physicians and other staff. The staff model environment allows pharmacists to work with staff physicians and other health care professionals as part of a healthcare team to ensure that the most appropriate and cost-effective drug treatment options are considered. Take, for example, the asthma patient. Pharmacists work with physicians to monitor the overuse or underuse of bronchodilators as well as the proper use of corticosteroids. In many staff model

HMOs, these aggressive drug therapy management techniques have significantly reduced patient use of other, more expensive treatment options (e.g., office visits or emergency room visits).

As part of the operation of some in-house pharmacies, pharmacists become involved with other aspects of the clinic operation. For example, pharmacists may be involved with injectable medications and admixtures or physician specialists, such as dermatologists, who may require more compounded medications. Pharmacists working in staff model HMOs work on clinic committees to deal with issues ranging from operational efficiencies to more effective patient health therapies. Pharmacists in a staff model HMO also may help develop a community-based expansion of pharmacy services for members who desire expanded access.

PHARMACY PRACTICE IN THE COMMUNITY PHARMACY

Because in-house staff model pharmacies account for only a small percentage of all patients that obtain their prescriptions benefits from a third party, it is important to remember that almost all of the attributes of staff model medication management programs can be duplicated in the community pharmacy. Utilizing "pharmaceutical care" techniques to better manage patient drug therapy is becoming more and more common in the community pharmacy. Community pharmacists can work with a managed care organization to design effective medication management programs. In addition, programs can be introduced that will help monitor and educate patients with specific diseases (diabetics, asthma, etc.) As these programs become more common, methods of reimbursement for these additional pharmacist services will become more commonplace.

WORKING FOR A PBM

Some pharmacists who are interested in managed care careers will join a PBM. These pharmacists will probably not handle traditional dispensing of medications. Today, activities that involve pharmacists employed by PBMs can include the following:

- *Systems development*: helping to develop system logic to process and administer drug benefit claims in a manner that is both therapeutically sound and cost-effective
- *Drug benefit plan design*: developing the drug benefit plan design, such as parameters for exclusions (e.g., cosmetic or weight loss drugs), coverage guidelines (e.g., infertility drugs or growth hormones), and related issues (e.g., deductibles and benefit maximums)
- *Network development*: negotiating contracts with community pharmacies and other aspects of the PBM-pharmacy relationship, such as coordinating system links, establishing maximum allowable cost reimbursement for generic drugs, and communicating program requirements to participating pharmacies
- *Clinical pharmacy services*: supporting health plan clients by helping analyze drug benefit costs and assisting with decisions on drug benefit coverage as well as preparing drug therapy analyses

- *Clinical consultants*: serving as an academic detailer by calling on physicians to educate and discuss current drug therapy management. Usually provides profiles that compare the physician's prescribing patterns to those of local peer groups.
- *Clinical writers*: develop drug utilization reviews, prior authorization guidelines, and disease management programs.

PRACTICING PHARMACY IN A MAIL-ORDER FACILITY

A mail-order facility offers pharmacists a variety of ways to utilize their clinical skills. The primary emphasis for mail order is accurate and cost-effective medication dispensing. However, the following other opportunities exist:

- Purchasing of pharmaceuticals
- Computer system and operational responsibilities
- Telephone consultations with patients about their prescription regimens
- Telephone consultations with patients, physicians, or other healthcare providers about clinically appropriate, cost-effective alternatives
- Facility management

Each type of practice setting offers employment advantages to pharmacists. For example, PBM and mail-order pharmacists generally are not required to work weekends or evenings, as is common for community pharmacists and many in-house pharmacists. On the other hand, community pharmacy and in-house pharmacy offer the greatest opportunity for patient contact. Although PBM pharmacists are probably exposed to the greatest variety of employment options, all of the employment areas discussed here offer a wealth of opportunities for skilled pharmacy professionals.

IMPACT OF MANAGED CARE ON THE PROFESSION OF PHARMACY

The pharmacists' stereotypical role as medication dispensers is rapidly changing. More and more, pharmacists work with physicians and patients to manage drug therapy, while dispensing medication is commonly automated or performed by paraprofessionals. The patient care movement means that more pharmacists are actively involved with patients, monitoring drug therapy, identifying drug therapy issues, and developing patient care plans to correct problems.

The next few years will play a critical part in determining the future role of pharmacists in managed care. As pharmacists become more involved in working with physicians and patients to manage drug therapy, payers will demand evidence of the cost-effectiveness and impact of this change on overall patient health. Most important, payers will watch to see if the community pharmacy and mail-order pharmacy can respond to demands for drug therapy management, providing services that previously were available at only an in-house pharmacy. PBMs will be challenged to assist in this transformation by working with community pharmacies to ensure the development of cost-effective drug therapy management programs that can reduce overall health care costs.

IMPACT OF LEGISLATIVE AND REGULATORY ISSUES ON THE PROFESSION OF PHARMACY

Potential legislation and regulation that can significantly impact various aspects of pharmacy is always omnipresent. This can occur on the federal level or at the state level through either congressional legislation or through regulation by a governing body such as the board of pharmacy or department of insurance. Current and future issues that are likely to have a substantial impact on at least some aspect of the distribution channel are in the paragraphs below.

HIPAA This acronym represents the Health Insurance Portability and Accountability Act of 1996; HIPAA is administered by the Centers for Medicare and Medicaid Services (CMS). This legislation sets national standards for electronic healthcare transactions along with ensuring the security and privacy of health data. Its impact can already be seen at the POS of the pharmaceutical where the pharmacist must have documentation on file addressing certain aspects of privacy of their medication records.

Technician Ratios A state often times regulates the maximum number of pharmacy technicians that can be supervised by one pharmacist at any one time. Most states are either increasing or eliminating this ratio in order to allow maximum use of support personnel. This allows the pharmacist to spend more time in actual patient care as well as minimizing the impact of a national pharmacist shortage. The Department of Defense and Veterans Administration have used this approach for many years.

Technician Certification Most states are demanding that pharmacy technicians demonstrate the successful completion of a certified program along with mandatory minimum on-the-job training and passage of a national certification test.

Payment Formulas Most state Medicaid programs have a pharmacy reimbursement formula based upon the AWP. Many federal and state entities are currently reviewing this approach. Newly considered payment formulas may be based upon other national pricing guidelines such as Average Manufacturers' Price, Actual Cost, or similar acquisition price.

Most Favored Nations Some state Medicaid programs include a *most favored nations* clause in their pharmacy contracts, which usually states that the pharmacy must extend to the state the lowest of either the Medicaid contract price or the lowest contract price given to any other payer. Obviously, in these cases, the pharmacy must carefully analyze the impact of their Medicaid business along with extending that favorable pricing to the rest of their managed care business.

PBM Licensure and Regulation Several states have attempted to regulate PBMs under both the Board of Pharmacy and the Department of Insurance. In most cases, the board has concluded that any pharmacist employed by a PBM, whose job falls under their definition of the practice of pharmacy, is already registered by the state board.

Medicare Drug Legislation On December 8, 2003, President Bush signed the first Medicare legislation that includes a drug benefit. Speculation is that this legislation will be regularly fine tuned through additional rules and legislation. This benefit has increased prescription volume at most pharmacies as well as increased business for the PBM. Also, medication therapy management (MTM) is mandated by this legislation.

Artificial Parity Laws Several states have enacted laws that prohibit health plans from specifying different cost-sharing, days-supply, and/or other terms and conditions for retail and mail pharmacies in a pharmacy network. These laws are referred to as "artificial parity" laws because they attempt to artificially eliminate pricing and other differences between community and mail pharmacies.

Any Willing Provider Laws Most states have enacted "any willing provider" laws that require health plans and insurers to include in their pharmacy networks any pharmacy and/or pharmacist who agrees to meet the health plan's terms and conditions. In addition, the new Medicare legislation also includes an "any willing provider" requirement.

CONCLUSION

The pharmacy profession will continue to undergo a dramatic transformation. As the value of the services offered by pharmacists becomes quantified and documented, the following trends will become more apparent:

Time Allowed for Dispensing Dispensing time functions will shift to pharmacy care services. With the increased reliance on technology and technicians, fewer pharmacists will be necessary to provide the dispensing functions. Greater numbers of pharmacists will be educated, trained, and certified to provide comprehensive pharmacy care programs. This is consistent with the transition from a bachelor's degree to a doctor of pharmacy degree as the new entry level required degree for pharmacy practice.

Physical Pharmacy Changes Pharmacy sites will be retooled as the proliferation of pharmacy care services will change the physical layouts of pharmacies. Pharmacies will provide private consulting areas and information centers utilizing kiosks, videos, and other training materials that are separate from the dispensing and compounding areas.

Mainstreaming Care Services Pharmacy care services will become mainstreamed as increased numbers of demonstration projects prove their worth.

Improved Performance Service-based networks with an emphasis on performance will become the norm as pharmacies see the bulk of their revenue tied to patient care outcomes. Problem identification followed by intervention will be rewarded.

Credentialing National credentialing standards will be adopted to certify uniformity and quality in the capabilities of individual pharmacists.

National Drug Clearinghouse A national clearinghouse for drug therapy management services will be developed for use by patients in locating the appropriate service desired.

SUGGESTED READING

"Managed care in alternative site," in *Managed Care Pharmacy Lecture Series*, Alexandria, VA: Academy of Managed Care Pharmacy; 1996: 18-21.

Blissenbach H., "Pharmaceutical services in managed care," in Kongstvedt P., (ed.): *The Managed Health Care Handbook*, 2nd Ed. Gaithersburg, MD: Aspen Publishers, Inc; 1993: 142-160.

Christensen D.B., Holmes G., Fassett, W.E., et al., Pharmacy practice: Principal findings from the Washington State Cognitive Services Demonstration Project. *Managed Care Interface*, 1998; July: 60-62, 64.

Cipolle R.J., Morley P.C., Strand L.M., *Pharmaceutical Care Practice*. New York: Health Professions Division, McGraw-Hill; 1998.

Cranor C.W., Christensen D.B., The Asheville Project: short-term outcomes of a community pharmacy diabetes care program. *J Am Pharm Assoc.*, 2003; 43: 149-159.

Cranor C.W. and Shristensen D.B., The Asheville Project: factors associated with outcomes of a community pharmacy diabetes care program. *J Am Pharm Assoc.*, 2003; 43: 160-172.

Cranor C.W., Bunting B.A., Christensen D.B., The Asheville Project: long-term clinical and economic outcomes of a community pharmacy diabetes care program. *J Am Pharm Assoc.*, 2003; 43: 173-184.

Garrett D.G. and Martin L.A., The Asheville Project: participants' perceptions of factors contributing to the success of a patient self-management diabetes program. *J Am Pharm Assoc.*, 2003; 43: 185-190.

Hejna C., Pharmacy networks: origins, functions, and future directions, in Ito S., Blackburn S., (eds.): *A Pharmacist's Guide to Principles and Practices of Managed Care Pharmacy*. Alexandria, VA: Foundation for Managed Care Pharmacy; 1995; 119-128.

Navarro R., Reimbursement for cognitive pharmacy services. *Managed Care Interface*, 1998; July: 57-59.

Shellard S., Managing prescription drug benefits, in Shellard S (ed.): *Prescription Price Watch*. New Haven, CT: Midwest Business Group on Health; 1994: 9-19.

Sterler L., The effect of retail pharmacy intervention on improving patient compliance. *Cost & Quality Quarterly Journal*, 1996; October: 27-29.

Timm M., Pharmacy network strategies and development. *Medical Interface*, 1993; May: 90-96.

Weinberger M., Murray M.D., Marrero D.G., et al., Effectiveness of pharmacist care for patients with reactive airway disease: a randomized controlled trial. *JAMA.*, 2002; 288: 1594-1602.

Appendix

5-1

A SAMPLE PBM PHARMACY PROVIDER AGREEMENT (ABRIDGED)

This sample PBM pharmacy provider agreement contains the portions of the contract to address the requirements of the PBM and pharmacy provider as they relate to provision and reimbursement for contracted pharmacy benefits. This is not a complete contract and does not represent a contract for any specific PBM.

This Provider Agreement (the "Agreement") is entered into between PBM and the undersigned pharmacy provider ("Provider") and shall become effective, and binding on the Provider, as of the date PBM accepts the Agreement (the "Effective Date").

RECITALS

A. PBM offers pharmacy benefit management services to its customers and has established a remote electronic claims adjudication and processing system known as the CLAIMS ADJUDICATION System for verifying and processing claims and furnishing other related administrative and clinical services through a nationwide system of pharmacies and other facilities for its pharmacy benefit management services. B. PBM's customers sponsor, administer, or otherwise participate in prescription benefit and related programs. C. Provider wishes to provide pharmacy and related services in connection with PBM's customers' programs.

AGREEMENTS

For valuable consideration, the receipt and sufficiency of which are acknowledged, PBM and Provider agree as follows:

1.   Responsibilities and Rights of Provider.

1.1   Services and Standards. Provider will render or cause to be rendered to all Eligible Persons the Pharmacy Services to which the Eligible Person is entitled in accordance with the Prescriber's directions, the applicable Plan, the PBM Documents and applicable Law (including, without limitation, licensing, certification, and continuing education requirements). Provider and its employees and agents, in providing Pharmacy Services under this Agreement, will exercise their own professional judgment, to the best of their ability, on all applicable questions.

1.2   Verification of Eligibility. Provider will require each person requesting Pharmacy Services under a Plan to verify that he or she is an Eligible Person.

1.3   Prior Authorization. For prescriptions requiring a "prior authorization" as indicated in the CLAIMS ADJUDICATION System, Provider will (a) contact PBM or its designee to receive prior authorization, (b) inform the Eligible Person that prior authorization from the Plan Sponsor is required and (c) provide PBM or the Eligible Person with such other information as PBM shall reasonably require.

1.4   Collection of Copayment. With respect to each Covered Item submitted through the CLAIMS ADJUDICATION System, Provider will collect the copayment as indicated in the CLAIMS ADJUDICATION System from the Eligible Person and Provider will not waive, discount, reduce, or increase the copayment indicated in the CLAIMS ADJUDICATION System.

1.5   Documentation; Signature Log. Provider will have each Eligible Person (or his or her designated agent to whom prescriptions may be dispensed) sign a log (in such form as may be required by PBM from time to time) that contains all information required by a Plan Sponsor or PBM, including, without limitation, the date, the prescription number, pick-up date, authorization for the release to PBM and Plan Sponsor (and each of their designees) of all information contained in the signature log related to Pharmacy Services and pharmacy benefit management services. Provider will maintain documentation evidencing that any (i) counseling required by Law occurred and (ii) the correct DAW code was transmitted.

1.6   Record Retention. PBM and Provider will maintain for a minimum of three years (or longer if required by applicable Law) after the respective record is created, in original form, fiche or on electronic media, the claims and claim forms supporting the in voices and other records sufficient to verify Covered Items dispensed, claims processed, payments made to Provider, and documentation and logs. Notwithstanding the foregoing, Provider shall keep hard copies of prescriptions, and updates thereto, as required by applicable Law and the PBM Manual.

1.7   Electronic Communication. Provider agrees to maintain the capability to send, receive, and display electronic messages to and from PBM in accordance with (i) NCPDP standards, including such new standards from time to time, and (ii) the PBM Documents and program requirements. Provider shall receive and display all messages transmitted by PBM and take appropriate professional action upon receipt of such messages. Provider will use software that has been certified by PBM as meeting both the NCPDP standards and PBM program requirements.

1.8   Compliance with Drug Formulary. Provider shall use reasonable efforts to comply with the PBM or applicable Plan Sponsor formulary to the extent such formulary applies to Pharmacy Services provided to an Eligible Person. Notwithstanding the foregoing, in no event shall Provider be required to comply with the PBM or applicable Plan Sponsor formulary if Provider or the Prescriber, physician or the dispensing pharmacist, deems such compliance contrary to his or her professional judgment.

1.9   Limitation on Collection. Provider agrees that in no event, including, without limitation, non-payment or bankruptcy by a Plan, will Provider seek compensation in any manner from an Eligible Person for Pharmacy Services with respect to a Covered Item provided under this Agreement. This provision does not prohibit Provider from collecting the applicable copayment, coinsurance or deductible amounts that are indicated in the CLAIMS ADJUDICATION System, which amount Provider is obligated to collect and agrees not to waive.

1.10   Insurance. Provider will maintain general and professional liability coverage in such forms and amounts as are reasonable for the industry and for a provider of Pharmacy Services of the type and size of Provider which shall in no event be less than required by applicable Law. Provider will provide PBM with a copy of all professional liability insurance policies in effect from time to time upon request.

1.11   Credentialing. Provider agrees to provide PBM with the necessary information required from time to time to complete PBM's credentialing programs.

1.12   Drug Utilization Review. Provider acknowledges and agrees that the information generated in connection with Drug Utilization Review is intended as an economical supplement to, and not a substitute for, the knowledge, expertise, skill, and judgment of Prescribers and pharmacists, including Provider and its employees and agents. Provider and its individual employees and agents are responsible for acting or not acting upon information generated and transmitted through Drug Utilization Review and for performing Pharmacy Services in each jurisdiction consistent with the scope of their respective licenses.

1.13   Nondiscrimination. Unless Provider's professional judgment dictates otherwise or Provider is being asked to provide Pharmacy Services to an Eligible Person covered by a Plan participating in the CLAIMS ADJUDICATION Network, Provider shall not (i) serve only some Eligible Persons of a particular group and not other Eligible Persons of the same group or (ii) provide only certain Covered Items to Eligible Persons of a particular group unless Provider does not provide such Covered Items to any Eligible Persons of the same group.

1.14   Eligible Persons Complaint Procedures. Provider shall cooperate with the administration of complaints by Eligible Persons. Provider shall make every reasonable effort to resolve all com plaints in an informal process and keep written records of events and actions surrounding each complaint that is not resolved to the Eligible Person's satisfaction.

2.   Transmission of Claims to PBM for Reimbursement. Provider will submit claims for payment in accordance with the PBM Documents and the following:

2.1   CLAIMS ADJUDICATION Submission. Provider will submit online claims through the CLAIMS ADJUDICATION System within fourteen (14) days from the date of fill. As to those claims, Provider will have the transmission capability to make online claim reversals. Provider will submit claim reversals before the close of the cycle following the cycle in which the claim was originally submitted.

2.2   Other Submissions. Upon PBM's prior approval, Provider may submit any claims not submitted through the CLAIMS ADJUDICATION System to PBM (whether in a paper, tape, or electronic format) within twelve (12) months of the date of fill. In the case of a PBM National Network or any Plan that may reimburse Provider at the Usual and Customary Price, Provider shall not be permitted to submit a claim in a format that does not provide for the transmission of Usual and Customary Price. Provider shall not be permitted to submit claims in a format that is not authorized by the Plan Sponsor.

2.3   Information. Provider will transmit with each claim the information requested by this Agreement, the PBM Documents or the CLAIMS ADJUDICATION instructions. Each claim submitted by Provider through the CLAIMS ADJUDICATION System shall constitute a representation by Provider to PBM that Pharmacy Services were provided to the Eligible Person and the information submitted is accurate and complete.

3.   Participation in the Plan Sponsor Networks.

3.1   Termination of Network Participation. Except as otherwise may be required with respect to a specific Network or Plan participating in the CLAIMS ADJUDICATION Network, Provider may terminate participation in any Network or any Plan participating in the CLAIMS ADJUDICATION Network by giving PBM ten (10) days' prior written notice specifying the date of termination and the names of the Network(s) and Plan(s) in which Provider will no longer participate. Absent the prior written consent of PBM, Provider may not elect to participate in a Network or Plan that is part of the CLAIMS ADJUDICATION Network for thirty (30) days following Provider's termination of participation in such Network or Plan.

3.2   Reimbursement to Provider.

3.2.1   Plan Sponsor Networks. Claims submitted for a Plan participating in a Plan Sponsor Network will be reimbursed at the lower of (i) AWP less the applicable Plan Sponsor AWP Discount plus the applicable Plan Sponsor Dispensing Fee less the applicable copayment, (ii) HCFA MAC plus the applicable Plan Sponsor Dispensing Fee less the applicable copayment, (iii) Ingredient Cost submitted by Provider plus the applicable Plan Sponsor Dispensing Fee less the applicable copayment or (iv) Usual and Customary Price less the applicable copayment. The "Plan Sponsor AWP Discount" shall mean the AWP percentage discount that (i) with respect to Plan Sponsor Networks established after the date of this Agreement, is set forth in this Agreement, an addendum hereto, the Enrollment Form or any subsequent enrollment form, each as may be amended from time to time, or (ii) with respect to Plan Sponsor Networks that were established prior to this Agreement, is set forth in the applicable Prior Agreement. A Plan Sponsor AWP Discount contained in a Prior Agreement may hereafter be amended as provided for in Section 1.3. The "Plan Sponsor Dispensing Fee" shall mean the dispensing fee that (i) with respect to Plan Sponsor Networks established after the date of this Agreement, is set forth in this Agreement, an addendum hereto, the Enrollment Form or any subsequent enrollment form, each as may be amended from time to time.

3.2.2   Non-CLAIMS ADJUDICATION Submissions. Claims submitted by means other than CLAIMS ADJUDICATION System will be reimbursed in accordance with the applicable reimbursement methodology provided for above. Provider acknowledges that claims that are not adjudicated through the CLAIMS ADJUDICATION System and verified as a Covered Item may not be reimbursed by PBM on behalf of one of its Plan Sponsors due to the non-payable nature of the claim (e.g., the individual is not an Eligible Person or the dispensed item is not a Covered Item).

3.3   Timing of Reimbursement: Reports. PBM will process Provider's claims and pay Provider in accordance with PBM's current schedule of processing and payment and will provide Provider with a report showing the record of all claims submitted, processed, and paid in each processing cycle.

4.   Responsibilities and Rights of PBM.

4.1   Inspection Rights: Discrepant Claims. PBM may inspect all records of Provider relating to this Agreement including, but not limited to, original signed Prescriber's orders, telephoned Prescriber's orders, signature logs, computer records, and invoices showing purchase or receipt of Covered Items. PBM may also inspect such other documents and items that reasonably relate to Provider's compliance with the PBM Documents.

4.2   Help Desk. To assist in resolving Provider's questions or issues, the PBM Pharmacy Help Desk will provide access to Provider to both its Voice Response System and PBM representatives. The PBM Pharmacy Help Desk will use its reasonable efforts to assist Provider while the Eligible Person is still at Provider. During PBM's normal business hours, a licensed pharmacist will be available to answer questions beyond the scope of the PBM Pharmacy Help Desk representatives' knowledge; provided, however, such licensed pharmacist will not provide any professional advice with respect to the provision of Pharmacy Services.

5.   Intellectual Property Rights; Confidentiality.

5.1 Advertising and Trademarks. PBM retains exclusive rights to, among others, the names "PBM," "CLAIMS ADJUDICATION," "DRUG UTILIZATION REVIEW," together with any distinctive trademarks and service marks that have been used by PBM or may be adopted or used by PBM in the future. Provider may not advertise or use any name, symbol, or trademark of PBM in any advertising other than as specifically permitted in the PBM Documents without the prior written consent of PBM. PBM may (i) use the name and address(es) of Provider in the Provider Directory, informational brochures or other publications provided to Plan Sponsors and Eligible Persons, (ii) use information regarding Provider's services that is provided to PBM by Provider in publications provided to Plan Sponsors and Eligible Persons, and (iii) provide Plan Sponsors with Provider's credentialing information.

5.2 Confidentiality. Any information or data supplied by PBM or Plan Sponsor to Provider under this Agreement, including, without limitation, HCFA MAC list or any proprietary MAC list used on behalf of a Plan Sponsor, must be maintained in confidence and may not be sold, assigned, transferred, or given to any third party. This information may be disclosed to employees, agents, or contractors of Provider only to the extent necessary for them to perform their duties and then only if they have undertaken like obligations of confidentiality. No information or data supplied by PBM to Provider may be quoted or attributed to Provider or PBM without the prior written consent of PBM. PBM and Provider must use all necessary security procedures sufficient to ensure that all data transmissions are authorized and to protect their business records and data from improper access.

SCHEDULE OF TERMS

AWP or Average Wholesale Price means the current wholesale cost of a given drug as defined in the latest edition of the First DataBank Blue Book (with supplements) or any other similar nationally recognized reference that PBM may reasonably select from time to time.

CLAIMS ADJUDICATION Network means a network of providers that have contracted with PBM to provide Pharmacy Services to Eligible Persons of certain Plans, which Pharmacy Services are reimbursed by the Plan Sponsor.

CLAIMS ADJUDICATION System means PBM's proprietary remote electronic claim adjudication process system that provides Provider with, among other things, eligibility and drug pricing information.

Copayment means the amount an Eligible Person must pay to Provider at the time a Covered item is dispensed as indicated by the CLAIMS ADJUDICATION System.

Covered Item means any drug or device covered, in whole or in part, in accordance with and subject to the terms of a Plan covering an Eligible Person.

DRUG UTILIZATION REVIEW means PBM's automated, non-discretionary drug utilization review system designed to provide to the Provider at the time of dispensing, certain information in the CLAIMS ADJUDICATION System that may help manage the costs of prescription drug programs and improve the quality of drug therapy provided to patients.

Eligible Person means a person entitled to a Covered Item pursuant to a Plan.

HCFA MAC or Maximum Allowable Cost means the maximum allowable cost of a drug pursuant to a Plan's list that establishes an upper limit reimbursement price for certain multiple-source drugs dispensed under the Plan without regard to the specific manufacturer whose drug is dispensed.

NCPDP means the National Council for Prescription Drug Programs.

Network means the Plan Sponsor pharmacy provider Network and the CLAIMS ADJUDICATION Network.

PBM Manual means the manual containing claims processing and program guidelines provided by PBM to Provider, as amended from time to time at PBM's sole discretion.

Pharmacy Services means all services usually and customarily rendered by a provider licensed to provide pharmacy services in the normal course of business, including services mandated by applicable Law.

Plan means that portion of Plan Sponsor's drug benefit plan that relates to Covered Items with respect to a group of Eligible Persons.

Plan Sponsor means the entity that contracts with a PBM for prescription benefit management services, which entity could be, among other things, an insurance company, self-insured group, health maintenance organization, preferred provider organization, multi-employer trust, or third party administrator.

Prescriber means a person who is licensed to prescribe drugs in accordance with applicable Law.

Usual and Customary Price means the lowest price the Provider would charge to a particular customer if such customer were paying cash for an identical prescription on that particular day. This price must include any applicable discounts offered to attract customers.
Additional Required Attachments and Information

- Drug Enforcement Administration (DEA) Number
- Federal Tax Identification Number
- State Board of Pharmacy License Number
- State Medicaid Number
- Liability Insurer
- Liability Insurer Policy Number

Copies of DEA Certificate, State License Certificate, and Liability Policy.

Appendix

5-2

ACRONYMS

AWP	average wholesale price (drug)
CMS	Centers for Medicare and Medicare Services
DAW	dispense-as-written
DUE	drug use evaluation
DUR	drug utilization review
GIS	geographic information systems
HIPAA	Health Insurance Portability and Accountability Act
HMOs	health maintenance organizations
MAC	maximum allowable cost
MCOs	managed care organizations
OBRA '90	Omnibus Budget Reconciliation Act of 1990
PBMs	pharmacy benefit managers, pharmacy benefit management (companies)
POS	point-of-service (pharmacy)
PPOs	preferred provider organizations
PSAO	Pharmacy Service Administrative Organization
R/A	remittance advice
Rx	prescription (drug)
U&C	usual and customary (retail price)

SPECIALTY PHARMACEUTICALS

KJEL A. JOHNSON
JOAN M. SIEGEL

INTRODUCTION

Although specialty pharmaceuticals are used in a relatively small portion of managed care lives, they represent the single most explosive segment of the prescription drug benefit in terms of growth and cost. Spending on specialty drugs grew by 20.4% in 2004, a rate 3.5 times that of the overall market (with 5.6% growth).[1] Four years later, this trend continued, with specialty pharmaceuticals accounting for more than 20% of the total pharmaceutical spend at $56.2 billion in 2006, which is a 16% increase from 2005.[2]

As such, these products have emerged as the largest category driving drug trends, contributing more to spending growth than lipid-lowering and diabetes drugs combined.

IMPORTANCE OF SPECIALTY PHARMACEUTICALS

The cost of specialty pharmaceuticals is high, and so is the level of care required by the patients that use such medicines. Many of these products provide sophisticated therapy for patients with rare or chronic conditions demonstrating significant morbidity and mortality. Specialty pharmaceutical products typically share several characteristics, including, but not limited to, the following:

- A chronic disease target, such as multiple sclerosis (MS), hepatitis C, cancer, hemophilia, pulmonary arterial hypertension, etc.
- A high cost; prescriptions average $1,200 to $1,500 per month
- Special handling requirements, such as refrigeration
- Reimbursement complexities, including the manner in which reimbursement is directed

- Clinical support essential to the effective outcome of the treatment regimen
- Customized dosing, including weight-based dosing and compounding
- Quantities typically supporting a small patient population
- Complex delivery methods that are primarily subcutaneous injection, intramuscular injection, and intravenous infusion; however, an increased amount of oral products are moving into the specialty channel by virtue of the above listed characteristics

One of the most significant challenges presented by specialty pharmaceuticals lies in the reimbursement for these products, because they can frequently be paid through either the medical or pharmacy benefit. This distinction can also be used to *define* specialty pharmaceuticals, where many characteristics may be used to determine what should and should not be considered a specialty product, beginning with the product's distribution channel. Specialty pharmaceuticals can be either provider-administered or self-administered; however, neither of these channels of administration determines the distinction of "specialty pharmaceutical." For example, oncology injectables and vaccines are both administered by the provider and paid through the medical benefit, but of these two, only oncology injectables are considered specialty pharmaceuticals. Conversely, rheumatology injectables and insulin are both self-administered and paid through the pharmacy benefit, but of these two, only rheumatology injectables get the specialty pharmaceutical distinction. While most provider-administered injectables are paid through the medical benefit and most self-administered injectables are paid through the pharmacy benefit, there are some exceptions to this rule in both directions. For example, intravenous immunoglobulin (IVIG) and luteinizing hormone-releasing hormone (LHRH) agonists are provider-administered products that may be paid through either the medical benefit or pharmacy benefit. For further elucidation of this matter refer to **Table 6-1**.

As mentioned earlier, other challenges in the management of specialty pharmaceuticals include the special handling and clinical support requirements of these products. Many specialty pharmaceuticals have a short shelf life, often requiring refrigeration and overnight delivery. In addition, these products commonly feature a high incidence of adverse events and compliance issues, along with complex dosing requirements, necessitating relatively intensive clinical intervention and guidance.

These cumulative characteristics of specialty pharmaceuticals present obvious challenges for traditional distributors and community-based retail pharmacies. As a means to more effectively manage these products, specialty distributors and specialty pharmacies were born.

EVOLUTION OF SPECIALTY PROVIDERS

In the 1970s, the healthcare landscape was dominated by the hospital. In addition to serving as the overall center of care, the hospital was likewise the center of care for both acute and chronic conditions that required an advanced level of clinical support for both

TABLE 6-1   Common Inclusions and Exclusions of Specialty Drugs

Definition	Provider Administered (Medical Benefit)	Self Administered (Pharmacy Benefit)
Included	Oncology	Rheumatology
	Oncology support	Factor
	Rheumatology	MS
	IVIG	Growth Hormones (hGH)
	LHRH Agonists	Hepatitis
		Anti-coagulants
		Infertility
		Oral chemotherapy
		Hemophilia factor
Excluded	Vaccines	Insulin
	Hydration	Bee sting kits
	Other low-cost or low use infusions	Glucagons
	Depo-Provera	

injections and infusions. In the 1980s, alternate sites for healthcare treatment emerged. In this era of significant change, injections and infusions could now be administered in the physician's office or clinic or at home (when appropriate) through the emergence of home healthcare nursing. These alternate administration sites were a welcomed change, because they were considerably more cost-efficient than the previous facility-based drug administration.

The early 1990s brought the advent of a select group of wholesale distributors, called *specialty distributors*. These distributors offered a streamlined and cost-effective process for ordering the small quantities of specialty pharmaceutical products necessary to successfully service chronically ill patients in office, clinic, and home healthcare settings. By the late 1990s, these specialty distributors had become a significant service provider for an evolving market.

During this emergence of specialty distributors, specialty pharmacies began offering an enhanced retail offering to patients who were now learning to self-inject at home in support of both a lower cost of care and better quality of life. Similar to the rapid growth of specialty distributors, by the late 1990s such specialty pharmacies were quickly expanding in number and breadth of services as new biotech products began to surface in support of a better quality of life and patient care for certain complex disease states.

With an increasing number of players entering the specialty pharmaceutical market, widespread consolidation had become the next logical step during the early 2000's.

Pharmacy benefits managers (PBMs) in particular were strongly positioned to compete in this market consolidation because virtually all of their assets were capable of being leveraged for specialty pharmacy. Specifically, PBMs possess an established membership base, mail-order capabilities, relationships with payors and manufacturers, historical data, and data analysis capabilities, all of which make these organizations prime for involvement in the specialty market. As such, a wave of specialty pharmacy acquisitions by PBMs has taken place since the late 1990s. Of note were specialty pharmacy management and distribution service leaders, Priority Healthcare and Accredo Health, which subsequently were acquired by PBMs such as Express Scripts and Medco as the concentration of efforts in this market segment intensified through the mid-2000s (**Figure 6-1**).[3] These acquisitions, in turn, led the transformation of these PBM mail order services into specialty focused distribution programs.

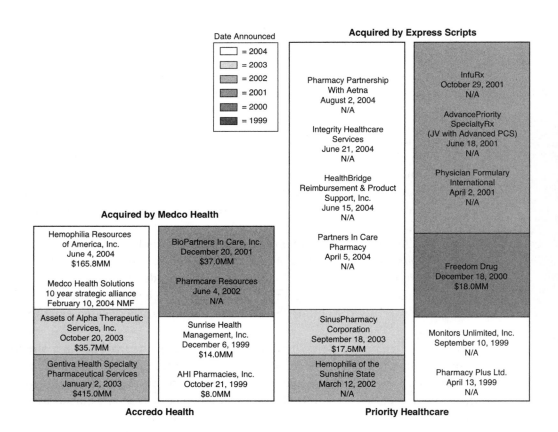

FIGURE 6-1   Acquisition History of Large Pharmacy Benefit Manager-Owned Specialty Pharmacies.

Source: Priority Healthcare and Accredo Health Companys' reports, 1999–2004.

CURRENT SPECIALTY PHARMACEUTICAL MARKET

A relatively small number of therapeutic areas drive the current specialty pharmaceutical market. Cancer leads these areas, contributing $25.3 billion to the $56.2 billion total spent on specialty pharmaceuticals in 2006.[2] The high cost of oncology within the specialty segment can be attributed to a number of factors, including the prevalence of cancer compared with other disease states and the elevated cost of therapy for patients with cancer (**Table 6-2**).[4] Other key therapeutic areas contributing to the total specialty pharmaceutical spend include renal, HIV/AIDS, rheumatoid arthritis (RA), multiple sclerosis (MS), hemophilia, transplant, hepatitis C, growth hormone, and respiratory syncytial virus (RSV) prophylaxis.[2]

Because specialty pharmaceuticals can be purchased under either the medical or pharmacy benefit, the contribution of these different therapeutic areas to the spend under the different benefits may vary greatly according to the most common distribution channel for agents in each area at a given managed care plan. For example, while oncology products account for nearly half of the overall (medical + pharmacy benefit) spend for specialty pharmaceuticals, this class only contributes 15.5% to the spend under the pharmacy benefit alone.[1] This is the result of the majority of cancer therapies being provider-administered and billed under the medical benefit. In fact, for some plan sponsors, up to 70% of specialty pharmaceutical spending may be billed under the medical benefit.[1]

As mentioned previously, spending on specialty pharmaceuticals is growing at an accelerated rate compared with the overall market. Estimates predict this trend will continue well into the foreseeable future, with specialty injectable drug sales expected to reach $73 billion in 2008, which is 26% of total prescription sales.[5] Chemotherapy will remain

TABLE 6-2 Prevalence, Cost per Therapy, and Estimated Drug Costs per 1M Lives

Disease State	Prevalence (per 1M lives)	Average Annual Cost Per Therapy Per Patient	Estimated Annual Drug Costs 1M lives
Oncology	1700	$25,000	$42,850,000
Rheumatoid Arthritis	1500	$10,000	$15,000,000
Hepatitis C	250	$15,600	$3,900,000
Multiple Sclerosis	980	$11,000	$10,700,000
Hemophilia	80	$80,000	$6,400,000
Respiratory Syncytial Virus (RSV)	800	$4,000	$3,200,000
Growth Hormone	80	$15,000	$1,250,000
Total	5390 (0.5%)		

Source: The Pharmacy Group, 2004.

a cost driver for the specialty segment, with an increasing number of novel, high-priced oral agents adding to the base of existing oral and injectable chemotherapy agents. Despite the traditionally modest impact of specialty chemotherapy on the pharmacy benefit, these newer oral chemotherapies carry elevated costs that have already impacted spending in this segment, where they are typically purchased. In fact, newer oral chemotherapies can be credited for cancer leading all therapeutic classes contributing to the specialty drug trend under the pharmacy benefit, accounting 30.6% of the total increase in plan costs (**Figure 6-2**).[1]

In addition to the recent introduction of costly oral chemotherapy agents, oncology will likely continue as a key cost driver in the specialty segment due to the breadth of the injectable chemotherapy pipeline. Oncology dominates the specialty pipeline, with more than four times the number of agents in development than any other therapeutic area.[6] As the late-stage pipeline matures and new oncology products are approved, cancer therapy will likely contribute to the specialty pharmaceutical spend more significantly than ever before.

Beyond the therapeutic areas of the products, the chosen distribution channels of specialty pharmaceuticals also may have a significant impact on costs in the current market, specifically for payors. As previously discussed, specialty pharmaceuticals reach the patient

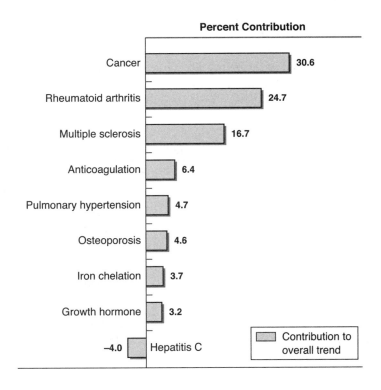

FIGURE 6-2 Top Therapeutic Classes Contributing to Specialty Drug Trend Under the Pharmacy Benefit.

via numerous distribution channels: specialty pharmacies, home health care, outpatient facilities, and physicians. Self-administered products delivered through the specialty pharmacy or home health care channels currently feature the lowest allowed dollars per-member-per-month (PMPM).[7] While all other distribution channels have demonstrated increasing allowed dollars PMPM since 2002, this statistic actually has been declining for specialty products delivered via the home health care distribution channel since 2004.[7] Conversely, provider-administered specialty products delivered via the physician and outpatient distribution channels have featured steadily increasing allowed dollars PMPM since 2004.[7] The physician distribution channel has demonstrated the most dramatic increase in allowed dollars PMPM, and is currently the largest contributor to the total allowed dollars PMPM for specialty products (**Figure 6-3**).[7]

A spend model of specialty drug spend for a 1 million life commercial payor by benefit and distribution channel serves to further elucidate the breakdown of costs in the current managed care environment (**Figure 6-4**).[8] For a plan with $205M in total specialty pharmaceutical spend, approximately $170M is allocated to specialty drug costs with $35M in administration costs.[8] These administration costs are paid under the medical benefit for provider-administered injectables, with $88M and $28M of the specialty drug spend allocated to provider- and facility-administered agents, respectively.[8] Breaking down the $88M of provider-administrated drug spend further, approximately $77M is office-administered, with the remaining $11M being administered in the home healthcare setting.[8] Approximately one-third ($54M) of the plan's annual specialty drug spend goes to self-administered drugs paid under the pharmacy benefit, with $17M in retail claims and $37M (~20% of the total specialty drugs spend) in specialty pharmacy purchases.[8]

Using this example, it becomes apparent that high specialty drug and administration costs in the current market are key in driving the medical cost ratio (MCR) toward

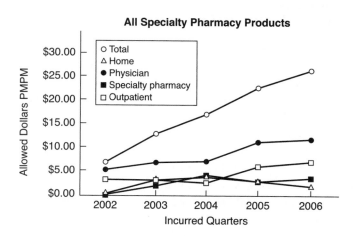

FIGURE 6-3 Impact of Specialty Drug Distribution Channels on Commercial Payor PMPM.
Source: ICORE Healthcare, 2008.

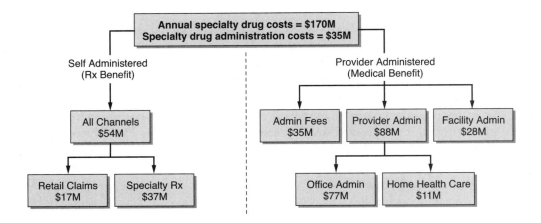

FIGURE 6-4 Estimated Specialty Drug Spend by Benefit and Distribution Channel.
Source: ICORE Healthcare estimates, 2008.

undesirable levels. Because nearly $200M in specialty products is spent annually across this example, these products represent approximately 10% of total medical and pharmacy costs combined. Because the annual specialty trend is more than 20%, one can see that a 2% annual increase in MCR is due to specialty products alone. From this realistic estimation, it is easy to see the difficulty in maintaining profitability of an at-risk payor given today's specialty pharmaceutical market.

SPECIALTY PHARMACY PROVIDERS

At the center of any discussion of specialty pharmaceuticals are the specialty providers: the distributors and pharmacies. At first glance, specialty providers may be seen as "middlemen"; however, these providers serve a critical step in the delivery of specialty pharmaceuticals to those with a medical need for such products. Specialty distributors offer a simplified and affordable means for acquiring the small quantities of specialty pharmaceuticals needed for managing patients in personalized settings. Similar to their retail pharmacy counterparts, specialty pharmacies offer direct patient services for those planmembers able to self-administer their specialty therapies.

Specialty pharmacies deal with both manufacturers and purchasers via three main specialty distribution models (**Table 6-3**). These models are designed and implemented based on a myriad of factors centered on the type of specialty pharmaceutical being distributed. Open or "traditional" distribution is ideal for both branded and multisource oral/solid products or for injectables that are administered in hospital or outpatient facilities. As their name implies, these distribution models offer the path of least resistance for purchasers,

TABLE 6-3   Types and Examples of Specialty Pharmacy Wholesale Drug Distribution Models

Metric	Open "Traditional" Distribution	Limited "Controlled" Distribution	Closed "Exclusive" Distribution
Best suited for	Branded and multi-source oral/solid products. Injectables if administered in hospital or outpatient facilities.	Branded and multi-source products. Primarily used for physician administered high cost injectables with limited sites of care.	High profile, branded products only that have unique attributes including but not limited to administration, shelf life, cost, or availability.
Product examples	Neulasta, Rituxan	Lucentis, Synagis	Iressa, Actimune
Physician relationship	Owned by the distributor and managed by distributor's customer service. Manufacturer must drive sales.	Owned by the distributor and managed by distributor's customer service. Manufacturer must drive sales.	Owned by manufacturer. Distributor acts as an agent for the manufacturer. Joint promotion with manufacturer and distributor.
Customer experience control	Limited	Limited	Enhanced
Pricing control	Limited to established WAC and direct contracting with providers.	Enhanced control based upon limited product access. Easier to dictate terms to distributors based upon desirability of distribution rights.	Absolute control. Exclusivity allows for establishing firm pricing parameters.
Promotional control	Limited. Distributors are typically brand neutral.	Enhanced control based upon limited product access and desirability of limited distribution rights.	Absolute control. Distributor acts as agent for manufacturer. Manufacturer dictates distribution policies and procedures.
Data capture	Typically restricted to distributor level data only. Limited visibility once product leaves distribution facility.	Enhanced data capture based upon limited product access and desirability of distribution franchise. Manufacturer can require capture and reporting of physician level data. Important for managing uptake and directing sales efforts at product launch.	Absolute control. Distributor acts as agent for manufacturer. Manufacturer dictates distribution policies and procedures. Important for managing uptake and directing sales resources for product launch.

(continues)

TABLE 6-3 (continued)

Hassle factor for purchasers	Path of least resistance. Product widely available from most sources. No impact on purchasing process for physician.	Path of limited resistance. Product available from multiple sources, but not all sources. Some physicians will need to alter purchasing processes to obtain product.	Often creates supply channel challenges, as product only available from a single source. Likely requires physician to alter purchasing processes. Creates barrier to purchasing.

Source: Courtesy of A. Gellman, 2008.

with products widely available from most sources and no impact on the purchasing process for the physician. Limited or "controlled" distribution is again ideal for both branded and multisource products but is primarily employed for physician-administered, high-cost injectables with limited sites of care. Limited distribution models are characterized by modest resistance for purchasers, with products available from multiple, but not all, sources. In addition, some physicians will need to alter their purchasing processes to obtain products in these distribution models. However, these distribution models offer enhanced control over pricing and enhanced data capture capabilities. For high-profile, branded products that have unique characteristics, such as complex administration, limited shelf-life, an extraordinarily high cost, or extremely limited availability, closed or "exclusive" distribution models are best suited. While these models offer absolute control over pricing through exclusivity and absolute control over data capture, these positive attributes come at a cost to purchasers. Closed distribution models often create supply chain challenges, as the products are only available from a single or very few sources, and likely necessitate physicians and payors to alter their purchasing and contracting processes, creating a barrier to purchasing.

Specialty pharmacies likewise use varying strategies, but these providers determine their strategies by focusing on different types of customers in managed care. This strategic focus may be directed towards manufacturers, payors, or physicians. Focusing on these three different key groups of stakeholders results in varying characteristics for the specialty pharmacies in terms of product portfolios and marketing direction. Manufacturer-focused specialty pharmacies serve as a "contract pharmacy" for certain drug manufacturers and, as a result, have a narrow product portfolio. These pharmacies work to create product preference among physicians on behalf of the manufacturers they represent. Payor-focused specialty pharmacies serve as an injectable-drug management carve-out for managed care organizations (MCOs) and therefore have a much broader product portfolio. These pharmacies work to create preferences of formulary products among contracted payors. By building relationships with high-volume prescribers, physician-focused specialty pharmacies strive to gain distribution business. These pharmacies also have a broad product portfolio and work to gain specialty drug dispense referrals as well as provide physicians with buy-and-bill drugs. The strategic focus of key specialty pharmacies is illustrated in **Figure 6-5**.

Regardless of strategic focus, today specialty pharmacies represent a significant portion of specialty product sales. In 2006, specialty pharmacies accounted for $33B in sales.[9] Among the leaders in specialty prescription dispensing were the specialty pharmacy operations of Caremark, Medco, and Express Scripts, holding 16%, 11%, and 8% of the total market, respectively.[8]

In addition to independent pharmacies in the specialty market, some large payors have chosen to invest in their own "in-house" specialty pharmacies to streamline the acquisition of services and control costs. Examples of these payor-owned specialty pharmacies include WellPoint's PrecisionRx Specialty Solutions, Aetna's Aetna Specialty Pharmacy, and CIGNA's Tel-Drug Specialty Pharmacy. A consortium of Blue Cross Blue Shield plans own Prime Therapeutics as a joint venture, and this company in turn owns and manages a specialty pharmacy.[9] The number of lives that payors have needed before pursuing this in-house specialty pharmacy strategy is typically 10 million or more: Wellpoint has approximately 35 million members; Aetna, approximately 15 million: CIGNA, approximately 11 million: and the partners of the Prime Therapeutics joint venture, collectively about 16 million.[9]

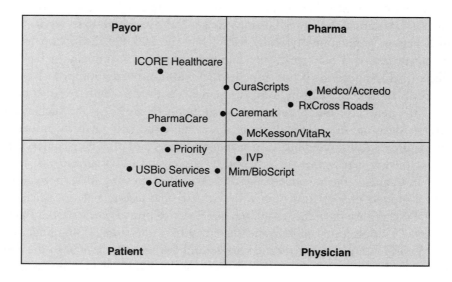

FIGURE 6-5   Strategic Focus of Key Specialty Pharmacies.

Source: Adapted from PBMI *Prescription Drug Benefit Cost and Plan Design Report, 2007.* Available at http://www.pbmi.com/2007report/pdfs/2007_Cost_and_Plan_Design_Report.pdf. Accessed 4 June 2008.

SELF-ADMINISTERED SPECIALTY PHARMACEUTICAL PRODUCTS

GOALS OF A SPECIALTY PHARMACY

Goals of the specialty pharmacy are primarily threefold: help manage and contain cost, provide dispensing accuracy, and support all clinical and special handling of the products in the channel. Achieving these goals requires a number of interventions, which specialty pharmacies specialize in executing.

Purchasing Options To help manage and contain the costs of specialty products, specialty pharmacies access the products through direct contracts with manufacturers, utilization of group purchasing organizations (GPOs), or utilization of both general and specialty wholesalers.

Direct contracts with manufacturers serve to secure pricing and may be necessary for volume pricing of agents in limited supply, such as hemophilia and IVIG products, due to manufacturer production challenges. In these cases, the grams in which the products are provided may have allocation requirements to assure the medications are available when needed by the end user. The allocations in some cases are tiered to help manage the high cost of producing or acquiring certain short-market, plasma-derived medications.

Orphan and "Mini-Bulk" Quantity Drugs In addition, direct manufacturer contracts may be necessary for products that are provided in what is referred to as a *limited drug distribution (LDD)* channel. LDD medications are generally very high-cost, service an extremely small patient population (typically well below the 200,000 distinction used to define orphan drugs), and may treat only hundreds of patients annually or have severe side effects (including death) if not dispensed and administered appropriately. Natalizumab (Tysabri), an infused agent indicated for patients with MS who have failed or not experienced the benefit of more traditional or common therapies, is one such example of an LDD medication. In order to dispense this agent, a specialty pharmacy must meet rigorous requirements for handling, dispensing, reporting, and providing clinical support. The goal of quality management is achieved by dispensing LDD agreements, as each pharmacy in the network must document and show the following: that they can provide the clinical support of specialists trained in the particular disease state in which the medication falls; that they have the technology necessary to provide the data the FDA has mandated the manufacturer collect; and that they have the storage, shipping, and tracking capabilities to ensure the medication arrives in both a timely fashion to the end user and at the temperature to which the medication must be maintained to meet stability requirements for use.

The use of GPOs and/or wholesalers may help manage acquisition costs for a specialty pharmacy when the GPOs and/or wholesalers can buy these high-cost products in "mini-bulk" quantities from the manufacturer. These "mini-bulk" quantities are greater than what the specialty pharmacy requires but are priced lower, allowing the specialty pharmacy to take advantage of the overall lower acquisition cost of the medications without purchasing unnecessary amounts.

MANAGING SELF-ADMINISTERED SPECIALTY PHARMACEUTICAL SAVINGS DRIVERS THROUGH A SPECIALTY PHARMACY

Stakeholders have identified six key specialty drug cost savings drivers for managing these products through the specialty pharmacy. These include: preferred product positioning, benefit design optimization, distribution channel management, reimbursement optimization, medical management, and operational improvements (**Table 6-4**).

Product Positioning and Preference Preferred product positioning is essentially promoting the use of lower cost, equal or higher quality alternatives to specific high-cost therapies. Product preferencing programs for specialty pharmaceuticals are similar to those for traditional pharmacy products but are complicated to a greater degree by implementation barriers. In addition, bioequivalence, a key concept in product preferencing based upon drug concentration levels, is challenging to establish for many biotechnology drugs/specialty pharmaceuticals.

TABLE 6-4 Key Specialty Drug Cost Savings Drivers, Initiatives, Implementation Speed, and Savings Size

Savings Driver	Related Initiatives	Implementation Speed	Size of Savings
Preferred Product Positioning	Formulary and rebates, when market shares improve	Moderate	Large
Benefit Design Optimization	Optimize medical benefit	Slow	Large
	Optimize pharmacy benefit	Slow	Large
Distribution Channel Management	Develop and optimize a specialty pharmacy network	Slow	Moderate
	Eliminate costly site of service changes	Moderate	Moderate
Reimbursement Optimization	Optimize network fee schedules	Rapid	Large
	Improve fee schedule adoption rates	Moderate	Large
Improve Operations	Eliminate billing errors	Rapid	Small
	Eliminate clinically impossible	Rapid	Small
Medical Management	Establish prior authorization where appropriate	Rapid	Moderate
	Develop stepped-care programs	Rapid	Moderate

Product preferencing is facilitated by a relatively low number of providers in a geographical area who actually prescribe specialty products for a given therapeutic area; this is key because providers ultimately control prescribing. To insure success, these programs should be targeted at key therapeutic areas, specifically those with large cost therapies (**Table 6-5**). Furthermore, efficient product preferencing programs should be implemented in less than six months, should be designed and implemented in a way as to prevent provider backlash, and should demonstrate measured substantial savings as opposed to percentage savings. A list of preferencing initiatives to optimize a specialty product formulary can be found in **Table 6-6**.

Supply Strategies One issue that typically arises in the implementation of product preferencing programs is channel conflicts that result between PBM-owned and distributor-owned specialty pharmacies. For example, PBM-owned pharmacies that purchase specialty therapies from a manufacturer often are limited in their ability to preference or disadvantage these products because such initiatives will affect the contracts of oral products purchased from the same manufacturers. Therefore, little to no rebates may be available to the payors who comprise their specialty pharmacy customers. Because of these channel conflicts, many specialty pharmacies had not historically used product preferencing programs. One exception, ICORE Healthcare, was launched in 2003 to focus solely on optimizing the use of the lowest cost alternatives for specialty injectables by using a nationally consistent specialty drug formulary.

Although self-administered injectables commonly come from a specialty pharmacy, varying costs for payors exist depending on the specific distribution channel used. As such, payors need to manage these distribution channels to maximize savings and they

TABLE 6-5 Key Therapy Classes of Specialty Products that Lend Themselves to Preferencing Programs

Therapy Class	Available Products
Anti-Arthritics	Remicade, Enbrel, Humira, Orencia, Rituxan, Kineret,
Multiple Sclerosis	Rebif, Avonex, Betaseron, Copaxone, Tysabri
Hepatitis	Pegasys, Peg-Intron, Rebetron, Infergen
Anemia	Aranesp, Procrit
Infertility	Follistim AQ, Bravelle, Repronex/Menopur, Gonal-F, Ganirelix, Pregnyl
Hyaluronic Acids	Hyalgan, Supartz, Synvisc, Euflexxa, Orthovisc
LHRH Agonists	Eligard, Lupron, Trelstar, Zoladex
Growth Hormones	Norditropin, Nutropin, Humatrope, Protropin, Saizen, Tev-Tropin, Genotropin

can do so by adjusting reimbursement for the different channels. However, this strategy can work against the payor's favor if not carefully thought out. An example of this occurred when one payor aggressively reduced reimbursement for leuprolide (Lupron), an LHRH agonist, administered in the physicians' offices, which drove distribution towards the costly hospital channel and resulted in a higher cost per dose (**Table 6-7**).[6] While this was an unintended consequence, it demonstrates the ability for reimbursement levels to drive the prescribing physician's choice of distribution channel.

Streamlining Benefit Design Benefit design likewise can have a significant impact on cost in the specialty channel and is hence considered a key savings driver. Generally, self-injected specialty drugs paid under the medical benefit are 20% to 30% more expensive on average than those paid through the pharmacy benefit. A move for better cost management has been observed with the push to steer specialty products into the pharmacy benefit and

TABLE 6-6   List of Preferencing Initiatives to Optimize a Specialty Product Formulary

Savings Driver	Common Initiatives
Preferred Product Positioning	1. Formulary placement and copay differentials NDC block
	2. Field medical director training
	3. Field visits to high prescribers
	4. Plan branding of pharma collaterals
	5. Provider segmentation and outreach (calls, mailings, fax)
	6. Provider report cards
	7. Medical EOB messaging
	8. Pharma representative outreach
	9. Web postings and messaging
	10. Outbound calls to providers
	11. Newsletters to providers
	12. Member communication
	13. Broker group communication
	14. Provider services visits
	15. PA and case mgmt scripting
	16. Fax order form preferencing
	17. New Rx or member steerage
	18. Proactive communication with high prescribers who are likely to, but have not yet, written Rxs for plan
	19. Distributor sends preferencing materials to members
	20. Distributor representatives visit targeted providers

TABLE 6-7 Site of Service Changes Associated with Aggressive Reductions in Reimbursement for Physician Office Administration of a Provider-Administered LHRHa Drug

Provider Type	Baseline Costs*	New Costs*	Baseline Claims	2003 Claims	2004 Claims	2005 Claims
Ancillary	$599	$599	140	156	173	158
Hospital	$1,130	$1,130	84	216	427	646
Physician	$599	$180	1,346	1,105	778	518
Specialty Rx	$601	$585	-	43	154	221
Total Claims			1,570	1,520	1,532	1,543
Cost per three month period			$1,882	$1,108	$1,598	$2,036

Source: ICORE Healthcare, 2007.

also through the specialty pharmacy as part of the benefit design. As a result, more specialty drugs are moving under the pharmacy benefit, and traditional cost-control measures are being applied, such as bulk-purchasing, copayments, and closer scrutiny of use and outcomes. Significant benefit design improvements exist for self-injectable drugs used in RA and MS, as a substantial portion of these prescriptions continue to be dispensed through retail rather than specialty pharmacies, an issue that can readily be addressed by appropriate benefit structures.

Payors should consider utilizing the following when developing benefits that include specialty products[12]: a) member cost-sharing; b) tiered injectable benefit structure; c) biologics as medical benefit versus migration to pharmacy benefit or a "mandatory" injectable benefit; d) differential patient copayment or coinsurance based on type of products (e.g., life-saving drugs, drugs that alter disease course vs. lifestyle enhancement drugs); and e) a preferred drug list for injectables.

Ultimately, a balance between shifting higher cost to the patient, requiring employers or plan sponsors to use narrower networks to obtain medications, and tighter utilization controls is needed. This ensures that patients who need these high-cost, high-touch medications will have access at an affordable price and, in turn, reduce the relative cost of care associated with unchecked chronic disease.

Operations: Reducing Errors and Fraud Operational improvements drive savings in the specialty pharmaceutical segment by reducing avoidable financial sinks in the system. Reducing claim submission and payment errors and fraud are two operational improvements that can result in significant cost savings. Special Investigative Units (SIUs) can be used to identify and manage the 5% of specialty pharmacy claims that are estimated to be fraudulent, and proper coding practices can ensure fewer errors in payment. For self-administered injectables, all claims should be paid on National Drug Code (NDC) codes to avoid confusion and reduce errors.

PROVIDER-ADMINISTERED SPECIALTY PHARMACEUTICAL PRODUCTS

Provider-administered specialty injectables are currently trending at ~26%, with ~70% of costs being oncology related (i.e., for chemotherapy or chemotherapy support). The costs associated with administering these products represents an additional 30% of the actual drug costs for a total office-based provider spend of drug and drug administration of about $125M per million lives).[12] In addition to this, an incremental 20% to 25% of provider administered injectables are provided in facilities, making the contracting strategy for these products integral to the total hospital contracting process.

GOALS OF MANAGING PROVIDER-ADMINISTERED PRODUCTS

Similar to self-administered specialty injectables, the goals of management of provider-administered specialty products are threefold: improve the quality of care, reduce the cost of care, and measure the improvements in care.

Improve the Quality of Care Improving the quality of care begins with identifying and developing medical management opportunities to ensure the most appropriate drug therapy is used for a given plan member requiring an infusible specialty drug. This end is achieved by ensuring laboratory tests are used, when appropriate, to guide the drug selection process. Furthermore, maintaining a provider network density ensures that members have access to the best specialists in any given geographical region. Finally, improving the quality of care in managing provider-administered specialty injectables includes support during all stages of life; therefore, enlisting hospice care to provide comfort to members who are deemed terminal is part of the quality care continuum.

Effective Cost Management Reducing the cost of care in an area as traditionally costly as provider-administered specialty pharmaceuticals can be a significant task. As stated, cancer care drives spending in this area, with oncology drugs accounting for about two-thirds of total cancer care costs. Validating this being a leading cost-driver, oncology-related direct costs are dramatically rising and estimated to reach ~$100 billion by 2010.[13] Furthermore, plan members with cancer and other chronic conditions requiring provider-administered injectables feature low member attrition rates, meaning that payors who provide quality cancer care will reap the benefits in the years to come (**Figure 6-6**).[14]

Managing these costs begins with the providers themselves and the rationalization of reimbursement, or equitably paying physicians for their services and drugs that they have had to carry in inventory. Contrary to some misconceptions, payors and specialty pharmacies generally should strive to keep provider-administered injectables in the physician's office, with appropriate management, education, and surveillance reporting, because the acquisition cost of most provider-administered injectables is lowest for physicians at the time of this writing. However, to control costs, stakeholders should ensure that physicians

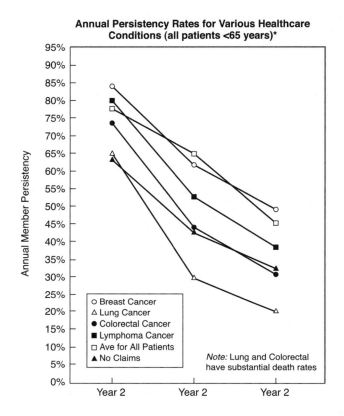

FIGURE 6-6   Members with Chronic Illnesses Requiring Provider-Administered Injectables Have Low Turnover Rates.
Source: Managed Care Oncology 2007; 4:7.

are compensated through reimbursement of all drugs, drug administration, and services. In the process, unnecessary costs such as overutilization or off-label use must be eliminated. For example, bevacizumab and erythropoietins are two specialty products that are commonly identified as use-management targets and are sometimes managed as such, on top of appropriate reimbursement strategies. Furthermore, costly chemotherapy agents are commonly administered to patients nearing end-of-life who are no longer benefiting from therapy: 20% die within 14 days and 43% die within 30 days of their last chemotherapy administration. Finally, identifying and resolving payment errors are crucial to reducing the cost of care for provider administered specialty injectables. With confusing units, doses and dosing ranges, and dosing schedules, payment errors are common among the provider administered specialty products, so it is difficult to pay and reimburse correctly.

In order to gauge progress, stakeholders must effectively measure improvements in care and cost management of these specialty pharmaceuticals. While this is an area where health plans are traditionally challenged, the complications of this market further cloud the issue. The Healthcare Common Procedure Coding System (HCPCS) language used for claims paid under the medical benefit is very broad in that it includes multiple NDC codes under a single HCPCS code, making provider-administered injectables difficult to code correctly, track, and measure. Of note is while the three "dump" codes (J3490, J3590, and J9999) used for miscellaneous therapies have been presented to payors as an enormous management opportunity, but do not yet have a specific HCPCS code, the reality is that less than 1% of costs lie in such HCPCS codes. This example illustrates the various misconceptions that exist in coding provider-administered injectables.

MANAGING PROVIDER-ADMINISTERED SPECIALTY PHARMACEUTICAL SAVINGS DRIVERS

The same six savings drivers used to manage the costs associated with self-administered specialty pharmaceuticals can be used to manage provider-administered product costs through a specialty pharmacy. To review, these are: product positioning, benefit design optimization, distribution channel management, reimbursement optimization, medical management, and operational improvements.

Product preferencing initiatives should be centered on therapies that represent a large portion of the drug costs and have more than one product per therapeutic area. For provider-administered injectables, product preferencing opportunities exist in RA and erythropoietin stimulating agents (ESAs), because they meet both of these criteria. Other areas include anti-emetic agents, LHRH agonists, and hyaluronic acids, which represent 3%, 1%, and 1% of the total provider-administered spend, respectively (**Table 6-8**).

In order to design successful product preferencing programs, payors must first have a well-defined review process, including a medical policy review committee that includes specialists who practice in the therapeutic areas of each preferencing program. In implementing the program, medical benefit controls, such as reimbursement, prior authorization (PA), medical benefit co-share tiers, and/or a well-defined provider communication process, should be put in place. Strong relationships between the payor and its providers are keys to the success of these programs. One challenge is that providers may stand to profit more from administering high-cost drugs with larger margins. In such cases, only compelling, clear-cut clinical evidence will serve to encourage providers to administer low-cost alternatives.

Current medical injectable benefit design includes: out-of-pocket maximums for 42% of members; co-shares and copays averaging 21% and $35, respectively; PA for 71% of medical benefits; and 15% of plans limiting specialty drug prescribing to relevant specialists only. Benefit design must be sold to employers/plan sponsors upon renewals, so strategic thinking is crucial. While effective, redesigning benefits can be a somewhat lengthy process, taking 12 to 18 months from conception to implementation (**Figure 6-7**).

TABLE 6-8 Twenty Provider-Administered Drugs Represent Nearly Two-Thirds of All Provider-Administered Injectable Costs

Drug	Type	Code	Percentage of Total
Remicade	Rheumatoid Arthritis	J1745	10%
Neulasta	Colony Stimulating Factors	J2505	9%
Aranesp	Erythropoietins	J0881	6%
Avastin	Chemotherapy	J9035	5%
Herceptin	Chemotherapy	J9355	4%
Rituxan	Chemotherapy	J9310	4%
Eloxatin	Chemotherapy	J9263	4%
Multi-Source	Hemophilia	J7192	4%
Procrit	Erythropoietins	J0885	3%
Xolair	Asthma	J2357	2%
Erbitux	Chemotherapy	J9055	2%
Gemzar	Chemotherapy	J9201	2%
Camptosar	Chemotherapy	J9206	1%
Sandostatin	Somatostatin	J2353	1%
Rocephin	Antibiotic	J0696	1%
Alimta	Chemotherapy	J9305	1%
Botox	Cosmetic	J0585	1%
Multi-Source	Hyaluronic Acids	J7317	1%
Neupogen	Colony Stimulating Factors	J1441	1%
Cerezyme	Gaucher's Disease	J1785	1%

Source: ICORE Healthcare, 2007.

The same distribution channel management principles hold true for provider-administered specialty pharmaceuticals as they do for self-administered specialty pharmaceuticals. As such, payors must closely manage the site of care in order to optimize savings. Provider-administered injectables can nearly double in price when administered in certain high-cost settings, such as hospitals, versus alternate settings, such as home health care (**Table 6-9**). Commonly, when payors reimburse based upon average sales price (ASP) rather than average wholesale price (AWP), physician office administration is less costly than specialty pharmacy distribution. This stresses the need for a cogent reimbursement approach, such that untoward effects in channel management do not occur. Ultimately, payors need measurement vigilance to detect where improvement opportunities exist and where unintended consequences may be manifested.

Generally, Medicare guides the reimbursement of provider-administered injectables. On January 1, 2005, Medicare moved from an AWP −15% reimbursement model to an

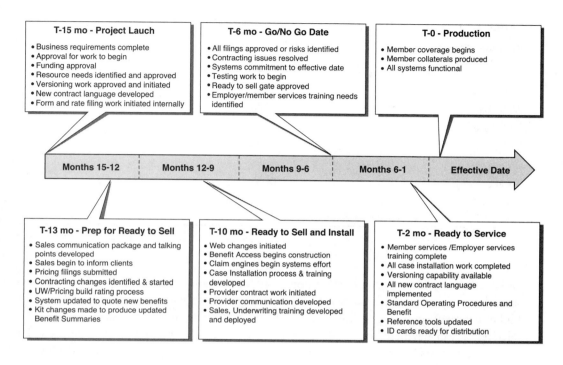

T-15 mo - Project Lauch

- Business requirements complete
- Approval for work to begin
- Funding approval
- Resource needs identified and approved
- Versioning work approved and initiated
- New contract language developed
- Form and rate filing work initiated internally

T-6 mo - Go/No Go Date

- All filings approved or risks identified
- Contracting issues resolved
- Systems commitment to effective date
- Testing work to begin
- Ready to sell gate approved
- Employer/member services training needs identified

T-0 - Production

- Member coverage begins
- Member collaterals produced
- All systems functional

| Months 15-12 | Months 12-9 | Months 9-6 | Months 6-1 | Effective Date |

T-13 mo - Prep for Ready to Sell

- Sales communication package and talking points developed
- Sales begin to inform clients
- Pricing filings submitted
- Contracting changes identified & started
- UW/Pricing build rating process
- System updated to quote new benefits
- Kit changes made to produce updated Benefit Summaries

T-10 mo - Ready to Sell and Install

- Web changes initiated
- Benefit Access begins construction
- Claim engines begin systems effort
- Case Installation process & training developed
- Provider contract work initiated
- Provider communication developed
- Sales, Underwriting training developed and deployed

T-2 mo - Ready to Service

- Member services /Employer services training complete
- All case installation work completed
- Versioning capability available
- All new contract language implemented
- Standard Operating Procedures and Benefit
- Reference tools updated
- ID cards ready for distribution

FIGURE 6-7 **Benefit Enhancements Implementation Timeline.**
Source: ICORE Healthcare, 2007.

ASP +6% approach; this was to address the large spread in office-based provider purchase price versus AWP-based reimbursement for certain drugs. Although physicians purchase provider-administered injectables at a lower cost than any other channel, this change in reimbursement model has led to a new challenge where perverse incentives exist for providers to use the highest cost medicine; a higher sales price translates into higher absolute income. This has had a significant impact on commercial payors, because approximately 17% of lives are ASP-reimbursed today (**Table 6-10**). Another strategy—

TABLE 6-9 **Avastin and Herceptin Cost per Channel for a Commercial Payor**

	Avastin	Herceptin
Place of Service	$ Paid/Unit	$ Paid/Unit
Home Healthcare	$57	$63
Hospital Outpatient	$128	$123
Physician Office	$58	$62
Specialty Pharmacy	$94	$121

Source: ICORE Healthcare, 2007.

TABLE 6-10 Reimbursement Models Employed by Commercial Payors

Reimbursement Model	% of US Commercial Payor Lives
ASP Based	17%
AWP Based	37%
VFS Based	34%
Risk	6%
Other	6%
Total	**100%**

Definitions: ASP = Average Sales Price; AWP = Average Wholesale Price; VFS = Variable Fee Schedule

Source: ICORE Healthcare Assessment of 921 U.S. Commercial Payors, 2007.

variable fee schedules—present an opportunity for providers to be appropriately compensated but help to manage costs for payors. In this reimbursement approach, there is a higher payment on therapeutically equivalent products with lower acquisition costs, and a relatively lower payment for the drugs with higher acquisition costs. By this way, payors can manage costs through the reimbursement of physicians by encouraging the use of lower cost, higher quality alternatives.

Medical management, or utilization management, serves several purposes. This savings driver optimizes the use of preferred products, mitigates inappropriate use, such as off-label use, and can optimize the use of preferred distribution channels. Different types of utilization management activities include PA, step therapy, case management, and disease management, which are described in greater detail in Chapters 2, 9, and others.

Perhaps the most popular of these provider-administered injectable management methods is PA; by example, more than 50% of plans have a PA for the provider-administered specialty injectable product infliximab (Remicade). Other widely employed PA programs include those for ESAs and for trastuzumab (Herceptin) for *HER-2*-positive breast cancer. For this drug, United Healthcare found that 12% of women receiving the specialty pharmaceutical were not tested for *HER-2*-gene expression or had inadequate levels of gene expression, rendering the drug potentially useless and in need of a PA intervention to improve the quality of care for these treated women.*

Step therapy is another utilization management technique enjoying widespread use. Examples of step therapy management include a required self-injectable trial and failure prior to authorized use of the provider-administered infliximab for RA; this intervention is used by 12% of health plans today. Another example, lapatinib (Tykerb) for breast cancer,

---

* *Source:* Personal communication. Kjel Johnson with Lee Newcomer, MD, of United Healthcare, January 14, 2008.

is sometimes authorized only when the payor's claim system finds a history of trastuzumab use in *HER-2*-positive women.

All payors employ case management in the form of a catastrophic care management program to make sure specialty drug uses are reasonable and cost effective for patients with complex chronic and terminal conditions. These types of utilization management programs are common in patients using *ultra-orphan drugs* such as Cerezyme (Imiglucerase), Fabrazyme (agalsidase beta), Aldurazyme (Laronidase), and others. In these programs, case managers coordinate the patients' care.

The use of IVIG presents a special case for utilization management programs since the agent is used "off-label" in more than 80% of cases. To properly manage the utilization of IVIG and drugs in a select few other classes, payors must assign an expert in provider-administered injectables to manage the use of these specialty products. For further discussion of utilization management, see Chapter 8.

One way to quickly reduce the costs associated with provider-administered specialty products is to address overpayments due to operational issues. These operational errors are most commonly found in the physician office channel, and it is common for a payor to reduce the costs of provider-administered injectables by ~1% by addressing these payment errors. One payor demonstrated a significant number of overpayments associated with the use of infliximab in their member population (**Figure 6-8**). In this histogram, the red box represents the plausible dosing range of the drug, with the blue dots to the right of this box indicating overpayments for doses that could not have been administered due to clinical dosing constraints; some have referred to the practice of implementing such payment limits as placing "Medically Unbelievable Edits." In implementing programs to correct operational errors, processes must be developed to pay units correctly and eliminate claims with units too high, as was the case in this example.

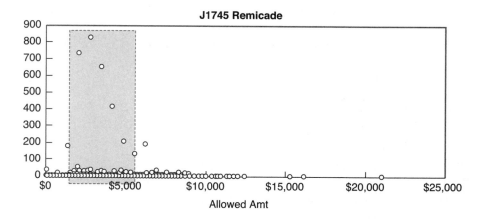

FIGURE 6-8 Significant Overpayments Occur Beyond the Clinically Possible Claim Costs of Certain Provider-Administered Specialty Products.
Source: ICORE Healthcare, 2008.

SPECIALTY PHARMACY OPERATIONS

An efficient way to discover the operational needs of specialty pharmacy for a payor customer is to review the request for proposal (RFP) requirements of a savvy health plan. Payors need specific information from a specialty pharmacy before contracting services from that specialty pharmacy. This information is provided in the form of an RFP featuring standard components such as company information and information on the pharmacy's clinical programs, specialty injectable drug distribution channels, customer service, eligibility, implementation, information system requirements, claims processing and administration, reporting, and formulary management and rebate programs (**Table 6-11**). In addition, the RFP features a cost summary so that the payor is aware of what the pharmacy will be charging (generally in AWP) for their specialty pharmaceutical products.

First, a payor needs information regarding the ownership of the specialty pharmacy. This information clearly outlines the specialty pharmacy's parent companies/owners, thereby demonstrating any potential conflicts of interest or channel conflicts that may be in play.

TABLE 6-11   Typical Payor Request for Proposal Requirements

1.	Company Background
1.1	Ownership Information
1.2	General Company Information
1.3	Liability and Insurance
1.4	Account Information
1.5	Customer References
2.	Clinical Programs
2.1	Drug Utilization Review
2.2	Prior Authorization
2.3	Disease Management
2.4	Other Programs
3.	Specialty Injectable Drug Distribution Channels
3.1	Mail Distribution
3.2	Other Distribution Channels
4	Customer Service
5	Eligibility Administration
6	Implementation
7	Information System Requirements
8	Claims Processing and Administration
9	Reporting
10	Formulary Management and Rebate Program
11	Cost Summary

Company information also provides payors with specifications regarding the overall size and general capacity of a specialty pharmacy. Usually, a payor will not give a specialty pharmacy prescription volumes that would initially represent more than a 25% increase in that specialty pharmacy's own volume; ultimately, the payor needs to know if the specialty pharmacy is capable of handling the volume of business they expect to direct to any pharmacy.

Payors also need to gather information regarding the clinical programs that a specialty pharmacy features before contracting the pharmacy's services. This section of the RFP provides information on the type of programs the pharmacy offers, such as step therapy, PA, pay-for-performance, etc., as well as data demonstrating the success of these programs.

In looking at the specialty injectable drug distribution channels of a specialty pharmacy, payors need information beyond simply the mail order channel. Payors want to know if a specialty pharmacy can provide them with home infusion assistance (e.g., nurses), facility assistance, etc. The customer service section of an RFP outlines the basic customer service oriented activities of a specialty pharmacy. A specialty pharmacy typically does not win new business because of this category, but can easily lose business because of this category if their customer service is lacking.

Contrary to the customer service category, the implementation, information system requirements, and claims processing and administration information provided by a specialty pharmacy *can* and do win them new business. These are the functional components of a specialty pharmacy and can differentiate one pharmacy over another as streamlining the lengthy contracting process can decrease the length of time before the first claim is processed. For more information on this process, see Chapter 7. Payors also look to the RFP for information regarding the reporting processes and capabilities of a specialty pharmacy. Whereas reporting was once relatively simple, with a basic operational report broken down by physician, drug class, setting, etc., it is now much more sophisticated and may be the deciding factor between a specialty pharmacy getting the contract or not getting the contract. Payors ideally want reports that show the adjudication cost of the claim: the drug cost after discounts, minus rebates, minus member contribution. This shows payors the actual drug cost that they will incur.

The most significant savings a specialty pharmacy can offer a payor come from optimizing the specialty formulary: promoting use of the lowest cost, highest quality therapy alternatives. Every RFP shows the cost-savings realized by taking a drug out of a retail pharmacy and moving it to a specialty pharmacy, but specialty pharmacies that can demonstrate effective optimization methods will inevitably win more payor business.

IMPLEMENTATION PROCESS OF A SPECIALTY PHARMACY AT A PAYOR

After a payor has reviewed the RFP provided by a particular specialty pharmacy and the specialty pharmacy has been chosen, implementation must take place before the relationship is operational.

There are several types of specialty pharmacy opportunities. A payor may contract with a PBM that owns a specialty pharmacy (e.g., with Express Scripts [a PBM] that owns CuraScript [a specialty pharmacy]). Conversely, a payor may contract directly with an independent specialty pharmacy (e.g., with BioScrip) and/or own an in-house specialty pharmacy (e.g., Aetna owns Aetna Specialty Pharmacy). Regardless of which of the aforementioned scenarios a specialty pharmacy represents, the set-up and implementation process for the use of a specialty pharmacy has a number of similarities.

First, the specialty pharmacy services must be "packaged" and sold as a benefit to a plan sponsor/employer. The dispensing and support services provided by a specialty pharmacy that are packaged as part of this benefit have been previously discussed in this chapter. Specialty pharmacy services may be sold as part of an overall health care benefit if the specialty pharmacy is owned by the health plan, sold as a pharmacy benefit if the specialty pharmacy is owned by a PBM, and/or sold as a carve-out or stand-alone benefit if the specialty pharmacy is independent.

Typically, a specialty pharmacy has both inside and outside sales associates who sell the specialty pharmacy services. The inside sales associates usually direct their sales efforts at physicians' offices utilizing specialty products to provide both written and verbal materials providing an overview of the services the specialty pharmacy has to offer. In addition, inside sales associates outline the value proposition for the physician when encouraging a move from a traditional buy-and-bill model to the use of a specialty pharmacy. Inside sales associates also may call on health plan members if the specialty pharmacy is owned by a plan to provide sales information on the services the specialty pharmacy can provide for the patient in need of specialty products. These sales calls may provide information to differentiate traditional retail pharmacy services from the "extra care" provided by a specialty pharmacy. A health plan that owns a specialty pharmacy may arm their sales associates calling on employers/plan sponsors with marketing and sales materials that describe the value proposition and support services the specialty pharmacy can provide their employees. These support services help the employees obtain access to high-cost medications in an easier and more cost-effective manner as well as promote a more positive health outcome. In addition, the value proposition supports enhanced cost-savings for the plan sponsor through lower overall health care dollar spend when their employees utilize the specialty pharmacy services to enhance compliance with their medication treatment regimen.

As mentioned previously, a payor may own a specialty pharmacy, choose to have a preferred specialty pharmacy, have a select number of specialty pharmacies in their network, or have a large number of specialty pharmacies, each of which has a unique disease state service offering. The current trend is either to limit the number of specialty pharmacies in the payor network or have a preferred or exclusive specialty pharmacy to better manage cost through tighter distribution controls.

Today's specialty pharmacy must feature technology as a primary platform to service the current market. The specialty pharmacy must be able to utilize technology for the following: data reporting and customization, integration of data and information, customized data collection, electronic medical records, e-prescribing opportunities, benefits verification, clinical intervention programs, compliance programs, billing, claims adjudication, shipping and tracking, call center capabilities, and Web site interactive opportunities. The broader the technology services and integration opportunities, the more value a specialty pharmacy may bring to the patient, physician, and plan sponsor/employer in providing usable data and knowledge for treatment best practices, reportable outcomes, and overall patient supportive care.

There are two primary periods for benefit plan changes and enrollment by employers/plan sponsors. The first is in January, with about 65% of the plan changes occurring here, and the second is in July with the majority of the remaining changes. A sparse number of changes may take place each month over the rest of the year, depending on the employers'/plan sponsors' fiscal years. Usually a sales cycle for a plan design or benefit opportunity may be anywhere from 12 to 24 months, depending on the size of the employer, the scope of plan design, the current benefit contract timeframe, and the available technology platforms and customization requirements for the plan sponsor/employer and/or health plan.

The contract itself may have a timeframe and implementation plan as part of the sale. Once a contract is signed, complete implementation can be consolidated down to as little as 30 days to 90 days, depending on the scope and customization of the services.

TYPICAL FLOW OF A SPECIALTY CLAIM

The process for a prescription to be received and processed by a specialty pharmacy may differ slightly dependent on the individual pharmacy provider. The following model process describes most of the core processing and dispensing activities of a typical specialty pharmacy provider:

1. A prescription/referral form is faxed into the specialty pharmacy by the physician or payor (Web-based or telephone prescriptions may be available also).
2. The prescription/referral is reviewed for completeness of information required to fill the prescription. This information may include the weight of the patient, the insurance carrier, the prescribing physician's signature, and other relevant information.
   a. If all the appropriate information is not included, a call to the prescribing physician may be necessary to complete the prescription/referral.
   b. If all the appropriate information is included and accurate, the prescription/referral will continue through the process.
3. Prior authorization requirements for the prescription are determined.
   a. If no PA is necessary, the prescription will be reviewed by a reimbursement team to determine the benefit verification (i.e., is the prescription covered under the

pharmacy or medical benefit?). The specialty pharmacy reimbursement team with then follow the payor guidelines as to where the benefit applies.

    b. If the drug requires PA, the specialty pharmacy reimbursement team will contact the payor to initiate the pre-certification. The specialty pharmacy team will contact the physician and patient to make them aware of the PA process initiation and communicate that a case or utilization management representative may contact the physician's office if any additional information is needed. If the specialty pharmacy is owned by the payor or contracted to perform these services on behalf of the payor, the specialty pharmacy may provide the PA on-site and/or the process will be streamlined as the records are available to the specialty pharmacy in an integrated fashion, avoiding the need for numerous phone calls back-and-forth to the payor.

4. If a PA is outstanding, the specialty pharmacy reimbursement team will check daily to see if the PA has been approved or denied and the team keeps in communication with the patient and/or physician to keep them abreast of the standing.

    a. Once approved, case management (or specialty pharmacy reimbursement if the pharmacy is payor-owned) will contact the specialty pharmacy reimbursement team, and this team in turn contacts the patient and/or physician to confirm a delivery date.

    b. If PA is denied, payor case management (or specialty pharmacy reimbursement if the pharmacy is payor-owned) will contact the physician regarding the denial and the appeal process. The specialty pharmacy reimbursement team will contact the patient to make them aware of the process.

5. An approved and verified prescription will continue through the process.

6. The prescription is adjudicated (processed).

7. The patient will be notified of any payment responsibility they may have and arrangements for their share will be handled, either by a credit card, referral to patient assistance program if financially necessary, or provided resources to help them obtain financial support from local avenues.

8. The patient is provided a nursing assessment to provide any product administration training he or she may need; this may include information on the disease state, answers to clinical questions within the scope of the nurse specialist, and/or triage to a pharmacist if there are drug-specific questions.

9. Delivery of the specialty product is arranged and verified.

10. The pharmacist provides up to four checks throughout the process to assure that the appropriate product, dose, and supplies for the patient are packed and shipped.

Obviously, this complex and varied multistep process requires the coordinated interaction of numerous parties, making integration and information technology crucial. Specialty pharmacies have evolved along with this process to provide safe, clinically effective, and cost-effective specialty therapies to patients. Today, efficient specialty pharmacy providers have automated or Web-enabled many of these steps.

FUTURE OF SPECIALTY PHARMACEUTICALS

In the late 1990s and early 21st century, specialty pharmacies were experiencing very large operating margins. During the last four to five years, there has been significant margin compression in the specialty market, as specialty providers attempt to capture increasing distribution market shares. This margin compression has a barricade to creativity and the extent to which specialty providers can invest in new quality and cost of care programs. As a result, large, PBM-owned specialty providers are moving away from non-benefit manager customers in an attempt to avoid this margin compression.

Whereas savings were once realized by moving the specialty drug distribution channel from retail to specialty providers, this opportunity has been ostensibly tapped; in the current market, only a small portion of the overall savings opportunity may be achieved by this measure. Now, providing quality care at the lowest cost is the only viable business for specialty pharmacies, although this is clearly easier to describe than to implement. Still, as the specialty market has evolved, specialty pharmacies have improved the quality of care through member drug compliance programs, appropriate use programs (e.g., step therapy), and duration of therapy programs. Health plans are realizing that squeezing another percentage point from the margin is not the answer to the cost-savings question. The real savings are now found by improving utilization rates of preferred products through formulary management and other internal controls, and by ensuring that the appropriate patient receives the right drug through the most efficient distribution channel for an adequate period of time.

While large payors have begun building their own specialty pharmacies, this process takes significant time and is only effective for plans with the largest member populations (>10 million lives). Building an in-house specialty pharmacy takes far longer than a year to complete, and several more years will likely pass before any savings are realized due to delays in realizing any operational efficiencies of a new pharmacy. Rather than building a specialty pharmacy from the ground up, large health plans looking to improve member care and save money in the specialty segment are best served by developing a relationship with an existing specialty provider, or by acquiring a fully operational specialty pharmacy that is available for purchase. Even so, the operational costs for a specialty pharmacy to support a single payor are 50% to 100% greater than costs the associated with contracting with an existing specialty provider, challenging the cost-saving benefit of this approach.

In the future, a broader view of costs will be adopted, as cost measures move from drug costs to total cost of care. While 40% of the costs in the specialty segment are spent on self-injected specialty pharmaceuticals, 60% is generally left unmanaged, as most specialty pharmacies and only some payors are involved in managing medical benefit injectables. From a wider perspective, in terms of total costs, payors will increasingly invest in specialty programs that have clearly demonstrated improvements in care, such as fewer hospitalizations and reduced rates of disease progression as well as management capabilities across all benefits. In order to stay competitive in this changing market, specialty pharmacies will need to play a part in patient care and demonstrate savings in *total* cost per patient, not merely in drug costs alone. In the process, risk agreements will need to be developed between payors, physicians, and specialty providers, and these arrangements will cover total cost of care. As a result, specialty pharmacies will become skilled in actuarial assessments.

Today, health plans do not generally have the infrastructure, time, and expertise to develop the types of intricate specialty programs necessary to manage total costs in this increasingly complex market segment. Providing the necessary components of effective specialty pharmaceutical management, specialty pharmacies have not yet demonstrated all of the ways that they can improve care or save costs. The future is bright for specialty providers and payors who are able to accomplish and measure these results.

Acknowledgment
The authors recognize and appreciate the content contributions of Andrew Gellman, Chief Operating Officer, ICORE Healthcare. The opinions expressed in this chapter are those of the author and do not necessarily reflect those of ICORE Healthcare, LLC, or its affiliates.

REFERENCES

1. Medco Drug Trend Report 2005. Available at http://www.medco.com/art/pdf/Drug_Trend_2007.pdf. Accessed 4 June 2008.
2. AIS Pharmacy Benefit homepage. "Specialty Pharmacy. Specialty Pharmacy Spending Still Increasing, As New Drugs Make Big Splash," Express Scripts analysis of IMS Health data. Available at http://www.aishealth.com/DrugCosts/specialty/SPN_Specialt_Pharmacy_Spending_Increasing.html. Accessed 4 June 2008.
3. Priority Health Care and Accredo Health Companys' reports, 1999–2004.
4. Meropol N.J. and Schulman K.A., Cost of cancer care: issues and implications. *J Clin Oncol.*, 2007; 25: 180-186.
5. Specialty Drug Costs Continue To Rise; Employees Hit With Higher Premiums. *Biotechnology Healthcare.* 2005; December: 18-19. Available at: http://www.biotechnologyhealthcare.com/journal/fulltext/2/6/BH0206018.pdf. Accessed 4 June 2008.
6. ICORE Healthcare, 2008. Available at http://www.icorehealthcare.com/mhs/icore/index.asp. Accessed 4 June 2008.
7. ICORE Healthcare estimates, 2008. Available at http://www.icorehealthcare.com/MHS/ICORE/education/trends.asp?leftmenu=2&sub=none. Accessed 4 June 2008.
8. Medco, Caremark, Express Scripts, BioScrip, and Option Care 10-k Company Annual Reports, 2007.
9. ICORE Healthcare, 2007.
10. American Cancer Society homepage. Available at http://www.cancer.org/docroot/home/index.asp. Accessed 4 June 2008.
11. *Managed Care Oncology*, Spring 2007. Available at http://www.managedcareoncology.com/elements/archive/MCO_summer_07.pdf. Accessed 4 June 2008.

ACRONYMS

ASP	average selling price
AWP	average wholesale price (drug)
ESAs	erythropoietin stimulating agents
FDA	Food and Drug Administration
GPOs	group purchasing organizations
HCPCS	Healthcare Common Procedure Coding System
IVIG	intravenous immunoglobulin
LDD	limited drug distribution
LHRH	luteinizing hormone-releasing hormone
MCR	medical cost ratio
MS	multiple sclerosis
NDC	National Drug Code
PA	prior authorization
PBMs	pharmacy benefit managers, pharmacy benefit management (companies)
PMPM	per-member-per-month
RA	rheumatoid arthritis
RFP	request for proposal
RSV	respiratory syncytial virus
SIU	Special Investigative Unit

MANAGED CARE PHARMACY INFORMATION SYSTEMS

GARTH E. BLACK
JOHN H. ROMZA

INTRODUCTION

Health care is a one and one-half trillion-dollar business in the United States. According to statistics compiled by National Health Statistics Group of the Centers for Medicare and Medicaid Services health care in 2004 accounted for 16.0% of the gross domestic product of the United States. Given this astonishing amount, controlling the costs associated with healthcare has become a primary focus of employers, governmental agencies, insurers, and all other organizations that are in any way responsible for budgeting and paying for health care. In this highly-charged, very competitive, and even distrustful environment, it is very clear that information is the key to understanding how health care is being used and how and where the healthcare dollar is being spent. Acquiring timely and accurate information and managing that information is also the key to improving the healthcare delivery process. Organizations that can best manage their information will make better decisions, drive efficient delivery processes, and be able to compete most effectively in the marketplace for the healthcare dollar.

The retail pharmaceutical distribution channel has the opportunity for more face-to-face encounters between a single healthcare professional and patients than potentially any other healthcare delivery channel. At the patient encounter, the pharmacy healthcare professionals must rely upon the most up-to-date and accurate information when they provide care. The amount of demographic, financial, and clinical information that pharmacists need to acquire and manage about their patients is staggering and only growing in complexity. The patient's desire for information on the latest products, spurred by direct-to-consumer advertising by the manufacturers, only increases the information burdens on the pharmacist and healthcare professional. Coupled with new government regulations and more complex financial arrangements for receiving payment for pharmaceutical products and services, it is obvious that this is a job that simply cannot be done effectively without state-of-the-art information systems.

Adding urgency and importance to cost of pharmaceuticals issue is the fact that, over the last few years, the pharmacy benefit and overall cost of drugs has surged and taken an even larger proportion of the healthcare dollar. This surge in pharmaceutical costs and utilization has made its way into the nightly news, headlines, *Wall Street Journal* articles, political campaigns, and even into international relations. It has forced pharmacy benefit sponsors to find new ways to control costs and new ways to share the costs of the pharmacy benefit with the consumers. It has caused drug manufacturers to examine their marketing plans and to re-examine their pricing policies. It has caused those who pay for pharmaceuticals to search for lower cost medications and lower cost providers and delivery methods. This cost trend has also found its way into the systems and information that all parties in the pharmaceutical delivery system use.

Only intensifying the situation are new government programs and legislation designed to help individuals better manage the cost of their healthcare and pharmaceuticals in particular. Flexible Savings Accounts and Health Savings Accounts are two examples of Consumer Directed Health strategies. These programs demand additional information management resources to adequately administer and to interface with other systems. For the senior population in the United States, it is no longer a question of *if* the government should provide improved pharmaceutical benefits, but *when* and *how* the assistance programs should be constructed each year.

Dealing with changes like these has fallen squarely upon the information technology departments to implement new and innovative programs to assist both the healthcare provider and the consumer. From an information technology standpoint, these rapidly changing markets and business practices have accelerated product life cycles, forcing systems to adapt and change more rapidly. Users of the new technology have had to adapt also. As technology has become available and familiar, the expectations on the role of the pharmacist and the pharmacy technician have grown. Patients and payors alike assume that the pharmacist is going to be equipped with technology to help them with their growing roles and to be able to navigate through these new challenges.

From a historical perspective, pharmacy information and claims processing systems have evolved significantly in recent years. In the 1970s, pharmacists used typewriters and completed manual claim forms. Today, interactive, online, real-time systems maintain detailed electronic records and permit pharmacists to submit a claim to a payor or payors and have a response back in seconds. This enormous change has resulted from advances in computing, information management, and telecommunication technology. Inclusion of pharmacy benefits as a component of managed health care also has greatly contributed to the adoption of this new information paradigm into the practice of pharmacy. The entire practice of pharmacy has been immutably altered through automation and the introduction of information processing and information management technology into nearly all aspects of the delivery process. This chapter describes the development and essential elements of pharmacy information and claims processing systems. It also discusses how pharmacy automation has and continues to augment the business and patient care aspects of pharmacy practice, dispensing, and pharmacy claim adjudication within managed care.

SCOPE OF PHARMACY INFORMATION MANAGEMENT

An important factor that accelerated the adoption of electronic pharmacy commerce was the presence of an accepted electronic data interchange standard. This standard, maintained by the National Council for Prescription Drug Programs (NCPDP), permits the submission of pharmacy claims and the adjudication of those claims in a real-time interactive mode. This standard has allowed the pharmacy profession an unparalleled position in electronic commerce that other segments of the healthcare industry are still striving to achieve, even after it has been commonplace in pharmacy for more than a decade. This standard, which allows communication between pharmacies and hundreds of payors, permits over 95% of all prescription claims to be processed electronically. In 2005, it was estimated that over 3.4 billion prescriptions were processed by pharmacies under this standard. From an information perspective, the NCPDP communication standard provides a common, comprehensive, well-defined set of data elements to feed the various information systems now present in the pharmaceutical distribution channel.

The majority of online transactions submitted by pharmacies to payors are currently being transmitted in the NCPDP 5.1 standard. The move to this electronic telecommunication standard version was spurred on by the Federal legislation known as HIPAA (Health Insurance Portability and Accountability Act) in 2003. This Act mandated standard transaction code sets with the intent to simplify the administration of systems handling electronic transmission of certain healthcare information and to protect confidential patient information. The date for the adoption of the NCPDP 5.1 transaction set was August 2002 and the adoption of the privacy rules, protecting patient confidentiality, was May 2003. The legislative bodies are now reviewing updates to the NCPDP 5.1 standard that if adopted would mandate a new transmission standard around 2010.

As pharmacists continue their evolution as respected providers in the managed care arena, they are in a unique position to capitalize on the incredible advances in electronic commerce and computing technology. The pharmacist is the key to providing accurate data to assist in managing a patient's care. Pharmacists are the healthcare professionals most frequently and regularly engaged by the patient. For this reason, they have an unparalleled ability to gather and submit real-time, accurate, and comprehensive information about the patient's health state and drug regimen. They are also in the best position to intervene and catch medication errors with proper systems support. The online transmission standard (NCPDP 5.1) recognizes this fact and includes fields for the defining and reimbursing of pharmaceutical care services rendered during the dispensing act. The standard also allows for the submission and adjudication of claims for pharmaceutical care services outside of a dispensing event.

However, there are several confounding factors and pressures that challenge the pharmacist's unique position. New drugs are coming onto the market faster and in unprecedented numbers. This challenge is compounded by the flood of new drugs that have names that sound alike or are spelled closely to the names of drugs already on the market. In addition, managed care organizations (MCOs) and other payors are constantly developing new models for pharmaceutical care, disease management, and prescription drug benefit programs. An example of the evolution of the pharmaceutical benefit program revolves around copay. At the turn of the century (the year 2000) three-tier copay plans were considered innovative. (A three-tier copay plan is one in which there is a different copay amount or different copay calculation depending upon the type of drug being dispensed. A three-tier copay plan organizes drugs into three different groups, with each group having a different copay amount or calculation.) Today three-tier plans are commonplace. N-tier plans (where N is greater than 3) exist, and dynamic or variable tier plans based on therapeutic classes are now considered the latest innovation. The retail pharmacist is being asked to dispense an ever-increasing number of prescriptions while providing counseling and other pharmaceutical care services to patients, in addition to being expected to explain to consumers their copay. Each of these dispensing activities may require a unique financial transaction with a third party payor that may or may not have similarities to earlier transactions conducted for that same patient. Information systems are now imperative in helping pharmacists efficiently and accurately perform and bill for this expanding list of routine tasks and an equally expanding list of different financial rules and/or roles. New advances in computer hardware and software will continue to be required to assist in the automation of other aspects of the dispensing process. These system advances are necessary to increase pharmacy efficiency and reduce the potential for human error and/or financial risk for either the patient or pharmacy. All of this needs to take place while the consumer is in front of the pharmacist to manage a patient's pharmaceutical regimen and overall health state.

The various e-prescribing systems permit the physician to electronically check to see if a drug is covered by the patient's benefit plan and at what formulary level a product is listed, transmit prescriptions to pharmacies, and retrieve a patient's drug history from a pharmacy's prescription record database or another central patient record repository. The electronic connectivity available to the pharmacy continues to improve the mechanisms that allow the communication of pharmacy claims to the various organizations that process them. Even now, advancing communication technology and Internet technology allows even the smallest or most remote pharmacies to send their prescription claims to processors and receive a response back in seconds. Third party processors continue to advance their claim adjudication systems, adding new functionality, benefit designs, and cognitive value to the dispensing process, while calculating the financial claim for the dispensed product and services. The Internet also has become a vehicle for pharmaceutical care claims submissions and communications between pharmacies, processors, payors and even the pharmacy manufacturing industry. The Internet is also a mode for the pharmacist and pharmacy benefits managers to communicate with their patients. The ability to order refills of prescriptions over the Internet or World Wide Web (*Web*) is commonplace. The ability for a patient to gain access to his or her medication profile for purposes of verification or as a financial record is also becoming commonplace. The right of the consumer to gain access to critical information over the Web about the drug products that he or she is using, such as drug precautions and or common side-effects, is now a tool that the pharmaceutical channel uses to empower and educate their patients.

These advancements in technology and the resulting pharmacy systems are now speeding information to claims processors, MCOs, drug manufacturers, and other entities in seconds. These data can be transformed and analyzed almost instantly, providing limitless opportunities to improve pharmaceutical care. The technology explosion in pharmacy has given pharmacists the ability to decrease the amount of time necessary to dispense a prescription, increase the accuracy of the task, and to increase the amount of data captured and retained. Technology has made it possible for the pharmacist to communicate with the prescriber at her or his place of business and with the patient at their home or work without using old fashioned paper-based systems or even the "old fashioned" telephone. Technology has also made it possible to analyze drug usage patterns and "mine" the data for fraud detection, disease state management, outcomes studies, patient outreach programs, and information vital to new drug research and development.

PHARMACY INFORMATION MANAGEMENT SYSTEMS

By embracing information system technology, pharmacists have made dispensing more efficient, instituted new standards of practice, greatly enhanced the cognitive capabilities of a pharmacist providing patient care, and fueled research by the medical and pharmaceutical manufacturing industries. Undoubtedly, the competitive pressures in the retail pharmacy drug industry and the managed care pharmacy practice setting have played a major role in advancing these information systems. Competition for the patient and the value that the patient's purchasing power brings to the rest of the store have encouraged attempts to reduce operational costs, improve the quality of the dispensed pharmaceutical product, and attract patients by offering new levels of service and convenience. Competition to attract and retain qualified pharmacists, especially in areas where multiple employment options exist, is another area of competition, especially among pharmacy chains. The system technology that is available to a pharmacist can be a critical factor in the recruiting process.

However, forces other than competition have played equally important roles in the adaptation of information technology. The relatively rapid expansion of the availability of pharmaceutical coverage as part of the expected medical benefit package has imposed new paradigms for marketing, dispensing, pricing, and reimbursement. The increased pace of new drugs entering the marketplace and the rapid rate of drug price changes have challenged the industry also. Finally, with more complicated drug therapies, regimens and unique packaging becoming common place, the need for information system technology to process and store great volumes of data to facilitate and record the required dispensing, counseling, and monitoring procedures has become paramount.

HISTORY

Centralized Computing Systems The first computers used by pharmacists in the dispensing of pharmaceuticals were usually computer terminals and printers attached to a large, centralized computer system that provided information services to an entire organization such as a university medical center, a major hospital, or a large retail drug chain. These systems were first introduced in the early 1970s and were designed to maintain patient demographics, track prescriber and drug information, and print prescription labels and simple prescription activity reports. These systems mostly replaced typewriters and some of the paper-based recordkeeping that previously occupied pharmacy personnel for decades. These first systems gave pharmacists the ability to maintain a database of patients, prescribers, and drugs as well as use this database to reduce errors and to speed the handling of subsequent prescriptions and refills (**Figure 7-1**). For example, when refilling a prescription, these systems were able to print an accurate label for the refill without much more than a few keystrokes on the part of the dispensing professional. This relatively simple process offered huge labor savings on a significant percentage of the dispensing operations and undoubtedly reduced label-based prescription errors by a significant percentage.

Once the advantages of computerization were realized, the centralized computer system was brought to the community pharmacy by the introduction of time-sharing computer services. Community pharmacies were linked to organizations that owned and operated these large, centralized computer systems using relatively expensive (by today's standards) private telecommunication lines and proprietary communications equipment. While these systems provided great benefit over paper-based systems and the typewriter, they also had reliability problems and were relatively slow. When telecommunication lines went down or the central system experienced hardware or software problems or just heavy utilization, the functionality of these systems suffered to the point that the pharmacist using the system probably had trouble viewing it as an asset. Moreover, the data collected by these systems were not available to the community pharmacist for anything other than the day-to-day, prescription-by-prescription functions that these systems supported. The data collected by these systems were "locked up" in proprietary database systems and organized in a way so that only the functions, features, and reports provided by the software vendor/developer were available. These systems did make pharmacies generally more efficient but did not expand the role of the pharmacist, improve patient care, empower the pharmacist with information about the business, or provide data for research.

Minicomputers In the late 1970s and early 1980s, information technology changed significantly. Many pharmacy organizations could now afford the less expensive "minicomputers" as an alternative to the large central systems. Small retail pharmacy chains and even many independent pharmacies were able to purchase the first true pharmacy management systems (PMSs), which became available with this technology. The minicomputer and the

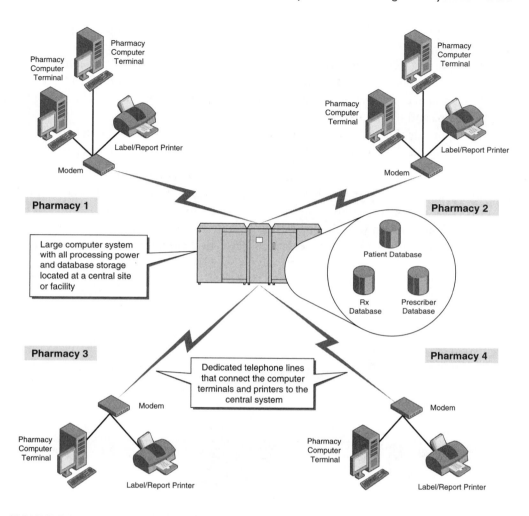

FIGURE 7-1 Pharmacy Management Systems Based on Centralized Computer System and Database Technology.

PMS offered the advantages of the large, centralized systems and added a host of new features that allowed the pharmacist to better operate the pharmacy business and serve patients. PMSs offered features such as the following:

- Drug-to-drug interaction detection in real time while the pharmacist was entering data about the patient and prescription into the computer system
- More sophisticated drug and prescription pricing algorithms
- Access to drug information services offering automatic updates of the system's information on drug prices, new drugs on the market, and drug interaction data

- Inventory management reports (stock movement, inventory valuation, purchase advice report, etc.)
- Reporting features that offered profit analysis, sales trends, and the ability to develop custom reports that allowed the pharmacist to identify key customers and key providers
- Automated production of third-party prescription claims and the ability to reconcile claims and payments
- Reporting and packaging capabilities tailored to specialized areas such as pharmaceutical home delivery and support for nursing homes and skilled care centers

Equally important, the minicomputer offered greater reliability, more consistent performance, and much greater flexibility in deployment of terminals (work stations) and printers in the pharmacy than previously available from the earlier generation of centralized computer systems. Additionally, minicomputers allowed pharmacists a higher degree of control and protection over the data collected in their pharmacy practice (**Figure 7-2**).

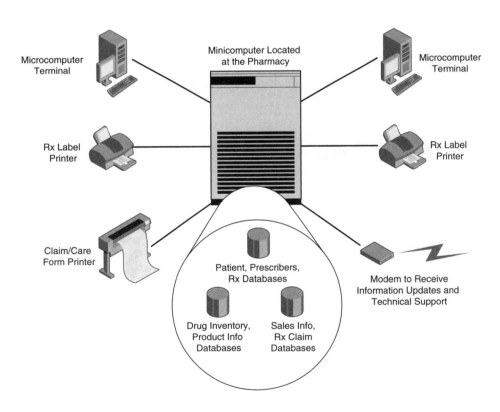

FIGURE 7-2 Pharmacy Management Systems Based on Minicomputer Technology.

Microcomputers In the mid-1980s, microcomputers such as the International Business Machine's personal computer (IBM PC) and various models from Apple Computer became the first really affordable computers for individuals and companies. These machines quickly became widely used in PMSs. They replaced the minicomputer as the technology of choice for PMSs, and PMSs became even more affordable and widely used. Since the mid-1980s, there has been a swift and consistent advancement in microcomputer technology and closely associated leaps in printer and telecommunication technology. The advances included the following important features (**Figure 7-3**):

- Microcomputers add greater speed, reliability, and cost-effectiveness than had been possible with minicomputers.
- Relational database technologies allow improvements in reporting and give pharmacy personnel the ability to query their data to their own specifications. Data no longer need be locked up and unavailable to the pharmacist. With even a little bit of training or through the use of easily understood software tools, pharmacy personnel could begin to design their own reports or to explore their data in ways that could benefit their patients and their business.
- Improvements in prescription labels and receipts make the product delivered to patients more readable and more professional looking. More patient-directed information can appear on the label. It is now possible to even print a picture of the product being dispensed on accompanying documentation, which enhances the safety of the dispensing process and can eliminate confusion for patients (and their caregivers) on multiple drug regimens. Not to be ignored is that the laser and inkjet printer technologies also have

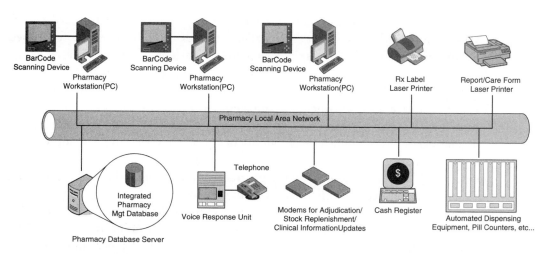

Typical Microcomputer/Network Pharmacy Management System Integrated with Automation and POS Equipment

FIGURE 7-3 Pharmacy Management System Based upon Microcomputer Technology.

made pharmacies much quieter places. These locations are no longer subjected to the sounds generated by the printing technologies used in typewriters and earlier generation computer printers.

- Signature capture devices, like those used commonly in retail credit card transactions, now allow pharmacies to collect patient signatures to acknowledge product delivery and the receipt of required counseling during the dispensing operation. These devices also allow pharmacies to record patient acknowledgment of the pharmacy's policy on privacy and for patients to document their consent to participate in a variety of health-related and marketing programs. This electronic signature can also now become a part of the electronic record available to the pharmacist and can be used to identity the patient and to prevent product loss or potential abuse situations.

- Drug utilization review (DUR) has expanded to include algorithms that check compliance, detect duplicate therapies, validate dosages and the duration of therapies, compare drug regimens to health state conditions, and screen for prior adverse reactions.

- Databases for patient education about drug therapy and patient directed monographs are now available.

- Scanning technologies improve dispensing efficiencies and reliability by the use of bar codes to identify products and prescriptions. Scanning technologies even allow for authentication of pharmacy personnel when they wear wristbands or badges that contain barcode identification. Scanning technologies also can make inventory management simpler and more precise. It can certainly also assist in product loss prevention.

- Voice response technology allows further dispensing efficiencies and conveniences for patients. Voice response technology allows for humans to give orders to computers using the numeric keypad on their phone or in even more advanced systems by recognizing the commands the human voice is giving by a technology called speech recognition. These systems now allow patients to order refills or check to see if their prescriptions are ready for pickup by using just their telephone at any time.

- Some PMS systems may include programs to ensure patient compliance with drug regimens. The PMS can identify non-complaint patients and provide information to the pharmacist to assist in contacting and counseling patients.

- Automated interfaces to the stock replenishment systems of drug wholesalers allow the pharmacist to determine the availability of a product at the supplier and to speed product ordering. These interfaces also give the system the ability to perform precise inventory purchasing and to allow the pharmacist to determine the exact acquisition and replenishment costs of pharmaceuticals.

- Improvements have been made to the system to more precisely track the products that are dispensed to patients. Many systems track products including the dispensed lot number of the product. This provides valuable information and a mechanism for contacting patients if a product recall occurs or if a product is withdrawn from the market.

- Interfaces to electronic prescribing systems (commonly called *e-prescribing*) help speed the entry of patient demographics and prescription data with information provided directly by the prescriber. These interfaces can minimize prescription errors by eliminating problems caused by illegible handwriting or errors introduced by the confusion caused by similarly named products. The e-prescribing systems also allow for communication with the prescriber for authorizations of prescription changes or additional refills. These systems cannot only eliminate the time-consuming phone calls and the frustrations that result when the appropriate personnel at the prescriber office are not available, but they offer improved accuracies, more security, and automatic essential documentation for these critical dispensing activities.

- Microcomputers allow online access (via modem or other telecommunication technologies) to up-to-the-minute drug price information, clinical drug information, and knowledge bases that can drive DUR.

Pharmaceutical Dispensing Applications Specialized PMSs have emerged for specific pharmaceutical dispensing settings also. Mail-order pharmacies, for example, typically dispense an extremely high volume of prescriptions from a single pharmacy site. These pharmacies often break down the tasks involved with prescription order fulfillment into a number of discrete, well-defined, reproducible component processes that ensure a high degree of quality and safety, despite the high volumes. Examples of these component processes might be data entry, product counting and packaging, prescription labeling, quality assurance, and prescription order shipment. These component processes, and the movement of pharmaceutical product between the various locations within the pharmacy where these processes take place, are often candidates for automation and additional functionality provided by the mail-order PMS. Prescription orders are placed in cardboard cartons or plastic bins that are referred to as *totes*. This tote will serve to hold all the prescription items and related documentation as the prescription order is filled within the pharmacy. The totes often contain a bar-code or an RFID (Radio Frequency Identification Code) tag that is read by sensing equipment as the tote passes a location on a conveyor belt system that runs throughout the pharmacy. Once the carton or tote is identified by the sensing equipment, it can direct the tote along a path on the conveyor that will take the tote into dispensing stations within the pharmacy that have been designed for efficient product counting, packaging, and labeling operations for exactly the product being dispensed. In some cases, these dispensing stations are equipped with tablet- and capsule-counting machines that automatically prepare the correct quantity of the desired medication and then insert the medication directly into the appropriate vial or bottle. Often this equipment can automatically apply the prescription label at this point in the process. These counting operations and packaging decisions are all driven by the computing resources of the PMS. At other times, robots (or *picking machines*) are employed at the dispensing stations to quickly assemble all the products required for a particular product order. These robots automatically retrieve prepackaged, exact quantities of the desired pharmaceutical from aisles holding thousands of products. Again, the PMS controls the robots and delivers to the pharmacist at the dispensing station the products that are needed for the orders currently at the station. Also delivered is the necessary information to ensure that the proper product and quantity is being dispensed. This may be delivered via the automatic printing of this documentation or the display of the information on computer monitors located at the dispensing station.

Imaging Technology   In addition, PMS systems in high-volume pharmacies have incorporated a computer technology called *imaging*. Imaging is basically taking a computerized picture (similar to pictures produced by digital cameras) and passing that digital picture (or image) through the pharmacy rather than passing the paper documents (prescription, patient order form, patient payment information, etc.) to the pharmacy personnel who require them in the dispensing process. This paperless system can improve efficiencies and eliminate errors because the documentation is consistently organized, always available, and easily reproducible for whoever needs it. Imaging can have other cost and time saving benefits. Retrieval of electronic documents is usually much faster and more accurate than paper-based retrieval.

Imaging can be a significant tool for the pharmacist in other ways. For example, electronic images of a particular medication and its identifying characteristics can be available to a quality control pharmacist at a dispensing station in a high-volume pharmacy to allow a quick, secure check that the proper medications are being dispensed. The PMS can make these product images and even the images associated with the paper-based prescription document appear at the dispensing station as soon as the tote containing the order arrives at that station. This instantly gives the pharmacist the tools they need to perform the dispensing and quality assurance processes required at that station.

Patient Support Technology   Some PMSs specialize in supporting pharmaceutical care and treatment programs. This functionality allows for the collection and tracking of patient care data (pulse, blood pressure, blood glucose levels, etc.), and the management and associated documentation of care programs directed at specific patient populations. These pharmaceutical care system additions to the PMS can assist the pharmacist in managing specialized programs for the control of asthma, hypertension, diabetes, or other medical conditions. These systems can assist the pharmacist in monitoring and documenting a patient's drug therapy, compliance, complications, and vital signs, while providing the pharmacist with additional tools to maintain a high level of patient-pharmacist interaction for program education and counseling. These systems can extend the reach of the pharmacist as a healthcare professional and increase the well-being of the patients in such programs.

PHARMACY MANAGEMENT SYSTEMS AND ELECTRONIC DATA INTERCHANGE

The information technology used within the pharmacy also has been heavily influenced by the increasing prevalence of pharmaceutical benefit programs. While these programs were growing in popularity for a number of years before electronic claim submission became commonplace, online adjudication of pharmacy claims at the point-of-service

(POS) for these benefit programs has certainly fueled their growth and acceptance. This electronic adjudication of pharmacy benefits from the POS allowed for the determination of eligibility, benefit information, and reimbursement amounts, and introduced new financial models, new market opportunities and, of course, some technological challenges.

ADJUDICATION

The first adjudication programs required the use of an adjudication terminal, a device similar to the financial terminals that process credit card transactions at most retail outlets. These terminals used a standard telephone line to transmit claims electronically. To adjudicate a prescription claim online (i.e., to electronically submit the claim at POS to the claims processor), the pharmacist had to enter information about the patient, the drug, the quantity dispensed, and the prescriber. Of course, this was an extra, time-consuming, mostly redundant step in the dispensing process, but the ability to submit the claim and to immediately determine the status of the claim was viewed as a huge advantage. These POS adjudication programs not only eliminated much of the financial risk associated with accepting payment by assignment from a third party payor, but it eliminated problems with determining the proper patient payment (or copayment) for the prescription and reduced the number of days the pharmacy had to wait for payment. With paper-based claims systems, determining co-payment and claim status was much more difficult and receiving payment had taken much longer.

PMS developers quickly realized that the information needed for online adjudication was already present in their systems when the pharmacist prepared the prescription. These developers quickly coupled their systems with a modem and a standard phone line and then modified their systems to replace the adjudication terminal. The PMS gathered the necessary information and submitted the claim to the claims processor as part of the dispensing process. The systems then incorporated information returned by the claims processors directly into their databases. The databases were automatically updated with the eligibility information, revenue information, patient payment responsibilities, and the DUR data provided by the claims processor. Additionally, documents such as the patient's receipt and the pharmacy log produced by the PMS now automatically contained this critical information. This innovation in PMSs eliminated the additional data entry steps and the need to separately record claim status information. This made the adjudication process less time-consuming and allowed pharmacy personnel to better keep pace with the rapid market changes that resulted from the growth of prescription benefit programs.

Besides technology, another very important factor that fueled the success of the POS adjudication process was that both pharmacies and claims processors quickly realized that adherence to a common electronic claim standard was of utmost importance. While the NCPDP had some previous success with promoting a standard pharmacy paper claim form with the NCPDP Universal Claim Form (UCF) since the late 1970s, many different paper-based claim forms were still present in the marketplace throughout the 1980s. Online POS adjudication was viewed as the way to eliminate these differences and the inherent inefficiencies associated with multiple standards, forms, and methods.

The NCPDP organization continues to play a key role in keeping its electronic claim standard relevant to new developments in the industry and almost universally accepted by industry participants and the governmental agencies that promote the efficiency, safety, privacy, and security of these transactions.

ROLE OF SWITCHING COMPANIES

Organizations known as national pharmacy claim switch vendors (national switches) evolved to act as a focal point for pharmacy claims that were destined to go to the hundreds of different claims processors that entered the market. These national switches, empowered by the NCPDP standards for pharmacy claim format and content, provided a common phone number, a common communication protocol, a source for technical support for telecommunication problems, and a consistent level of service and availability to the pharmacy. The national switches also contributed to the growth of the pharmacy claims processors and pharmacy benefits managers (PBMs) by allowing them to offer adjudication services without having to support the communication needs of thousands of different pharmacies.

Other Communication Technologies Communication technology continues to improve and offer new options for the exchange of claim data between pharmacies and claims processors. For example, when a modem and standard telephone line is used for adjudication, the process may take from 30 to 60 seconds to complete. Dialing and establishing a data connection between modems take up most of this time. The actual time to process the claim at the processor is usually under five seconds. Communication technologies that are "always on" such as frame relay (a virtual, private network connecting the pharmacy to a claims switching organization), Digital Subscriber Line (DSL), cable-modem connection to an Internet Service Provider (ISP), or even satellite communications (similar to the technology now employed to deliver video entertainment to homes) are now priced (and available) so that almost every pharmacy can choose one of these technologies to reduce the time consumed by the adjudication process to 10 seconds or less per claim transaction (**Figure** 7-4). Today the national switches offer their services through the "legacy" dial-up communication mechanisms and through these more modern, higher speed technologies. With these high-speed, high-capacity communication technologies, more data can be exchanged between the pharmacist and other parties in the drug distribution process. In addition, the dispensing process is improved; there is access to increased information, improved drug utilization review algorithms, and other pharmaceutical care and managed care initiatives. NCPDP and other standard-setting organizations have used the successful model developed for the submission of pharmacy claims to bring the advantages associated with electronic data interchange to other dispensing processes. One prime example of this is electronic prescribing as described above. The national switches and other organizations are offering connection services between prescriber offices and pharmacies so that electronic prescribing can become a viable tool in the prescribing process.

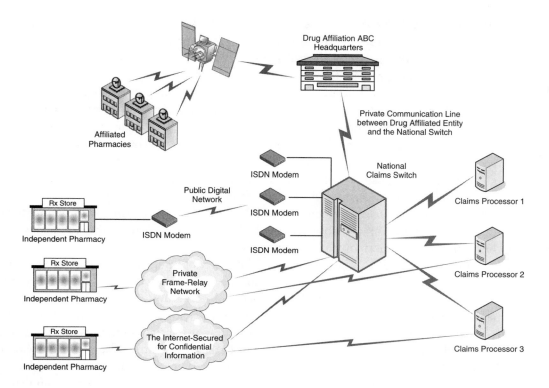

FIGURE 7-4 **High Speed, High Capacity Technologies Employed for Electronic Data Interchange.**

INTERNET TECHNOLOGY

The Internet has increasingly become a pervasive factor in almost every area of public communication. More information becomes available via the Internet every day and Internet technologies are improving to provide easier access, more universal availability, higher speeds, and greater data capacities. It is certain that this technology will have a greater impact than even the microprocessor did on Pharmacy Information Systems. We have already seen much evidence of the Internet's influence in pharmacy. Internet technology is not only improving the capabilities of current pharmacy systems and processes, but is responsible for the development of new delivery paradigms and for changing the roles of the prescriber, pharmacist, and patient in the pharmaceutical delivery chain.

The Internet simply put is one great set of enabling technologies. The Internet allows people all over the world to get access to the same information or the same computer application at the same time using universally available tools and near universally accepted conventions for the presentation of this information. The Internet browser is perhaps the most visible software product that is both a tool and a standard for a user interface for the presentation of the information available over the Web. Other important technologies include a common protocol to connect computers together known as TCP/IP (Terminal Control Protocol over Internet Protocol). Another enabling technology is known as HTML (Hyper Text Markup Language). HTML is a standard way to organize information and to provide instructions to the Internet browser on how the information is to be displayed to a user. However, there are dozens of other major technology components that have come together to make the Internet the most powerful influence in defining what information systems can do today and what they will do in the future. Cost effective ISPs, Internet information search engines (e.g., Yahoo and Google), electronic marketplaces (e.g., eBay), and content providers (e.g., MSNBC or AOL) are setting high standards for functionality and enabling further technical advancements built upon the technology that they can bring to almost any home or business.

Some very well established examples of the power of Internet technology in pharmacy have already unfolded. The Internet has enabled a new means of communication between patients, prescribers, pharmacies (mail-order and community retail), and prescription benefit managers. Pharmacy Web sites have been developed to allow patients to order refills or to inquire on the status of their prescription using the Internet. While these sites offer similar conveniences to voice response technology, often they also provide advanced features like price comparison information, access to detailed consumer-directed drug information, comparisons between drug products, automated patient compliance reminders via e-mail, and access to a pharmacist via e-mail or Internet chat functions on a 24-hour-per-day basis. Patients who belong to managed care organizations may have the ability to connect to the MCO's Web site (or the Web site for the MCO's PBM) to look at formulary drug choices and examine the details of their pharmacy benefit plans. Even more astounding is the idea that many Web sites allow the patient to pre-adjudicate a transaction before taking their prescription to a pharmacy or submitting it to a pharmacy online. This allows the patient to know exactly what the patient's responsibility for payment will be for the prescription or to allow patients to "shop" between similar drugs or even pharmacies for the most advantageous benefits or prices. This is particularly important as attempts to control pharmacy costs focus on more consumer-driven heath care choices and the use of defined contribution health plans. Finally, patients can even track their own drug prescription history that was adjudicated against various PBM's systems, fueling the personal health record.

The Internet also provides patients access to drug information from sources other than their local pharmacists. Universities and pharmacy schools are now maintaining drug information databases on their Web sites and making this information available to the general public. Drug manufacturers have established their own Web resources to provide patients with clinical information on their drug products (along with coupons for sample doses and sales and marketing materials). Even the federal government has realized that the Internet is a tool for information and change. In 2004, the Centers for Medicare and Medicaid Services (CMS) established a Web site to help Medicare recipients make best use of a federally-sponsored drug discount program. The CMS Web site offers pricing and competitive information on discount program sponsors, pharmacies, drugs, and drug prices.

The Internet also provides new tools for the pharmacist. Web sites provided by drug manufacturers have sections dedicated to pharmacy professionals. These sites can provide the latest information on drug products and can act as an online reference library replacing the common package insert information or the "old fashioned" published reference books, which can quickly become out of date. Likewise, the pharmacist can use the Internet to connect to the drug wholesaler or other supplier to check on the status of a drug order or the availability of a drug product. PBMs are also offering online contact (e.g., "chat line" real time e-mail) as an alternative to calling a help desk to gain access to services for problem determination and claim payment status.

Another well-established example of the influence of the Internet as a driver of change is in the area of interaction between the pharmacist and patient. A new pharmacy distribution model is evolving. Acceptance of Internet technology by patients in the very personal world of health care, coupled with the workload pressures of community pharmacists, have resulted in a situation in which patients no longer expect as much face-to-face interaction with pharmacists as they once did. This has led to the creation of online pharmacies (termed *virtual pharmacies*) located anywhere in the world. Dozens of these pharmacies have appeared on the Internet since 2000. They offer patients the ability to order prescription drugs via the Internet for home delivery. The difficult step in the evolution of this process has been to get the patient's prescription into the hands of the unknown pharmacist, who is often practicing in another state or even another country. The prescription as a primarily paper-based document still is a bit cumbersome to deliver to such a virtual pharmacy. But even this logistic hurdle can often be offset by the fact that online pharmacies are always open and offer patients ready information about their medications, health states, and related lifestyle and over-the counter products. Online pharmacies also have the ability to send reminders to patients via e-mail, offer "instant" coupons for health-related products, and provide patients with links to other pertinent and interesting Web pages based on their prescription profile. While the technology and systems exist today to support this business model, we cannot discount the fact that clinical and legal issues have and will cause challenges in the evolution of this business model. These challenges limited the independent virtual drugstore to servicing just patients who were very price-sensitive or were confident that this model served their needs well as a means for refilling familiar prescriptions.

Given these challenges, many of these virtual pharmacies went out of business when the speculative financing associated with the Internet technology bubble burst in 2000. However, the concept was quickly recognized, adopted, and advanced by the more traditional brick and mortar pharmacies that started their own virtual pharmacies as the natural complement to their retail outlets. The national chains and large regional pharmacy chains realized the importance of Internet portals to their patients and their marketplace. These organizations made the virtual pharmacy just another "front door" for the more traditional corner retailer. This was an advancement over the original concept of the strictly virtual pharmacy. The brick and mortar players with an Internet presence have the advantage of name recognition. They also can permit patients to order maintenance medications and refills online and offer these same patients the option to order their acute care medications for preparation and pickup right at the patient's local pharmacy.

Another Internet-powered business paradigm known as the *central refill facility* also evolved from these virtual "front doors." The central refill facility uses technology like that of the virtual pharmacy to collect refill orders for patients from many geographic areas and then couples this with the high prescription volume technologies and efficiencies often used in mail order pharmacies. Prescription refills from the central refill facility can then either be shipped directly to patient's homes or can be sent to the local pharmacy for pickup. This system provides conveniences for the patient and can make operations at the local pharmacy more efficient by moving some of the prescription fulfillment process to the central facility. The central facility can become a "third hand" for the local pharmacist. Personnel and technology at the central refill center can handle counting and packaging operations for the local pharmacist. The central refill center also can provide a convenient source for infrequently ordered products or for products whose high price or limited availability makes them impractical to inventory at every dispensing location within a pharmacy chain. Additional time-consuming tasks, like contacting physicians for refill authorizations or prescription changes, or researching problems with third party prescription claims, can also be offloaded to the central refill facility: this allows the local pharmacist to be more productive and permits more time to focus on patient care.

In the not too distant future, the Internet will also be used by the pharmacy as a cost-efficient way to perform new tasks or to dramatically improve the efficiency of "traditional" computerized functions. Switching claims to a third party processor or sending/receiving electronic prescription documents will become even more efficient, secure, and less expensive using Internet technology. Just as the Internet established a common way to display information to a user using HTML, a similar technology known as XML (eXtensible Markup Language) is being used to establish the *de facto* standard to transmit information between systems. XML promises to make the interchange of information between pharmacy information systems and other healthcare systems more prevalent and productive in the future. The ability to exchange information about prescriptions, prescription claims, drug orders, and even entire patient medical records will be commonplace using this type of technology. The security of these types of information transactions will be ensured by the passing of digital signatures or certifications that identify the requestor and provider of information in a way that is more secure than ever possible with paper-based or telephone-based systems. Digital signatures are very much like the personal signature that has long served as an indicator of authenticity on a document.

Once everyone (patient, prescriber, pharmacist) has a widely-accepted personal digital signature, it will serve not only to authenticate the electronic document, but it will secure it by encrypting it so that only the author and the intended recipient will be able to use the document. The authenticity, security, accuracy, and speed of delivery of these electronic documents will make paper-based systems nearly obsolete. The pharmacist, prescriber, and patient will all be better informed and, more importantly, will be able to make better clinical and financial decisions.

PRESCRIPTION BENEFIT MANAGEMENT ADJUDICATION SYSTEMS

In the mid-1970s, when prescriptions were filled and a prescription claim was to be generated, the claim form was usually completed by hand. In the late 1970s and early 1980s, PMSs (as noted above) became capable of printing these forms automatically, greatly advancing the speed and the ability of pharmacies to communicate claims to payors. However, these paper-based processes allowed for no immediate feedback from a payor on either the eligibility of a patient, the claim's status, or any clinical protocols. In addition, the pharmacist was usually responsible for collecting a single, relatively small, fixed-amount copayment from the patient when dispensing the prescription. There simply was not enough information present at the point of dispensing for the pharmacist to do anything more than these elementary claim procedures. The situation changed dramatically in the mid-1980s with the advent of the microprocessor, standardized modem technology, and improvements in the public phone network to carry data traffic. These advancements, along with the strong efforts of standard-setting organizations such as the NCPDP, ushered in the era of pharmacy point of service systems communicating in real-time with payor prescription benefit management systems (PBMSs).

The first online systems did little more than verify eligibility. This helped to keep the response time between the pharmacy and payor reasonable. They were valuable in that they instantly answered information about the patient's eligibility and confirmed the exact copayment amount. However once the online adjudication technology became accepted, and expected, by most pharmacies, the capabilities of these online claim adjudication systems evolved quickly. Their use of the available technology followed *Moore's Law of Computing*, which states that every few years computing power increases exponentially, with a corresponding drop in the cost to provide that computing power. As the adjudication systems raw processing power increased, they could perform their tasks faster and for a wider variety of benefit programs. However, very predictably, another law of computing came into play, *Moore's Compliment*, which states that as business learns to exploit each new generation of technology, it does so with ever more complicated sets of processing tasks. This second law has never been more valid than within the pharmaceutical adjudication arena. The cost pressures associated with the pharmacy benefit have quickly introduced new business concepts to assist with the cost sharing of pharmaceuticals and extending the processes to the Internet. The evolution in computer and database technology has provided the capability to not only verify eligibility but check complicated pharmacy benefit plan designs, perform claims adjudication, and prospective DUR. All these tasks as well as basic online claims adjudication can be accomplished while still keeping online transaction systems' response time to a few seconds.

FINANCIAL AND DELIVERY CONSIDERATIONS

The adjudication systems evolved quickly into a second generation in a very short period of time. The first generation of these systems, as stated above, verified eligibility and rudimentary payment information. As the technology advanced, more edits (transaction test conditions for adjudication) were added. These edits perform sophisticated pricing algorithms and were focused primarily on managing claims to achieve the lowest possible cost for the benefit program based on broad clinical guidelines or to design a benefit program for a unique segment of the population. Today, the second-generation adjudication systems are able not only to evaluate claims based on general clinical guidelines but to evaluate each submitted encounter for cost-effectiveness and appropriate drug usage based on a patient's pharmaceutical history. The push for greater online prospective DUR and auditing has forced the second generation of systems to design sophisticated edits, requiring more computing power to enhance a patient's total health state. These new systems aim to reduce side effects, dispensing errors, interactions with other nutritional supplements, and the improper use of medications. Frequently, systems encourage drug compliance through messaging or other forms of communication directed at the dispensing pharmacist. Although improved compliance may increase drug costs, the goal is to reduce long-term overall medical costs for the patient. These system advances can also be used to enforce formulary compliance and other non-clinical goals of MCOs. All these improvements have been made possible by faster, more stable hardware and creative programming.

Second-generation adjudication systems are able to select appropriate pharmaceuticals based on submitted diagnosis codes, patient drug histories, or other specific clinical guidelines. Today's prescription benefit system can evaluate each submitted patient encounter against specific clinical guidelines and a patient profile instead of just applying broad guidelines to a submitted transmission. Specific evaluations of encounters (not available in the first-generation systems) can enable the pharmacist to encourage patient drug utilization and compliance or provide patient-specific counseling strategies. These advances can target small high-cost patient populations. For example, a strategy could focus on the familiar 80/20 rule where 20% of the patient population will incur 80% of the costs. This relatively small population can be the target of increased auditing and/or retrospective DUR processes to ensure financial and clinical goals are being met. This allows the technology to be applied where it should yield the greatest benefit. Second-generation capabilities are the result of technological hardware and software advances featuring greater history review, more complicated algorithms, and pharmacist-directed software design.

Armed with this new computing power and processing ability, the systems work for the most cost-effective drug prescribing and patient utilization of pharmaceuticals. Adjudication systems are no longer the domain of only PBMs. They are now used to administer and manage drug benefit programs for chain pharmacies, manufacturers, governmental agencies, wholesalers, health maintenance organizations, insurance companies, and other MCOs. As these systems have become more mainstream, many MCOs that once outsourced these functions, or carved the pharmacy benefit out, are now able to bring these functions and their associated systems in-house to gain greater control and then create unique informational interfaces to other key systems in their organizations.

All the adjudication systems can provide similar basic functions, regardless of who administers them. First, they offer administrative or recordkeeping contract functions, including eligibility validation, pharmacy network maintenance, pricing algorithms, help desk support, payment functions, and creation and update processes of product databases. Second, they offer clinical control functions, including drug utilization edits, formulary management, and drug substitution programs. These two major functional areas are the essence of adjudication and the evolution of these systems has caused the lines between them to become blurred. Everyone in the claims adjudication channel should understand these functions. A description of a typical adjudicated transaction follows.

When a pharmacy submits a claim to a claims processing system via a modem, leased line, satellite connection, or the Internet, the electronic claims transaction is evaluated for adherence to a standard format and, within that format, for a set of required submitted data elements necessary for the claim's adjudication. If the claim fails either of these two basic checks, the system will reject the transaction prior to beginning the adjudication process. Once the transaction has been verified to contain a valid pharmacy claim, the adjudication process begins in earnest. The adjudication process is where the administrative, clinical, and financial edits that form the heart of the pharmacy benefit plan are carried out. Even if the claim has been verified for a valid format, the claim can still be rejected at any point for violating a clinical or administrative system edit.

Typically, one of the first steps is to check the member's eligibility. If the patient is shown on the system as being eligible for pharmacy benefits, the claim is directed to the benefit plan. Note that adjudication has evolved to the point that patients can even be enrolled dynamically by the adjudication system when their first claim is submitted for a benefit program. Once the eligibility had been verified the transaction locates the benefit plan that governs decisions and edits to be conducted with regard to the where, what, when, how much, patient responsibility and clinical details of the claim.

BENEFIT PLAN EDITS

"Where" is often a network of contracted physicians who may prescribe prescriptions and/or the network of pharmacies under contract with the managed care organization (MCO) or PBM to fill prescriptions for their patients. The advances in system technology now allow a specific drug to be evaluated for a specific physician and pharmacy network. For example, claims for lifestyle drugs for impotence may only be properly adjudicated if they have been prescribed by a physician that has a urology specialty or other specialty deemed appropriate in plan setup and are being dispensed by a pharmacy specializing in these types of drugs.

"What" are the products or services that are covered (or eligible for reimbursement) based on the member's benefit plan. With three-tier or multi-tier drug copays, the "what" question has become a complicated proposition. The system intends to "steer" patients to drugs that may help control cost or to those drugs that clinical experts may feel are most effective through economic incentives like lower copays or products that bypass a deductible. The adjudication process may also help the patient and the physician by providing information on the formulary benefits (and cost) available to a patient via Web sites. However, in many instances this involves a pharmacist's intervention at the point of dispensing to inform the patient of the lowest cost alternative available to the patient. The pharmacist may obtain this information by examining messages that may be contained in the response to the claim that they filed electronically on behalf of the patient. Pharmacists may even try to file electronic claims for multiple drug options until the lowest cost alternative is determined. As e-prescribing matures and consumers have more access to benefit information the lowest cost alternative should be clearer to all parties involved in the transaction. These "what" type of edits also evaluate if over-the-counter (OTC) medicines and related medical devices will be covered by the benefit.

"When" edits involve whether the drug is currently covered or how often the patient can receive the pharmaceutical product. The duration and conditions surrounding the quantity and days supply of the product being dispensed have become more complex with new drug therapies with starter doses, maintenance doses, and maximum limits placed on certain products by the benefit sponsors for non-essential therapies. Simple "when" edits may scan for refill-too-soon conditions. More complex "when" type of edits may restrict a product to those patients in a certain age group. They may even limit products to a once-a-year or even once-a-lifetime dispensing that will be covered under benefit. Examples of these might include weight-control and smoking-cessation products.

"How much" refers to the quantity of the product that is permitted under the plan benefit. The quantity edit in these systems has become more complicated from a medical and financial perspective. The adjudication systems have become smarter and if an incorrect or illogical quantity is submitted the system may attempt to correct it or send a message back regarding what an acceptable quantity of the product might be. The "how much" question can also be related to which pharmacy is performing the dispensing operation. Larger quantities and longer duration of therapies will typically be available to patients who use mail order pharmacies or retail pharmacies designated for this type of fill. These types of quantity related "how much" benefit restrictions have also become more commonplace as certain lifestyle drugs have become more popular.

"Patient responsibility" or out-of-pocket expenses refers to the patient's financial responsibility as part of the financial transaction, and the total reimbursement due the dispensing pharmacy. In this area the complexity can be enormous. Not only do benefit plans use the aforementioned multiple tiers for copayment to determine the "patient responsibility" question, but they can also include in these calculations factors such as:

- A patient or family deductible that must be met for out-of-pocket drug spend before a benefit is available
- A patient or family maximum benefit for a period that once exceeded eliminates or greatly reduces the benefit available
- Patient incentives in terms of lower copayments to use favored products, favored pharmacies or even favored delivery methods such as mail order
- Limits on the number of prescription claims allowed for the patient on a monthly or annual basis
- Whether the benefit plan being used is the primary plan for the individual patient or has been designated as a secondary or even "stop-gap" benefit plan
- Limits on benefits paid on behalf the patient for other medical claims (hospital care, doctor care, dental care, etc. . . .) also may be considered in determining benefit available or the patient's responsibility.

The financial calculation also involves how much the pharmacy will be reimbursed for the product and associated dispensing fees. This calculation involves not only commonly available price data (i.e., the drug's Average Wholesale Price [AWP], Wholesale Average Cost [WAC], Average Manufacturer's Price [AMP], or future price basis) but also the contractual relationship between the pharmacy and the PBM or other organization processing the claim. Pharmacy total reimbursement amounts usually involve calculations centered on pre-negotiated discount amounts and dispensing fees. However, other factors may be involved in the final calculations:

- Comparisons to Usual and Customary (U&C) retail pricing
- Point of sales rebates
- Patient copay incentives to move patients quickly to new market available generics
- Maximum reimbursements for some drug products available generically
- Pharmaceutical care, where pharmacies may be compensated for providing additional consulting or providing special services like home delivery or 24-hour availability
- Pharmacy dispensing performance, such as pharmacies that dispense high percentages of generics or strictly adhere to tight formularies, may be entitled to higher dispensing fees

As the above illustrates, the claims adjudication system is now a highly complex system that enables the administration of pharmacy benefit plans that would be impossible, without its POS availability and the vast amounts of data that the system considers during its claim adjudication activities.

CLINICAL MANAGEMENT

Much of the discussion above has focused on the financial and delivery aspects of the claims adjudication systems. Clinical management functions are an increasingly important factor. Clinical management functions start with prospective DUR edits. These edits evaluate the claim to make essential decisions. Drug-to-drug interaction checking, duplicate therapy detection, and validating the dosage of the drug and the duration of therapy are all commonly performed edits. Another clinical edit can evaluate a drug in relation to the patient's health condition, age, gender, or prescription history. A message may be generated that warns that the prescribed drug may be contraindicated for a patient's known or inferred health state. An inferred health state is an educated guess that can reliably be made based upon the patient's current or past medical and drug history. For example, a patient whose drug history includes insulin may reasonably be assumed to be diabetic. All of these edits can cause a claim to be rejected or just trigger informational messaging to be sent to the dispensing pharmacist. These reject and informational messages are formatted in a standardized manner within the NCPDP 5.1 claim standard. These prospective drug utilization programs have a definite advantage over the manual systems of the past, as they can prevent drug-to-drug interactions, minimize dispensing errors, and avoid inappropriate drug usage. They even offer advantages over the technology available within the pharmacy, because the system can consider prescription activity from multiple providers and may even be able to include other medical information about the patient while performing these edits.

Other forms of clinical management are also available in the adjudication systems. Contingency therapy, or step therapy edits may require that a patient try a first line of drug therapy before progressing to a more expensive or more potent second-line drug. More sophisticated clinical edits, referred to as *prior authorizations*, may restrict certain drug therapies dispensed by specific pharmacies or prescribed by particular physicians. With the advances in technology and business practices, many of these prior authorizations have become automatic. The adjudication system, by examining a patient's historical drug profile, may dynamically create a prior authorization that a clinician in an organization would routinely approve. The system may even generate documentation automatically as to why the authorization was given, to be used in subsequent utilization reviews. Many MCOs have pursued this evolution of the smart prior authorization in order to provide convenience in the dispensing process while minimizing labor costs and retaining the desired controls over the pharmacy benefit that prior authorization offers. In the past, MCOs needed to have large staffs dedicated to considering and processing prior authorizations. Now organizations can apply more sophisticated formulary controls and facilitate the application of clinical protocols embedded and invoked during the claims adjudication process.

This new generation of systems also can focus on clinical guidelines based on specific conditions or disease states. The guidelines are generally developed by using the vast amounts of pharmaceutical data collected from online systems. Pharmaceutical and medical professionals can design patient management and compliance programs that target small, high-risk populations that are driving healthcare costs. Special programs targeted to patients identified with asthma, diabetes, hypertension, and other conditions can effectively be managed through the capabilities of the modern adjudication systems. Clearly, the ability to analyze increasing volumes of information online and in a near-instantaneous fashion has been a key in the evolution and success of claims adjudication systems.

A relatively recent development is the extension of the PBM's systems to the patients via the Internet. This might be classified as the third generation of claims adjudication systems. These systems extend the capabilities of the first and second generation systems to the consumer. The patient access to these systems is generically called a *Patient Portal*. Through this portal, the MCOs and other organizations have extended their systems to permit their members to model their claims history to enable them to choose the most appropriate drug benefit for their situation. In addition, the extension of these systems has enabled patients to become smarter consumers with their benefit dollars and lower the cost of their overall health care. Through the portal, a patient can submit test claims to the adjudication system over the Internet. The patient can now determine how much a drug will cost before they reach the pharmacy or can even discuss the clinical and financial benefits of their drug regimen with their physician or pharmacist by printing their history or saving it to a portable storage device. Recent pharmacy and healthcare benefit plans, broadly labeled as defined Consumer Driven Health Plans (CDHPs), have given the consumer the power to spend the limited funds in these accounts based on their own informed choices. These extensions of the adjudication process are an outgrowth of consumerism and allow consumers with an Internet connection to shop for their best deal. Consumers can examine price differentials between brand and generic products, and also compare competing drugs in a drug therapy class. They can evaluate the different costs associated with their selected drug but consider the use of different providers in a pharmacy network. Again, without the advancing technical sophistication of the claims adjudication systems and the advancements in technology, these important evolutions in consumerism and cost-control would not be possible.

OTHER MCO INFORMATION SYSTEMS

The pharmacy systems and technological advances in pharmacy systems, switching, and third-party adjudication programs are integral to patient care and to the cost-effectiveness of pharmacy practice. With the majority of Americans now enrolled in some form of managed care, MCO management information systems now store unprecedented amounts of data regarding member functions, provider functions, claims administration, clinical management, rebate administration, and financial details. These systems and those discussed above fall under the general heading of online transaction processing (OLTP) systems.

In a very real sense, the OLTP systems and advances in technology have made it possible to collect billions of prescription records every year. While handling this great volume, today's systems must also effect changes in prescribing and patient drug usage patterns to benefit the affected patients and perhaps reduce the costs of drug therapy and improve the overall health care for a particular patient or patient population. Some of these challenges have been met by the advances in the pharmacy management systems and the PBM systems, but further challenges remain. Even more effective clinical and financial systems can be developed, once new challenges and goals are discovered and targeted. To discover these new opportunities will depend squarely upon creating systems that take the online real-time data and present them to the clinical pharmacist or other healthcare knowledge worker in a way that advances prospective DUR, disease state management, incentive-based cost management (rebate programs), and other emerging business models. This analysis requires the systems to reduce huge amounts of data to simple, understandable information for decision-makers. The challenge is to "mine" the information to detect fraud, unanticipated facts, discover trends and patterns, and to organize and present the data for other healthcare and benefit professionals.

The differences between an OLTP system and an online analytical processing (OLAP) system are straightforward. OLTP systems are efficient operational systems that adjudicate claims and collect data, while OLAP systems transform the data collected by the OLTP systems into decision support tools (**Figure 7-5**). These decision support tools then enable the clinical pharmacist to concentrate on the information being gathered and to act upon the data by making changes to the OLTP system, by interacting with the affected patient population, the prescribing population, or by designing outcomes studies to further explore health situations.

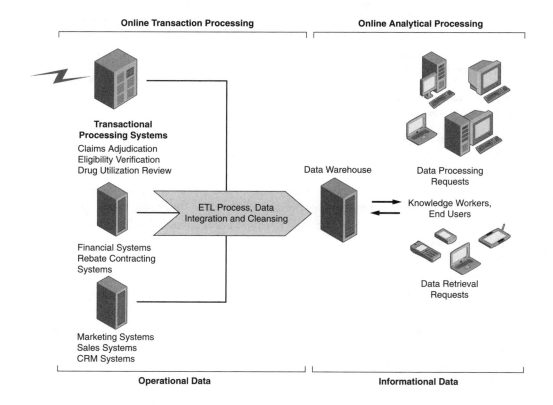

FIGURE 7-5 OLTP to OLAP.

OLAP systems are often called *data warehouses* or *data marts*. The graphical presentation of the relational or multidimensional views of these data repositories are often termed *decision support systems* or *executive information systems*. A data warehouse is a process whereby data from transaction-based systems are collected, integrated, and delivered to end users expressly to support data or clinical analysis activities. An OLAP system assembles the data, transforms the raw data into a form suitable for analysis, distributes the data, and provides access to the information store. Today, virtually every MCO has some type of data repository and many have several tailored to capitalize on unique opportunities.

This idea of extracting the data from disparate systems, transforming it, and delivering it to the end users is popularly known as "business intelligence." Simply put, these systems are a home for second hand data for utilization data, customer relationship management (CRMs) data, marketing data, and rebate data. The transformation of all these data from different systems involves checking them for gaps, missing values, business rules, and looking at the data for reasonableness (**Figure 7-6**).

In addition, the transformation process may add values for the end users, like tagging a utilization record with a disease state. The goal of business intelligence is to deliver the right amount of information and analytical power to fit the user. One of the tenets of business

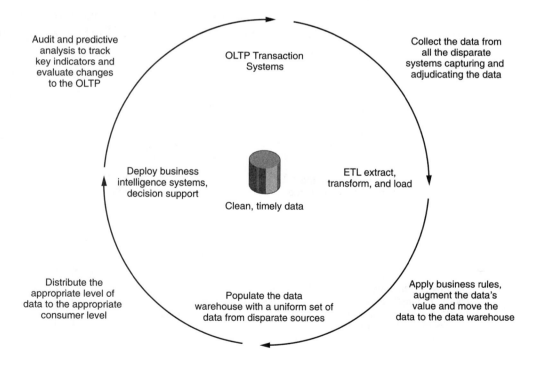

FIGURE 7-6   Data Warehousing Process.

intelligence is the fact that not all users of data have the same sophistication or the same goals. Users can range from a dedicated power user like a data analyst to the casual user or a report consumer. The distribution of these consumers resembles a pyramid with a small number of report authors to a large number of report consumers or readers (**Figure 7-7**). The tools employed can range from simple reports to business intelligence tools that require months of training and a strong educational background in mathematics, statistics, and the appropriate clinical disciplines. These are known as the *power users*. Coupled with delivering the right amount of information to the right users is also the ability to secure the information. Allowing for legal and appropriate access to the correct level of information by user class is just another challenge facing businesses dealing with the technology and information explosion. This security issue is critical to HIPAA and must be considered in protecting the rights of patients, while still permitting the analysis of information critical to the advancement of all related disciplines.

Managed care organizations define key metrics from the data repositories to measure their organization's progress. Examples of key metrics are per-member-per month (PMPM) pharmacy cost, average number of prescriptions per thousand members (Rx/1,000 members), and member cost share percentage. This ability to use metrics to score card or present a management dashboard is an important trend in all industries today. OLAP is a key technology putting these informational tools together.

OLAP systems are typically run on different computer hardware and software than OLTP systems, so the performance of the operational systems (OLTP) is not affected by

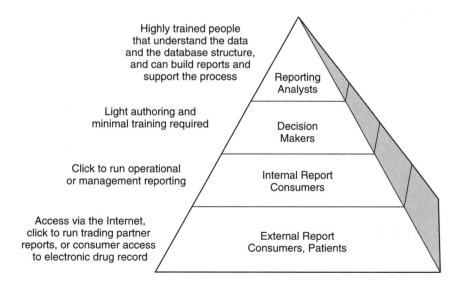

FIGURE 7-7 **Pyramid of Reporting Roles.**

OLAP processing. The tuning of the hardware and software systems can be set up specifically to support the unique needs and processing requirements of OLAP. The analytical systems also can integrate data from a variety of sources. For example, it is possible to integrate patients' drug history information with their medical and lab claims information to get a complete picture of their health state.

Forecasting based on accurate information in these data repositories is an area receiving a lot of attention. Using predictive modeling to provide an organization links to patients needing case management, modeling historical benefit information, and predicting drug costs and rebates is a vital and growing outgrowth of the OLAP systems. This predictive modeling is based on the use of algorithms and supporting technology to focus on appropriate clinical programs to match the population. The processes and programs can be used to identify high risk patients before they reach a crisis and assist with care management. This predictive technology is also being applied to project the future cost of new benefit designs by analyzing copay tiers, deductibles, benefit maximums, and healthcare spending accounts to derive new benefit plans to achieve specified objectives. Software tools exist that allow the testing of a yet-to-be-tried benefit plan against great volumes of historical data. The success of the plan can be tested before it is introduced into the marketplace. Other software tools are designed to "mine the data" or to look for hidden relationships in the data instead of making assumptions about the data. These mining activities can lead to innovative ideas and the discovery of clinical and financial relationships between drug utilization, health state, future patient drug spend trends, and other important measurements. Of course, the key to predictive analytics and data mining is having clean data in the source data repository and the right tools and personnel to exploit the data.

Information can be an important force in changing patient behavior, educating physicians, and modifying online transaction-based systems. Using OLAP-powered informational systems in tandem with the claims adjudication engines and transaction systems can empower an MCO to use the pharmaceutical channel to become a quality supplier of healthcare services.

CONCLUSION

The pharmaceutical delivery and claims adjudication channel has exploited and adopted emerging computer and communication technology spurred on by new electronic data interchange standards. In just decades, pharmacy systems have evolved from paper-based, manually intensive systems that took long periods of time to process claims, to sophisticated and powerful electronic recordkeeping systems that can exchange data to adjudicate a claim or gather information for pharmaceutical care in seconds.

The early adjudication systems have evolved from offering simple eligibility verification and basic transaction editing to providing full-fledged pharmaceutical care influencing patient and physician behavior. These systems will probably always manage drug costs but also will continue to evolve to encompass clinical guidelines developed from analyzing billions of transactions from online analytical systems and offering information to the consumers to make more cost-effective benefit decisions.

Influences of government policies and programs will continue to have a major impact on the function and expense of the pharmacy information systems. The last few years of government regulations around PART D, HIPAA, and National Provider Indicator (NPI) have resulted in regulation fatigue for many healthcare information departments. The other driving force to watch is the innovative cost-sharing plans between employers and benefit recipients. Pharmacy systems are now being interfaced with medical systems for single (or integrated) deductible programs. They also are being designed to support and interface with increasingly available patient-flexible spending accounts. They are even being interfaced with credit card systems in today's ever increasingly cashless world. These interfaces and programs make it easier for the patient to assume an equitable cost share and obtain needed medications quickly and easily. Continued evolution of these systems will continue to require information technology resources and dedicated pharmacy professionals to design and adapt technology to the future challenges of these systems.

Recent drivers in systems design have concentrated on meeting the demands of new government programs that favor consumer-driven healthcare benefits and the need to provide seamless integration with other healthcare or finance systems. These drivers have been the largest factors impacting the adjudication systems in recent years. Significant cost pressures due to increases in pharmacy costs have forced information technology staffs to push more data out to the consumer. The new consumer-driven health plans demand that patients have the information to make intelligent decisions regarding their own healthcare dollars.

The government regulations like HIPAA have forced information technology staffs to redesign their pharmacy systems both in the pharmacy and on the payor side to accept new transaction sets. In addition to changing transaction sets, the privacy regulations have placed a daunting burden on system designers. Data must be secured and access constantly documented. However, locking down the systems can only go so far before it interferes with business operations. Therefore, a balance must be struck in the organization between operational efficiency and security, while still respecting all patients' rights. It is imperative that technology be coupled with new procedures and training on these new regulations throughout all parts of healthcare administrative and provider organizations.

Use of these pharmacy informational systems will continue to advance, driven by cost containment, consumerism, new government regulations, new business practices, competition, and technology. Pharmacists will assist in designing innovative benefit plans, analyzing clinical issues from the OLAP systems, and improving patient care prospectively by designing new edits placed in the online transaction systems and interfacing with the dispensing pharmacy systems. To continue to deliver comprehensive pharmaceutical care, pharmacists will be required to analyze the captured transactions in data warehouses, assist in the engineering of new pharmacy systems, and ultimately shape the future of the pharmaceutical care channel with information technology.

ACRONYMS

AMP	average manufacturer's price
AWP	average wholesale price (drug)
CDHP	consumer-driven health plans
CMS	Centers for Medicare and Medicare Services
CRM	customer relationship management (data)
DSL	Digital Subscriber Line
DUR	drug utilization review
HIPAA	Health Insurance Portability and Accountability Act
HTML	Hyper Text Markup Language
ISP	Internet Service Provider
MCOs	managed care organizations
NCPDP	National Council for Prescription Drug Programs
NPI	National Provider Identifier
OLAP	online analytical processing
OLTP	online transaction processing
PBMSs	prescription benefit management systems
PBMs	pharmacy benefit managers, pharmacy benefit management (companies)
PMSs	pharmacy management systems
POS	point-of-service (pharmacy)

TCP/IP	Terminal Control Protocol over Internet Protocol
U&C	usual and customary (retail price)
UCF	Universal Claim Form
WAC	wholesale acquisition cost
Web	World Wide Web

Chapter 8

DRUG UTILIZATION REVIEW STRATEGIES

ANDREW M. PETERSON

VICKY CHAN

MARCUS D. WILSON

A major emphasis in today's healthcare system is balancing the quality of care with the cost of care. Hospitals, healthcare systems, managed care organizations (MCOs), and pharmacy benefit managers (PBMs) struggle to achieve this balance daily. Central to this theme is the appropriate use of medical services, including drugs. Pharmacy practitioners are charged with evaluating how drugs are used in individuals as well as in populations. One method of evaluating how drugs are used is through a systematic process called *drug utilization review (DUR)*.

Other terms often considered synonymous to DUR are drug use evaluation (DUE), medication use evaluation (MUE), and medication use management. In this chapter, we will use the term DUR unless the situation requires an alternative term. Regardless of the terminology, DUR programs can save money and improve quality of care by curtailing the use of unnecessary or inappropriate drugs and by preventing the adverse effects of misused medications. This chapter describes the role of DUR programs in pharmacy benefit management and discusses programs that use prescription claims data to accomplish DUR objectives.

HISTORY AND CURRENT ROLE OF DUR

DUR has matured into a quality assurance and improvement activity and is now mandated by the Joint Commission on Accreditation of Healthcare Organizations (Joint Commission), the National Committee for Quality Assurance (NCQA), and the federal government. DUR is intended to ensure appropriate drug therapy. In 1972, Brodie published an important paper that defined the DUR process as the "ongoing study of the frequency of use and cost of drugs, from which patterns of prescribing, dispensing, and patient use can be determined."[1] In 1976, Brodie and Smith published a conceptual model for DUR based on five utilization review principles.[2] These principles outlined are the basic structural components of all DUR programs then and now (**Table 8-1**). In essence, these principles suggest that a DUR program must have the authority to review the use of drugs through available information and that the results of the review must be compared to standards put forth by knowledgeable professionals. A year later, Brodie and colleagues published a model description of DUR programs based on these criteria.[3]

Stolar furthered the concept of DUR by stating that for a DUR program to ensure the quality of drug use, it had to be authorized, structured, and continuous. DUR programs must measure the use of drugs against predetermined criteria and initiate changes in drug use patterns that do not meet these criteria.[4] The added criteria of continuous review and change initiation helped transform DUR from simply a study of drug usage patterns to a full evaluation of clinical drug use.

A complete DUR program is "the system by which quality drug use is defined, measured, and ultimately achieved."[4] DUR programs are qualitative studies with corrective action, prescriber feedback, and reevaluation. This not only achieves the improved patient care objective but also provides substantial benefit to the pharmacist and prescriber.

Early in the 1980s, the Joint Commission focused on evaluating antibiotics because of their growing cost and use in hospital settings. From 1981 to 1985, the term *antibiotic utilization review* appeared in the Joint Commission accreditation standards several times, placing the responsibility only on the medical staff, with the assistance of the department of pharmacy. These standards required the medical staff to review the appropriateness, safety, and effectiveness of the prophylactic, empiric, and therapeutic use of all antibiotics in all patient care areas based on established criteria. In 1986, the emphasis on antibiotics was broadened; hence, DUE became a more popular term. It was not until the 1994 standards were published that "DUE" was removed from the standards and replaced by "MUE."[5] MUE is similar to DUE except that the Joint Commission requires a multidisciplinary approach to improving patient outcomes. This reflects the variety of users (nurses, physicians, and pharmacists) involved in using medications. **Table 8-2** lists the important processes evaluated in DUE and MUE.

TABLE 8-1 DUR Structural Principles

- Authority derived from an appropriate source
- Availability of operational and demographic characteristics of the delivery system and population served
- Availability of existing profiles of drug usage
- Standards of appropriateness against which drug usage can be reviewed and judged
- A scheme of evaluation through which the impact of review can be measured

Source: Brodie, D.C., Smith, W.E., Constructing a conceptual model of drug utilization review. *Hospitals.* 1976; 50: 143-150.

TABLE 8-2 Processes Evaluated in DUE and MUE

- Prescribing medications
- Preparing medications
- Dispensing medications
- Administering medications
- Monitoring efficacy and safety

Pharmacists and other practitioners generally accept the definition of MUE used by the Joint Commission and the American Society of Health-System Pharmacists. Recently, the NCQA promulgated new standards for utilization management incorporating the tenets of DUR.[6] These organizations state that DUR is a criteria-based, ongoing, planned, and systematic process designed to continually improve the appropriate and effective use of drugs. This definition applies whether DUR is focused on an individual drug or is looking at various drugs used to treat a specific disease. In addition, it is important to note that the responsibility for drug use does not rest solely with physicians or pharmacists, but falls on all persons that are involved in the use of medications (e.g., nurses, respiratory therapists, and patients). In 1990, the federal government enacted the Omnibus Budget Reconciliation Act (OBRA '90), which required a review of drug utilization in the ambulatory care setting. The law requires the prospective and retrospective review of drug utilization, specifically for Medicaid patients.[7]

Today, the distinction among MUE, DUE, and DUR is based mainly on the origin of the terms, not the process. DUE is used by NCQA, MUE is used by the Joint Commission, and DUR is used in OBRA '90. However, the goal of each of these endeavors is the same: to measure and enhance the use of medications.

Benefits of DUR to the pharmacist include expanding the opportunity to identify and resolve drug-drug interactions, therapeutic duplications, and under- and overdosing problems, all on the patient's behalf. Most pharmacists act as patient advocates whenever a new prescription is filled. However, using a comprehensive DUR program, pharmacists can further identify trends in prescribing and drug utilization for an entire population and improve drug therapy within groups of patients, not just individuals. Moreover, complete DUR programs require documentation of the intervention(s) and thus provide a mechanism for pharmacists to demonstrate their value as professionals.[8]

Prescribers benefit from DUR as well because the process not only improves the quality of care for their patients but also allows comparison among prescribers regarding their use of drugs in treating specific disease states. This comparative information is often effective in changing physician prescribing patterns in an effort to improve patient care.[9] For example, many healthcare plans use DUR to encourage physician compliance with formulary drugs and use of generics.

TYPES OF DURs

Assessment of drug use can be performed through a retrospective, concurrent, or prospective study design.[10] Each type has its advantages and disadvantages. Retrospective studies evaluate drug therapy that has already been given, concurrent studies evaluate drug therapy being presently administered, and prospective studies evaluate drug therapy prior to administration.

RETROSPECTIVE REVIEWS

A retrospective review is the simplest to implement and perform. Data regarding drug therapy that has already been administered to a patient are reviewed to determine if that therapy met approved criteria. This is often a screening step in identifying potential problems requiring increased scrutiny and intervention. Retrospective studies are not time-dependent and require limited resources. **Table 8-3** outlines some of the items that can be identified using retrospective DUR.

Curtis et al. published the results of a retrospective DUR analyzing the extent of potentially inappropriate outpatient medications prescribed to elderly patients. The data were retrieved from a large pharmacy benefit manager and showed approximately 21% of patients filled a prescription that may be of concern based on the revised Beers list. This analysis is beneficial in that it identifies which medications of concern are most routinely prescribed in practice for future physician detailing and intervention opportunities.[11]

The disadvantages of retrospective review include issues around timing and reliability. Because by definition the event being reviewed has already occurred, the ability to immediately impact patient care is limited. In addition, using historical data may make it difficult to draw strong conclusions. Hennessy and colleagues challenged the validity of retrospective DUR required by state Medicaid programs when results obtained from six Medicaid programs showed no reduction in the rate of potential prescribing errors or hospitalizations. While these endpoints appear appropriate, it is unknown whether all retrospective DUR programs will result in the same outcome or if DUR programs offer other clinical

TABLE 8-3   Items Commonly Identified Using Retrospective DUR

- Abuse/misuse
- Appropriate generic use
- Drug-drug interactions
- Drug-disease contraindication
- Inappropriate duration of treatment
- Incorrect dosage
- Over- and underutilization
- Therapeutic appropriateness
- Therapeutic duplication

Source: American Pharmaceutical Association special report. Opportunities for the community pharmacist in managed care. Washington, DC: American Pharmaceutical Association; 1994.

benefits that were not analyzed. Additionally, not all DUR programs are designed with decreased hospitalizations as an endpoint, which may be difficult to achieve utilizing these methods, further complicating how these results should be applied.[12]

Retrospective reviews of drug use patterns can assist plans in developing strategies for more comprehensive and relevant prospective DUR. For example, Wilson and associates retrospectively studied pharmacy claims data of patients with hypertension from six managed care plans.[13] Data were extracted, integrated, and subsequently examined to determine the modification patterns by physicians managing these patients and the subsequent impact on economic endpoints and the need for subsequent therapy. The basic findings were that certain drug therapy modification paths appeared to result in better outcomes (i.e., less need for subsequent modifications to therapy). In addition, it was found that patients requiring modification to their regimen had higher subsequent drug costs than those who did not, and that as the number of modifications increased, drug costs rose in a linear fashion.

A subsequent study utilizing a three-year longitudinal, integrated pharmacy/medical claims database not only confirmed these findings with respect to drug costs but also showed a rise in medical costs. Interestingly, it was also found that nonadherent patients (> 80%) had a modest increase in antihypertensive drug costs than adherent patients (9%) but had dramatically higher medical costs (42%) (unpublished data, HealthCore, Wilmington, DE). These findings may contradict the current Zeitgeist that the economic "payoff" for disease management efforts in patients with hypertension is not realized until years later. Instead, they suggest that allocating more resources to educating physicians to make better antihypertensive drug modification decisions may "pay off" almost immediately. In addition, patient education efforts to improve medication adherence could also, in theory, decrease drug costs and could certainly decrease medical costs within the first 12 months of therapy.

CONCURRENT REVIEWS

A concurrent review, often done in the institutional setting, provides the opportunity for corrective actions to be taken during the time the patient is receiving the medication. Such reviews can be conducted through a periodic search of patient profiles for drug-drug interactions or therapeutic duplication. Although the patient may be receiving the medication combination, this type of review allows therapy for a patient to be altered if necessary. This method has the advantage of affecting patient care more directly than retrospective review. However, the logistics of identifying and resolving the problem are more complex than in retrospective reviews. Computerized review of medication profiles assists in the concurrent review process. However, the key physician(s) prescribing the medication must be contacted and the situation discussed for the DUR to be effective. Often this step can be difficult, even disheartening, if a physician is reluctant to change therapy.

Table 8-4 lists some items that can be addressed using a concurrent DUR system. Though the process they used was similar to a concurrent review, Burch and Rascati published a report on the use of "retrospective" DUR to decrease the concurrent use of H_2 antagonists and sucralfate, a therapeutic duplication. In a control group design using physician-directed intervention letters, they saw an absolute difference of 17.9% decreased

TABLE 8-4 Items Commonly Identified Using Concurrent DUR

- Drug-disease contraindications
- Drug-drug interactions
- Drug-gender precautions
- Drug-pregnancy precautions
- Incorrect dosage
- Over- and underutilization
- Therapeutic interchange

Source: American Pharmaceutical Association special report. Opportunities for the community pharmacist in managed care. Washington, DC: American Pharmaceutical Association; 1994.

use of concurrent agents in the experimental group.[14] Though no statistics were provided, the concept that concurrent DUR has positive contributions in the promotion of health is still valid.

PROSPECTIVE REVIEWS

A prospective review occurs before the patient has received the medication. The primary advantage to this type of analysis is that problems are identified and resolved before medication is dispensed. Another advantage to this method is that it serves as an excellent teaching opportunity for pharmacists. However, the potential for conflict between physicians and pharmacists exists and may hinder good patient care if not handled skillfully. A major disadvantage to prospective evaluation is that a very organized and well-defined approach to identifying specific criteria for evaluation and communicating those criteria to all involved is required. Immediate access to patient information is required, making the system more difficult to implement.

The practice of pharmacy inherently involves the prospective review process. Medication orders are reviewed at the time they are received, and if a problem exists, the medication is not dispensed until the problems are resolved. **Table 8-5** outlines some of the items

TABLE 8-5 Items Commonly Identified Using Prospective DUR

- Abuse/misuse
- Drug-allergy interactions
- Drug-disease interactions
- Drug-drug interactions
- Inappropriate duration of treatment
- Incorrect dosage
- Therapeutic duplication
- Therapeutic interchange

Source: American Pharmaceutical Association special report. Opportunities for the community pharmacist in managed care. Washington, DC: American Pharmaceutical Association; 1994.

that can be identified and resolved using prospective DUR. Further discussion of prospective drug use evaluation is found later in this chapter.

STEPS IN CONDUCTING DURs

Various individuals describe the process of conducting a DUR with remarkable similarity. **Table 8-6** outlines the steps in a quality related DUR program. These are based on the Joint Commission 10-step process for conducting MUE programs.[5] A sample DUR is also included to help illustrate how a DUR may be applied in practice. Patients with

TABLE 8-6   Steps in Conducting a DUE/DUR

Step	Discussion
1. Gain organizational authority and assign responsibility	A PBM offers an asthma DUR to one of its HMO clients
2. Delineate scope of DUR	The goal of the DUR is to promote the use of inhaled corticosteroids for members who have consistently filled a prescription for a beta-2 agonist.
3. Identify important specific drugs to be monitored and evaluated	List all beta-2 agonists and all inhaled corticosteroids
4. Identify indicators	Identify members with an ICD-9 code for asthma in their medical claims data. The PBM builds an algorithm to target all members who were dispensed more than three canisters of a beta-2 agonist within the last three months but who have not received an inhaled corticosteroid in the same time period using a database link pharmacy and medical claims
5. Establish thresholds	Identify the expected percentage of members meeting or not meeting the indicators identified
6. Collect and organize data	Apply the algorithm and identify members who fit the criteria for DUR inclusion and organize based on clinical and/or financial considerations
7. Evaluate drug use when thresholds are reached	Determine if the use of the medications is appropriate based on clinical knowledge or mitigating circumstances
8. Take actions to improve drug use	Contact the physician through a DUR letter that includes the latest asthma guidelines and the concern regarding their patient's asthma control
9. Assess effectiveness of actions	Generate a report after the DUR period with the number of canisters of beta-2 agonists and inhaled corticosteroids for the members identified
10. Communicate relevant information to appropriate individuals	Report these findings to the P&T committee

Source: Modified from Joint Commission on Accreditation of Healthcare Organization (JCAHO), *Comprehensive Accreditation Manual for Hospitals (CAMH)*. Oakbrook Terrace, IL: 1996.

asthma who use an inhaled beta-2 agonist more frequently than recommended may have suboptimal asthma control and may require an inhaled corticosteroid. An asthma DUR program implemented at a managed care organization can help improve the care of patients by helping physicians identify those with suboptimal control.

The first step in constructing a quality DUR program is gaining authority from the parent organization and designing an appropriate structure incorporating all potential stakeholders. This should include the PBM, the MCO, and the associated medical and pharmacy staff. While it is difficult to incorporate all participants in a PBM's efforts, it may be helpful to start with a utilization management committee or even a pharmacy and therapeutics (P & T) committee. Within this context, the objectives of the program should be clearly defined. Most often in the managed care environment the DUR objectives are part of the contract for any full-service pharmacy benefit management organization.

Step two is delineating the scope of DUR for a disease state within an MCO's population. Underpinning this is a comprehensive search and critique of peer-reviewed scientific literature, relevant clinical practice guidelines, manufacturer, and collegial information. In many cases, the focus for the evaluation needs to match the type of data available in a medication-only database. It is essential to consult with people experienced in data evaluation and extraction and clinicians experienced with the medications and medical conditions reviewed. The clinicians must then agree on the use of appropriate surrogate markers from the available data.

Third, the drugs to be reviewed must be identified. Again, the clinicians involved as well as the administrative stakeholders must decide on the drug or drugs to be surveyed. Information from retrospective DUR and the medical and pharmacy literature can be used. In addition, new drugs or diseases of recent interest may trigger a DUR study.

The fourth step is for the stakeholders to discuss and decide upon the appropriate measures of quality. Constructing these measures using a medication-only database is often difficult. Surrogate markers of disease or outcomes often must be used because the PBM or MCO may not have access to medical claims or medical chart data on individual patients (patient-level data). In a medication-only database, there exists a vast amount of information: drug class, drug name, dose, frequency, quantity dispensed, supply (number of days), refill history, prescribing provider, dispensing pharmacy, cost, and other demographic data. One could easily construct a profile of regional or population drug use patterns, employer group-specific use patterns, individual patient use patterns, and even provider prescribing patterns.

Fifth, thresholds for optimal use must be established. Thresholds are the standard against which performance is measured. It is not necessary to set absolute standards (e.g., 0% therapeutic duplication or 100% adherence with dosage recommendations) because individual variation should be taken into account, and clinical reasons for one or more of these aberrations may exist. Clinical pharmacists and physician specialists should be involved in the development of thresholds because of their clinical experience with the medication and help establish these reasonable yet optimal limits.

Sixth, data must be collected and organized. Retrospective DURs are best accomplished via computer retrieval of medication use history and claims data. However, because of the vast amount of information available and the old maxim "garbage in—garbage out," having a clear plan for collecting the data is essential. The use of information systems (IS) experts familiar with the data source is essential in this step. Often, the pharmacy specialist must work closely with the IS specialist to develop a realistic and usable data retrieval method.

Seventh, once the data are collected, clinicians compare and evaluate the results against the predetermined thresholds. While this step is often conducted well by experienced pharmacists, care must be taken not to interpret the results too strictly. A discussion of the results with all clinicians involved in the criteria and threshold development would prove a valuable process to ensure that patterns or trends have not been overlooked. Often the criteria themselves must be revised because of an oversight or because of new and emerging yet appropriate trends in the use of the drugs being evaluated.

The next three steps in the process relate to using the information to improve drug use. After the differences between actual and optimal drug use are identified, the authorized body of clinicians must decide what steps need to be taken to correct or change the aberrant patterns of use, assess the effectiveness of these actions, and communicate the findings, actions, and follow-up information to the appropriate individuals. These individuals may be the patients, the providers, or the MCOs.

APPLICATION OF DUR IN PHARMACY BENEFIT MANAGEMENT

Health policy and professional responsibilities have changed during the years since DUR was introduced into the healthcare system. Federal regulations are based on the performance of DUR in the ambulatory setting. Hospitals and healthcare systems are bound to conduct MUE and DUR programs to maintain accreditation. Law has now mandated pharmacist professional responsibilities, such as identifying and resolving drug-related problems. The impact of DUR on today's healthcare system is enormous and continues to grow.

Effective DUR programs became required for all Medicaid patients January 2, 1993, secondary to OBRA '90.[15] This act provides legislation for federal financial participation payments to be made for covered outpatient drugs under the Medicaid program. Each state must have a DUR program. The DUR program must consist of a prospective DUR, a retrospective DUR, application of explicit predetermined criteria, and an educational program. Coupled with this, the state must have established a DUR board consisting of at least one-third physicians and one-third pharmacists. This board is to make recommendations regarding the mix of the interventions (prospective, retrospective, criteria-based, and educational programs) that would most effectively lead to improved drug therapy. The key is that the intervention programs must be based on data reviewed by the board directed at solving or improving an identified drug-related problem. Although OBRA '90 was developed for the Medicaid population, it has since been expanded to all populations because creating a two-tiered system of care would be unethical and potentially generate legal challenges.

The application of a DUR program in pharmacy benefit management, within either a health maintenance organization (HMO) or a PBM, may be intuitively clear to the reader, but a brief discussion is warranted. HMOs that manage their pharmacy benefit through an internal program will develop their own DUR programs. However, as we have discussed in previous chapters, many HMOs and other MCOs contract for the services of PBMs. In providing broad pharmacy benefit management services to a variety of MCOs, PBMs are charged with managing the medication use of one or more populations of patients. As such, they are responsible for understanding and improving the prescribing, administration, and use of medications for their customers' patients. To accomplish this, they must perform a variety of DUR studies as part of a comprehensive DUR program.

In addition to these requirements, OBRA '90 strongly recommends the use of an electronic claim management system to improve the billing and data collection of drug-related dispensing information.[15] These widely used point of sale (POS) systems are important in collating and sorting data used in retrospective and prospective DUR programs.

In the late 1970s, Mount Sinai Medical Center used an electronic data process for DUR. Within his 1979 report, Mehl contends that the "sheer volume of activity in a large institution would necessitate programming and ready availability of even basic information so that drug utilization can be accomplished on a large enough scale to be worthwhile."[16] PBMs may be responsible for millions of members, resulting in tens of millions of prescriptions annually. To evaluate patterns of drug use in this environment, computers are indispensable.

Since the introduction of POS systems, five distinct management functions have arisen for the PBM. They are: 1) eligibility verification; 2) prior authorization for certain drugs; 3) claims submission; 4) claims adjudication; and 5) prospective DUR. Eligibility verification, claims submission, and claims adjudication are beyond the scope of this chapter but are discussed in Chapters 2, 4, 5, and 6. Prior authorization and prospective DUR are inherent in any PBM DUR program and will be discussed below.

PRIOR AUTHORIZATION

Prior authorization programs are intended to prevent the prescribing of certain medications unless defined and specific criteria are first met. Often these agents subject to prior authorization are expensive or dangerous medications with a potential for misuse or abuse. As a result, the PBM or HMO has determined that it will approve these medications for only selected individuals, certain indications, or defined treatment durations. The dispensing pharmacist is alerted to the prior authorization requirement for certain medications through the online POS pharmacy edit messages. For example, a pharmacist may attempt to enter the National Drug Code of a prescribed medication into the pharmacy computer for a given patient. At the POS the claim is transmitted to the PBM for online adjudication. If the medication requires a prior authorization, an online message is transmitted on the screen to the pharmacist indicating a special authorization is required before the medication may be dispensed and reimbursed. The pharmacist then has the responsibility to contact the prescriber and resolve the issue by either changing the medication or having the prescriber obtain authorization for dispensing from the HMO or PBM.

Smalley and associates studied the effect of a prior authorization program on the Medicaid expenditures for nonsteroidal anti-inflammatory drugs (NSAIDs) in Tennessee.[17] Their results showed a reduction of $12.8 million in two years, primarily due to the increased use of generic NSAIDs and a decrease in overall use of NSAIDs. In an analysis of the operational performance of prior authorization, Phillips and Larson noted that the average response time for a prior authorization was 52.4 minutes in the Iowa Medicaid prior authorization program.[18] Using the online verification system, a POS system can further reduce the time needed for authorization. The POS system not only enables quicker processing of claims and fewer charge backs for denials but also assists in prospective DUR by alerting the pharmacist to potentially inappropriate drug use.

PROSPECTIVE DUR

Prospective DUR involves providing guideline information to the prescriber. Prospective DUR occurs before the patient receives the medication; therefore, it must occur before the pharmacist fills the prescription. The pharmacist is required to conduct a review of the drug order before dispensing and proactively resolve any detected or potential drug use problems for the patient. The legislation requires pharmacists to review and resolve problems as listed in Table 8-5.

Prospective DUR occurs when an authorized medication is entered into the computer and alerts the pharmacist of a drug-drug interaction, drug-disease interaction, or other potential problem. Some authors consider these interventions concurrent because the prescribing has occurred. However, because the patient may not have received the medication, other authors consider these interventions prospective.

True prospective DUR programs involve educating the prescriber on the appropriate prescribing of targeted drugs. Because PBMs can generate comparative profiles of physician prescribing, they can design various educational interventions targeting selected physicians who demonstrate inappropriate prescribing history or encouraging all physicians to proactively prevent problems. These targeted interventions take the form of counterdetailing, telephone calls, letters, newsletters, and educational symposia; all of these interventions are designed to improve rational prescribing, formulary compliance, and patient adherence.

Monane and associates prospectively studied the impact of a DUR database linked to a pharmacy telephone intervention program on medication use in the elderly.[19] Using explicitly defined criteria and a computerized alert system, they found 43,007 medication-related problems in 23,269 elderly patients in a 12-month period. They contacted 19,368 physicians regarding the interventions, and the physicians accepted 24% of the recommended changes. The authors concluded that the integrated pharmacist, physician, and computerized alert system improved the prescribing patterns and quality of care for geriatric patients. The success of this DUR program may be attributed to a well designed algorithm to distinguish which medications warranted an intervention as well as relying on pharmacists trained in geriatrics and physician detailing.

In a survey of decision-making tools used by HMOs, Barner and Thomas found that the results of prospective DUR ranked relatively high in frequency and importance for drug decision making, eclipsed only by retrospective DUR and counterdetailing of physicians.[20] (*Counterdetailing* is the use of evidence-based medicine for decision-making rather than "detailing" practices used by pharmaceutical sales representatives to encourage prescribing of a particular drug in their pharmacopoeia.) As stated earlier, this type of intervention results in improved drug therapy because the intervention occurs before the patient receives the medication.

PHYSICIAN EDUCATION PROGRAMS

Because prescribers are often the targets of DUR interventions, appropriate follow-up must be made. The P & T committee should review the results of a DUR program, and the results should be shared with the providers evaluated. The dissemination of information can easily be accomplished through newsletters and direct physician communication. Avorn and Soumerai discuss the concept of *academic detailing*, in which physician prescribing behavior is altered after one-on-one education by doctoral-level trained clinical pharmacists.[21] In this study, 435 physicians were targeted through a review of 12 months of Medicaid prescription claims data. In a random fashion, the physicians were assigned to three groups: 1) physicians that received face-to-face education by a clinical pharmacist; 2) physicians who received printed educational materials by mail; and 3) a control group of physicians who received no intervention. The print material did not produce a significant change in prescribing, but the one-on-one intervention improved the prescribing of targeted drugs by 14%.

In addition to educational interventions, feedback on performance is key to an effective DUR process. Feedback includes providing physicians with descriptions of their past prescribing behaviors, which may or may not include a comparison of these patterns with those of peers or predefined criteria. For example, Groves reported on the Florida Medicaid program, which used computer-generated mail notification of overuse or underuse of medications, contraindications, and adverse reactions.[22] The results showed a 50% change in prescribing behavior as a result of the feedback to physicians.

Early involvement of respected peers throughout the implementation and evaluation phases in the DUR program is likely to be important to the program's success, because opinion leaders have been shown to positively influence physician practice patterns. Other data suggest that clinicians prefer receiving brief manuals, executive summaries of guideline recommendations, or synopses of the supporting evidence and quantification of the expected benefits.[23]

PERFORMANCE MEASUREMENT OF DUR PROGRAMS

As noted earlier, DUR programs focus on the quality of care and the resultant cost savings associated with improved quality. Defining quality in the pharmacy benefit management context means focusing on the various customers of the PBM: patients, clients, providers, and other stakeholders. Therefore, the goal of each individual DUR program depends on the customer being served. **Table 8-7** outlines potential DUR goals and associated customers.

DUR has been useful in identifying areas for potential cost savings in pharmacy practice. Studies have shown its efficacy in uncovering medication problems and improving drug therapy.[19,24,25] The impact of DUR on cost is easier to quantify than is DUR's effect on quality of care. Cost reduction (in dollars spent on drugs) is a common variable used when reviewing drug use. Changes in the quality of care are more difficult to measure.

Quality measures most often involve clinical and humanistic (quality of life) measures. Claims data systems were initially constructed without consideration to their eventual use as assessment tools for non-economic factors.[26] Given that currently the most common data sources for DUR activities are pharmacy (and sometimes medical) claims databases, noneconomic outcome measures involve a great number of assumptions if claims data are used. These databases can detail what happened to the patients and when, but they cannot tell why. For example, in the study by Wilson and associates, a careful review of the claims data revealed that more than 50% of patients adherent with hypertension therapy had no modifications to their drug regimen over a 12-month period.[13] While this implies patients had reached their "goal" blood pressure, this cannot be definitively determined from the claims data. Many of the patients could be at a blood pressure that is considered satisfactory by the patient and provider but may be well above 140/90 mmHg. Thus, the percent of patients with controlled blood pressure, defined as less than 140/90 mmHg, cannot be determined in using only claims data.

In cases such as this, validation studies can be accomplished to increase the accuracy of interpreting claims findings. Using the above example, there could be a study comparing the levels of blood pressure control of the patients with no modification to therapy with the levels of blood pressure control of those with one or more modifications to therapy. This would provide a clinical basis for future claims evaluation using an identical approach.

EVOLUTION OF DUR

There are several large issues that will affect the future of DUR. Improved data systems and software applications and the growing use of relational databases and data warehouses are drastically improving the capabilities and efficiencies of claims-based analyses. MCOs have adopted the idea of sharing their results, as evidenced by the growing number of recent published literature with DUR data. This type of health outcomes research has

TABLE 8-7 DUR Goals and Customers

Goal	Customer
Cost reduction	Patient, Client MCO
Improved quality of care	Patient, Client MCO
Education of providers	Client MCO, Provider

grown as MCOs continue to strive for the most cost-effective care for their members. In addition, the methodology for merging claims data with clinical outcome markers is evolving. As noted by Bowman, this marriage of data is necessary to make the leap from DUR to a more comprehensive "healthcare utilization evaluation" (HUE).[27] The evolution of DUE/DUR into HUE is the next logical step, because drugs are such an integral part of medical care and affect the economic, clinical, and personal outcomes of patients.

CONFIDENTIALITY

One major issue associated with integrating and using these large databases is the debate around patient confidentiality. In December 2000, the Department of Health and Human Services released the final version of the privacy regulations, thus paving the way to continue DUR programs as long as they are in support of the organizations core services and the organization takes all necessary precautions. Many MCOs have taken action to protect patient confidentiality while still fulfilling their responsibilities to members.[28] Of note, research of any type is not considered a "core" service and each study is subject to different requirements under the regulations. For the purposes of research, for example, patient identifiers must be removed by specified methods prior to the conduct of research on the data. If information protected under the HIPAA provisions is deemed necessary for the completion of the research project, the investigators are required to gain informed consent from each patient or have the protocol reviewed by an Institutional Review Board (IRB), which must grant to the investigator a waiver of this consent prior to working with the data.

Pharmacists must continue to be patients' rights advocates but must also consider the need for access to drug and medical information, with the ultimate goal of improving patient care. Warholak-Juarez et al.'s study showed that pharmacists can make better decisions when they have greater access to patient information. The quality of their DUR decisions were heavily influenced by how much information was provided, demonstrating the need to access pertinent patient information.[29]

CONCLUSION

Pharmacists have always been involved in analyzing the effect of drug therapy when they have had the ability to collect data or interact with a patient. Managed care presents both challenges and opportunities for DUR. Managed care provides greater access to data and the legal responsibility to identify and correct aberrant drug use patterns. However, the managed care system also can prove frustrating due to the large number of patients to monitor, the enormous amount of data generated, and the lack of resources required for interacting with prescribing physicians. System automation will allow the process to be performed more expeditiously. DUR will only grow in importance as the quest to optimize drug therapy becomes more acute, and pharmacists will have the opportunity to be population-based pharmacotherapy managers.

REFERENCES

1. Brodie D.C., Drug utilization review/planning. *Hospitals.* 1972; s46: 103-112.

2. Brodie E.D. and Smith W.E., Constructing a conceptual model of drug utilization review. *Hospitals.* 1976; 50: 143-150.

3. Brodie D.C., Smith W.E. Jr., Hlynka J.N., Model for drug usage review on a hospital. *American Journal of Hospital Pharmacy.* 1977; 34: 251-254.

4. Stolar M., Drug use review: operational definitions. *Am J Hosp Pharm.* 1978; 33: 225-230.

5. Accreditation Manual for Hospitals. Chicago: Joint Commission on Accreditation of Healthcare Organizations; 1995.

6. Standards for the Accreditation of Managed Care Organizations. Washington, DC: National Committee on Quality Assurance; 1999: 55-68.

7. Palumbo F., Drug use review under OBRA 90. *US Pharmacist.* 1993; April: 84-94.

8. Sleath B., McCament-Mann L., Collins T., Hollarbush J., Response forms reflect pharmacists' participation in retrospective DUR. *J Am Pharmaceut Assoc.* 1997; 37: 77-84.

9. Edgren B., DUR and DUE in managed competition. *J Res.* 1996; 7: 117-127.

10. Kubacka R., A primer on drug utilization review. *J Am Pharmaceut Assoc.* 1996; 36: 257-279.

11. Curtis L.H., Ostbye T., Sendersky V., et al. Inappropriate prescribing for elderly Americans in a large outpatient population. *Arch Intern Med.* 2004; 164: 1621-1625.

12. Hennessy S., Bilker W.B., Zhou L., et al., Retrospective drug utilization review, prescribing errors, and clinical outcomes. *JAMA.* 2003; 290: 1494-1499.

13. Wilson M., Patwell J., Shoheiber O., et al., Clinical and economic implications of drug utilization patterns in the treatment of hypertension with ACE inhibitors and calcium channel blockers in a managed care setting. *J Manag Care Pharm.* 1998; 4(March-April): 194-202.

14. Burch C. and Rascati K., Promotion of the appropriate use of outpatient drug therapy in the Texas Medicaid program through retrospective drug use review. *Pharm Pract Manag.* 1995; 15(no. 2): 57-64.

15. Palumbo F.B., Drug use review under OBRA 90. *US Pharmacist.* 1993; 18: 86-90.

16. Mehl B., Use of electronic data processing for drug utilization review. *Orb Qual Rev Bull.* 1979; 5(Jan): 13-16.

17. Smalley W.E., Griffin M.R., Fought R.L., et al., Effect of a prior authorization requirement on the use of nonsteroidal anti-inflammatory drugs by Medicaid patients. *N Engl J Med.* 1995; 332(June): 1612-1617.

18. Phillips C.R. and Larson L.N., Evaluating the operational performance and financial effects of a drug prior authorization program. *J Manag Care Pharm.* 1997; 3 (November-December): 699-706.

19. Monane M., Metthias D.M., Nagle B.A., Kelly M.A., Improving prescribing patterns for the elderly through an online drug utilization review intervention. *JAMA.* 1998; 280: 1249-1252.

20. Barner J.C. and Tools T.J., Information sources, and methods used in deciding on drug availability in HMOs. *Am J Health-Syst Pharm.* 1998; 55 (January): 50-56.

21. Avorn J. and Soumerai S., Improving drug therapy decisions through educational outreach: A randomized controlled trial of academically based "detailing." *N Engl J Med.* 1983; 308: 1457-1463.

22. Groves R.E., Therapeutic drug use review for the Florida Medicaid program. *Am J Hosp Pharm.* 1985; 42(February): 316-319.

23. Greco P.J. and Eisenberg J.M., Changing physicians' practices. *N Engl J Med* 1993; 329(October): 1271-1274.

24. Keating E.J., Maximizing generic substitution in managed care. *J Manag Care Pharm.* 1998; 4(Nov-Dec): 557-563.

25. Phillips C.R., Larson, L.N., Evaluating the operational performance and financial effects of a drug prior authorization program. *J Manag Care Pharm.* 1997; 3(Nov-Dec): 699-706.

26. Schafermeyer K.W., Basics of managed care claims processing: from claims payment to outcomes management. *J Manag Care Pharm.* 1995; 1(no. 3): 200-205.

27. Bowman L., Drug use evaluation is DUE: Healthcare utilization evaluation is over-DUE. *Hosp Pharm.* 1996; 31(no. 4): 347-353.

28. Curtiss F.R., HIPAA effects on health research and PBM functions in drug utilization review. *J Manag Care Pharm.* 2003; 9(1): 95-97.

29. Warholak-Juarez T., Rupp M.T., Salazar T.A., Foster S., Effect of patient information on the quality of pharmacists' drug use review decisions. *J Am Pharm Assoc.* 2000; 40: 500-508.

ACRONYMS

DUE	drug use evaluation
DUR	drug utilization review
HIPAA	Health Insurance Portability and Accountability Act
HMOs	health maintenance organizations
HUE	healthcare utilization evaluation
MCOs	managed care organizations
MUE	medication use evaluation
NCQA	National Committee for Quality Assurance
NSAIDs	nonsteroidal anti-inflammatory drugs
OBRA '90	Omnibus Budget Reconciliation Act of 1990
PBMs	pharmacy benefit managers, pharmacy benefit management (companies)
POS	point-of-service (pharmacy)
P & T	Pharmacy & Therapeutics (Committee)

ROLE OF DRUG FORMULARIES IN MANAGED CARE ORGANIZATIONS

ROBERT P. NAVARRO

MICHAEL J. DILLON

JAMES E. GRZEGORCZYK

INTRODUCTION

Escalating pharmacy benefit costs and utilization of prescription drugs require a mechanism to support the appropriate use of the most cost-effective pharmaceuticals to achieve the desired clinical, economic, and quality of life outcomes. Managed care pharmacy directors have followed the lead of hospital pharmacies and adopted drug formularies to achieve these goals. Formularies have become an essential structural component of an effective managed care drug benefit. This chapter will briefly explore the development of drug formularies, discuss their use in managed pharmacy programs to support cost and quality of care objectives, and describe future changes in formulary development and enforcement.

GENESIS OF MODERN DRUG FORMULARIES

The concept of a pharmacopeia or drug formulary as a compendium of recommended drugs developed by healthcare facilities or regulatory bodies has existed for at least 200 years in the United States. Formularies are *de rigueur* in all hospitals, many long-term care facilities, and in most public and private third party prescription drug programs, including commercial insurance products, Medicaid, and Medicare Part D. Medicare Part D formularies must observe the drug coverage requirements of the Centers for Medicare Services (CMS)[1] and the U.S. Pharmacopoeia (USP) Formulary Model Guideline recommendations.[2]

Early formularies in the United States were primarily compilations of formulas and recipes used to prepare medicines. The first hospital formulary, the Lititz Pharmacopoeia (1778), attempted to standardize compounding and dispensing of medicines in military hospitals that were set up during the Revolutionary War.[3] The first civilian hospital formulary was the Pharmacopoeia of the New York Hospital (1816) and is worth mentioning in that it was the first attempt to incorporate the opinions of a hospital's medical staff in the development of an institutional formulary.[4]

The hospital formulary system, the progenitor of managed care formularies, began to significantly develop drug management systems in the 1920s.[5] In 1925, 45 physicians and a pharmacist at Syracuse University Hospital established a scientific basis for drug control and reduction of therapeutic duplications through its drug therapy program. The New York Hospital completed a similar project in 1932.[6]

During the 1960s, the formulary system was established in virtually every hospital in the United States. This process was aided by the publication of the American Hospital Formulary Service by the American Society of Hospital Pharmacists (ASHP) in 1959.[7] The so-called "service" was a loose-leaf binder that an institution could selectively adopt and not an unyielding national formulary.[3] The flexibility of the "service" allowed even the smallest hospital to incorporate a formulary system into its operating policies. Today, the ASHP has been transformed into the American Society of Health-System Pharmacists,[8] and remains a definitive source of drug formulary information and drug formulary system management resources.[9]

The hospital formulary had evolved into a model of control and standardization of drugs as well as the embodiment of the drug use policies of the pharmacy and therapeutics (P & T) Committee. The P & T Committee consisted primarily of physicians and pharmacists who were charged with reviewing available drugs and determining which drugs would be expected to provide the most cost-effective outcomes, and would be allowed to be prescribed. The functions of the P & T Committee are thoroughly reviewed in Chapter 13. The federal Health Maintenance Organization (HMO) Act of 1973 spawned the birth of many HMOs. Most of the early HMOs were staff and group model HMOs, and they often established their own on-premises pharmacies that dispensed drugs prescribed by HMO staff physicians or affiliated medical groups. These prescriptions were filled by the members in the HMO's own pharmacy, usually located within the medical building. This "captive" drug purchasing and dispensing process was remarkably similar to that of a hospital. HMO pharmacy directors used their hospital experience and created their own P & T Committees and proprietary drug formulary. Issues surrounding drug selection and inventory control in the HMO were very easily resolved using the hospital's model of a formulary system.

As managed care expanded from the staff and group model HMOs to the more prevalent independent practice association, network HMO, and preferred provider organization (PPO) models in the 1980s, the managed care formulary system continued to evolve and became an integral component of many health plans' pharmacy benefit management programs. No longer utilized primarily to manage the inventories of health plan-owned pharmacies, formularies and formulary systems in managed care serve as the foundation for today's prescription drug benefit. In 1989, just 39% of all HMOs reported using formularies. This statistic increased to 67% by 1992.[10] The number of HMOs with formularies grew to 80.6% in 1994 and 93% in 1997,[11] and today virtually all insurance companies, managed care organizations (MCOs), Medicaid programs, Medicare Part D plans, the Veterans Administration Hospitals, and even many physician group practices use a drug formulary to manage the cost and utilization of prescription drugs for which they have responsibility.

FORMULARY DEFINITIONS

The simplest definition of a drug formulary is that it is a list of recommended medications developed and updated by the issuing organization that applies to physicians who prescribe, pharmacists who dispense, and patients who obtain medications as a result of a relationship with the organization. The Draft ASHP Guidelines on Formulary System Management[9] define a drug formulary and formulary system as follows:

> "A formulary is a continually updated list of medications and related information, representing the clinical judgment of pharmacists, physicians, and other experts in the diagnosis and/or treatment of disease and promotion of health. A formulary system is an ongoing process whereby a healthcare organization, through its physicians, pharmacists, and other healthcare professionals, establishes policies on the use of drug products and therapies, and identifies those that are most medically appropriate and cost-effective to best serve the health interests of a given patient population."[12]

It is a uniquely dynamic system that represents the current body of pharmaceutical knowledge and medical community practice standards in the healthcare setting it serves. Formularies are regularly evaluated by a committee of experts, primarily physicians and pharmacists, working within the healthcare setting. This committee is most often called the P & T Committee, which is the body that is responsible for developing, managing, updating, and administering the formulary.[13]

Formularies have been defined as being "open" (covering a broad array of drugs) or "closed" (covering a more limited number of drugs), although the formulary type is highly dependent upon the MCO model and the insurance product. An open formulary (typical of many Blue Cross–Blue Shield health plans) implies that all or most drugs are available for reimbursement at some level, but that non-preferred brand drugs, or even some non-formulary drugs, are reimbursable on a higher copayment tier. Open formularies offer more choice, but as a result of fewer restrictions, the cost of an open formulary is often greater than of a closed formulary.

A closed formulary may be found more typically in a highly controlled staff or group model health plan, with in-house pharmacies and employee-physicians (e.g., Kaiser Permanente). Closed formularies often include fewer drugs but are a positive list of drugs that are reimbursed and drugs not included are not eligible for reimbursement. In a closed formulary, a non-formulary drug only can be reimbursed if a member pays cash for the drug at the pharmacy, or through an approved medical exception or appeal by the member's physician. This limitation in the number and type of drugs covered often frustrates community-based physicians as well as members. Health plans offering Medicare Advantage programs with a Part D drug benefit are at financial risk for medical and pharmacy costs and often, but not always, use a closed formulary to help contain drug costs.

The formularies of MCOs are highly individualized and dynamic, and are often somewhere between being open and closed, and may be described best as partially closed or selectively closed. Such formularies are hybrids, limiting prescribing choices within certain therapeutic categories and offering unlimited choice within most other categories. In some cases, such formularies are employed to direct prescribing to preferred agents within a therapeutic category, which may be included in a treatment protocol or clinical guideline. In other cases, entire categories may be closed to prevent payment of prescriptions that are excluded from coverage in a pharmacy benefit plan sponsor. For example, some employer groups may require their MCO or pharmacy benefit management (PBM) to exclude oral contraceptives from their drug formulary for moral or ethical reasons.

Managed care has found a method to combine broader choice allowed with more open formularies and the cost-containment of closed formularies by using open formularies with member copayment tiers that allow choice, but provide financial incentives for physicians to prescribe, and members to accept, the lower cost drugs when therapeutically appropriate. Formulary copayment tiers are discussed later in this chapter.

ROLE AND IMPACT OF DRUG FORMULARIES

From the earliest formularies established in Revolutionary War hospitals to today's electronic versions in managed care, all formulary systems have been most concerned with the safety, efficacy, and appropriateness of drug therapy. While today the federal Food, Drug and Cosmetic Act empowers the Food and Drug Administration (FDA) to evaluate all new drugs for safety and effectiveness, the FDA does not recommend specific new products as being superior to currently available prescription drugs, nor does the FDA monitor current drug use to recommend drug treatment protocols that identify the ideal drug or combination of drugs to use in a particular disease management program. P & T Committees and formulary systems build upon the FDA's findings, supplemented by peer-reviewed published medical and pharmacy research, highly regarded physician specialist recommendations, and centers of medical excellence to identify the most appropriate products to incorporate into their drug formulary.

When a formulary system is designed to balance cost management and clinical outcomes, the system enhances the quality of patient care. However, this result is not achieved by the use of a formulary alone. Formularies do not work in isolation. This effect on quality is most often noted when formularies are incorporated into clinical guidelines or treatment protocols. Formularies that are designed around disease management programs effectively contribute to the program's overall goals: to maximize patient outcomes, to reduce overall direct and indirect medical costs, and to improve the quality of patient care.

The formulary is a means to communicate the pharmacy program eligible drugs as well as the dispensing and reimbursement policies to physicians, pharmacists, and members. Formularies are communicated through various media, including paper (hard copy to physicians, pharmacists, or plan members) and/or electronically (e.g., plan or PBM Internet or Web site posting, email provider or member newsletters, physician e-prescribing systems), and pharmacy point-of-service online adjudication system. Most large health plans and PBMs post their primary drug formulary online for public review.

The formulary's primary goal—to promote safe, effective, and appropriate drug therapy—is often overshadowed by the public's perception of the formulary as a highly restrictive cost containment device. The formulary system's ability to achieve pharmacy program cost containment is viewed by detractors as the only reason for formularies' existence. Fueled by anecdotal claims that drug formularies are confusing, limit physician choice, and only cover the lowest cost products, formulary systems and policies are often criticized and challenged.[14–16] These findings contradict the experience of decades of formulary use. The fact remains that the studies conducted thus far "justify only cautious inferences about causation"[17] and that, to date, no study conducted in a managed care setting has demonstrated a direct cause and effect relationship between formulary limitations and higher health utilization.[18,19]

It is a fact that formularies do contain costs and have been doing so since their incorporation into hospital pharmacy practice. A key reason formularies were started was to control inventories. Now, managed care formularies control costs by ensuring appropriate healthcare outcomes while balancing cost with quality objectives. Formularies are necessary for two additional reasons: 1) enforcement of a "generics first" maximum allowable cost (MAC) policy, and, 2) implementation of a rebate or contracting relationship with pharmaceutical manufacturers.

The MAC program was discussed in Chapter 2. To summarize, the formulary is a vehicle through which generic drug use is encouraged with lower Tier I copayments (whenever clinically appropriate). Without a formulary structure, a MAC program cannot be enforced. The level of generic dispensing varies among plans depending upon their model type and level of generic use aggressiveness. Closed model plans are often able to achieve more than 90% of total prescriptions dispensed as generic drugs. Open model, individual practice association (IPA), or preferred provider organization (PPO) health plans may have 50% to 70% of prescriptions dispensed generically. An aggressive generic substitution program may reduce pharmacy program costs significantly compared with unmanaged prescription costs. The generic discount is obtained by reducing the pharmacy reimbursement on highly competitive generic drug products that are subject to significant wholesale and generic drug manufacturer discounts and incentives to community pharmacies. The role of generic drugs in a managed care drug formulary is discussed in greater depth later in Chapter 15.

An enforceable formulary system is necessary to obtain rebate or discount contracts from pharmaceutical manufacturers (see Chapter 15). Open model health plans and PBMs using a community pharmacy network may obtain rebates from pharmaceutical manufacturers in exchange for improving the formulary position of the rebated drug.

Closed model health plans or any organization that takes possession of drug products may obtain a similar rebate or chargeback discount. The rebate on branded drugs may average 8% to 12%, also some brand drugs are not rebated, and some have much higher rebates.

Therefore, with an enforceable drug formulary, the generic program savings and brand drug rebates can significantly reduce pharmacy program costs compared with an unmanaged system. However, formularies are, first and foremost, instruments to recommend the most cost-effective drug products. Formularies include more expensive drugs that may be expected to provide superior clinical outcomes, offer improved safety, or help reduce the use of more expensive medical resources.[19,20] In fact, the AMCP Format for Formulary Submissions version.2.1 helps clinical pharmacists and members of the health plan or PBM P & T Committees conduct a systematic review of the clinical, economic, and patient quality of life data to select the most cost-effective drugs for their formularies.[21] However, convincing head-to-head comparative clinical and economic data often are not available, and the physicians and the pharmacists must make decisions based upon meta analyses, comparing dissimilar clinical study methodologies, published literature, and the experience and recommendations of specialist colleagues. When there is no evidence that one product does not display significant statistical or clinical superiority, the less expensive product is usually chosen. Formularies induce competition among manufacturers and those drugs that are either well supported with strong clinical or economic data will prevail in a preferential drug formulary tier that may result in increased utilization. The result is that the drug formulary becomes a compendium of cost-effective drugs as determined by the P& T Committee. The role of the P & T Committee as well as the drug formulary review process and decision criteria are discussed in Chapter 13.

AUTHORITY OF THE DRUG FORMULARY

The drug formulary is an essential management component of the pharmacy benefit design purchased by the plan sponsor. The drug formulary is referenced in the Certificate of Coverage, the legal contract between the pharmacy benefit provider (e.g., health plan, insurance company, or PBM) and the purchasing plan sponsor. The Certificate of Coverage is often filed with the state healthcare regulatory agency, and in some states, the formulary itself is a component of the filed document. Some health plans and state Medicaid agencies refer to their drug formulary as a *preferred drug list* or *prescription drug list (PDL)*, although the purpose, function, and impact of either document are identical. Drug formularies among various health plans may vary widely in the number of drugs included, the specific drugs included in each therapeutic category, the member copayment structure, and specific drug reimbursement access rules (e.g., step edits, prior authorization, and mandatory generic use). Health plans, and especially PBMs, generally develop a primary or master drug formulary or PDL as well as other formularies customized to the specific needs of separate plan sponsor customers, all with subtle but important differences in drug coverage, formulary limitations, or copayment levels. Many health plans and PBMs post their primary formulary online for public review. A review of the Aetna Web site demonstrates the broad array of pharmacy benefits shown in the Aetna Preferred (Formulary) Drug List Information[22]. Other insurers, health plans, and PBMs post similar online information emphasizing the highly variable nature of managed care pharmacy benefits that seem almost infinitely dynamic and customizable.

As a result, the net health plan cost impact and the patient out-of-pocket copayment amount for the same drug may be vastly different among various formularies and benefit designs. For example, a large self-funded health welfare union trust may negotiate an open formulary with very low, two tier member copayments, which may result in relatively higher per capita pharmacy program costs. In contrast, a self-funded employer group may request a closed formulary with higher, multi-tiered copayments, which may result in lower per capita pharmacy costs. To remain competitive, health plans and PBMs must be willing and able to provide customized pharmacy benefits for their highly varied plan sponsor client base.

Health plans acknowledge the plan sponsor formulary differences within the formulary document. UnitedHealthcare, a national health insurance and MCO, defines its PDL, and acknowledges that plan-specific documents are the ultimate authority on drug coverage, and the pharmacy benefit and drug formulary may vary from the UHC 2007 Three-Tier Prescription Drug List Reference Guide available online:

"What is a Prescription Drug List?"[23]

"A Prescription Drug List (PDL) is a list of Food and Drug Administration (FDA)-approved brand-name and generic medications. The UnitedHealthcare pharmacy benefit is designed to provide you with coverage for a comprehensive selection of prescription medications. This guide lists the most commonly prescribed medications for certain conditions."

"Keep in mind that the benefit plan documents provided by your employer or health plan may include a Summary Plan Description or a Certificate of Coverage, and a Pharmacy Rider. These documents define your pharmacy coverage and may exclude coverage for certain medications listed in the PDL found in this guide."

The Coventry Health Plan 2006 Member Drug Formulary[24] refer the member to their plan-specific coverage documents for more definitive coverage information due to plan sponsor variability, and describe their drug formulary as follows:

"The Member Drug Formulary is an alphabetical list of approved medicines covered by your benefit plan . . ."

". . . Please consult your Plan coverage documents for more information on your specific benefit design. Some benefit plans allow you to get nonformulary drugs at the highest copay level. Some benefit plans do not cover nonformulary drugs."

Pharmacy benefit needs of plan sponsors are highly variable and dynamic. Sponsors interested in implementing strident cost controls often evolve to closed formularies and higher member cost sharing. Health plans and PBMs must respond or the plan sponsor will find another plan or PBM to accommodate their desires.

DRUG FORMULARY STRUCTURE

Managed care organizations and PBMs use a drug formulary or PDL as a public document to communicate the selective list of covered drugs, and rules for reimbursement (e.g., copayment level, quantity limits, use edits, or prior authorization), to prescribing physicians, dispensing pharmacists, plan sponsors, and individual members.

DRUG FORMULARY COPAYMENT TIERS

Most managed pharmacy programs require a member to pay a portion of the prescription cost when they access a prescription benefit. The member payment is generally termed a *copayment* and is a fixed dollar amount. There is a slowly growing trend to replace the fixed-dollar copayment with a percent of the total prescription cost. The percent payment is termed a *coinsurance*. At this time, coinsurance is more common with self-injectable or non-essential oral drugs. Comments made in this report about copayments also apply conceptually to coinsurance. Copayments (or coinsurance) serve two purposes:

1. Copayments represent a "user fee" and present an opportunity for the member using the pharmacy benefit to pay a portion of the use. By sharing the total prescription cost with the utilizing member, the program premium costs for all payors and members can be reduced. Copayments for brand drugs on average represent approximately 40% of the total prescription cost. That is, without a copayment total prescription costs and premium may increase by 60% overall.
2. Copayments are often linked to the relative price of the drug. That is, drugs are assigned to a specific copayment amount (termed a *tier*) based upon the drug net price to the health plan or PBM. Lower priced drugs are assigned a lower copayment. Very high net price drugs often are assigned the highest copayment. Drugs with a medium net price are assigned to a mid-level copayment tier.

Therefore, copayment tiers are designed to provide a financial savings for members who use lower tier (and lower cost) drugs. Of course, clinical value is of paramount importance, and physicians must prescribe the best drug for the patient. However, the copayment tier structure is designed to influence physicians to prescribe, and members to accept, the lowest priced drug that provides the necessary clinical outcome.

- **Tier I** is generally reserved for generic drugs that are expected to have the lowest net cost. However, some plans have placed some branded drugs on Tier I in several specific therapeutic categories to encourage use and discourage non-adherence that may be due to a high copayment. Some of these categories with brand drugs on Tier I include asthma and diabetes. While the copayments for Tier I vary widely among plans, it often averages $10 to $15 per prescription, although some plans have even lower Tier I copayments.
- **Tier II** generally includes preferred brand formulary drugs. Traditionally, Tier II was the best position a branded drug could be placed, and manufacturers would often

offer a rebate if their drug was placed on preferred Tier II. We have seen recent changes, prompted by Medicare Part D and multi-tiered commercial formularies, which have caused some manufacturers to offer rebates for Tier III placement (when the option may be Tier IV, with an even higher copayment, or not being covered). Tier II copayments are often in the $25 to $35 range.

- **Tier III** is often the position of any drug not placed in either Tier I (generic) or Tier II (preferred brand). That is, in a three-tier formulary, a non-preferred or non-formulary drug not placed in Tier I or Tier II would generally be placed in Tier III. In the past, Tier III drugs were not eligible for a rebate, but as described above, this is changing. The high copayment may cover the copayment differential between Tiers II and III, and the net cost of a Tier III product may be similar to a Tier II product. A drug may be moved from Tier III to Tier II as a result of a rebate, which will reduce the drug's net cost to the plan or PBM. Tier III member copayments are frequently in the $45 to $60 range.

Most prescription drug programs use a tiered formulary structure (some Medicaid programs may have a single tier copayment structure). The formulary tiers are associated with different member copayments which encourage the use of the least expensive drug that is clinically appropriate for the specific medical condition. While most large health plans and PBMs offer a variety of pharmacy benefit structures and formulary tiers, the three-tier formulary structures are the most common among commercial pharmacy programs at this time. Copayments have been successful in achieving cost-sharing with utilizing members and encouraging the use of cost-effective pharmaceuticals. The popularity of formulary copayment tiers has increased also among plan sponsors, who have requested higher copayment amounts. The increase in copayments over the recent past is shown in **Figure 9-1**.

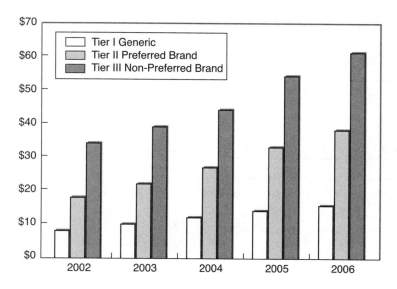

FIGURE 9-I **Copayment Trend in Managed Care Commercial Plans.**

More recently, many large health plans and PBMs offer formularies with four and five or more tiers that may be closed or open, and may or may not include injectables. Aetna, for example, includes ten different non-Medicare pharmacy benefit formulary options, including single open, closed, and injectable; two tier open, closed, and injectable; dual copay open; three tier open; four tier open; and a five tier open formulary.[25] Coinsurance is more often used on Tier IV and above than on Tiers I, II, or III. Although plan and PBMs formularies vary widely in structure and appearance, **Table 9-1** illustrates a typical formulary copayment tier structure.

DRUG FORMULARY DOCUMENT COMPONENTS

Drug formularies and PDLs are highly variable in content and copayment tier system, but often share a common organizational structure, including the following elements:

- **Formulary preamble** that defines and describes the purpose of a formulary or PDL, how it is developed and managed and changed, the basis of its authority, and rules for physicians to prescribe, pharmacists to dispense, and members to obtain eligible medications.
- **Formulary coverage policies** that describe formulary copayment tiers, coverage limitations or edits (e.g., quantity limits, step edits), the mandatory generic program, and the prior authorization process.
- **Extended medication days supplies** (if an option). Typical pharmacy benefits include up to a 30-day supply of medication for one copayment dispensed through a community pharmacy. Many health plans and PBMs offer an option that may offer up to a 90-day supply of medication for a reduced copayment (one or two copayments, rather than three). Extended duration prescriptions with lower copayments were originally used to encourage members to access mail service, which typically had lower prescription dispensing costs compared with retail as well as patient convenience. Today, the lower copayment, three-month prescriptions are offered through mail but also through retail pharmacies in a "90-day, same as mail" program. Some plans now have a higher percent of extended duration prescriptions being dispensed through retail pharmacies than through mail service pharmacies.

TABLE 9-1   Example of Drug Formulary Three Tier Copayment Structure

	Tier I	Tier II	Tier III
Type of Drug in Tier	Generic	Preferred Brand	Non-Preferred Brand
Relative Cost of Prescriptions	Usually the least expensive drugs	Usually subject to a pharmaceutical manufacturer rebate, resulting in a lower net cost.	Usually the highest cost drugs. Often not eligible for a pharmaceutical discount or rebate.
Patient Prescription Copayment Range	$10.00 – $15.00	$25.00 – $35.00	$45.00 – $60.00

- **Specialty pharmacy services**. Most pharmacy benefit programs include coverage of specialty medications (injectables, biologicals, and specialized oral medications). Injectables may be managed by the health plan pharmacy department, but may be financially covered under the medical benefit. Specialty pharmaceuticals often are dispensed through specialized pharmacy providers. Specialty pharmacies may be an independent entity (e.g., ICORE), a component of large health plans (e.g., Aetna Specialty Pharmacy) or PBMs (e.g., Express Scripts CuraScript Specialty Pharmacy) as well as chain pharmacy organizations (e.g., Walgreens Specialty Pharmacy). Specialty pharmacy services are discussed in Chapter 6.
- **Appeals or exception process**. Physicians may appeal for a patient-specific medical exception for authorization to use a non-formulary medication if formulary drugs have failed or are inappropriate for the patient.
- **List of covered drugs** ranked by copayment tier. Some formularies also provide covered drugs alphabetically or a list of common non-covered drugs with recommended formulary alternatives. Formularies and PDLs use a logical method of organizing and categorizing covered drugs within defined categories. Formulary categories are often organized by medical condition or indication, AHFS classification,[7] organ systems, or using a combination of organ systems and medical conditions. With each major therapeutic category, drugs are listed according to therapeutic class. For example, the proton pump inhibitor drug class is found within the gastrointestinal therapeutic category.

The formulary also will indicate (perhaps with an asterisk) if the drug molecule is subject to a MAC that limits reimbursement to a defined generic level for any brand drugs of the identical molecule. The MAC program was described in Chapter 2.

Formularies often provide a relative cost index for drugs within a category or class. Formularies often employ dollar signs with the number of signs indicative of a less expensive or more expensive drug. **Table 9-2** illustrates how the PPI category may appear using this structure, and **Table 9-3** is an example of a three-tier formulary structure.

TABLE 9-2 Drug Formulary PPI Class Example

Therapeutic Category: Gastrointestinal Agents

Drug Class: Proton Pump Inhibitors

Formulary Tiers	Drugs Included in Tier and Relative Cost Index*	Member Co-Payment
Tier I—Generic	$ Omeprazole**	$12.00
Tier II—Preferred Brand	$$$ Aciphex (rabeprazole)	$25.00
	$$$ Protonix (pantoprazole)	
Tier III—Non-Preferred Brand	$$$$ Prevacid (lansoprazole)	$50.00
Tier IV—Non-Essential Brand	$$$$$ Nexium (esomeprasole)	50% coinsurance

* The number of dollar signs is a relative cost index. The drug with the fewest dollar signs has lowest net cost.

** Omeprazole (generic and brand Prilosec) are subject to a maximum allowable cost (MAC).

TABLE 9-3 Example of a Drug Formulary or Preferred Drug List Therapeutic Category Organizational Structure

Number	Category
I.	Anti-infective and antiviral drugs
II.	Blood products and expanders
III.	Cardiovascular
IV.	Central nervous system and psychiatric
V.	Dermatological
VI.	Endocrine and metabolic
VII.	Gastrointestinal
VIII.	Genitourinary
IX.	Immunological
X.	Musculoskeletal
XI.	Opthalmic and otic
XII.	Respiratory system

ROLE OF GENERIC DRUGS IN DRUG FORMULARIES

The use of generic drugs is an important component in managed care prescription drug program formularies. Generic drugs typically have a published wholesale acquisition cost (WAC) of approximately 40% to 60% compared with brand drug equivalents, and with mandatory substitution in a MAC program, the actual net cost of a generic drug may be 70% to 90% less than a brand equivalent. A mandatory generic drug program may reduce pharmacy program costs by 10% to 25% compared with unmanaged prescription costs. Closed model plans may be able to dispense 80% of total prescriptions as generic drugs. Open model, IPA or PPO health plans may have a 50% to 70% generic dispensing rate. This generic fill rate is entirely controlled by the pharmacy benefit design purchased by the plan sponsor as well as the decision of the member to request a generic drug in place of a brand drug. Members can often pay one-half to one-third in out-of-pocket copayments for generics compared with the copayment of a brand drug equivalent (e.g., $10 generic copayment compared with a $60 copayment for a non-preferred brand equivalent).

The practice of "generic substitution" is the pharmacist dispensing of a bioequivalent generic drug in place of a therapeutically identical brand drug for the purpose of reducing prescription costs for the plan sponsor and member. All state board of pharmacy laws allow a pharmacist to dispense a bioequivalent generic drug when allowed by the patient's medical condition, and if not prohibited by the prescribing physician, and if accepted by the patient. Pharmacists generally consult the FDA *Approved Drug Products with Therapeutic Equivalence Evaluations* (27th edition; referred to as the "Orange Book")[26] to determine generic equivalence and substitutability. Some states require the pharmacist to dispense a generic equivalent product whenever possible, unless prohibited by physician, not accepted by the patient, or not contraindicated by a medical condition.

Many generic drugs are available from several manufacturers, and as a result of the competition, the actual acquisition price is lower than the published list price (WAC). In specific situations, the first generic version of a brand drug is launched with 180 days of exclusivity before other generic competitors become available. During this period of exclusivity, the first generic's WAC is only slightly discounted (often 10%) to the brand originator. However, when three or more generic products are available after the 180-day exclusivity period, the increased price competition among the generic manufacturers usually results in significant WAC reductions and volume purchase discounts. As a result, the AAC of such a heavily competitive and discounted generics may be 70% to 90% less than the published generic WAC. Health plans and PBMs are aware of such significant discounts on some highly competitive, multi-source generic products. In such situations, health plans and PBMs discover the AAC and assign an approximate MAC to take advantage of the significant costs savings in the distribution system, and pass these savings on to plan sponsors and members. Health plans and PBMs are aware of the existence of the heavily discounted competitive generic prices and, in an attempt to reduce costs for their customers and members, the pharmacy reimbursement is limited to the MAC. Generic drugs subject to a MAC will have a cap on reimbursement, regardless of the published WAC. Additionally, if there is a brand drug molecule identical to a generic drug subject to a MAC, many plans also limit the reimbursement for the identical brand drug to the generic MAC amount. In such cases, pharmacists will not dispense the identical brand drug unless the patient pays the reimbursement difference in cash (or they would lose money). Other health plans may eliminate reimbursement for brand drugs that have a MAC generic alternative on the formulary.

Pharmacists maintain a clinical responsibility to make certain a prescribed drug is not contraindicated for any reason, and if there is such a concern, the pharmacist must contact the physician to request a change to another formulary product. If a physician believes a patient must be prescribed a non-formulary product, the physician may request a patient-specific medical exception from the health plan or PBM.

Health plans and PBMs develop the drug formulary and specify the brand name of patent-protected pharmaceuticals. However, when listing a generic drug in the formulary, the health plan or PBM only specifies the generic molecule, dosage form, and strength in the formulary, and not the manufacturer. The selection of the generic drug manufacturer is determined by the dispensing pharmacists in the retail community, close-model health plan pharmacies, and mail service pharmacies, and not dictated by MCO or PBM drug formulary.

Pharmacists may purchase and dispense any legal generic drug product from any FDA-approved generic manufacturer (directly from the manufacturer or through an authorized drug wholesaler). Pharmacists will generally select and limit purchasing of a specific drug molecule to one manufacturer's product for the purpose of obtaining a significant volume purchasing incentive. However, they are free to change the manufacturer of the generic drugs whenever they may obtain a lower price from another FDA-approved manufacturer. The cost at which the pharmacy purchases a generic drug—the AAC—reflects the net price after discounts and purchase incentives are applied. The AAC, based upon discounted generic products, is often far less (up to 90% less) than the published WAC.

Health plans and PBMs attempt to discover the AAC and reduce reimbursement close to the AAC cost, rather than reimburse at the higher published WAC. Managed care establishes a MAC for a specific drug molecule and strength that approximates the AAC. The MAC is the highest reimbursement health plans and PBMs will reimburse pharmacies for a specific product subject to a MAC. For example, the WAC of a generic product may be $0.40 per tablet, but the AAC may be $0.10 per tablet from one wholesaler, $0.11 per tablet from another, and $0.13 per tablet from yet another wholesaler. Managed care does not dictate which wholesaler or generic manufacturer pharmacies must use and determine the MAC by averaging the AAC from three or four sources. In this example, the MAC may be $0.12 per tablet. When a MAC is established, this means the pharmacist will receive this MAC amount of reimbursement regardless of what generic product is used. Pharmacists have the incentive of greater profits if they can find a source with an AAC less than the MAC level of reimbursement.

In addition to pricing incentives from generic manufacturers, drug wholesalers often select and promote generic product lines that are offered to their customers at significant savings. For example, the wholesaler McKesson offers its One-Stop Generic program,[27] Amerisource Bergen has its PRxO Generics[28] program, and Cardinal Health has it PreferredSOURCE[29] generic program.

DRUG FORMULARY ENFORCEMENT

Health plans and PBMs must enforce physician, pharmacist, and member conformance with the drug formulary if they expect to achieve the cost and clinical drug management benefits from their formulary. Conformance with the formulary is often defined as the percent of formulary drugs dispensed divided by the total number of prescriptions. Drug formulary conformance can easily be 90% or higher if the formulary is strictly enforced (e.g., closed formulary) or if an open formulary is extremely liberal in the drugs it contains. Therefore, when evaluating the formulary conformance rate, one must also understand the type and scope of the drug formulary.

Closed drug formularies are more easily enforced as they simply block reimbursement for non-formulary products at the point of dispensing. The national drug code (NDC) of non-formulary drugs are coded into the pharmacy adjudication drug file as "not eligible for reimbursement" (without a medical exception). Closed formularies cause member and pharmacist frustration when prescriptions are denied for coverage when presented at the pharmacy.

As discussed above, the majority of open-model health plans and PBMs use open or selectively closed formularies, and use both passive and active enforcement strategies. Passive strategies include the following activities:

- Tiered formulary copayments that encourage the use of Tier I generic or Tier II preferred brand products.
- Physician, pharmacist, and member education via newsletters (paper, online) that describe the patient cost advantages of using Tier I generic or Tier II preferred brand products.

- Health plan or PBM formularies posted online for public access, and for physicians via a point-of-prescribing interface (computer or PDA, such as Epocrates®[30]).
- Physician formulary conformance incentives. Although they must be carefully structured, physicians may indirectly receive a financial incentive associated with a low rate of non-formulary drug prescribing.
- Pharmacist generic dispensing incentives. Pharmacists may receive a higher dispensing fee whenever they switch a patient from a brand drug to a generic, if clinically appropriate.

Active strategies for formulary enforcement are also commonly employed and may include the following:

- NDC blocks. Non-formulary drugs are simply not eligible for reimbursement without a patient-specific medical exception.
- Formulary step-edits, prior authorizations, mandatory generic (MAC) programs, and quantity limitations that place barriers to the use of non-preferred or non-formulary products.
- Therapeutic intervention programs, whereby physicians prescribing non-formulary products are notified (by letter or e-mail) that an alternative formulary product exists, and should be prescribed when appropriate.
- Pharmacist-to-physician personal academic counter-detailing, by which a plan or PBM pharmacist contacts a physician who prescribes non-formulary products in person or via telephone to discuss the preferred alternative formulary product.

Health plans and PBMs must enforce their formulary to demonstrate to their plan sponsor that they are able to successfully deliver the pharmacy benefit design and forecasted performance results that were purchased. Also, they must demonstrate formulary conformance to continue to be eligible for pharmaceutical rebates.

FORMULARY EXCEPTION PROCESS

Over ninety percent of prescriptions filled in managed care are filled using formulary drugs. This demonstrates the comprehensive nature of the formulary system. However, a small percent of members will legitimately require the use of a non-formulary drug. Patient-specific medical exceptions are often appropriate and necessary, and plans and PBMs have a mechanism to accommodate unique patient requirements. No formulary (with the exception of a completely open formulary) can account for every therapeutic eventuality or unique patient need, such as a rare allergy to the available formulary choices, or the occasional patient who has used every formulary drug without success. It is for these reasons that formulary systems must incorporate a patient exception process. There should be drug formulary and benefit design policies and procedures that clearly identify the exception process, recognizing the possibility of unsuccessful results using formulary choices, drug allergies, and drug sensitivities as basic reasons for physicians to prescribe outside the formulary. It is critical that the formulary exception process is clearly communicated to participating physicians and pharmacists.

The exception procedures to allow the prescribing of non-formulary medications must neither pose an insurmountable barrier to the prescribing physician nor hinder the patient's ability to receive necessary medication. Often referred to as *prior authorization procedures*, they typically provide a means for the prescribing physician to "prescreen" orders for non-formulary drugs and to justify to the pharmacist and to the health insurer the therapeutic basis for the choice before the patient arrives at the pharmacy. The entire exception process must remain transparent to the patient. Health plans and PBMs are reluctant to use prior authorization programs, as a fully-loaded prior authorization may cost $15 to $25 each. Thus, they are usually only used when there is a positive return on this investment, such as for very expensive pharmaceuticals with a potential for misuse or inappropriate use.

In the absence of a well-defined, clearly communicated exception process, and highly responsive process, patients are placed in the middle, among their physicians' desire to prescribe the necessary non-formulary drug, the pharmacists' inability to receive reimbursement for the non-formulary drug, and the health plan or PBM, which will not reimburse for the non-formulary product without explanation for the reason. These situations eventually do get resolved, but not without delaying the onset of therapy and causing patients to be less than satisfied with their prescription coverage and their health insurers.

It is important to note that prior authorization procedures should deal specifically with exceptions that are based solely on clinical need and therapeutic rationale. The pharmaceutical industry has focused a great deal of attention lately on advertising the benefits of brand-name drugs directly to members (direct-to-consumer [DTC] advertising). Based on the claims of television or magazine advertisements, many members request their physicians to prescribe specific brand-name drugs as a result of DTC advertising. If the requested drug is inappropriate for the member or is not included in the formulary, the physician must explain to the patient why the requested drug may not be the best choice. Formulary exception processes should not be created for this kind of situation. Prior authorization procedures should have criteria that are based upon the demands of science, not those produced by advertising.

DRUG FORMULARY INTERACTION WITH CLINICAL PROGRAMS

Drug formularies are but one important component in the comprehensive managed care prescription drug program. The formulary can promote cost-effective use of pharmaceuticals that is critical in medical therapy management (MTM) and disease management programs (both are discussed in Chapter 20).

DISEASE MANAGEMENT AND MEDICATION THERAPY MANAGEMENT PROGRAMS

The Disease Management Association of America (DMAA) defines disease management as ". . . a system of coordinated healthcare interventions and communications for populations with conditions in which patient self-care efforts are significant."[31] Many health plans have implemented disease or care management programs to address the top five high prevalence and high-cost medical conditions: ischemic heart disease, diabetes, chronic obstructive pulmonary disease (COPD), asthma, and chronic heart failure (CHF). The actual programs components are highly variable, and may range from screening programs to increase diagnosis to comprehensive patient case management. Drugs are perhaps the most cost-effective therapy for these five medical conditions, and the drug formulary must be comprehensive when addressing the corresponding therapeutic categories used to treat these conditions. All drugs within the categories and classes are not necessary, but all reasonable patient care needs must be addressed. Additionally, a critical component of disease management is the use of evidence-based practice guidelines.

Whether dealing with national guidelines (e.g., NHLBI NCEP for hyperlipidemia[32] NHLBBI NAEPP for asthma[33], and JNC VII for hypertension[34]) or clinical guidelines developed internally, it is important that the drug formulary include drugs recommended in utilized guidelines. Also called *critical pathways or treatment protocols*, clinical guidelines are recommendations to practitioners for treating a specific disease or medical condition. In the adaptation or development of clinical guidelines, one must take into account the role that pharmacotherapy plays in the treatment pathway. Often developed to minimize treatment variations and to improve outcomes for patients while reducing costs, it is easy to see how formularies support clinical guidelines.

Drug Use Evaluation   Drug use evaluation or drug utilization review (DUR) is a process designed to monitor and improve appropriate medication utilization and clinical outcomes. Formulary systems ensure that the most cost-effective drugs are available for prescribing, and drug use evaluation ensures that the drugs prescribed from the formulary are used appropriately. Through the evaluation process, patient prescription data are evaluated for the appropriateness, over- or underutilization of drug therapy. Clinical pharmacists at the health plan or PBM monitor the drug utilization or DUR reports and alert clinicians about prescribing and drug regimen problems, and identify patients who may require intervention by the physician. Drug use evaluation minimizes therapeutic failures caused by underutilization and poor adherence to prescribed therapy. Drug use evaluation criteria development is often the responsibility of the P & T Committee.

Drug Use Adherence   Drug adherence is comprised of compliance (taking the correct dose at the correct time and in the correct manner) and persistence (continuing to take the medication correctly until advised to discontinue by the prescribing physician). Members do not adhere to medication therapy for a variety of reasons, including cost (they may be unable to afford the copayment or out-of-pocket expense), fear of medication adverse effects, denial of the medical need, forgetfulness, misunderstanding of prescribed directions, religious or cultural reasons, physical impairment (poor vision or arthritis), or a combination of these and other reasons. Health plans, PBMs, and dispensing pharmacies often have adherence monitoring programs to intervene if non-adherence is suspected.

Medication Therapy Management Programs The Medicare Prescription Drug, Improvement, and Modernization Act of 2003 (Public Law 108–173, 8 December 2003) requires Medicare Part D prescription drug plans (PDPs) and Medicare Advantage prescription drug plans (MAPDs) to provide medication therapy management programs (MTMPs) as part of the Medicare beneficiary benefit. The act states that MTMPs are "furnished by a pharmacist [and] designed to assure . . . that covered part D drugs are appropriately used to optimize therapeutic outcomes through improved medication use, and to reduce the risk of adverse events, including adverse drug interactions."[35] Medicare Part D MTMPs concludes that the act bestows a large degree of flexibility to PDPs and MAPDs for the design and execution of MTMPs. The act suggests, but does not definitively describe, candidate beneficiaries for MTMPs as those with multiple chronic conditions, taking multiple medications, and having prescription drug expenses exceeding $4,000 per year. However, each PDP or MAPD may develop its own specific patient eligibility criteria for MTMP enrollment. The Academy of Managed Care Pharmacy has published the 2006 Consensus Document entitled, "Sound Medication Therapy Management Programs."[36] Successful MTMPs will support the appropriate use of formulary medications and also include drug utilization monitoring. MTMPs and disease management programs are discussed in Chapter 20. MTMPs appear to be a contemporary manifestation of clinical pharmacy programs and will support appropriate utilization of formulary medications. Medicare Part D recipients, either chronically ill, dual eligible or beneficiaries over 65 years of age, are expected to be high medication utilizing beneficiaries. Therefore, MTMPs seem to be necessary activities to help improve appropriate drug use to optimize clinical and economic outcomes. MTM Programs are discussed in Chapter 21.

FUTURE DRUG FORMULARY DIRECTIONS

Drug formularies will continue to evolve in response to health policy changes, new evidence-based guidelines and clinical research, plan experience, plan sponsor business, and patient care needs. Whereas formularies were novel, misunderstood, and highly criticized two decades ago, the concept of a limited and defined list of eligible prescriptions is now accepted by most commercial members as well as Medicaid and Medicare beneficiaries.

Comprehensive and responsive drug formularies will remain a benefit design cornerstone for cost-effective prescription drug management programs. As health savings programs and consumer driven health care become more popular, members will require more education and accountability as they navigate the drug formulary and attempt to obtain the greatest value when spending their out-of-pocket deductible amounts. To remain competitive, health plans and PBMs must monitor drug utilization and outcomes, and refine their formularies to include the best drugs and copayment levels to achieve the optimal cost and quality outcomes for their plan sponsors.

REFERENCES

1. Department of Health and Human Services, Centers for Medicare and Medicaid Services homepage. Available at http://www.cms.hhs.gov/PrescriptionDrugCovGenIn/. Accessed 19 June 2008.

2. U.S. Pharmacopoeia, Medicare Model Guidelines. Available at http://www.usp.org/hqi/mmg/. Accessed 19 June 2008.

3. King NM. *Pharmacopoeias and Formularies: A Selection of Primary Sources for the History of Pharmacy in the United States.* Madison, WI: American Institute of the History of Pharmacy; 1985: 9-11.

4. Iglehart J., Health Policy Report: The American health care system—expenditures. *N Engl J Med.* 1999; 340(1): 75.

5. Zellmer W.A., "Overview of the history of hospital pharmacy in the United States," in Brown T.R., (ed.): *Handbook of Institutional Pharmacy Practice*, 4th Ed. Bethesda: ASHP; 2006: 19-32.

6. Sonnedecker G., *Kremers and Urdang's History of Pharmacy.* Madison, WI: American Institute of the History of Pharmacy; 1976: 259.

7. American Society of Health System Pharmacists, AHFS homepage. Available at http://www.ashp.org/ahfs/index.cfm. Accessed 19 June 2008.

8. American Society of Health-System Pharmacists homepage. Available at http://www.ashp.org/s_ashp/index.asp. Accessed 19 June 2008.

9. Draft ASHP Guidelines on Formulary System Management. Available at http://www.ashp.org/s_ashp/bin.asp?CID=511&DID=6695&DOC=FILE.PDF. Accessed 19 June 2008.

10. *Managed Care Digest. HMO Edition.* Kansas City, MO: Marion Merrell Dow, Inc.; 1993: 33.

11. *Managed Care Digest Series. HMO-PPO/Medicare/Medicaid Digest.* Kansas City, MO: Hoechst Marion Roussel; 1998: 40.

12. "Principles of a Sound Drug Formulary System," in Hawkins B., (ed.), Best Practices for Hospital & Health-System Pharmacy: Positions and Guidance Documents of ASHP. Bethesda, MD: American Society of Health-System Pharmacists; 2006: 110-113.

13. *Concepts in Managed Care Pharmacy Series—Formulary Management.* Alexandria, VA: Academy of Managed Care Pharmacy; 1998.

14. Sansgiry S.S. and Sikri S., How Patients View Pharmacy Benefit Plans and Management Strategies. *Drug Benefit Trends.* Available at http://www.medscape.com/viewarticle/487254_3. Accessed 6 April 2007.

15. Shapiro R., "Drug formulary always changing." *Milwaukee Sentinal Journal.* 23 July 2006. Available at http://www.jsonline.com/story/index.aspx?id=474778/. Accessed 6 April 2007.

16. Drug Formularies. *DB's Medical Rants.* 16 June 2003. Available at http://medrants.com/index.php/archives/1253. Accessed 19 June 2008.

17. Horn S.D., Sharkey P.D., Phillips-Harris C., Formulary limitations and the elderly: results from the Managed Care Outcomes Project. *Am J Manag Care.* 1998; 4(8): 1105-1113.

18. Curtiss F., Drug formularies: real opportunities to improve MCO efficiency. *J Manag Care Pharm.* 1997; 3(3): 254-376.

19. Chung R.S., Taira D.A., Noh C., Alternate financial incentives in multi-tiered formulary systems to improve accountability for outcomes. *J Manag Care Pharm.* 2003; 9(4): 360-365.

20. Watkins J. Application of economic analyses in U.S. managed care formulary decisions: a private payer's experience. *J Manag Care Pharm.* 2006; 2(9): 726-735.

21. *Journal of Managed Care Pharmacy,* June 2005, Continuing Education Program. The AMCP Format for Formulary Submission V2.1. Available at http://amcp.org/data/jmcp/formatsupp.pdf. Accessed 19 June 2008.

22. Aetna® Preferred (Formulary) Drug List Information. Available at http://www.aetna.com/members/individuals/medicare/data/formulary.pdf. Accessed 7 August 2008.

23. UnitedHealthcare® 2007 Three-Tier Prescription Drug List Reference Guide. Available at https://host1.medcohealth.com/uhc/uhc_formu2007.pdf. Accessed 19 June 2008.

24. Coventry Health Plan Member Drug Formulary. Available at http://www.cvty.com/content/items/13468/AlphaFormulary.pdf. Accessed 19 June 2008.

25. Aetna® Plan Selection (non-Medicare). Available at http://www.aetna.com/FSE/planType.do?businessSectorCode=CM#. Accessed 19 June 2008.

26. *FDA Approved Drug Products with Therapeutic Equivalence Evaluations,* 28th Ed. Available at http://www.fda.gov/cder/orange/obannual.pdf. Accessed 19 June 2008.

27. McKesson OneStop Generics[SM]. Available at http://www.mckesson.com/en_us/McKesson.com/ For%2BPharmacies/Independent%2BRetail/ Rx%2BPurchasing%2BPrograms/McKesson% 2BOneStop%2BGenerics%253Csup%253ES M%253C%252Fsup%253E.html. Accessed 19 June 2008.

28. Amerisource Bergen Generics. Available at http:// www.amerisourcebergen.com/cp/1/markets/retail_ pharmacies/chain/inventory_man/progenerics/index. jsp. Accessed 19 June 2008.

29. Cardinal Health Rx Product Management. Available at http://www.cardinal.com/us/en/pharmacies/ community/distribution/rx/. Accessed 19 June 2008.

30. Epocrates® home page. Available at http://www. epocrates.com/?cid=GA_SM1_EPOC_2&gclid= CJ3wvL6F-ooCFSNCgQodMyBKkw. Accessed 19 June 2008.

31. Disease Management Association of America, DMAA Definition of Disease Management. Available at http://www.dmaa.org/dm_definition. asp. Accessed 19 June 2008.

32. National Hearth, Lung, and Blood Institute, National Cholesterol Education Program. Available at http://www.nhlbi.nih.gov/about/ncep/index.htm. Accessed 19 June 2008.

33. National Heart, Lung, and Blood Institute, National Asthma Education Prevention Program, Guidelines for the Diagnosis and Management of Asthma (EPR-3). Available at http://www.nhlbi. nih.gov/guidelines/asthma/index.htm. Accessed 19 June 2008.

34. National Heart, Lung, and Blood Institute, National Blood Pressure Education Program, Prevention, Detection, Evaluation, and Treatment of High Blood Pressure (JNC 7). Available at http://www. nhlbi.nih.gov/guidelines/hypertension/jnc7full. htm. Accessed 19 June 2008.

35. Public Law 108–173, Dec. 8, 2003, Medicare Prescription Drug, Improvement, and Modernization Act of 2003. Available at http://frwebgate.access. gpo.gov/cgi-bin/getdoc.cgi?dbname=108_cong_ public_laws&docid=f:publ173.108.pdf. Accessed 19 June 2008.

36. Academy of Managed Care Pharmacy, Sound Medication Therapy Management Programs, 2006 Consensus Document. Available at http://www.amcp. org/data/nav_content/websiteMTMdocument.pdf. Accessed 19 June 2008.

Chapter 10

MEMBER SATISFACTION STRATEGIES

JAMES M. WILSON

Health care is an increasingly competitive, consumer market-driven business. Purchase decisions regarding the types of health plan options offered to employees historically have been made by corporate health benefit officers. However, more and more insurers are now offering consumers more choice through the use of consumer-directed health plans (CDHP), making the decision process even more complicated. Price and quality of care are two of the most important decision criteria. Even after health insurance options are made at the corporate level, employees often have two or more health plan alternatives. In 2007, 62% of covered employees had more than one health plan option, according to the WilsonRx® Health Insurance Satisfaction survey conducted by Wilson Health Information, LLC.[1,2] Of those, 20% could choose from two plans, 19% from three plans, 8% from four plans, and nearly 15% from five or more plans. Employee decisions typically are based upon criteria similar to those used by their employers: price and quality of care as determined by the extent of benefits desired (**Figure 10-1**).

Ultimately, health plan members must be satisfied with their benefit choices or they complain bitterly during the contract year and will make different purchase decisions upon annual renewal. Like marketers in most businesses, healthcare marketers know that it is more expensive to recruit and enroll a new member than it is to retain an existing member. They also understand the public relations damage an unhappy or dissatisfied customer or member may cause.

Therefore, health plans are trying to understand the factors affecting member satisfaction and implement programs to ensure their delivery as well as measure those member services and quality of care and their resulting levels of member satisfaction. In the past, corporations were satisfied if their costs were reduced and member complaints were

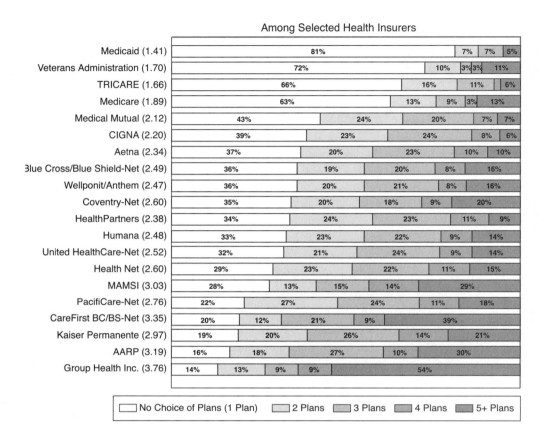

FIGURE 10-1   Health Plans of Selected Health Insurers from Which Members Have to Choose.
Source: © 2007, Wilson Health Information, LLC. New Hope, PA. All Rights Reserved.

minimized. However, today, many employers are more concerned about how fringe benefits, including healthcare benefits, affect employee retention and productivity.

Health plans can manage and improve only what they can measure. Therefore, most plans are actively involved in measuring member satisfaction and implementing programs to improve satisfaction if deficiencies are discovered. Studies reveal that satisfaction with the pharmacy benefit is an important driver of overall health plan satisfaction and member loyalty; on average, members access and utilize the pharmacy benefit more than any other covered benefit.

This chapter describes the importance of member satisfaction for re-enrollment, the factors that influence member satisfaction, the implementation of member satisfaction improvement programs, the measurement of such programs' performance, and the role of pharmacists in member satisfaction and services.

IMPORTANCE OF MEMBER SATISFACTION

Members' perceptions of their health plan—specifically, how satisfied they are with their plan—affect the perceived value of the plan, the likelihood that they will stay in the plan, and the chance that they will recommend the plan to a friend or coworker. Higher retention and recommendation rates lead to increased enrollment, lower marketing costs, and in some cases higher premiums.[3,4] The bottom line is that member satisfaction can ultimately lead to higher revenues and enhanced profit margins.

Health plan members are generally satisfied with their health plans. According to the same WilsonRx® Survey, 29.1% of plan members were highly satisfied with their plan in 2007 compared to 24.8% highly satisfied in 2001, an increase of 4.3 percentage points in the percentage of those who were highly satisfied with their plan overall (**Figure 10-2A**). Conversely, decreases were seen in the percentage of members who were either highly dissatisfied (2.1% in 2001 versus 1.4% in 2007) or dissatisfied (8.8% in 2001 versus 7.0% in 2007.[5]

The WilsonRx® survey found that TRICARE (U.S. military healthcare system) enrollees indicated the highest satisfaction with their health plans overall: 44% said they were "satisfied," and 52% said they were "highly satisfied." However, while more than 60% of respondents with employer-sponsored health maintenance organizations (HMOs) or self-sponsored HMO and preferred provider organization (PPO) plans related that they were "satisfied" with their health plans, less than a quarter of the respondents with those plan types said they were "highly satisfied" (**Figure 10-2B**).

These findings that higher levels of member satisfaction are more difficult to achieve are consistent with data from the National Committee for Quality Assurance (NCQA) survey, which indicate a somewhat lower, but still positive level of health plan member satisfaction. In 2002, 61.3% of commercial plan members (non-Medicare or Medicaid) surveyed by the NCQA rated their health plan an "8," "9," or "10," with "0" equaling "worst health plan possible" and "10" equaling "best health plan possible."[6]

Obtaining higher levels of member satisfaction is crucial to health plan re-enrollment. In 2007, 56% of health plan enrollees indicated that they "definitely" planned to re-enroll in their current health plan compared to 52% in 2003; and another 34% said they would "probably" re-enroll compared to 35% in 2003, according to the WilsonRx® survey (**Figure 10-3**).

However, health plan members who are "highly satisfied" with their health plan overall are more than twice as likely to have positive re-enrollment intentions compared to health plan members who are just "satisfied." More than 94% of "highly satisfied" health plan members reported that they "definitely" intended to re-enroll, while only 41% of all other members exhibited that same level of commitment to re-enrolling. Members who are "highly satisfied" with their plan are nearly six times more likely to recommend their plan to a friend or relative compared to those who are less than highly satisfied (**Figure 10-4**).

A

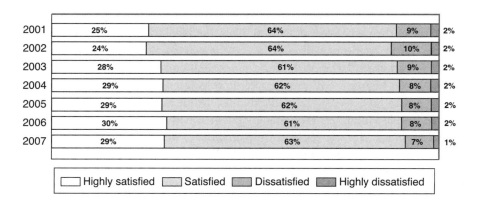

B

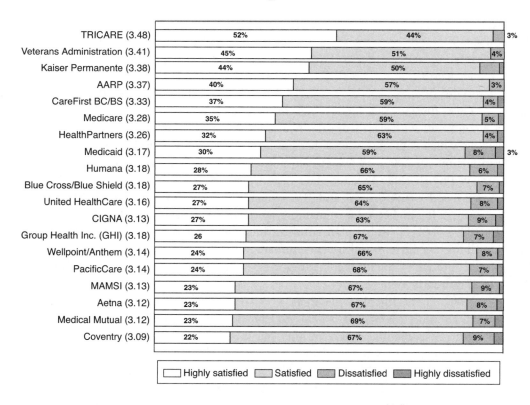

FIGURE 10-2 **(A) Overall Satisfaction with a Health Insurance Plan During the Years 2001 to 2007. (B) Overall Satisfaction with a Health Insurance Plan Among Selected Health Insurers (2007).**
Source: © 2007, Wilson Health Information, LLC. New Hope, PA. All Rights Reserved.

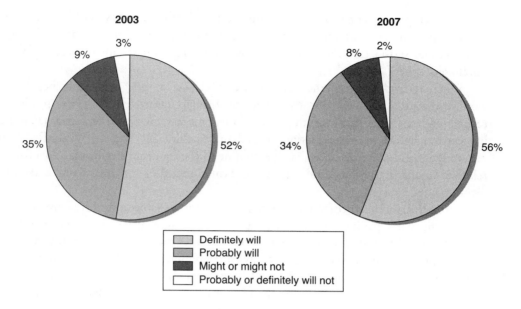

2003

2007

Definitely will
Probably will
Might or might not
Probably or definitely will not

FIGURE 10-3   Likelihood of Re-Enrolling in a Health Plan.
Source: © 2007, Wilson Health Information, LLC. New Hope, PA. All Rights Reserved.

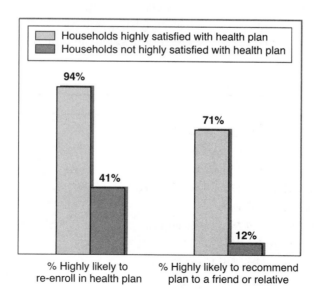

FIGURE 10-4   Impact of Satisfaction with Health Insurance Plan on Re-Enrollment and Recommendation Intentions.
Source: © 2007, Wilson Health Information, LLC. New Hope, PA. All Rights Reserved.

A growing number of employers, employees, and other purchasers of health plans are requesting member satisfaction reports to assist in their selection of plans. This means that member satisfaction data are becoming increasingly important to health plans and purchasers alike.

When individuals have the opportunity to choose among competing health plans, word-of-mouth assessments of satisfaction can strongly influence plan selection. However, research indicates that many health plans still must make some significant strides in improving word-of-mouth recommendations. Less than one-third (30%) of the WilsonRx® Survey respondents said they "definitely" will recommend their current health plan to a friend or relative. Slightly more than a third (34%) indicated that they "probably" will make such a recommendation.

Typically, member satisfaction programs currently available to health plans are components of the plan's quality improvement department. Most health plans monitor and evaluate member satisfaction at least annually. Other sources for evaluating member satisfaction within a plan may include complaint analysis, telephone monitoring, exit interviews, and focus groups. Senior management typically reviews analyses of these key indicators of service on a regular basis. Areas are identified for improvement, and a plan of action is incorporated into the strategic goals and objectives of the company.

According to the WilsonRx® Survey, the 10 most important issues to managed care enrollees (in descending order of importance) are shown in **Table 10-1**.

The top two most important issues—overall quality of the medical care received and overall quality of healthcare providers—remained the same in relative importance in 2007 as in 2002; they are also the top two issues with which health plan members were most satisfied.[5] The most significant changes in relative importance were seen with the importance ratings of out-of-pocket costs for health care, choice and coverage of primary care

TABLE 10-1   Top 10 Most Important Health Insurance Issues

	2003	CHG	2007
Overall Quality of Medical Care Received	1		1
Overall Quality of Health Care Providers	2		2
Choice of and Coverage for Primary Care Doctors (PCP visits)	5	++	3
Coverage and Availability of Diagnostic Tests and Services	4		4
Prescription Drug Benefit Coverage	6	+	5
Coverage and Availability of Medical Treatments	3	– – –	6
Out-of-Pocket Costs for Health Care	11	++++	7
Overall Ease and Convenience of Using Plan	10	++	8
Choice of and Coverage of Hospital Care	7	– –	9
Access to and Coverage of Referrals to Specialists	8	– –	10

Source: © 2007, Wilson Health Information, LLC. New Hope, PA. All Rights Reserved.

physician visits, the overall ease and convenience of using the plan, and the prescription drug benefit. In fact, the importance of out-of-pocket costs for health care did not even appear in the top 10 list in 2002 and is a reflection of the shift of costs to consumers in the form of higher co-pays, limited coverage and percentage co-pay plans, high deductible plans, and premium cost increases. Decreases in relative importance of health plan issues were seen in the coverage and availability of medical treatments, hospital care, and access and coverage of specialists.

Some issues ranked higher in member satisfaction than warranted by the importance they were given by health plan members. The fifth most important issue, the prescription drug benefit, placed twelfth in member satisfaction. Likewise, issue #7, out-of-pocket costs for health care, showed the highest ranking increase, but was seventeenth in terms of member satisfaction.

Other areas that showed a gap between the relative importance and satisfaction rankings were satisfaction with the coverage and availability of diagnostic tests and services (satisfaction = #7; importance = #4) and coverage and availability of medical treatments (satisfaction = #8; importance = #6). However, issues that rated higher in relative satisfaction compared to lower relative importance included the overall ease and convenience of using the plan (satisfaction = #6; importance = #8); choice and coverage of hospital care (satisfaction = #4; importance = #9); and access and referrals to specialists (satisfaction = #5; importance = #10).

Comparing the various plan types, HMO and POS plans appear to have similar importance ratings; both plan types rank the prescription drug benefit coverage higher (#3) compared to other plan types. Hospital coverage and overall convenience of using the plan appear to be relatively more important to members enrolled in PPO and major medical type plans (**Table 10-2**).

TABLE 10-2 Top 10 Most Important Health Insurance Issues by Type of Insurance Plan

	HMO	POS	PPO	MM
Overall Quality of Medical Care Received	1	1	1	1
Overall Quality of Health Care Providers	2	2	2	2
Choice of and Coverage for Primary Care Doctors (PCP Visits)	6	4	3	4
Coverage and Availability of Diagnostic Tests and Services	4	5	4	3
Prescription Drug Benefit Coverage	3	3	9	12
Coverage and Availability of Medical Treatments	5	6	6	6
Out-of-Pocket Costs for Health Care	7	7	8	10
Overall Ease and Convenience of Using Plan	9	8	7	7
Choice of and Coverage of Hospital Care	11	10	5	5
Access to and Coverage of Referrals to Specialists	8	11	10	8

Source: © 2007, Wilson Health Information, LLC. New Hope, PA. All Rights Reserved.

NATIONAL COMMITTEE FOR QUALITY ASSURANCE AND HEALTH PLAN EMPLOYER DATA AND INFORMATION SET

Member service programs of managed care organizations (MCOs) have focused on the promotion of health and wellness. Many of these programs were developed as a direct response to the Health Plan Employer Data and Information Set (HEDIS) reporting measures. These standardized performance measures, developed by the not-for-profit National Committee for Quality Assurance (NCQA), stipulate how health plans collect and report performance data in numerous areas, allowing healthcare purchasers and consumers to compare the performance of MCOs. More than 90% of U.S. MCOs use HEDIS as a performance measurement tool, according to the NCQA.

Some of the health and wellness programs offered by MCOs include:

- Screening mammography for early detection of breast cancer
- Immunization programs for children, with tracking and periodic reminders sent to parents
- Men's and women's preventive health programs, including:
    - Screening for coronary artery disease risk factors and annual well woman exams (an incentive may be given to the patient in the form of a birthday card with a coupon to waive the office visit co-payment)
    - Disease state management programs, such as those established to deal with asthma and diabetes, which encourage members to seek services to prevent illness and manage their own chronic conditions.

If they are directly involved in one of the above programs, members may recognize that these programs increase the quality of their health care. This realization often leads to increased member satisfaction.

Other member service programs typically offered by health plans are designed to meet perceived member needs and marketed with the goal of increasing member satisfaction, which is recognized as a key driver of member retention. These member service programs include welcome letters with follow-up telephone calls to explain health plan benefits, mail and e-mail reminders, wellness and patient education programs, and patient newsletters.

The NCQA currently asks plans to submit information on various member satisfaction measures for inclusion in its annual HEDIS report. HEDIS measures are incorporated into the NCQA health plan accreditation process for HMO and point-of-service plans; however, public reporting of the measures is voluntary.

The data categories included in HEDIS cover eight majors areas of measurement:

1. Effectiveness of care
2. Access and availability of care
3. Satisfaction with the experience of care
4. Health plan stability
5. Use of services

6. Cost of care
7. Informed health services
8. Health plan descriptive data

The data are reported by health plans and voluntarily submitted to NCQA for inclusion in the Quality Compass Program for calculating benchmarks and producing comparative information for healthcare purchasers. The member satisfaction measures included in HEDIS are based upon the Consumer Assessment of Health Plan Survey or CAHPS. They include:

- Overall satisfaction
- Problems receiving necessary care
- Problems with referrals to specialists
- Delays in waiting for approved services
- Number of doctors to choose from
- Length of time between request for appointment and visit
- Availability of information
- Ease of making appointments

A number of other organizations combine quantitative member service information with consumer satisfaction information to develop managed care report cards for use by consumers and purchasers. The report cards publish comparative data submitted by competing health plans to give potential corporate purchasers and individual patients information on how each of the plans rate on predetermined measurements. For example, NCQA's HEDIS measures ask plans to report the percentage of their diabetic patients who receive yearly retinal exams.

Employer coalitions, national publications, and state regulators track the report card activity. Employer coalitions, formed to use the participants' collective wisdom in evaluating health plans, include such innovative groups as the Pacific Business Group on Health, the Greater Detroit Area Health Council, and Maryland and New Jersey.[7] *Newsweek* and *U.S. News & World Report* publish an annual health plan rating based upon plan-reported HEDIS and NCQA accreditation data, as does *Consumer Reports*. Plans can and do opt out of releasing their data to these publications, particularly when the ratings may not be complimentary.

SATISFACTION MEASUREMENT AMONG EMPLOYER GROUPS

Findings from a survey of employers indicate that NCQA accreditation and HEDIS reports play a growing but still fairly minor role in employers' health plan selection decisions. According to a 1998 survey of more than 1,500 large employers conducted by KPMG Peat Marwick,[8] the top three factors that were important to employers when selecting a health plan were:

1. Number and quality of physicians
2. Employee satisfaction
3. Cost of the service

More recent studies show little improvement overall in the use of NCQA accreditation. In total, only 15% of U.S. firms are familiar with the two most-used types of health plan accreditation [NCQA and the Utilization Review and Accreditation Committee (URAC), which does business as the American Accreditation HealthCare Commission], according to the *Employer Health Benefits 2003 Annual Survey* by the Kaiser Family Foundation and Health Research and Educational Trust.[1]

However, while accreditation still plays a limited role at smaller firms, it has gained an increasingly stronger foothold in the decision-making process of larger employers. Just 14% of small U.S. firms (three to 199 workers) are aware of NCQA or URAC accreditation, according to the Kaiser Family Foundation survey. However, 36% of midsize companies (200 to 999 workers) and 52% of large firms (1,000 to 4,999 workers) are acquainted with NCQA or URAC accreditation. Finally, 71% of jumbo firms (5,000 or more workers) are familiar with NCQA or URAC accreditation.

Similarly, only 7% of all U.S. firms were familiar with HEDIS as of 2003, according to the Kaiser Family Foundation survey. However, the size of the firm is again a factor. Only 6% of small firms were aware of HEDIS, but that percentage jumped to 17%, 36%, and 62% for midsize, large, and jumbo firms, respectively.

NCQA studies have shown that health plans that choose to publicly report performance data deliver recommended care at much higher rates than those who do not.[6] So as employers gain a better understanding of the tie-in between cost-savings and quality of care, they are likely to increasingly use publicly-reported comparative data such as HEDIS and NCQA accreditation as a basis for choosing a health plan.

A number of employers do provide employees with information on health plan quality so that they can make better decisions about which coverage will best meet their needs. According to a report by the Employers' Managed Health Care Association, some employers provide their workers with the following quality criteria for health plans:

- *Administrative quality*, based on accessibility, service, and responsiveness
- *Customer satisfaction*, based on enrollees' experiences with plans and providers
- *Clinical quality*, based on the structure of the plan, the frequency of preventive care services, and outcomes

Reports of plan quality and satisfaction can be communicated through distribution of plan report cards during open enrollment and electronically available information. According to the 1998 KPMG study, only 9% of employers provided information to employees on their health plans' NCQA accreditation status. One of five employers with 5,000 or more workers provided this information to employees. In addition, KPMG found that only 1% of employers provided HEDIS data to their employees to assist in plan selection (**Figure 10-5**).[8]

However, more recent surveys reveal a growing awareness of health plan reporting systems on the consumer side of the equation. According to a Kaiser Family Foundation survey conducted in 2000, 27% of all consumers indicated that they had seen compara-

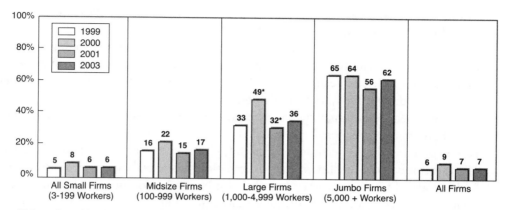

*Estimate is statisitically different from the previous year shown: 1999-2000, 2000-2001, 2001-2003.

FIGURE 10-5 Percentage of Firms that Are Familiar with HEDIS, by Firm Size, 1999–2001 and 2003.
Source: "Employer Health Benefits 2003 Annual Survey" (#3369), The Henry J. Kaiser Family Foundation & HRET, 2003. Data are from the Kaiser/HRET Survey of Employer-Sponsored Health Benefits: 1999, 2000, 2001, and 2003. This information was reprinted with permission from the Henry J. Kaiser Family Foundation. The Kaiser Family Foundation, based in Menlo Park, California, is a nonprofit, private operating foundation focusing on the major health care issues facing the nation and is not associated with Kaiser Permanente or Kaiser Industries. © 2007, Wilson Health Information, LLC. New Hope, PA. All Rights Reserved.

tive quality information for health plans and providers within the last year.[2] These findings are consistent with a 2002 national telephone survey conducted by Harris Interactive Inc., which found that millions of consumers have seen report card–type ratings of health plans, hospitals, and physicians.[9]

This increased knowledge base is possibly due in some part to the availability of report card information on the Internet. The Kaiser Family Foundation Survey found that 28% of respondents "very likely" would access the Internet to find quality-of-care information. Responding to this surge in Internet use, many organizations have developed Web sites that use HEDIS and other data to offer health plan report cards. For example, the NCQA has created an interactive Web-based tool called the *Health Plan Report Card* (available at http://hprc.ncqa.org/index.asp; accessed June 20, 2008) that allows consumers to obtain comparative data on NCQA-accredited health plans.

Yet even when Americans are aware of health plan report cards, they rarely use them at this point as the basis for healthcare decision-making. The Harris Interactive survey found that only 1% or less of all adults had decided to make a change based on those ratings. Further, a comparison of 2001 and 2002 data showed a slight increase in the number of consumers who were aware of ratings, but no increase whatsoever in the number of consumers who used ratings in their decision-making process. Likewise, the Kaiser Family Foundation survey found that only 9% of respondents said they would personally use comparative information about health plans, even though 87% believed the data would be useful in healthcare decision-making.

Instead, consumers are still taking a very personal approach to assessing quality, relying on friends and family (70%) and healthcare providers (65%) rather than more impersonal resources such as health plans (37%), printed booklets (21%), and state agencies (20%), according to the Kaiser Family Foundation.[1]

Consumer decision-making has changed little over the past few years despite the continued growth of report-card systems. A 1996 survey done jointly by the Kaiser Family Foundation and the Association for Health Care Policy also indicated that consumers did not use comparative quality-of-care information when making a decision about their health plans. This earlier survey found that 69% of Americans regard their family and friends as trusted sources of healthcare information despite the fact that 87% of respondents thought comparative quality information was useful.[10]

Other companies (including Wilson Health Information, LLC) independently collect health plan member satisfaction information. Because the studies are independent, excellent member satisfaction ratings and quality awards are highly valued by plans that use the ratings in their marketing programs to attract new members. Plans typically use the information for competitive intelligence and market positioning to help identify their competitive strengths and weaknesses.

MEMBER SATISFACTION WITH PHARMACY BENEFITS

Offering a prescription drug benefit to employees and retirees as part of the plan benefit package is crucial to attracting and retaining members. According to a 2003 Kaiser Family Foundation survey, 99% of covered workers had a prescription drug benefit.[1] According to a 2007 WilsonRx survey, those who were least likely to have prescription drug benefit coverage were those who purchase their own health insurance or were self employed, with as many of 23% without PBM coverage, and Medicare recipients with as many as 17% without prescription drug benefit coverage (**Figure 10-6**).

However, many drug benefit plans have undergone substantial changes in the past few years to combat escalating drug prices. For example, there is a growing use of three-tier cost-sharing arrangements, with one consumer co-pay for generic drugs, a higher co-pay for preferred drugs, and a third, even higher co-pay for non-preferred drugs. The Kaiser Family Foundation found that 63% of covered workers had a three-tier pharmacy benefit in 2003, up from 55% in 2002.

Pharmacy benefit managers (PBMs) are a resource to which many health plans have turned in their quest to lower costs while providing value-added pharmacy services. According to a June 2002 Issue Brief prepared by the Pharmaceutical Care Management Association, PBMs managed roughly 70% of the 3 billion prescriptions dispensed annually in the United States, which involved nearly 190 million people.[11]

Since 2006, Medicare Part D has grown significantly as a new source of prescription drug benefit coverage. Prior to the introduction of Part D coverage, most Medicare

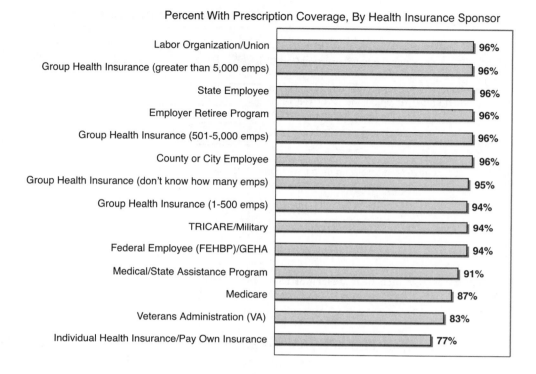

FIGURE 10-6   Prescription Drug Coverage.
Source: © 2007, Wilson Health Information, LLC. New Hope, PA. All Rights Reserved.

recipients received whatever drug coverage they had as part of a plan from their current or former employers or from the Department of Veterans Affairs (VA), TRICARE, or a union plan with a smaller percentage receiving medical and drug coverage through a Medicare HMO product. As of 2007, the majority of Medicare recipients (42%) were enrolled in a Medicare Part D plan and 37% in a drug plan sponsored by current or former employers, union, VA, or TRICARE, and 14% through a Medicare HMO. Only 5% of respondents reported that they had Medicare and no prescription drug benefit coverage (**Figure 10-7**).

While very few member satisfaction instruments, including HEDIS, currently measure levels of satisfaction with the pharmacy benefit, the role of the pharmacy benefit in member satisfaction and choice of plans will grow as benefit design initiatives such as restrictive formularies, higher and tiered co-payments, and maximum annual benefit amounts become more prevalent. Managed care pharmacists and health plan executives need to ensure that they are measuring the impact of benefit design changes on the perceived levels of satisfaction, not only with the pharmacy benefit but also with the overall plan.

Health plan members in PBMs are generally satisfied with their pharmacy benefit plans, with 91.5% of members expressing some form of overall satisfaction in a Wilson

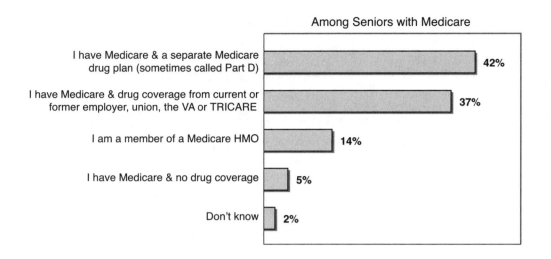

FIGURE 10-7 Which Best Describes Your Medicare Coverage?
Source: © 2007, Wilson Health Information, LLC. New Hope, PA. All Rights Reserved.

Health Information, LLC survey. Of those, however, only 30.2% said they were "highly satisfied" with their prescription drug benefit overall (**Figure 10-8**).

As with overall health plan satisfaction, TRICARE led the pack in terms of prescription drug benefit satisfaction. More than 96% of TRICARE enrollees expressed satisfaction: 52% were "highly satisfied" and 44% were "satisfied." But only one-quarter or fewer of the enrollees in employer-sponsored HMOs or self-sponsored HMO and PPO plans reported being "highly satisfied" with their prescription drug benefits. These plan types, however, did manage to rate "satisfied" among 63%, 58%, and 62% of members, respectively.

Once again, studies show that the degree of satisfaction is of paramount importance in predicting re-enrollment. Overall, fewer than half of the Wilson Health Information, LLC respondents indicated that they would "definitely" re-enroll in their pharmacy benefit plan, and only about one-quarter said they would "definitely" recommend their pharmacy benefit plan. However, PBM members who were "highly satisfied" with their pharmacy benefit plans were five times more satisfied with their overall health plan, twice as likely to have definite health plan re-enrollment intentions, and more than three times more likely to make a positive recommendation to friends and family, compared to PBM members who were simply "satisfied" (**Figure 10-9**).

In many cases, health plans and pharmacy benefit managers implement significant changes without measuring the impact on satisfaction or re-enrollment intentions. Yet the same plans would not consider changing physician or hospital visits or co-payments without measuring the impact of the change. Clearly, managed care pharmacists have an incentive to study the impact of pharmacy benefit design features on member perceptions and levels of satisfaction.

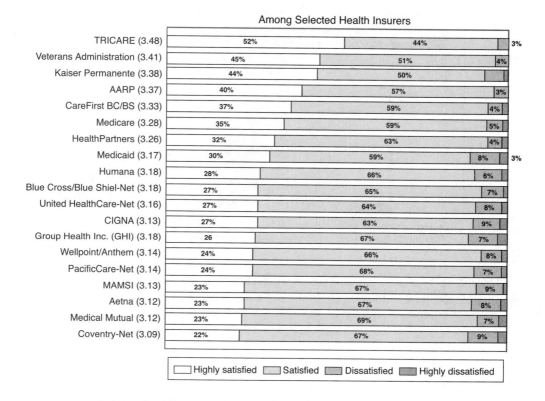

FIGURE 10-8   Overall Satisfaction with Health Insurance Plan.
Source: © 2007, Wilson Health Information, LLC. New Hope, PA. All Rights Reserved.

According to a survey conducted by Wilson Health Information, LLC, the top 10 PBM issues that concern health plan members with pharmacy benefit coverage are (in descending order of importance; **Table 10-3**): The ability to get the expected prescribed medication remains the single most important pharmacy benefit issue among PBM members. Coverage of generic medications significantly rose in relative importance from #9 to #4 during the same period. Satisfaction with out-of-pocket costs for prescription drugs increased slightly from #3 to #2 in relative importance between 2003 and 2007. Also increasing in importance were satisfaction with coverage of retail prescription drugs, branded medications, and satisfaction with having easy-to-understand benefit and coverage information. Falling in relative importance were availability of participating pharmacies (from #7 to #9), resulting from the availability of most retail pharmacies within most PBM networks and satisfaction with the ease and ability of having prescriptions filled and refilled (from #2 to #3), and notification of plan changes and changes to coverage (falling from #5 to #6).

Health plans use member satisfaction surveys internally to identify opportunities for improvement in service to their membership. Members' satisfaction with the ability to

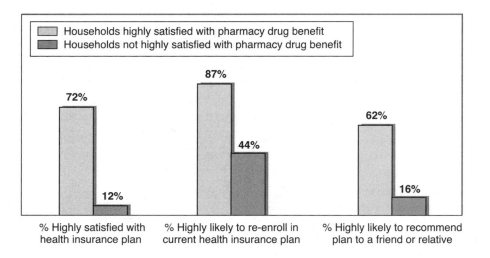

FIGURE 10-9 Impact of Pharmacy Drug Benefit Satisfaction on Health Insurance Plan Satisfaction, Re-Enrollment Intentions and Recommendation Likelihood.
Source: © 2007, Wilson Health Information, LLC. New Hope, PA. All Rights Reserved.

access physicians or pharmacies influences a plan's decision regarding the expansion of existing networks. Customer service improvements that health plans have added based on member satisfaction responses include such practices as phoning new members to inform them of how to access services within the plan and asking members to select new primary care physicians or pharmacists when there is a change in the plan's network. Another example is the 24-hour telephone helpline offered by many plans. Healthcare providers are available 24 hours a day by telephone to provide advice and authorize referrals for members who may need emergency services.

A recent survey of patients in a primary care clinic highlights the need to expand pharmacy services beyond traditional dispensing to boost member satisfaction. Eighty-six percent of patients surveyed expected to be able to discuss medication-related problems with a pharmacist, 82% wanted the pharmacist to interact with the physician to optimize drug therapy, and 58% wanted to discuss medication needs regularly with the pharmacist. Patients also requested that a pharmacist monitor their response to medications by performing blood pressure, blood sugar, and lipid level tests.[12]

It appears that although members desire "clinical" pharmacy services, price continues to be a major focus when making decisions. There are two potential explanations for this seeming contradiction. First, members want clinical pharmacy services, believe they should be included in the basic prescription price, and are unwilling to pay an additional fee for these services. Second, members "desire" clinical pharmacy services but are unwilling to pay more for them. If pharmacists wish to obtain additional reimbursement for

TABLE 10-3   Top 10 Most Important Pharmacy Benefit Issues

	2003	CHG	2007
Ability to Get the Expected Prescribed Medication	1		1
Out-of-Pocket Costs for Prescription Drugs	3	+	2
Ease of and Availability to Get Prescriptions Filled and Refilled	2	–	3
Coverage of Generic Medications	9	+++++	4
Easy to Understand Benefit and Coverage Information	6	+	5
Notifications of Plan Changes and Coverage	5	–	6
Coverage of Branded Medications	8	+	7
Retail Prescription Drug Coverage	10	++	8
Availability of Participating Pharmacies	7	– –	9
Information Provided About My Medications	10		10

Source: © 2007, Wilson Health Information, LLC. New Hope, PA. All Rights Reserved.

clinical services, pharmacists must demonstrate the value of these services to members in a manner that is meaningful and convincing.

Primary care clinics that have in-house pharmacies (such as the VA, Public Health Service, and staff-model HMO pharmacies) have traditionally met many of these patient expectations and consistently continue to reflect high satisfaction ratings. For example, pharmacists routinely perform a medication history and review on all new patients. Medication history reviews are evaluated for drug interactions, polypharmacy, and therapeutic duplication. Drug allergies and prior adverse drug events are documented in the patient's record. A report with recommendations on drug therapy is prepared and made available to the patient's physician prior to the initial visit.

In addition, many clinics offer pharmacist-run patient monitoring services for such medications as coumadin and lipid management. The pharmacist is responsible for monitoring lab values, side effects, drug interactions, and adverse events. The pharmacist adjusts the patient's drug therapy according to prescribing protocols or by recommending drug dose changes to the treating physician. The pharmacist then evaluates patient outcomes to ensure appropriate pharmaceutical care has been given.

In many managed care plans, pharmacists have been removed from the pharmacy. The role of filling and dispensing prescriptions has been automated or contracted out to PBMs. This approach allows pharmacists to take an active role as part of the healthcare team. The pharmacist may see the patient immediately before a physician visit to:

- Evaluate the patient's current drug regimen.
- Develop an optimal drug therapy treatment plan.
- Monitor the patient for compliance, side effects, drug interactions, and adverse events.
- Counsel the patient on proper use of medications to encourage positive outcomes.

Most importantly, with shifting political winds and the prospect of national health insurance, more will need to be done to eliminate the gaps in insurance for the low income and elderly households. The 2007 WilsonRx Health Insurance Survey found that the highest percentage of households without health insurance were those with low incomes (**Figure 10-10**) as well as senior and elderly households (**Figure 10-11**).

CONCLUSION

Member satisfaction measurement has not yet expanded to all areas of health care. However, satisfaction with pharmacists and the pharmacy benefit will begin to play an expanded role in measuring member satisfaction. A service that is very visible to members, the pharmacy benefit will continue to grow in importance as a measure of the level of satisfaction among employers and consumers. Health plans and pharmacists are in a position to expand services to meet member needs. These services can improve quality and be marketed as valuable member service programs. Consumers will want to know how their plan rated and will want to choose the plan with the highest scores. Employers will insist that the plans that they offer their employees will continue to satisfy employee needs and keep turnover to a minimum. Furthermore, improved outcomes among members' health and productivity can play a significant role in satisfying patients and ultimately the bottom line of the business.

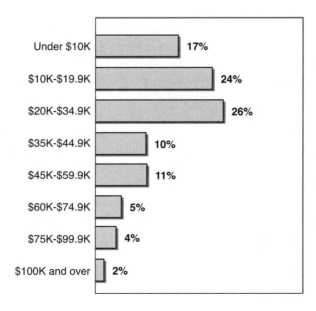

FIGURE 10-10   Respondents Without Health Insurance, by Income.
Source: © 2007, Wilson Health Information, LLC. New Hope, PA. All Rights Reserved.

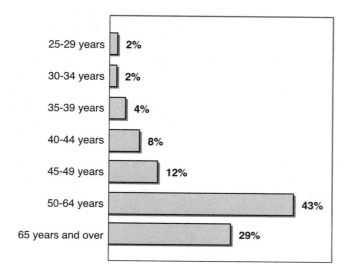

FIGURE 10-11 Respondents Without Health Insurance, by Age.
Source: © 2007, Wilson Health Information, LLC. New Hope, PA. All Rights Reserved.

REFERENCES

1. The Henry J. Kaiser Family Foundation and Health Research and Educational Trust, *Employer Health Benefits 2007 Annual Survey.* Available at http://www.kff.org/insurance/7672/index.cfm. Accessed 20 June 2008.
2. The Henry J. Kaiser Family Foundation, *Trends and Indicators in the Changing Health Care Marketplace.* Available at http://www.kff.org/insurance/7031/ti2004-1-1.cfm. Accessed 29 October 2008.
3. Tai-Seale M., Does Consumer Satisfaction Information Matter? Evidence on Member Retention in FEHBP Plans. *Med Care Res Rev,* Jun 2004; 61:171–186.
4. Wood S.D., Strategies for Improving Health Plan Member Retention—1999 HFM Resource Guide. *Health Financial Management,* Dec 1998.
5. Wilson Health Information, LLC, *Health Insurance Report by Plan Sponsor and Type of Insurance.*

Available at http://www.wilsonrx.com/health_ins_type.htm. Accessed 29 October 2008.
6. National Committee for Quality Assurance, *The State of Health Care Quality 2003: Industry Trends and Analysis.* Available at http://www.ncqa.org.
7. Pennsylvania Health Care Cost Containment Council, *Managed Care: A Strategy for Data Collection and Reporting* (1998). Available at http://www.phc4.org/reports/issue_briefs/docs/managed.pdf. Accessed 20 June 2008.
8. Gabel J.R., Hunt K.A., Hurst K., *When Employers Choose Health Plans: Do NCQA Accreditation and HEDIS Data Count?* (Report to the Commonwealth). Montvale, NJ: KPMG Peat Marwick; 1998.
9. Harris Interactive Inc., Quality Ratings Have Almost No Influence on Consumers' Choices of Hospitals, Health Plans, and Physicians. *Health Care News.* 2002; 2(19). Available at http://www.harrisinteractive.com/news/newsletters/healthnews/

HI_HealthCareNews2002Vol2_Iss19.pdf. Accessed 20 June 2008.

10. Robinson S. and Brodie M., "Understanding the Quality Challenge for Health Consumers: The Kaiser/AHCPR Survey," *Joint Commission Journal on Quality Improvement.* 1997; 23(5): 239-244.

11. Pharmaceutical Care Management Association, *Issue Brief: PBMs Deliver Value to Patients and Payers.* June 2002. http://www.pcmanet.org/issuebrief_pdfs/issue_brief.pdf.

12. Galt K., Skrabal M., Abdouch I., et al., Using Patient Expectations and Satisfaction Data to Design a New Pharmacy Service Model in a Primary Care Clinic. *J Manag Care Pract* 1997; 3(5).

SUGGESTED READING

Employee Benefit Research Institute. 1996. Sources of health insurance and characteristics of the uninsured: Analysis of the March 1996 Current Population Survey. *EBRI Issue Brief* N. 179.

Employers use varied communications to give employees health plan quality information. 1997. *Employee Benefit Plan Review* 52: 24-28.

Agency for Healthcare Research and Quality. *National Healthcare Quality Report.* 2007 DHHD, AHRQ Publication N. 08-0040, Rockville, MD: February 2008.

Chapter 11

AMCP FORMAT FOR FORMULARY SUBMISSIONS

A Format for Submission of Evidence-Based Clinical and Economic Data in Support of Formulary Consideration by Healthcare Systems in the United States

RICHARD N. FRY

The AMCP Format *was developed with the considerable assistance of many people whose names are listed in the* Format *document available at http://www.fmcpnet.org. The Academy of Managed Care Pharmacy and the Foundation for Managed Care Pharmacy are deeply indebted to the members of the FMCP Format Executive Committee for their continuing support of the* Format: *Sean D. Sullivan, Peter J. Neumann, Pete Penna, Kerri Miller, Pete Fullerton, Joseph A. Gricar, Eric Klein, Bryan R. Luce, Eric Racine, and John B. Watkins.*

INTRODUCTION

The AMCP Format for Formulary Submissions promises to change the paradigm of formulary decision making with a simple yet powerful idea: Pharmacy and Therapeutics (P & T) committees' decisions could be improved if health plans *requested* that drug companies submit to them a standardized set of clinical and economic evidence. Rather than passively receiving information and worrying about biased or poor quality evidence, health plans could follow the example of health reimbursement authorities worldwide and develop their own expertise and procedures for evaluating effectiveness and cost-effectiveness information.

The *Format* is above all a tool of empowerment for P&T committees, one that levels a playing field traditionally favoring drug manufacturers. It urges plans to request formally that drug companies present a standardized "dossier," which contains detailed information not only on the drug's effectiveness and safety, but also on its overall economic value relative to alternative therapies. The *Format* further prescribes the layout for the submission, recommending that companies include unpublished studies, data on off-label indications, information on the drug's place in therapy, related disease management strategies, and an economic model to provide evidence of the product's value.

The AMCP *Format* has the potential to serve as a national unifying template for P & T committees to consider clinical and economic information in a systematic and rigorous fashion. It is a welcome development for a U.S. health system that is in need of more rigorous evaluation of evidence.

FOUNDATION OF A SOUND FORMULARY SYSTEM

Rational product adoption decisions employing clinical, economic, and humanistic data are built on the foundation of a sound formulary system. Newly approved pharmaceutical, biological, and vaccine products should be subjected to a rigorous clinical review (and periodic re-review) based on evidence from the clinical literature. Evidence-based assessment of product efficacy, safety, effectiveness, and value provide the foundation for such a review. This process has gained additional attention and importance given recent concerns about drug safety relative to incremental effectiveness.

These precepts are affirmed by the National Committee for Quality Assurance (NCQA) managed care organization accreditation standard, "Procedures for Pharmaceutical Management," and by the *Principles of a Sound Drug Formulary* developed and endorsed in August 2000 by The Academy of Managed Care Pharmacy and the Alliance of Community Health Plans, the American Medical Association, the American Society of Health-System Pharmacists, the Department of Veterans Affairs, Pharmacy Benefit Management Strategic Healthcare Group, the National Business Coalition on Health and the U.S. Pharmacopeia.[1]

The goal of the formulary review process is to provide a quality pharmaceutical benefit, determined through an evidence-based decision-making process, taking into account the reality of constrained healthcare budgets. Where feasible, health systems should make product comparisons relative to existing competitor products as well as to placebo. For products with similar safety and efficacy profiles, they may reasonably make such decisions primarily on net acquisition cost, unless manufacturers can support reasonable product value or other program efficiency arguments with pharmacoeconomic evidence. When two or more products have similar indications but different acquisition costs, pharmacoeconomic analyses—which consider total costs and value for expenditure—may be particularly relevant to those who must make formulary status decisions, including issues designed to limit coverage to areas with maximum value for expenditure (e.g., prior authorization, copays).

GUIDELINES AND DRUG COVERAGE DECISIONS

Healthcare professionals and healthcare systems worldwide are challenged daily to set priorities in an environment where demand for healthcare services outweighs the supply of resources allocated to provide it. In the absence of widely accepted models for legitimate and fair priority-setting in health care, healthcare professionals must rely on the best available evidence to reach consensus about what constitutes the best allocation of resources to meet competing healthcare needs. For example, healthcare systems frequently conduct formulary decision-making under uncertain conditions due to the variability of available evidence on safety, effectiveness, and appropriateness of particular interventions. Gibson et al. stated, "In the absence of consensus on guiding principles, the problem of priority-setting becomes one of procedural justice—legitimate institutions using fair processes."[2] Therefore, health systems need tools to support product evaluation and selection with clinical outcomes as the most important consideration, while avoiding the use of low acquisition cost and rebates as the primary basis for selection.

In recent years, P & T committees have begun to move away from a narrow focus on the impact of pharmaceuticals on the pharmacy budget to broader considerations of "value for money." Simply stated, value in health care relates to whether a medical intervention (e.g., drug, device, program, surgery), improves health outcomes enough to justify the additional dollars spent compared to another intervention. To determine value, healthcare systems are increasingly utilizing formulary guidelines that standardize the format for clinical and economic information submitted to the P & T committee by product manufacturers. While the United States has not adopted national formulary guidelines, Australia (in 1992) became the first country to require pharmaceutical and biopharmaceutical companies to submit evidence of their products' cost-effectiveness to national authorities as a condition for consideration on the national formulary.[3] Other countries, including Canada, the United Kingdom, Sweden, Italy, and the Netherlands have adopted their own version of reimbursement and pricing guidelines.[4]

However, with the exception of guidelines developed by The Regence Group in the United States in 1994 and substantially revised in 1998,[5] no standardized format for the submission of product clinical and economic information by manufacturers existed in America. In an attempt to fill this vacuum, the Academy of Managed Care Pharmacy published the AMCP *Format for Formulary Submissions* in October 2000 and revised it in 2002 (version 2.0). AMCP Leadership and its members were motivated to develop these guidelines by a growing need to ensure that any increased utilization of medications, biopharmaceuticals or vaccine products was appropriate, and that newer products would bring added clinical and economic value to covered populations. To satisfy this need, the Academy recognized that it had to provide its members with the means to: 1) promote the concept of combining efficacy, safety, effectiveness and economic evaluation for the formulary decision-making process; 2) provide a consistent and direct means for manufacturers to supply information directly to health systems in order to support use of their products; and 3) break down cost silos and emphasize that simple acquisition cost reduction is not the best approach to controlling overall healthcare expenditures and achieving overall health objectives.

The AMCP *Format's* requirements mirror those of other countries by requiring manufacturers to provide product dossiers that contain sufficient detail to give transparency to study design, research protocols, analytical methods, and presentation of results. Although the *Format* suggests a formalized system, users should view it as a dynamic and individualized, rather than static, process. AMCP and FMCP anticipate that increased standardization of information will lead to progressive improvement in the quality of submitted evidence over time, and provide health systems with data often unavailable in the past. As feedback is integral to the process, AMCP welcomes comments on its most recent version of the *Format*.

RECOGNITION OF THE AMCP *FORMAT*

The AMCP *Format* has been recognized at the national and international level. In a February 2003 speech at the Resources for the Future conference, "Valuing Health Outcomes," Mark McClellan, then Commissioner, Food and Drug Administration (FDA) stated, ". . . FDA does recognize that industry is responding to many requests for economic information from payers and others, and in doing so industry seems to be increasingly following standards created by the Academy of Managed Care Pharmacy in formulary submissions of clinical and economic data. We hope that the influence of these standards for economic data is increasing the quality and the reliability of economic data in medical studies, and it certainly seems to be an interesting basis for potential guidance."[6]

Under the Medicare Modernization Act, PBMs and MCOs administering the Medicare drug benefit will need to adopt decision-making processes that are more transparent, consistent, and evidence-based. Many of these entities adopted the AMCP *Format* as a national model for formulary decision-making. Indeed, the Centers for Medicare and Medicaid Services (CMS) has publicly stated that it intends to look to existing national standards and guidelines such as those established by AMCP to develop a framework for formulary management.[7]

ROLE OF THE *FORMAT*

The *Format* and other formulary submission guidelines support the informed selection of pharmaceuticals, biologicals and vaccines by:

1. Standardizing and communicating product and supporting program information requirements
2. Requiring projections of product impact on both the organization and its enrolled patient population
3. Requesting information on the value of products being evaluated
4. Making evidence and rationale supporting all choice(s) more clear and evaluable by the health system decision-makers

These guidelines emphasize that, while cost-effectiveness analysis and economic modeling are important elements in the value equation, they are secondary to the principal clinical concerns of safety and efficacy. Clearly, the benefits to patients as reflected in safety and efficacy must underlie any projected economic value.

The AMCP *Format's* process is designed to maintain a high standard of objectivity to achieve two important goals. First, it is intended to improve the timeliness, scope, quality, and relevance of information available to a health system's evaluators and ultimately to its P & T Committees. Further, by assessing the health system impact of using a product, the data requested can improve the P & T Committee's ability to compare the effects of formulary alternatives on clinical outcomes, value, and economic consequences for the entire health system. According to Neumann, the type of rigorous clinical and economic analysis called for in the *Format* "forces and focuses discussions about the value of health and medical services within a clear theoretical framework. It generates a more careful consideration of available evidence and sheds light on how to target resources to particular clinical practices or subgroups of patients."[8] However, it is important that this information is weighed in the context of other values such as equity, social justice, and the health of individuals as opposed to populations, the "rule of rescue" and democratic decision-making.[2,9,10]

Second, the AMCP *Format* streamlines the data acquisition and review process for health system staff pharmacists. By clearly specifying the standards of evidence implicit in the existing formulary process, the submission guidelines furnish pharmaceutical manufacturers with consistent direction concerning the nature and format of information that is expected. In addition, the standardized format allows clinical staff to formally evaluate the completeness of submissions received and to easily add the results of the health system's own literature reviews and analysis. Manufacturers should understand that submission of information in the format recommended does not guarantee approval of their product for formulary listing. Manufacturers and health systems should view discussion about, and subsequent submission of a dossier, as a process to improve the quality and layout of information provided, but not as a formula for approval. The guidelines offer a clear, shared vision of the requirements to facilitate the collaboration necessary between health systems and manufacturers to support drug product evaluation. Recognizing that manufacturers may not have all the requested information, especially for new products, the document describes the minimum information requirements necessary to support a comprehensive assessment of the proposed product.

AMCP is not a standard setting organization. Therefore, the Academy has always viewed the AMCP *Format* as a template or guide, not a mandate or standard. As such, it does not claim to establish a standard of practice for managed care pharmacy. It is up to individual healthcare systems to decide how they will implement the AMCP *Format* and how they will operate their formulary review processes.

ADVANTAGES FOR THE MANUFACTURER

Using the AMCP *Format*, the pharmaceutical and biopharmaceutical industry will have the opportunity to present a full and scientific portfolio of clinical (benefit and safety data) and economic evidence to support formulary consideration. Thus, manufacturers are given the opportunity to supply information (e.g. adherence data, patient satisfaction, indirect and non-medical cost impacts) to demonstrate the broad value of their products when compared to usual treatments. In addition, manufacturers will have the opportunity to present economic evidence to justify the price of a new agent in terms of its overall value to the health system. The economic data requested must be broadly applicable to a health system's population and address the system-wide impact of formulary changes on both clinical outcomes and resource utilization and costs. Early planning by manufacturers will help ensure that their product value message is supported by credible evidence. Therefore, planning for dossier development should start early in the drug development program (Phase II or III), depending on how much data generation is required. The general goal for manufacturers should be to have completed dossiers ready six to nine months prior to product launch.

CONFIDENTIALITY ISSUES

The AMCP *Format* contains the following statement in the Unsolicited Request Letter Template:

> "By submitting this request (the health system) recognizes that confidential information may be provided. (The health system) recognizes the need to respect and honor commercial-in-confidence information and may be willing to sign necessary confidentiality agreements under agreed circumstances."

As public agencies such as state Medicaid agencies and the Department of Defense (DoD) have begun to adopt the AMCP *Format*, some pharmaceutical companies have raised concern about the need for confidentiality. For example, manufacturers have expressed considerable concern over the decision of Oregon's Medicaid agency to make dossiers available to any interested parties upon request. Concern also has been raised about dossiers submitted to the DoD, which could be obtained under the Freedom of Information Act. However, the DoD now has a committee review the dossiers and prepare a brief report summarizing the key points contained in the dossier. The committee's summary reports are made public, while the dossiers presumably remain confidential. The Academy has counseled public agencies that are considering the use of the AMCP *Format* to develop procedures that will allow them to keep the dossiers confidential. AMCP encourages any organization that begins using AMCP's *Format* to hold a presubmission meeting with pharmaceutical companies, which is called for in the AMCP *Format,* to disclose the level of confidentiality that will be possible and to ascertain what level of data can be expected to be furnished.

It is important to point out that the issue of confidentiality is not unique to the United States, as product evaluations in Australia, Canada, and the United Kingdom are available to the public and often downloadable over the Internet.[11–14]

DIALOGUE WITH THE FOOD AND DRUG ADMINISTRATION

A distinguishing feature of the AMCP *Format* is its use as an unsolicited request from a health system to a manufacturer for all possible clinical and economic information necessary to assess the overall clinical utility—in particular safety—and value that a product brings to a specific patient population and healthcare system. In response to this Unsolicited Request, manufacturers are asked to submit all available published and unpublished studies and information regarding both FDA-approved indications and anticipated off-label uses of the product (permitted under Section 114(a) of the Food and Drug

Administration Modernization Act of 1997), should such information exist.[15] Therefore, this request attempts to improve access to material that has been difficult to obtain in the past. It also enables manufacturers to submit such data within regulatory constraints mandated by the FDA. While no explicit FDA guidance regarding unsolicited requests exists, FDA officials have repeatedly stated their intention to issue such guidance in the future.

Because the FDA closely regulates the information a pharmaceutical company can provide regarding their products, there has been apprehension that complying with the AMCP *Format* information requirements may raise concerns at the FDA. Beginning long before the AMCP *Format's* publication, the Academy has maintained an ongoing dialogue with the FDA to keep the agency apprised of the project's progress and to seek their guidance. FDA officials have stated on several occasions that they are comfortable with the Academy's position that the AMCP *Format* represents an unsolicited request from a health system to a pharmaceutical company for all possible published and unpublished studies and information regarding both FDA-approved indications and anticipated off-label uses of the product. FDA officials have stated they have four areas of concern regarding this process: 1) that requests for off-label product information are truly unsolicited and unprompted; 2) that the information provided is not false and misleading; 3) that the response from manufacturers is specific to the requestor; and 4) that pharmacoeconomic models are transparent and model assumptions are clearly stated.

Regarding the first concern, health systems must initiate the request and clearly identify the information they desire. The AMCP *Format* is a template designed specifically for this purpose. AMCP recommends that health systems also submit a signed request letter to accompany the AMCP *Format*. Regarding the second concern, FDA regulations require pharmaceutical companies to provide accurate information. The pharmaceutical industry takes this responsibility seriously, and the AMCP *Format* recognizes the importance of these requirements. Issues regarding the third and fourth concerns are covered in more detail in the *Format* section on Customizing the Economic Model and in Section 3 of the Evidentiary Requirements, respectively. However, FDA officials have stated that, regarding AMCP *Format*-based dossiers, pharmaceutical companies must refrain from taking any proactive steps that could be construed as marketing and promotion, such as preparing identical formulary submission documents (dossiers) for a product with the intent of soliciting health system pharmacist's requests for the dossiers or informing health system pharmacists that an updated dossier is available. In these scenarios, the request would not be truly unsolicited nor would the contents of the response (the dossier) be specific to the requestor.[16]

THE IMPORTANCE OF CLINICAL INFORMATION

There has been a misperception among some users and potential users of the AMCP *Format* that it is merely a tool for presentation of a pharmacoeconomic model. Consequently, some health systems with less expertise in appraising economic models have been hesitant to utilize the *Format*. A careful examination of the AMCP *Format* document will clearly show that these guidelines, first and foremost, require the health system staff to perform a thorough clinical evaluation of the product based on all possible available information obtained from the manufacturer and other sources. If the evaluation concludes that the effectiveness of the product does not outweigh safety concerns or there are better alternatives, an economic review would be unnecessary. It is imperative to determine the potential clinical impact of a drug on its target patient population before considering the economic consequences.

The field of pharmacoeconomics is relatively new. Therefore, the current number of individuals in this country with significant training and experience in analyzing the type of cost-effectiveness information required by the AMCP *Format* is limited. While pharmacoeconomic models and outcomes research have become increasingly accepted as tools for helping healthcare systems to make formulary decisions, many health systems do not have a pharmacist on staff with sufficient experience to analyze this information. This is a concern often expressed by pharmaceutical manufacturer officials and some health plan managers. There are at least two solutions to this problem. One solution would be for one or two staff pharmacists to acquire the training in pharmacoeconomic evaluation. Numerous organizations around the country provide this type of training, including the Foundation for Managed Care Pharmacy, the International Society for Pharmacoeconomics and Outcomes Research (ISPOR) (http://www.ispor.org), several colleges of pharmacy, and the American College of Clinical Pharmacy.[17] Another solution is to engage an outside consultant to perform the reviews of the pharmacoeconomic modeling. Private consultants, faculty and students at colleges of pharmacy, and experts in the public health arena can help meet health system needs. Writing about training opportunities, the late Bernie O'Brien, PhD stated, "Part of the solution, as FMCP has been quick to understand, is offering training workshops on the AMCP *Format*. But it may also make good business sense for the pharmaceutical industry to help subsidize the continuing education of MCO dossier reviewers in contemporary methods of modeling and cost-effectiveness. Helping to create the skilled receptors in managed care for the evidence and analyses submitted is almost as important as the studies themselves."[18]

CONTENT OF A FORMULARY SUBMISSION DOSSIER

A complete formulary submission dossier for pharmaceutical, biological, and vaccine products should include the following sections:

1. Disease and Product Information
2. Supporting Clinical and Economic Information
3. Cost-Effectiveness and Budget Impact Model Report
4. Product Value and Overall Cost
5. Supporting Information: Reprints, Bibliography, Checklist, Electronic Media, and Appendices

These guidelines are not intended to restrict the content, presentation of data, and the research methods of studies that comprise the dossier. Rather, they are intended to specify evidentiary requirements for product review. However, in preparation of the evidence, the approach and methodology adopted by the manufacturer and the techniques employed should be consistent with the formulary evaluation objectives of the MCO receiving the dossier. It is recommended that the manufacturer consult with MCO representatives to determine appropriate sources for data and to agree on specific requirements and model assumptions.

1. PRODUCT INFORMATION

1.1. Product Description   Manufacturers are required to provide detailed information about their product. They should compare the new product with other agents commonly used to treat the condition. The product description consists of information that traditionally has been incorporated in a product monograph or formulary kit and includes the following:

   a. Generic, brand name, and therapeutic class of the product
   b. All dosage forms, including strengths and package sizes
   c. The National Drug Code (NDC) for all formulations
   d. A copy of the official product labeling/literature
   e. The AWP and WAC cost per unit size (if available, the contract price should be included as well)
   f. AHFS or other drug classification
   g. FDA approved and other studied indication(s): Must include a detailed discussion of the approved FDA indications and the date approval was granted (or is expected to be granted)
   h. Information on current and pending off-label indications and other non-labeled uses, if available
   i. Pharmacology
   j. Pharmacokinetics/pharmacodynamics
   k. Contraindications
      i. Warnings/precautions, adverse effects
      ii. Interactions, with suggestions on how to avoid them
         1. Drug/drug
         2. Drug/food
         3. Drug/disease
   l. Dosing and administration
   m. Access (e.g., restrictions on distribution, supply limitations, anticipated shortages)
   n. Current or anticipated product market share information
   o. Co-prescribed/concomitant therapies, including dosages
   p. Concise comparison with the primary comparator products in the same therapeutic area, to include: dosing, indications, pharmacokinetic/pharmacologic profile, adverse

effects, warnings, contraindications, interactions, and other relevant characteristics (expand as appropriate for the therapeutic class). The material may include a discussion of comparator product(s) or services that the proposed product is expected to substitute for, or replace.

1.2. Place of the Product in Therapy   This section includes two parts: disease description and approaches to treatment.

1.2.1. Disease Description   The disease description should include the disease and characteristics of the patients who are treated for the condition. Manufacturers should provide a description of specific patient subpopulations in which the drug is expected to be most effective. Include clinical markers, diagnostic or genetic criteria, etc., which can be used to identify these subpopulations. Present a brief summary of information from the literature for each topic. When information from studies is presented, the manufacturer should compile the results in detailed evidence tables.

Disease-specific descriptive information should include, but not be limited to:
  a. Epidemiology and relevant risk factors
  b. Pathophysiology
  c. Clinical presentation
  d. Societal and/or economic impact

1.2.2. Approaches to Treatment   The key questions are twofold: how is the disease/condition treated and how does the new product fit in therapy?

Present a brief summary of information from the literature for each topic:
  a. Approaches to treatment: principal options/practice patterns
  b. A description of alternative treatment options (both drug and non-drug)
  c. The place and anticipated uses of the proposed therapy in treatment (e.g., first line)
  d. Proposed ancillary disease or care management intervention strategies that are intended to accompany the product at launch
  e. Relevant treatment guidelines from national or international bodies
  f. The expected outcomes of therapy
  g. Other key assumptions and their rationale

Next, an attempt should be made to generalize these findings to the populations of the MCO. Discuss the implications of any differences that exist between the literature and typical practice patterns and patient populations. When more than one disease is addressed, complete the description for each separate condition.

1.3. Evidence for Pharmacogenomic Tests and Drugs   In considering the appropriate use of genetic testing to guide drug therapy (variously referred to as *pharmacogenomics, pharma-*

cogenetics, individualized medicine, or *targeted therapy*), clinicians and healthcare system decision-makers must consider the accuracy with which a test identifies a patient's genetic status (analytic validity), clinical status (clinical validity), and the risks and benefits resulting from test use (clinical utility).[19] The following evidence should be presented as appropriate in support of submissions involving pharmacogenomic testing, or drugs for which pharmacogenomic testing is available.

2. SUPPORTING CLINICAL AND ECONOMIC INFORMATION

2.1. Summarizing Key Clinical and Economic Studies Submit summaries of the key clinical and economic studies that have been conducted, whether published or not, in each of the following categories:

1. Pivotal safety and efficacy trials
2. Relevant published and unpublished safety, efficacy, and effectiveness trials regarding off-label uses
3. Prospective effectiveness (e.g., large simple) trials
4. Additional prospective studies examining other non-economic endpoints such as health status measures and quality of life. If the instruments utilized in these studies are supported by previous validation and reliability studies, also reference these studies.
5. Retrospective studies
6. Systematic reviews and meta-analyses (no more than 3–4 pages per study + evidence table). Place particular emphasis on the inclusion and exclusion criteria and main outcome measure(s) for studies analyzed. When a Cochrane Collaboration systematic review or Agency for Healthcare Research and Quality (AHRQ) evidence summary is available and relevant, manufacturers should include the major conclusions.

Studies reported in this section should be summarized in a clear, concise format and include all relevant positive and negative findings. Summaries of trial results of key comparator products are desirable but not required. Systematic reviews or meta-analyses may be referenced in item (6). In the Appendix, include a reprint or unpublished manuscript of each study discussed or referenced.

All of the following items that apply should be included in the study summaries:
a. Name of the clinical trial or study, location, and study date
b. Trial design, randomization, and blinding procedures
   i. Research question(s)
   ii. Study perspective;
c. Washout, inclusion and exclusion criteria
d. Sample characteristics (demographics, number studied, disease severity, comorbidities)
   i. Treated population (actual or assumed)
e. Patient follow-up procedures (e.g., If an intention-to-treat design is used, were drop-outs followed and for what time period?)
   i. Treatment period

f. Treatment and dosage regimens
  i. Treatment framework
  ii. Resource utilization classification
  iii. Unit costs
g. Clinical outcome(s) measures
  i. Outcomes evaluated
  ii. Delineate primary vs. secondary study endpoints and their corresponding results
h. Other outcome measures (e.g., quality of life)
  i. Principal findings
i. Statistical significance of outcomes and power calculations
j. Validation of outcomes instrument (if applicable)
k. Compliance behavior
l. Generalizability of the population treated
  i. Relevance to enrolled populations of the MCO
m. Publication citation(s)/references used
n. Relevant data and findings from the Center for Drug Evaluation and Research's Office of Drug Safety
o. Manufacturers should state whether trials for the product are registered in a public trials registry, and if so, provide access information (e.g., http//:www.clinicaltrials.gov)[20]

2.1.1. Evidence Table Spreadsheets of All Published and Unpublished Trials Information from all known studies on the product should be summarized in evidence tables (spreadsheet format) noting which studies were presented previously (items 1–6). Include negative or null findings as well as positive findings.

A standard evidence table should include the following data elements:

- Citation, if published
- Sample size
- Primary endpoints
- Secondary endpoints
- Treatments

- Design
- Inclusion/exclusion criteria
- Statistical significance
- Results
- Study dates

2.2. Outcomes Studies and Economic Evaluation Supporting Data Many researchers have expressed concern over the quality of some published economic evaluations.[21,22] Because the focus of this portion of the dossier is a comprehensive assessment of available evidence, the number of studies considered will not be restricted by imposing methodological standards. However, the MCO and its consultants will judge the merit of individual studies based on published standards for conducting and reporting these analyses.[23–29]

Provide summaries addressing items a through o (see Section 2.1) for all studies in each of the categories listed below (items 1–6). Studies reported in this section should be summarized in a clear, concise format and include all relevant positive and negative findings. MCOS are particularly interested in head-to-head comparison studies between the proposed product and the principal comparators. Analyses that focus on actual outcomes rather than intermediate endpoints are preferred. Summaries of principal trial results of key comparator products when these data are referenced or used in economic models are extremely helpful, but not required. Discuss important study findings and comment on their implications for the patient populations of the MCO. In the appendix, include a reprint of each study discussed or referenced.

1. Prospective, trial-based cost-effectiveness studies
2. Economic modeling studies
3. Cross-sectional or retrospective costing studies and treatment pattern studies
4. Systematic review articles
5. Quality of life studies
6. Patient reported outcomes (PRO) studies, including quality of life studies

2.2.1 Evidence Table Spreadsheets of All Published and Unpublished Outcomes Studies Information from all relevant outcomes studies on the product should be summarized in evidence tables (spreadsheet format) as indicated in Section 2.1.1, noting which studies were presented previously (items 1–6 above). Include negative or null findings as well as positive findings.

3. MODELING REPORT

3.1. Model Overview The ISPOR's task force on good modeling practices states: "Although evidence from randomized clinical trials remains central to efficacy testing, taken alone it can be misleading if endpoints are not translated into measures that are valued by patients, providers, insurers and the general public."[32] When comparing two or more interventions, properly constructed model-based evaluations can combine evidence on health consequences and costs from many different sources, including data from clinical trials, observational studies, claims databases, case registries, public health statistics and preference surveys, and a measure of uncertainty in any estimates. The goal is to evaluate the value of the product and project the health and economic consequences of potential formulary changes to the health plan.

Manufacturers are strongly urged to provide cost-effectiveness models. They are the best means to accomplish this goal because they establish the value of a new technology relative to the most clinically appropriate comparator(s). They are disease-based and take into account the impact of the new technology on the clinical outcomes for the target population, and include evidence on the incidence of the disease or condition in the target population, the medical care required to diagnose and treat the disease, the relative and absolute risk reductions offered by the technology, survival and quality of life impacts, and the costs of the interventions.

The reader should consult the full description of the *Format for Formulary Submissions* for more details on economic modeling.

4. PRODUCT VALUE AND OVERALL COST

This section of the submission requirements represents the principal opportunity for a manufacturer to communicate the value of its product to the MCO. The manufacturer should briefly summarize all clinical and economic information presented previously and state the expected per unit product cost. Based on this information, the manufacturer should articulate a value argument to justify these expected expenditures for this product in the context of its anticipated effects on the clinical and other outcomes, and the economic consequences for the MCO and its clients and members. Through this process, product value is redefined as both parties move beyond cost containment to focus on optimizing drug utilization in an environment of limited resources.

5. SUPPORTING INFORMATION

5.1. References Contained in Dossiers   Submissions should list and provide copies of all relevant clinical and pharmacoeconomic references made in Sections 2 and 3 above.

CONCLUSION

The persistent rise in healthcare expenditures, particularly prescription drugs, can be readily attributable to an unwillingness to accept real-world limitations. This is also a major factor contributing to resistance to the use of cost-effectiveness analysis in the United States as an important policy making tool.[10] Other contributing factors such as a lack of understanding about the conceptual approach, a mistrust of methods and motives, and regulatory and legal barriers may be more easily overcome. However, Daniels and Sabin, writing in *Health Affairs* in 1998 stated, "To change that culture requires a concerted effort at education, and education requires openness about the rationales for a managed care plan's decisions."[31] By adhering to careful and thoughtful decision-making processes that provide the rationales for limits, health care systems will be able to show, over time, that "arguably fair decisions are being made and that those making them have established a procedure we should view as legitimate."[31] AMCP and FMCP believe that the AMCP *Format* is a valuable tool that will help health systems establish a record of commitment to rational evidence-based decision-making, thus gaining the confidence of patients, clinicians, payors, and members.

REFERENCES

1. Consensus document. *Principles of a Sound Drug Formulary.* Alexandria, VA: Academy of Managed Care Pharmacy, October 2000. Available at http://www.amcp.org/data/nav_content/drugformulary.pdf. Accessed 19 Aug 2008.

2. Gibson J.L., Martin D.K., Singer P.A., Priority setting for new technologies in medicine: a transdisciplinary study. *BMC Health Serv Res.,* 2002; 2: 14.

3. Neumann P.J., Evidence-based and value based formulary guidelines. *Health Affairs.* 23; 1: 124-134.

4. Hjelmgren J., Berggren F., Andersson F., Health economic guidelines—similarities, differences, and some implications. *Value Health.* 2001; 4(3): 225-250.

5. Mather D.B., Sullivan S.D., Augenstein D., Fullerton D.S., Atherly D., Incorporating clinical outcomes and economic consequences into drug formulary decisions: a practical approach. *Am J Manag Care.* 1999; 5(3): 277-285.

6. McClellan M., *Valuing health outcomes: an assessment of approaches.* Speech at the Resources for the Future Conference, Valuing Health Outcomes: Session I: The Policy Context. February 13, 2003. Available at http://www.rff.org/rff/Events/Valuing-Health/Valuing-Health-Outcomes-An-Assessment-of-Approaches.cfm. Accessed 22 June 2008.

7. United States Department of Health and Human Services, Centers for Medicare and Medicaid Services. Medicare Modernization Act Guidelines—Formularies, CMS Strategy for Affordable Access to Comprehensive Drug Coverage, Guidelines for Reviewing Prescription Drug Plan Formularies and Procedures. December 3, 2004. Available at http://www.cms.hhs.gov/PrescriptionDrugCovContra/Downloads/FormularyGuidance.pdf. Accessed 22 June 2008.

8. Neumann P.J., Why don't Americans use cost-effectiveness analysis? *Am J Manag Care.* 2004; 10: 308-312.

9. Daniels N., Four unsolved rationing problems. *Hastings Cent Rep.* 1994, 24: 27-29.

10. Richardson J. and McKie J., The rule of rescue. Working paper #112 (2000). Centre for Health Program Evaluation, Health Economics Unit, Monash University, Australia. Available at http://www.buseco.monash.edu.au/centres/che/pubs/wp112.pdf. Accessed 22 June 2008.

11. Australia Pharmaceutical Benefits Scheme. Guidelines for the pharmaceutical industry on preparation of submissions to the pharmaceutical benefits advisory committee: including major submissions involving economic analyses. Canberra, Australia: Department of health and Ageing: Australian Government. Available at http://www.health.gov.au/internet/main/publishing.nsf/Content/health-pbs-general-pubs-guidelines-index.htm. Accessed 19 Aug 2008.

12. Canadian Coordinating Office of Health Technology Assessment. *Guidelines for Economic Evaluation of Pharmaceuticals.* Ottawa, Ontario, Canada: Canadian Agency for Drugs and Technologies in Health (CADTH); 1997. Available at http://www.cadth.ca/index.php/en/hta/reports-publications/search/publication/35. Accessed 22 June 2008.

13. National Institute for Clinical Excellence, *A Guide for Manufacturers and Sponsors Contributing to a Technology Appraisal.* London: The Institute; 2004. Available from http://www.nice.org.uk/processguides/contributing_to_a_technology_appraisal_a_guide_for_manufacturers_and_sponsors_reference_n0518.jsp. Accessed 22 June 2008.

14. Drummond M., Should commercial-in-confidence data be used by decision makers when making assessments of cost-effectiveness? Editorial. Applied Health Economics and Health Policy. 2002; 1(2): 3-4.

15. United States Food and Drug Administration. *FDA Modernization Act of 1997.* Available at http://www.fda.gov/oc/fdama/default.htm. Accessed 22 June 2008.

16. Foundation for Managed Care Pharmacy. Response to comments for AMCP's *Format for Formulary Submissions* version 2.0. Alexandria, VA. October 2002. Available at http://www.fmcpnet.org/cfr/waSys/f.cfc?method=getListFile&id=A2D3AAB3. Accessed 22 June 2008.

17. American College of Clinical Pharmacy. *Pharmacoeconomics and Outcomes: Applications for Patient Care,* 2nd Ed. Kansas City, MO: ACCP; 2003.

18. O'Brien B.J., Academy of Managed Care Pharmacy *Format*: relevance, rigor, regulation, and realism. *Value Health* 2003; 6(5): 501-502.

19. U.S. Department of Health and Human Services, Food and Drug Administration, Center for Drug Evaluation and Research, Center for Biologics Evaluation and Research and Center for Devices and Radiologic Health. *Guidance for Industry: Pharmacogenomic Data Submissions.* March 2005. Available at http://www.fda.gov/cber/gdlns/pharmdtasub.pdf. Accessed 22 June 2008.

20. DeAngelis C., Drazen J.M., Frizelle F.A., et al. Clinical trial registration: a statement from the international committee of medical journal editors. *Ann Intern Med.* 2004; 141(6): 477-478.

21. Hillman A.L., Eisenberg J.M., Pauly M.V., et al., Avoiding bias in the conduct and reporting of cost-effectiveness research sponsored by pharmaceutical companies. *N Engl J Med.* 1991; 324: 1362-1365.

22. Johannesson M., Jönsson B., Göran K., Outcome measurement in economic evaluation. *Health Econ.* 1996; 5: 279-296.

23. Agro K.E., Bradley C.A., Mittmann N., et al., Sensitivity analysis in health economic and pharmacoeconomic studies: an appraisal of the literature. *Pharmacoeconomics.* 1997; 11(1): 75-88.

24. Detsky A.S., Guidelines for economic analysis of pharmaceutical products: a draft document for Ontario and Canada. *Pharmacoeconomics.* 1993; 3(5): 354-361.

25. Drummond M.F., Stoddart G.L., Torrance G.W., *Methods for the Economic Evaluation of Health Care Programs.* Oxford: Oxford University Press; 1987.

26. Glick H., Kinosian B., Schulman K., Decision analytic modeling: some uses in the evaluation of new pharmaceuticals. *Drug Inf J.* 1994; 28: 691-707.

27. Henry D., Economic analysis as an aid to subsidisation decisions: the development of Australian guidelines for pharmaceuticals. *Pharmacoeconomics.* 1992; 1: 54-67.

28. Kassirer J.P., Angell M., The journal's policy on cost-effectiveness analyses. *N Engl J Med.* 1994; 331: 669-670.

29. Sheldon T.A., Problems of using modeling in the economic evaluation of health care. *Health Econ.* 1996; 5: 1-11.

30. Weinstein M.C., O'Brien B., Hornberger J., et al. Principles of good practice for decision analytic modeling in health-care evaluation: report of the ISPOR task force on good research practices—modeling studies. *Value Health.* 2003; 6(1): 9-17.

31. Daniels N., Sabin J.E., The ethics of accountability in managed care reform. *Health Affairs.* 1998; 17(5): 50-64.

PHARMACOECONOMIC RESEARCH AND APPLICATIONS IN MANAGED CARE

DIANA I. BRIXNER

JOSEPH E. BISKUPIAK

VIJAY N. JOISH*

HEMAL SHAH

INTRODUCTION

Healthcare costs have been rising for several decades. National health expenditures in the United States were nearly $1.9 trillion in 2004 (or 16% of gross domestic product [GDP]), almost two and a half times the $696 billion spent in 1990 (12.0% of GDP). Though the percentage of the GDP spent on health care leveled off earlier in the 1990s, the percentage is again rising. Total healthcare expenditures grew at an annual rate of 7.3% between 2002 and 2003, slower than in the previous five years, but still outpacing inflation and the growth in national income (**Figure 12-1**).

In addition, employers and managed care organizations (MCOs) have yet to demonstrate their ability to manage costs across the spectrum of care for their employees and members. Since 2000, employer-sponsored health insurance premiums have increased by 73%, while the proportion of Americans with employer-based insurance has declined from 63.3% in 2002 to 61.9% in 2003. Employers are increasingly shifting costs to their employees in the form of higher premiums, deductibles, and copayments. Employees' wages are growing at a much slower rate than healthcare costs and many are beginning to face difficulties affording the growth in out-of-pocket spending. In addition, the percent of the nonelderly population without insurance rose from 17.3% in 2002 to 17.7% in 2003 (44.7 million uninsured).[1,2]

---

*At the time this work was completed, Vijay Joish was a Research Assistant Professor at the University of Utah.

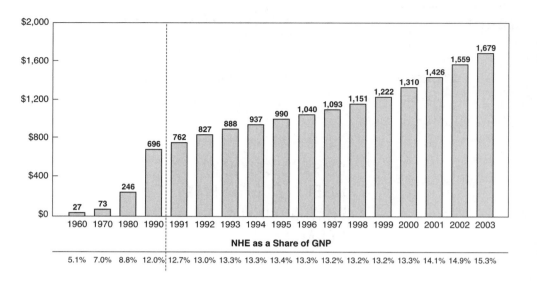

FIGURE 12-1 U.S. National Health Expenditures, 1960-2003.

Source: Centers for Medicare and Medicaid Services, Office of the Actuary, National Health Statistics Group. Available at http://www.cms. gov/statistics/nhe/default.asp (2003 National Health Care Expenditures Data Files for Downloading, file nhegdp03.zip). Source of actual graph: http://www.umassmed.edu/uploadedfiles/HealthPolicyPracticeMedicine_January2006MATjh.pdf.

Medicare and Medicaid program spending also have been rising but at lower rates than private employer plan premiums. With the enactment of Medicare Modernization Act of 2003, Medicare spending increased when the prescription drug benefit was implemented in January 2006. Spending in the Medicaid program now represents one of the largest items in most state budgets; many states report that it is leading to financial strains and are implementing cuts in eligibility or benefits.

As the balance of the payor moves from private to public, the scrutiny on drug prices will continue to increase. Therefore, the value of the increased benefit gained versus the increase in cost will become more important. Pharmacoeconomic research assesses the overall value of pharmaceutical products in the treatment or prevention of disease. There are many cases where the appropriate use of pharmaceuticals decreased overall healthcare costs. One of the first such examples is the changing treatment of ulcers over the past 15 years.[3] Prior to the advent of H2 antagonist therapy in 1977, over 97,000 ulcer surgeries were performed each year. By 1987, that number had dropped to about 18,000. The average annual cost of drug therapy per person amounted to about $900 compared to $28,000 for surgery. The discovery that the *Helicobacter pylori* bacterium is the principal cause of ulcers led to the use of antibiotics in combination with H2 antagonists to treat ulcers. At a cost of about $140 per patient, combination therapy now decisively eradicates the cause of most ulcers.

Another example is the case of low-molecular-weight heparins (LMWHs), which are used as a prophylaxis against and treatment for diseases involving thrombosis. The challenge that pharmacists must face is making decisions between budgetary concerns and patient outcomes. With the help of pharmacoeconomic data, scientific methods, and principles, pharmacists can evaluate the impact that new drugs (like LMWHs) have on a pharmacy budget or overall hospital expenditures.[4]

As treatment changes, the way in which healthcare costs are distributed changes also. **Figure 12-2** shows the distribution of healthcare costs in 2003. As expenditures on ulcer surgery and hospitalization decline, expenditures on drugs to treat ulcers rise, but the total treatment expenditures for ulcers shrinks. This same principle applies across the continuum of health care. If pharmaceuticals are used effectively, then overall healthcare costs should decrease.

The use of pharmaceuticals also affects overall employer expenditures. Use of prescription drugs saves money for employers by reducing disability and absenteeism and increasing productivity while improving the quality of life for employees. An example is

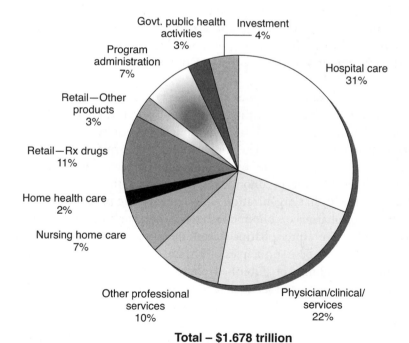

Total – $1.678 trillion

FIGURE 12-2   U.S. National Health Expenditures, 2003.
Source: Centers for Medicare and Medicaid Services, Office of the Actuary, National Health Statistics Group, at http://www.cms.hhs.gov/NationalHealthExpendData.

the growing availability and effectiveness of pharmaceutical products to treat migraine headaches. Migraine headaches not only cause pain to those who suffer from them but also increase absenteeism and decrease employee productivity. A study by Legg et al.[5] found that the total costs of treating patients for migraine headaches declined 41% as the result of a new drug treatment. Another study showed that the drug Sumatriptan saved employers $435 per month per employee due to a reduction in lost productivity costs, while the monthly cost of the drug per employee was only $44.[6] A third example of the positive impact of pharmacoeconomic data is shown in a study examining the relationship of work loss associated with gastroesophageal reflux disease (GERD) and peptic ulcer disease (PUD).[7] This study looked at the impact of both direct and indirect costs using an employer's claims database. A significantly higher rate of sickness-related absenteeism was observed in the diseased group than the controls. Pharmacoeconomic data were used to calculate an incremental economic impact cost as applied to a hypothetical 25,000 employee firm (**Table 12-1**). A $125 per day average wage was applied the pharmacoeconomic data to achieve an incremental total cost of an employee with the disease. In Table 12-1, these costs show an economic impact of $3,441 per employee per year for an employee diagnosed with GERD and $1,374 for an employee with PUD. An employee suffering from both GERD and PUD was estimated to have an economic cost impact to the employer of $4,803 compared to an employee with only one or no disease.[7] Information on how pharmaceuticals can affect employer costs is particularly important when contracts between MCOs and employers are being reviewed or initiated.

These types of examples have made MCOs take a more comprehensive approach as they decide which pharmaceuticals to add to their formularies. Pharmacoeconomic information has become as important as clinical and safety information in the formulary decision-making process. The highest-quality pharmacoeconomic information is evidence-based on the literature, observational or clinical study results, or retrospective database analyses. Pharmacoeconomic research done within an MCO often can provide the greatest value in that organization's decision-making process.

Evolution of pharmacoeconomic research has had an impact on the role of the pharmacists as well. To interpret pharmacoeconomic information, pharmacists must be adequately trained in the basic principles of pharmacoeconomics. Then, they can judge the quality and thoroughness of published pharmacoeconomic research and integrate this information with clinical and safety data to make sound decisions as to what drugs should be made available, when, and to which patients.

This chapter discusses pharmacoeconomic methodologies and applications in pharmaceutical development. In addition, this chapter demonstrates how pharmacoeconomics can affect product value, strategic product marketing, and managed care formulary decision making by pharmacy and therapeutics (P & T) committees. It also describes opportunities and challenges involved in pharmacoeconomic data collection and integration, research projects with managed care, and the role of the pharmacist in conducting and applying pharmacoeconomic research.

TABLE 12-1 **Economic Impact of GERD, PUD and GERD + PUD on a 25,000-employee population***

Parameters	GERD	PUD	GERD+PUD
Prevalence of Disease[1]	10% (± 2.5%)	2% (± 0.5%)	2% (± 0.5%)
Size of Firm[2]	25,000 (± 6,250)	25,000 (± 6,250)	25,000 (± 6,250)
Average Daily Wage[3]	$125 (± $31)	$125 (± $31)	$125 (± $31)
Incremental Median Medical Costs[4]	$2,672 (± $668)	$593 (± $148)	$3,984 (± $996)
Incremental Average Absenteeism rate[4]	1.20 (± 0.30)	1.30 (± 0.33)	1.60 (± 0.40)
Presenteeism rate[5]	15 (± 3.75)	15 (± 3.75)	15 (± 3.75)
Prevalence of Presenteeism[5]	33% (± 8.3%)	33% (± 8.3%)	33% (± 8.3%)
Incremental Economic Impact			
Incremental Direct Cost Impact to Employer (D)[6]	$6,680,000 ($2,818,125 – $13,046,875)	$296,500 ($125,086 – $579,102)	$1,992,000 ($840,009 – $3,890,625)
Incremental Absenteeism Cost Impact to Employer (I_A)[7]	$375,000 ($118,652 – $915,527)	$81,250 ($25,708 – $198,364)	$100,000 ($31,641 – $244,141)
Incremental Presenteeism Cost Impact to Employer (I_p)[8]	$1,546,875 ($367,081 – $4,720,688)	$390,625 ($99,124 – $1,142,502)	$409,375 ($105,057 – $1,188,278)
Incremental Total Economic Impact ($D+I_A+I_p$)	$8,601,875 ($3,303,858 – $18,683,090)	$687,125 ($224,210 – $1,721,603)	$2,401,375 ($945,432 – $5,078,903)
Incremental Total Cost/Dx Employee[9]	$3,441 ($2,349 – $4,783)	$1,374 ($797 – $2,204)	$4,803 ($3,362 – $6,501)

* All parameters are annualized rates/dollars and have been varied ± 25% of their base case value, and shown in parentheses.

[1] Prevalence of GERD derived from Dean et al. (2003); prevalence of PUD from Graham et al. (1999); prevalence of GERD+PUD assumed by authors.

[2] Hypothetical numbers of employees.

[3] Average daily wage rates were derived from the U.S. Department of Labor, Bureau of Labor Statistics for 2000.

[4] Incremental median medical care costs and average absenteeism rates were derived from the MedStat database and were calculated as the difference between the costs of the disease group minus controls. Cost data were highly skewed with extreme values compared to the absenteeism rates. Thus, it was assumed that median costs and average absence rates were more "typical" of the population

[5] Presenteeism rate and prevalence of presenteeism were derived for GERD from the Dean et al. study and assumed to be the same for PUD and GERD+PUD cohorts.

[6] Incremental Direct Cost Impact to Employer (D) = Direct Medical Costs = Prevalence of Disease × Size of Firm × Incremental Median Medical Cost.

[7] Incremental Absenteeism Cost Impact to Employer (I_A) = Prevalence of Disease × Size of Firm × Incremental Absenteeism Rate × Average Daily Wage

[8] Incremental Absenteeism Cost Impact to Employer (I_p) = Prevalence of Disease × Size of Firm × Average Daily Wage × Presenteeism Rate × Prevalence of Presenteeism

[9] Incremental Total Cost/Dx Employee = [($D+I_A+I_p$) ÷ (Prevalence of Disease × Size of Firm)]

Source: Economic Impact of GERD, PUD and GERD + PUD on a 25,000-employee population (Source: Joish VN et al, "The economic impact of GERD and PUD: examination of direct and indirect costs using a large integrated employer claims database." Curr Med Res Opin. 2005 Apr;21(4):535-44).

BASICS OF PHARMACOECONOMIC RESEARCH

Pharmacoeconomic analyses are full economic evaluations as both costs and consequences are measured. There are four types of research methodologies used when conducting pharmacoeconomic research:

1. Cost-minimization analysis (CMA)
2. Cost-benefit analysis (CBA)
3. Cost-effectiveness analysis (CEA)
4. Cost-utility analysis (CUA)

Cost-of-illness (COI) analysis is a type of evaluation frequently used in health economics to quantify the economic burden of a specific disease. It provides information on the cost structure related to a disease for a specific population. Because there are no consequences or outcomes measured, it is not a full economic evaluation. COI often is used as a first step in cost identification (i.e., direct and indirect costs) that may lead to a full economic evaluation. For example, economic evaluations of immunization programs involve estimating the cost of the disease that a vaccine would eradicate. Results of COI are thus important, but they do not answer questions related to the most effective option for treating a disease or disorder.

To answer questions concerning optimal resource allocation, CMA, CBA, CEA, and CUA pharmacoeconomic methods are used. All four methods attempt to weigh costs and consequences of alternative medical or pharmacotherapeutic actions logically. Where the methods differ is in the way outcomes are valued, and whether the resource allocation issue in question is one of *allocative* efficiency or *production* efficiency.[8] Allocative efficiency is concerned with given scarce resources and deciding which goals are worth achieving, and thereby determining which programs are worthwhile. On the other hand, production efficiency is concerned with how best to deliver a program once the decision already has been made to allocate resources toward it. CBA and CUA are appropriate techniques to answer the question of allocative efficiency, whereas CMA and CEA evaluations would be fitting where the efficiency in question is that of production.

CMA is the simplest of the five evaluation methods because it compares only costs between the interventions or drugs. The effectiveness of treatments is assumed to be clinically identical or similar, so the goal of CMA is therefore to identify the least costly treatment. For example, in a study by Howard and colleagues, a cost-minimization analysis was conducted to compare costs between intravenous azithromycin and erythromycin for treating community-acquired pneumonia.[9] As the effectiveness profiles of the two drugs were assumed to be equivalent, costs in terms of medication use and treatment of adverse events were compared. Two challenges are often faced when conducting a CMA: establishing therapeutic equivalence and determining equi-effective doses.[10] Thus, even though CMA appears to be the most straightforward of the five types of pharmacoeconomic analyses, there are only a relatively small number of published CMA studies in the literature.

CBA values all costs and consequences of treatments or programs in monetary units.[11] For example, cost of a health program may include direct medical (e.g., cost of therapy), direct non-medical (cost of conveyance to a pharmacy), and indirect costs (cost to a patient as forgone wages). The challenge in conducting a CBA is to quantify health and non-health benefits that patients derive from a program. There are three general approaches to the monetary valuation of outcomes: 1) human capital; 2) revealed preferences; and 3) stated preferences of willingness-to-pay.[1,12] The human capital method values the gains in a person's health due to an intervention by using market wage rates, as utilization of a program is viewed as an investment in a person's human capital. Revealed preference is based on the wage-risk approach and on individual preferences regarding the value of increased or decreased health risk as a trade-off against increased or decreased income. It is based on actual and not hypothetical consumer choices involving health versus money. Finally, stated preferences of willingness-to-pay approach uses survey methods to present respondents with hypothetical scenarios about a new intervention or health benefit under evaluation and elicit their maximum willingness to pay for such a benefit, given an existing program or therapy. All three evaluation methods have limitations. The advantage of CBA in general is that by converting all inputs and outputs to monetary units, comparisons are not restricted to treatments for a particular disorder but can be used to inform resource allocation decisions both within and between sectors of health care and of the economy in general (e.g., investing in a vaccination program vs. industrial safety program). However, the major disadvantage of CBA is its requirement of valuing human lives in monetary units, which for many healthcare decision-makers is difficult and unethical; therefore, they are mistrustful of such analyses.

CEA is the most popular form of pharmacoeconomic method. Resources (i.e., inputs) are valued in monetary units and consequences in natural efficacy/effectiveness units (e.g., years of life saved, disability days avoided). It is important that the reader appreciate the difference between the efficacy and effectiveness. Although sometimes erroneously used interchangeably, *efficacy* refers to the success of a drug in a randomized clinical trial (i.e., controlled environment), whereas *effectiveness* refers to the success of a drug in the real world (i.e., natural environment). When a CEA is performed alongside a clinical trial, the ratios reported are cost-efficacy ratios (CERs), and when CEA is performed using real world clinical outcomes data, they are referred to as cost-effectiveness ratios. CEA is used when a choice needs to be made between two or more competing pharmacotherapeutic options for which the expected health gains are measured in terms of a common clinical measure. For example, when choosing between two or more oral triptans for migraine headaches, a measure of effectiveness may be the complete relief of migraine headache within two hours. Thus, a CER in such a study would be reported as the cost per relief of migraine headache within two hours. The choice of an efficacy or effectiveness measure is usually made either from the primary end-point used in a clinical trial (which is always reported in the package insert for a drug) or from the most popular clinically and economically meaningful outcome reported in the literature. Generally, two ratios are calculated as an average or absolute CER (ACER), and the incremental CER (ICER). When the CER is calculated relative to no treatment, it is referred to as the ACER. On the other hand, the ICER represents the change in costs and health benefits when one intervention is compared with an alternative. ACER captures the average costs of resources spent per unit of benefit. Although an interesting measure, the ACER calculated in isolation is of limited usefulness. In most cases, decision makers are interested in knowing the net cost-effectiveness of an intervention compared to some alternative. For example, if drug A offers an additional benefit compared to drug B but at a higher cost, then the question of interest is whether the extra benefit gained is worth the additional cost. In order to attempt to answer this question, one calculates the ICER, which expresses the additional cost required to gain an incremental unit of benefit. A limitation of the CEA is that in comparing CEA ratios, the benefit or outcomes need to be identical for both interventions to compare the cost-effectiveness of the interventions validly.

CUA may be used when different interventions treating varying diseases need to be compared. In CUA, resources are measured or valued in dollars whereas benefits or consequences are expressed in terms of a subject's preference for a given health state, and the most common measure being quality adjusted life year (QALY). Thus, CUA attempts to summarize the effects of a health intervention on both survival (i.e., quantity of life) and health-related quality of life (HRQoL) in a single index. Just like CEA, both average cost-utility and incremental cost-utility ratios are calculated. Results are expressed in terms of cost per QALY gained. CUA is recommended to be used when: 1) the main impact of a health intervention is upon HRQoL rather than survival; 2) a program affects both morbidity and mortality and a common index is needed to capture the trade-off between these effects; and 3) there is a need to standardize health benefits across different outcome measures, disease contexts and interventions.[8] The controversy surrounding CUA is often due to the way preferences are measured. In brief, there are two key aspects of the measurement of preferences. One is the way in which the question is framed, that is, whether the outcomes in the question are certain or uncertain. Second is the way in which the subject is asked to respond, specifically, whether the subject is asked to perform a scaling task based on introspection or to make a choice.[8]

CUA is one of the newest forms of pharmacoeconomic analysis and can be the most controversial because of the way utilities are measured. The standard gamble and time trade-off are some of the techniques used to establish utilities. Utilities are the distinct values placed on a health status as measured by the preferences of individuals or society.[13] All utility values are between zero and one, where zero is equal to death and one is equal to perfect health. The measurement of these utility values is necessary for the calculation of the most commonly used outcome measure in CUA, quality-adjusted life-years gained.

Despite the controversy, CUA has certain features that other pharmacoeconomic analyses do not. It is able to incorporate multiple outcomes simultaneously from the same intervention and evaluate the overall quality of the health outcome achieved.[13] It is most appropriate to use CUA when quality of life is an important outcome. For example, CUA is most valuable in comparing interventions that predominantly affect a patient's satisfaction, function, and well-being. CUA also may be beneficial in comparing a wide range of potential outcomes and in situations where a common unit of outcome is necessary for comparison.[8]

Each of the different types of cost effectiveness analyses are used to determine the value of a particular drug or healthcare option and is dependent on several factors. The audience receiving the information is critical, whether it be from a societal, individual, provider, or payor perspective. In this chapter, the perspective is that of managed care, trying to utilize health and pharmacoeconomic information to determine the value of a pharmaceutical. Within this determination, the choice of study type can vary between the phases of drug development, drug category, therapeutic area, and the specific research question being asked.

APPLICATION OF PHARMACOECONOMICS IN PHARMACEUTICAL COMPANIES

Pharmacoeconomics are used in numerous ways by the pharmaceutical industry. The central question has been and continues to be: "When is it appropriate to include a cost-effectiveness perspective?" Utilizing this research methodology across all therapeutic areas in all stages of drug development would be cost prohibitive and inefficient.

In the early stages of drug development, one looks at certain disease states or therapeutic areas, and decisions are made based on the efficacy and value of bringing a new agent into the marketplace. From a clinical standpoint, this would primarily include the mechanism of action of the drug. Do the inherent properties of the molecule predict better efficacy or lower side effects than those of similar drugs on the market? Does the drug work through a novel mechanism of action and is therefore expected to have better results in clinical trials than the current therapy? While these questions are being answered through biological testing in animals and Phase I and II trials in humans are being planned, a pharmacoeconomics group would begin looking at the overall cost of illness for the particular disease state of interest and understanding the burden of the disease to society. This includes information on the proportion of time a patient would spend in emergency departments, outpatient treatment centers, physician's offices, long-term care, and time on drug therapy for the disease. With these data in hand, a pharmacoeconomics group can then do predictive modeling to determine the potential cost benefit of the new drug under consideration.

Consider the example of Alzheimer's disease. A new product in development may work through a different mechanism of action that may stabilize memory loss once diagnosis is made and treatment is begun. All current therapeutic alternatives slow the progression of disease but do not halt it. This new drug would halt the disease progression. From an economic perspective, one would consider this drug in the context of the overall cost of treating Alzheimer's disease and the impact on the caregiver, the MCO, and institutional care.

Based on early development work already completed, from both a clinical and an economic perspective, a decision then can be made to proceed to Phase II and Phase III clinical trials in humans. The pharmacoeconomic perspective now comes into play as experts ask what key endpoints will communicate the value of this product to the payer and the patient. In the Alzheimer's example, the early development modeling determined that the drug would significantly decrease institutional charges. However, the MCO may end up bearing the burden of increased pharmaceutical cost. The patient's quality of life is maintained as long as the progression of disease is postponed. With these economic endpoints in mind, one would want to be sure to measure the time to institutionalization, the cost of time in the institution, and both patient and caregiver quality of life.

A significant challenge at this stage can be the globalization of clinical trial protocols. Often, practice patterns vary in different countries, which impact the value profile of the drug as well as the desired economic endpoints in the clinical trial from a global perspective. Usually, the needs of the key country markets are met through a global health economic development plan, and the needs of individual countries are met through collecting additional endpoints at clinical trial sites within their country or through designing a country-specific trial. These country-specific trials often are designed as Phase IV studies, which are clinical trials that may be conducted outside the requirements of Food and Drug Administration (FDA) registration. Such studies may look at the impact of a new drug therapy across a large population with a less restrictive protocol to allow for a more realistic assessment of safety and efficacy. It may make sense to include quality of life or other economic endpoints in this type of study. Alternatively, a study may be designed with a primary endpoint that is economic or outcome oriented. Examples include evaluating the incidence and costs of gastrointestinal side effects for osteoporotic women on alendronate[14] or understanding the impact of onychomycosis on the patient's perception of pain and quality of life.[15]

USE OF PHARMACOECONOMIC DATA FOR EFFECTIVENESS CLAIMS

The standard for a cost-effectiveness labeling claim is that the efficacy denominator must be based on two well-controlled clinical trials. Few pharmaceutical products have cleared this hurdle. For health economic information to be of value to a decision maker, the new therapy must be compared to the current standard of practice. In most cases, the current standard of practice is an alternative drug therapy that is already on the market and not a placebo. Most clinical trials compare a new product to a placebo or to an older class of drugs because the larger the expected difference between two items being compared, the fewer the number of patients who need to be enrolled in the trial to demonstrate an efficacy endpoint. Using fewer patients lowers costs and decreases the time to market for a new product. Therefore, the goals of a clinical trial protocol are inherently different from the information a P & T committee member needs to make informed decisions about drug coverage for a health plan. When a product treats a specific disease for which no prior drug therapy existed, the goals of clinical trials and decision makers are more similar. In such a case, a placebo would more closely resemble the current alternative therapy.

Even so, there are few examples in the literature of economic endpoints collected and analyzed as part of a clinical trial protocol, resulting in an economic claim for the product at the time of launch. One example was a large international study by Genentech. The study compared the Genentech product, tissue plasminogen activator (tPA), against streptokinase.[16] The results of this trial led the FDA to change product labeling to include data on the life-saving benefits of the product.[17] Simultaneously, Mark and colleagues at Duke conducted a CUA based on the results from this trial.[18] Each dose of tPA cost $2,000 and each dose of streptokinase cost $270. Given the slightly higher life expectancy for patients who received tPA, an incremental cost-effectiveness ratio of $32,000 per life-year gained was achieved, on average. The results of this CUA were not included in the labeling, however. Dissemination of this information was left to publication and peer-to-peer scientific exchange. Nevertheless, some products may show potential for an extremely favorable cost effectiveness ratio per discounted life year gain as shown by Huybrechts et al.[19] in their study entitled, "Health and economic consequences of sevelamer use for hyperphosphatemia in patients on hemodialysis." The study results indicate that sevelamer has important clinical and economic consequences over the comparison drug, which in turn means good value for the money.[19]

Dissemination of health economic information is handled by those who create this type of information and those who use this type of information in decision making. In the early stages, the FDA considered information from pharmacoeconomic studies as part of ensuring that promotional materials involving pharmaceuticals were not inaccurate or misleading. Therefore, the FDA did not restrict publication of pharmacoeconomic information by the pharmaceutical company, but did regulate circulation of such a study for the purposes of promotion. This guideline still left a significant gap regarding the utilization of economic models and the presentation of these models to formulary decision makers. To address this gap, the enacted Section 114 of the Food and Drug Administration Modernization Act of 1997 (FDAMA) now allows manufacturers to provide healthcare economic information to a formulary committee or similar entity. Committees use this information as they select drugs for managed care or other organizations. "Healthcare economic information" is defined in FDAMA as, "any analysis that identifies, measures, or compares the economic consequences, including the costs of the represented health outcomes, of the use of a drug to the use of another drug, to another healthcare intervention, or to no intervention." According to this legislation, healthcare economic information provided will not be considered to be false or misleading if it directly relates to an FDA-approved indication and is based on "competent and reliable scientific evidence."

FDA USE OF RETROSPECTIVE DATA

Two principal sources of data for pharmacoeconomic analyses are meta-analysis of the literature and retrospective data from electronic claims databases.

In principle, meta-analysis is a good example of what could be referred to as "competent and reliable scientific evidence" for a pharmacoeconomic claim to be made to a formulary committee. This systematic, quantitative analysis statistically combines the data of multiple studies that address essentially similar research questions.[20] Information obtained via meta-analysis can be considered as an alternative to data from two well-controlled clinical trials. Results of meta-analyses can be used to advance further research and provide critical values and parameters for decision models. In a study by Marchetti et al.,[21] a meta-analysis was conducted to summarize current findings on onychomycosis and to statistically summarize available cure rate estimates of all available oral treatments for the disease. Cure rates and other relevant values obtained from the meta-analysis were used for the development of an onychomycosis cost-effectiveness model.[21]

Retrospective information from electronic claims can be obtained from a pharmacy claims–only database, such as that commonly found through a pharmacy benefit management company (PBM) or through the integration of medical and pharmacy claims. Such integrated data often are obtained from a disease management company, where the medical claims of a health plan may have been combined with the pharmacy claims from the affiliated PBM. Integrated data also are available from health maintenance organizations (HMOs), where complete care is provided to the patient through providers employed by or contracted by the HMO. Each data source offers advantages and disadvantages.

An HMO's information comes from one source, unlike information from a health plan and PBM, which can come from many different sources. But because a staff model HMO's providers are paid regardless of the specific service they provide, they do not have a significant financial incentive to promptly submit encounter data to administrative offices. When these data are submitted, they are more likely to accurately reflect care, because payment is not dependent upon the specific claim.

In a health plan or a PBM, the provider submits the claim to obtain reimbursement. These providers often are paid at a discounted fee for service. Providers are quick to submit claims because payment is dependent upon claim submission, which is a good aspect of such claims databases. The potential downside is that the diagnosis submission may not be accurate because providers may code a diagnosis to maximize reimbursement (upcoding) or enter a more general code instead of a specific one to ease the submission process. Although limitations exist with claims databases, they do offer some advantages. Often, databases can be used for longitudinal studies, as patient information can cover long periods of time. Some databases contain information on a large number of patients from diverse demographic and geographic backgrounds. This large body of information may allow researchers to conduct studies that will provide useful information to a wide audience and is universally applicable. Most important, these claims databases allow examination of the real-world use of different treatments and services.[22]

However, the use of retrospective data to change prescribing behaviors of physicians can become quite controversial. In 1995, Pasty and colleagues[23] published results of a population-based case controlled study assessing the risk of myocardial infarction in patients with hypertension on different therapeutic regimens. Their results indicated that short-acting calcium channel blockers (CCBs), especially taken in high doses, were associated with an increased risk (trend $P < 0.01$).[23] Many debates arose about the validity of these data and the assumption that the risk was truly due to the drug agents chosen. Based on published studies, the FDA agreed to a label warning against off-label use of short-acting nifedipine in patients with hypertension, acute myocardial infarction, or nonvasospastic unstable angina. Practitioners were encouraged to exercise caution when prescribing CCBs, especially to high-risk patients. They were told that long-acting CCBs should be used.[24] The market share of CCBs in general has been significantly affected by this controversy, even though the warning concerned only short-acting CCBs.

This example and other controversies with respect to retrospective research have led to the development of standards in the conduct of such research. In an effort to address the methodological challenges and assist decision makers with the evaluation of the quality of these published studies, a task force was organized by the International Society for Pharmacoeconomics and Outcomes Research (ISPOR). This task force organized a checklist of 27 questions to guide decision makers through the evaluation process of retrospective database studies including the study methodology and the study conclusion.[25]

Another up and coming source of retrospective data is the electronic medical record (EMR). This can be a compilation of records from local facilities or systems or a comprehensive national research consortium providing information on millions of patient lives. There are several advantages to conducting research in an EMR database, including access to vital sign statistics such as height and weight and clinical outcomes including blood pressure, glucose and lipid levels. Potential disadvantages are that the data are mostly primary care in focus, making the integration of hospital information difficult. Also, prescription information is collected through physician orders and not from claims data; therefore, assumptions are made related to patient adherence to their medications. There are many areas where the specific data available in an EMR database may be particularly beneficial in determining the value of a pharmaceutical. For example, in diabetes management, the trends on A1C levels across different drugs or drug classes can be measured. A 2005 study looked at the weight profile between patients on first and second generation antipsychotics in a naturalistic study using a national EMR database.[26] For the most part, the results in a real world setting validated those demonstrated in clinical trials, with aripiprazole and ziprasidone having less of an impact on weight than olanzapine and others. Clozapine did not show a significant impact on weight gain, although this was expected from earlier clinical trials. This could be a reflection of the real world use of this drug for several years where weight gain may have been experienced early on in the course of treatment.

Pharmaceutical companies are expanding the potential use of EMR databases to implement and measure disease management programs and to simulate clinical trial protocols to maximize patient selection.

RETROSPECTIVE DATA IN PHARMACOECONOMIC RESEARCH

There are many examples of how retrospective data can be used in pharmacoeconomic research. A study conducted by Gianfrancesco et al.[27] and published in a peer reviewed journal represents some of the data and statistical methods that should be incorporated into pharmacoeconomic studies that evaluate both drug costs and other treatment outcomes using retrospective insurance claims. Many of these data are available from government entities like Medicaid, Medicare, and the Veterans Affairs as well as healthcare insurers like Wellpoint, I3Magnifi, and Medstat.[28] The Gianfrescesco et al.'s study[27] was based on administrative data from 46 U.S. commercial health plans. The study evaluated claims in the period between January 1998 through April 2002 to determine the mental health resources used by patients diagnosed with bipolar disorder and treated with either risperidone, olanzapine, or quetiapine. The results showed that mental health costs outside of the cost of the prescribed drug was not different between the three. But the equivalent daily dose prescription cost appeared to be more significant for olanzapine than risperidone or quetiapine.[27]

Another study conducted by Lyman et al.[29] using retrospective data from a commercial healthcare company evaluated the economic burden of anemia in cancer patients receiving chemotherapy. The study found that 26% of the 2760 cancer patients meeting the study requirements had anemia and that direct medical costs associated with the anemia were substantial.

ROLE OF PHARMACOECONOMIC RESEARCH IN BRAND MANAGEMENT

As pharmacoeconomic impact and assessment of product value become integral elements of a brand strategy, brand management teams have begun to include pharmacoeconomic data in the marketing mix. The use of pharmacoeconomic information in the various stages of pre-launch activity for a drug was discussed earlier ("Application of Pharmacoeconomics in Pharmaceutical Companies"). This next section describes the use of pharmacoeconomic data for marketing purposes after the drug is FDA approved and launched by the pharmaceutical company for distribution to providers and patients.

SUPPORT OF BRAND MANAGEMENT BY OUTCOMES DIVISION

Within the pharmaceutical industry, there is an increasing interest in developing value propositions through health economic and outcomes data to inform both internal and external decision-making. Successful marketing of any product requires a key strategy, clear objectives, and a tactical plan that ensures the objectives are met. All aspects of the marketing plan need to be aligned with this strategy, the positioning statement, and key messages for the product. The development of marketing tools, the design and implementation of Phase IV trials, and other activities also need to conform to the marketing strategy for the product.

This principle holds true for the health economic and outcomes research strategy for a product as well. Take, for example, the launch of a new treatment for chronic obstructive pulmonary disease (COPD). This disease state presents some inherent marketing challenges. COPD is not high on the radar screen for managed care because it is perceived to be a disease of the elderly who are no longer working and, thus, not covered under the commercial benefit. In reality, however, seventy percent of COPD patients are under the age of 65. In addition, a large segment of the COPD market is either misdiagnosed or undiagnosed. To address these challenges, one of the key marketing strategies for the product might be to highlight the epidemiology and economic burden of COPD in a managed care population by conducting a burden of illness study.

More often than not, the key component of a pharmacoeconomic or outcomes strategy is the identification of the appropriate population for a specific therapy. In this case, that could involve the establishment of a predictive model for COPD patients that would determine which patients should be targeted for COPD treatment. Another major issue in this therapeutic area is that the main driver of healthcare costs is inpatient hospitalizations for COPD exacerbations. Treatments that improve a patient's lung function may result in reductions in COPD exacerbations and related hospitalizations. Thus, an economic model that extrapolates the clinical and economic impacts of a new treatment on reducing COPD exacerbations and related hospitalizations can be developed to demonstrate the medical cost offsets that may be achieved with a new treatment. The economic hypotheses would be that despite higher drug costs, the overall treatment costs for a patient who receives a COPD treatment may be lower due to reductions in COPD-related hospitalizations. The model would provide a key economic value message in support of the brand strategy.

A wide variety of health economics and outcomes data can be provided by pharmaceutical companies in order to demonstrate the value of new products from a payor perspective.

WHEN PHARMACOECONOMICS HELPS AND WHEN IT IS UNNECESSARY

When aligning a pharmacoeconomic strategy with an overall marketing strategy, it is critical to decide whether a pharmacoeconomic argument will influence the decision maker. New, high priced technologies might be expected to sell just because of their clinical benefit. But decision makers often want to understand how the drugs will impact patient therapy and outcomes in a particular disease state as well as how the drug will affect non-pharmaceutical healthcare costs. This decision is becoming more critical now in light of the proliferation of biologicals in the armamentarium of treatment options for disease. In treatment areas such as multiple sclerosis, psoriasis, rheumatoid arthritis, and Crohn's disease, the first drug to market often did not need a pharmacoeconomic study profile due to the vastly superior demonstrated efficacy to standard available therapies. However, as additional, high priced biologics enter the marketplace, the utilization of pharmacoeconomics to demonstrate the differentiation between drug therapies can be important. These products can be different enough in both structure and mechanism of action that both efficacy and tolerability differences can have an impact on drug and overall costs.

Pharmacoeconomics can play a dominant role in the new treatments for diseases that in the past have had few treatment options. For example, the many new expensive biologic drug therapies for multiple sclerosis have shifted the attention and focus of healthcare payors to the economic burden of the disease. A major task will be the collection of data on the impact of the new disease-modifying therapies in reducing disability progression over the long-term, independent of clinical trials. Gathering this kind of information is of critical importance in order to improve the precision of cost-effectiveness estimates in the future.[30]

Rheumatoid arthritis in the past has had limited options for treatment. Faced with the same situation of new expensive drug therapies becoming available, healthcare providers and/or decision-makers need evidence of relative efficacy and cost-effectiveness. These data will come from direct clinical and/or long-term pharmacoeconomics studies. Erkan et al.[31] conducted a study to determine whether pharmacoeconomic variables modified a physician's choice. Their study concluded that pharmacoeconomics appears to have a role in a rheumatologists' choice of disease therapy and physicians may choose a type of therapy based on cost, even though this may be contrary to their perception of the drug's effectiveness in treating rheumatoid arthritis.[31]

When two drugs from different classes are available to treat the same disease, a pharmacoeconomic analysis can be very helpful. The costs and outcomes due to adverse events, impact of dosing regimens, and clinical efficacy profiles should be compared for the drugs from both classes. Economic analysis is difficult when comparing two drugs of the same class. In this case, there may be a slight difference that may have economic consequences, but for the most part this difference is not enough to sway a decision maker. Ultimately, the choice between drugs in the same class often comes down to marketing savvy and price.

PHARMACOECONOMIC INFORMATION STRATEGIES WITHIN PHARMACEUTICAL COMPANIES

Conducting any type of pharmacoeconomic analysis requires accessing information and data. The quality of the data received will dictate the quality of the ultimate analysis. In a clinical analysis, the randomized controlled trial is typically the "gold standard" for comparing one drug with a treatment alternative. In an economic analysis, standards may be different. Economic studies can be based on data acquired during the clinical trial phase through adding specific questions relating to resource utilization or quality of life to the case report forms. This approach allows economic information to be presented along with clinical and safety information at the time of the drug launch. However, the drawback of this approach is that economic information obtained via a clinical trial is limited by the clinical protocol and therefore is less indicative of how a drug may impact patient outcomes or overall drug costs when utilized within a healthcare system. Also, the time needed to get the information is dependent on the length of enrollment and data analysis for the clinical trial. Because most clinical trials are still done via conventional form collection and data processing, this is an expensive way to collect data. Finally, if these economic analyses are conducted during early drug development, researchers still run the risk that the product may never reach the market.

Because of these limitations, economic data are usually collected in Phase IV trials, which can still be limited by strict protocols, or in a "naturalistic" or "observational" trial. In this type of study, a drug is usually compared to its most likely alternative within a healthcare system environment. Although the assignment of patients to certain treatments may be randomized, few other interventions are conducted other than enrollment into the trial. The physician tracks the natural outcomes of therapy via data collection forms during treatment of the episode of care. Typical endpoints that are collected include quality of life, compliance, drug switches, dose changes, and side effect profiles. This information can then be plugged into an economic model to compare outcomes and costs of different therapeutic options. Despite the fact that these types of trials and information are often most favored by decision makers, they can still be lengthy and costly because of their prospective design. Because these types of trials cannot be initiated until the FDA approves a drug, it may be a year or two before the information is available.

Retrospective data analysis remains a key source of information for economic studies. The data can be accessed rapidly and often at significantly lower costs than prospective data. Before using retrospective data, health plans should consider carefully what they want to learn from the data. A significant amount of data manipulation must go on before being able to conduct a sound research project in a retrospective database. A managed care plan or PBM may be collecting integrated claims data specifically for financial reasons, such as to calculate per member per month (PMPM) charges for drugs or medical services. The organization would want to capture data on patients enrolled for any amount of time within a given year to ensure it has the most accurate PMPMs for forecasting future year expenses. However, for a research project on compliance, the organization would want to exclude any patients who are not continuously enrolled for the full year to ensure that disenrollment is not mistaken for noncompliance.

Another important consideration is whether a project requires access to both medical and pharmacy claims or just pharmacy data. If one is conducting a study on the use of epileptic drug therapy in the treatment of epilepsy, medical claims are very important. One would want to make sure that patients are receiving drug therapy for epilepsy and not trigeminal neuralgia, for instance, because this would affect the frequency and dose of drug use patterns. However, if one were comparing two drugs' incidence of concomitant therapy with interacting drugs, pharmacy data would be adequate, because the diagnosis associated with the drug would not be important.

A final type of resource used to collect pharmacoeconomic information is the Delphi panel. Experts in the treatment of a specific disease or condition are brought together in a panel to gain consensus on how a condition is treated and at what cost to the primary care provider or specialists. A problem with this approach is that inherent biases appear in a small group of specific individuals. However, Delphi panels can often help fill in missing data in an economic analysis.

PHARMACEUTICAL INDUSTRY APPROACH TO THE GENERATION OF PHARMACOECONOMIC INFORMATION

From the industry perspective, the ideal strategy for gathering pharmacoeconomic information balances various resource options with the strategy and timing for a particular product. Until recently, most pharmacoeconomic analyses were conducted based on clinical information that had been collected in conjunction with information from expert panels to derive an economic model or hypotheses for a particular product's economic value. Pharmacoeconomics was still a young discipline, and economic endpoints were not incorporated into clinical trials. Pharmacoeconomics has now developed into a discipline that is integral to the drug development process. Therefore, a decision to include economic endpoints in a clinical trial is dependent on the economic profile of a product, the expense and timing of obtaining the data, and the potential impact on managed care decision makers at the time of launch for the product.

Within the pharmaceutical industry, pharmacoeconomic information is gathered as part of the development process, as appropriate. The needs of the U.S. market have a strong influence on the specific economic endpoints that may be collected in a global clinical trial. However, depending on the global launch plan of the product, the needs of other major markets, and the countries in which a clinical trial will be completed, the endpoints required for the U.S. market may or may not be incorporated into these global trials. In most global clinical trials in which the United States has a significant number of clinical trial sites, the inclusion of pharmacoeconomic endpoints to meet the needs of the U.S. market is commonplace.

Pharmacoeconomics efforts in the development process usually target products that are two to three years from product launch, that is, in Phase II to Phase IIIB. Pharmacoeconomics information is also used to support currently marketed products. The challenge here is to supplement information gathered during the development process with naturalistic data, when time allows. If time is short, retrospective data can be used to develop a pharmacoeconomic position. Pharmacoeconomic information also supports disease management or health management initiatives. If disease management is implemented appropriately, patient outcomes are measured before and after a particular intervention, be that an education program, a disease-specific clinic, case management, or physician intervention plans. Disease management involves measuring the outcomes and costs of pharmaceutical therapy, or pharmacoeconomic information, as a part of the treatment of disease. Compliance with drug therapy is also increasingly critical to disease management. Therefore, the collection of pharmacoeconomic information is also central to disease management initiatives.

The final necessary component for the use of pharmacoeconomic information in the pharmaceutical industry is the ability to communicate this information to the decision-maker in a professional and scientifically sound medium. This requires experts in the field that are knowledgeable about various customers, including MCOs, integrated hospital systems, physician practice groups, and PBMs. Experts should understand how each of these groups utilizes pharmacoeconomic information in making decisions on drug therapy.

PACKAGING PHARMACOECONOMIC DATA FOR USE BY P & T COMMITTEES

P & T COMMITTEES

P & T committees are established by most hospitals and MCOs and serve as the primary formal communication link among pharmacists, administrators, and medical staff. The basic objectives of a P & T committee are to specify drugs of choice and alternatives, based on safety and efficacy; to minimize therapeutic redundancies; and to maximize cost-effectiveness.[32-34] Decisions to include medications on a formulary are based on data provided from randomized clinical trials, extensive literature evaluation, clinical experience, and pharmacoeconomic studies.

In most hospitals and managed care organizations, the medical staff's bylaws establish the P & T committee as an advisory committee that makes recommendations to a medical staff executive committee.[35] Traditional P & T committee responsibilities include all matters related to the use of medications in the organization, including the development and maintenance of the formulary. An effective P & T committee has educational, communication, and advisory roles.[34] Members must be able to evaluate literature and assess the results of clinical and pharmacoeconomic studies to determine which medications should be included on the formulary list.

The P & T committee is composed of physicians, pharmacists, nursing representatives, administrative personnel, and consultants. The number of committee members usually ranges from 8 to 12. Most P & T committees meet monthly and have formal procedures for considering formulary additions.[36] Some organizations have subcommittees, such as an antibiotic usage review group, to manage specific drug categories.[37] In most cases, the chairperson and secretary are responsible for the determination and allocation of the committee work. Committee decisions are translated into work orders through development of the meeting agenda,[38] which contains supporting documents, copies of the previous minutes, and the schedule of events. It is important that P & T committees develop documents that describe the procedure for making formulary additions. Thus, the P & T committee serves as the primary formal communication link between the pharmacy and the medical staff and is the most important committee to the hospital's or MCO's pharmacy department.

FORMULARY SYSTEM

Formularies evolved as early as 1816 and have undergone considerable change in content and purpose. The basic formulary list consists of drug entities, dosage forms, strengths, and package sizes that reflect the current clinical judgment of the hospital or MCO. The formulary system is a method whereby the medical staff of an institution, working through the P & T committee, evaluates, appraises, and selects from among the numerous available drug entities and drug products those considered most useful for patient care.[39] Participants will evaluate medications with respect to their efficacy, effect on patient quality of life, cost, support system, and ease of use.

Formularies exist on a continuum; they have different degrees of exclusion and substitution. The open formulary is the most liberal and comprehensive formulary, putting few restrictions on providers. However, this formulary system has relatively little influence on the ability of hospitals and MCOs to manage expenses and drug utilization. Restrictions may be imposed on open formularies to curtail excessive medication use. For example, a partially closed formulary may not provide coverage for an entire class of medications (i.e., anorexients) or specific medications. An intermediate formulary is similar to an open formulary, but generic substitution for brand-name prescriptions is encouraged.[40] Some partially or selectively closed formularies restrict the use of brand-name products in certain categories and encourage generic substitution whenever possible. Other restrictions pertain to prescribing privileges: certain physicians, such as endocrinologists and pediatricians, have the prerogative to prescribe medications related to their field of specialty. A closed formulary is created by members of the P & T committee. The list may contain anywhere from 300 to over 1,000 medications. Additions to a strict or closed formulary are usually based on objective criteria: to gain admission, products must prove that they are superior to existing formulary drugs. Generic substitution and often therapeutic interchange or switching (with physician approval) by pharmacists are encouraged if not mandated.

The rising cost of pharmaceuticals and health care are hot topics among healthcare providers. Many providers use a combination of pharmacy budget cost-controlling strategies like closed, tiered or preferred formularies.[41] Gottlieb et al.[42] described events associated with a pharmacy advisory committee in an effort to demonstrate how improvements were made for better management of costs associated with psychiatric drugs in a Medicaid population. The study evaluated the pharmacy management process, its review of literature, how it conducted discussions regarding removal, and addition of specific drugs from formulary lists. Also, the study described the effort of the committee with regard to the enhancement of psychiatric drug availability and treatment, along with controlling costs. The study concluded that the P & T committee had enhanced the development of best-practices models for the region studied, in addition to contributing to the mediation of disputes that arise from the dual goal of providing quality care and controlling costs. Effective formulary decision making occurs in multiple stages. First, physicians use their knowledge and personal experience to evaluate products and make recommendations to P & T committee members. Second, P & T committee members evaluate the product's existing pharmacoeconomic data, clinical trial data, and outcome data, which in the third stage is given an economic review by a subcommittee. Evaluations from these three stages will serve as the foundation for evidence-, outcome-, or value-based drug formulary decisions. At the fourth stage, health plan partners and members from health plan alliances evaluate information provided to them by the committee for economic review. Finally, product inclusion on the formulary is endorsed by senior management. This process is complex, yet it allows maximum opportunities for healthcare professionals and senior management to make informed decisions about products.[43]

FORMULARY GUIDELINES: THE AMCP FORMAT

The drug formulary committees of some countries (Australia, New Zealand, Canada, and the United Kingdom) began using explicit value-based evidence guidelines beginning in the early 1990s. These guidelines typically state the type of pharmacoeconomic analysis to be conducted (commonly cost-effective analysis) and the methodology that must be used when comparing a new agent to existing medications. The absence of a single government payor in the United States has resulted in individual MCOs, each slowly adopting their own set of formulary guidelines. Pharmacoeconomic data are used informally and with great variation by MCOs in the United States and it is unclear how much impact these data have on the formulary decision-making process. As pharmaceutical manufacturers continued to generate these data in ever increasing amounts and provide them to MCOs for consideration in the formulary decision-making process, it became necessary for MCOs to adopt a more standardized approach to evaluating these data. In 1998, the Regence Blue Shield health plan in Seattle began asking pharmaceutical manufacturers to submit standardized packages of clinical and economic evidence as a condition for formulary review. The Regence guidelines served as the basis for the Academy of Managed Care Pharmacy (AMCP) endorsement of their own guidelines, the *AMCP Format for Formulary Submission* in 2000 (*AMCP Dossier*), which are regularly updated.[44]

The emergence of the AMCP *Format* represents a shift in the formulary review process conducted by MCOs because it stipulates that plans formally request that drug companies provide a standardized dossier that contains detailed information on the economic value of a new medicine relative to alternative therapies in addition to safety and efficacy data. The need for a standardized dossier is the consequence of P & T committees having to evaluate the economic data of new products without any input from the FDA. The FDA review of a new drug product focuses entirely on safety and efficacy with no regard to cost. An expensive drug with marginal clinical benefit relative to existing therapies will be approved by the FDA, resulting in MCOs having to determine if the new product's benefits are worth the added cost. Therefore, the *AMCP Dossier* details the information needed for formulary review recommending that drug companies include unpublished studies, off-label usage, drug's place in therapy, related disease management strategies, as well as a cost-effectiveness model that provides evidence of the value of the new product. A budget impact model (BIM), describing the impact of the new product on a plan's drug budget may be included as well; however, the BIM is optional and not meant as a substitute for the cost-effectiveness model, nor does a BIM serve to document the value of a new therapy.[44–46]

AMCP guidelines indicate that the concept of economic value is an important consideration for MCOs when evaluating a new agent for formulary inclusion. The guidelines also recognize the need for standardized methodology for evaluating economic value and should facilitate the adoption of cost-effectiveness modeling as a routine component of the formulary decision-making process. To date, it has been difficult to assess their impact on the decision-making process. Within just two years, more than fifty health plans, PBMs, hospitals, state Medicaid programs, and other public agencies (including the Department of Defense), which represent over 100 million covered lives, have adopted the AMCP format or some variation of it. AMCP, through its foundation (the Foundation of Managed Care Pharmacy) has undertaken a series of educational initiatives to inform MCO pharmacists, pharmaceutical personnel, and other interested professionals about the guidelines. Requesting the *AMCP Dossier* and understanding its content, however, do not indicate their role in the decision-making process.[44]

In March and April of 2004, two roundtable discussions were held evaluating a pharmacoeconomic model of the class of serotonin reuptake inhibitors as well as an *AMCP Dossier*. A group of representatives from MCOs involved in the P & T decision-making process and drug industry executives met to discuss the merits of the pharmacoeconomic model and the *AMCP Dossier* and their role in the formulary process. Based on these discussions, it was clear that the model was well accepted by MCO personnel because, as recommended by the AMCP guidelines, assumptions used in the model were realistic and clearly stated for all to examine. Further, the data that populated the model were transparent and could be modified by anyone using the model. The question that arose from the roundtable discussions was whether MCOs give any weight to financial considerations. As noted by the MCO participants, some P & T committees evaluated a drug solely on its clinical merits while others gave equal weight to financial considerations. Whether the financial considerations go beyond drug acquisition costs to considering total healthcare costs remains to be understood.[47]

ROLE OF PHARMACOECONOMIC DATA IN EVIDENCE-BASED DRUG FORMULARIES

In February and March 1998, the Zitter Group conducted a national study of managed care decision-makers, the Health Economics Leaders Study.[48] The study was designed to examine the attitudes and perceptions of managed care decision-makers regarding health economics and pharmacoeconomics research. The study reported that findings from health economics research conducted outside the MCOs were overwhelmingly used to make formulary decisions.

Use of evidence-based drug formularies is gaining acceptance by healthcare providers to assist in the evaluation, appraisal, and selection of drugs.[49] In the Health Economics Leaders Study, Suh et al. examined the value of pharmacoeconomics to formulary decision-making among MCOs and concluded that for managed care providers to remain competitive, they need to use existing pharmacoeconomic studies and conduct further studies to assist in their decision-making process.[49]

Brigham and Women's Hospital (Boston, MA) has a clinical division that focuses on pharmacoeconomics to ensure that the hospital remains on the cutting edge. Their division serves as a reservoir of expertise with a goal of providing ongoing formulary review and surveillance of current prescribing patterns in an effort to use medication appropriately while containing the drug budget.[50]

Formulary system effectiveness is based on the ability to provide appropriate therapy, control inventory, monitor drug utilization, and control drug use.[40] Rucker and Schiff suggest that the basic objectives of an effective formulary include (as noted above): 1) specification of drugs of choice and alternatives, based on safety and efficacy; 2) minimization of therapeutic redundancy; and 3) maximization of cost-effectiveness through the exclusion of expensive medications when the quality of care is not compromised.[51]

FORMULARY MANAGEMENT IS A NECESSARY PRECURSOR FOR FORMULARY EFFECTIVENESS

Studies have revealed that restrictive formularies have been reported to reduce drug product costs by using group, bid, and prime vendor purchasing agreements.[34] Pharmacists' use of generic substitution, therapeutic substitution, and consultation with physicians to implement the formulary system have been found to reduce healthcare costs.[52,53] An innovative approach to formulary management is exemplified by Health Plan of the Redwoods (HPR), a regionally based, nonprofit HMO that uses an independent practice association model.[54] A study was conducted at HPR to gain insight into the accuracy of dosing guidelines and the overall success of a therapeutic interchange program.[55] Specifically, the therapeutic interchange between angiotensin converting enzyme (ACE) inhibitors, which was prompted by the economic pressure of pharmacy expenditures, was evaluated via pharmacy claims data. Patients were switched from lisinopril, quinapril, ramipril, or enalapril to benazepril, which was the preferred ACE inhibitor. Overall, 70.2% of the conversions in the therapeutic interchange program corresponded with guideline recommendations.

Alternatively, other investigators report that formulary restrictions shift costs by increasing the use of other services.[56–58] To manage drug costs, which escalated beyond efforts to control costs through protocols and limited formulary selections, HPR adopted another concept to manage the formulary, a computer-assisted *step therapy*. Instead of a closed formulary, HPR developed a preferred drug list to ensure appropriate utilization of medications while allowing prescribing physicians the flexibility to employ other medications when medically necessary.[51] The success of the preferred drug list was dramatic. Although HPR had projected a 20% increase in trended year-end drug costs PMPM for 1996, they actually experienced a 9% decrease within six months of implementation.[51]

Formulary management based on PMPM data may capture the management process at a given time; however, simply evaluating a medication formulary system with process measures (e.g., restrictiveness, utilization, substitution, and redundancy) will not provide useful information about short- or long-term effects on patient outcomes. New approaches to formulary management should demonstrate how efficient management strategies are linked to positive patient outcomes. For example, data from retrospective studies can be used in Phase IV post-marketing studies to determine how well medications work in the general population. Moreover, community-based studies are important because patients can respond to questions about compliance, medication-taking behavior, and quality of life free from the constraints imposed by clinical trials.

Publication of the results from the Asheville Project showed remarkable costs savings to employers not only in healthcare costs but reduction in days of work missed.[59] One of the study's purposes was to evaluate the economic outcome of pharmaceutical care services provided by community pharmacists to patients with diabetes mellitus. The study found that patients with diabetes had consistently lower hemoglobin A1C levels, and their employers realized lower direct costs in insurance and medical costs even though the cost of prescriptions had increased over time.[59]

PHARMACOECONOMIC EDUCATION

The utilization of pharmacoeconomic information in making informed drug decisions based on value is not the end of the process. It is the responsibility of the P & T committee members to interpret their decision to providers, insurers, employers, and patients. This requires translation of pharmacoeconomic information into an explanation of why one ACE inhibitor in a category may be at a second tier copayment level and another may be at a tier three copayment level. Common ways to disseminate this information is through newsletters, electronic mail systems, and educational programs.[60] The formulary system itself can be used as an educational tool for providers and patients to assist in their understanding of how decisions on drug coverage are made. The process also serves as a method to stay current with the growing number of medications available.[61]

The education of pharmacists who are involved in formulary decisions begins with training that is part of the Doctorate of Pharmacy program. Many Colleges of Pharmacy provide courses and/or lectures dealing with the finances of the healthcare system and how formularies assist in providing the maximum benefit from pharmaceutical departments and organizations with restricted healthcare budgets. Some colleges also provide formal training in the principles of pharmacoeconomics, either as a component of drug information courses or as stand-alone electives. Post-graduate training is available through various Pharmacoeconomic Fellowship programs. Practicing pharmacists who are exposed to the use of pharmacoeconomic information in decision making quickly learn these techniques. There are also programs provided through many of the pharmacist professional societies such as the American College of Clinical Pharmacy (ACCP) and the AMCP.

The need for pharmacoeconomics reaches globally. Although the concepts and methods of pharmacoeconomics can be standardized, the specific applications differ internationally, nationally, and by region.[62] In an effort to recognize the need for standards and coordination, the International Society for Pharmacoeconomics and Outcomes Research (ISPOR) assists in educating pharmacists and others by offering conferences, workshops, and seminars that raise awareness of concepts and application of methods to healthcare issues on a regional and global level.

MCOs and hospitals provide educational services for patients through the drug information system, the Internet, and telemedicine. Most important, however, is information conveyed through pharmacists and other healthcare professionals, who serve as "gatekeepers" for the healthcare system. Pharmacists become primary service providers in rural areas and are responsible for channeling patients to appropriate care providers.

RESEARCH OPPORTUNITIES FOR MCOS AND PBMS

Research opportunities for MCOs and PBMs are found by first identifying mutual goals. Both types of organizations want to lower costs by encouraging providers to pursue effective and efficient strategies. For example, both MCOs and PBMs want to know if the early detection that comes from offering health-related screening programs to the public will save healthcare dollars. To assess the effectiveness of these programs, both providers must consider the number of individual health problems that are likely to be discovered through active screening and determine if this number justifies the investment. The most important opportunity to work together will involve the storage and exchange of clinical data for research purposes. Additional opportunities associated with this type of collaboration are discussed in the next section in this chapter.

A partnership between MCOs and PBMs can be very beneficial because both types of organizations want to maximize efficiency; just because something works does not mean it is the most efficient option. The big question is whether the activities, programs, or services produced yield results that are in proportion to the effort expended. Both providers would be interested in knowing if the same service can be streamlined without compromising quality, be performed with less skilled personnel, or be substituted for a less expensive service that will achieve the same goals. Efficiency criteria are also important for large screening programs that must be assessed for reliability, validity, yield, cost, and acceptance. Each provider can contribute to this process based on relative strength, resource availability, geographical coverage, and provider capability.

However, the differences in infrastructure between PBMs and MCOs need to be considered when evaluating pharmacoeconomic research within these institutions. Because PBMs are primarily interested in drug costs and the pharmacoeconomic impact of drug choices within a class, research done by these organizations often focuses on compliance differences between drugs that may be dependent on variance in efficacy or tolerability. An MCO, however, is truly interested in the total healthcare costs, and the pharmacoeconomic impact of a drug in reducing physician or hospital visits can be very beneficial. Another perspective that MCOs are interested in is the impact on outcomes and costs of disease management programs, which often incorporate the appropriate use of pharmaceuticals. One study demonstrated the value of disease management on patient quality of life at the Lovelace Health System in New Mexico.[63] A second research project took the disease management guidelines developed at Lovelace and adapted them to a primary care perspective through a national consensus panel.[64] Future research will be directed towards understanding the pharmacoeconomic benefit of following treatment guidelines in epilepsy.

ROLE OF PHARMACOECONOMICS IN DECOMPARTMENTALIZING PLAN MANAGEMENT

Managed care organizations rely on restrictive drug formularies to curtail rising drug costs. However, formulary decisions are becoming more difficult because many pharmaceutical products are used to treat chronic conditions in which clinical and economic outcomes of therapy are not immediately apparent.[38] This is particularly true with biologics that often are brought to the market for one specific indication, but while other indications are being pursued, the product is being used by physicians in the marketplace for all indications of a disease. This practice is potentially risky for the patient and has a significant impact on the pharmacy budget. Another issue for the management of biological costs is under what portion of an insurance plan the product is covered. Currently, injectable products are covered under the Part B section of the Medicare drug plan and are not a concern to the pharmacy budget. Other insurance plans cover injectables under the medical (versus Pharmacy) portion of the plan and therefore does not impact drug cost. However, under the Medicare Modernization Act, injectable drug prices moved to an average sales price, which is a disadvantage for an individual physician purchasing small quantities and, therefore, more are being sold as part of a specialized pharmacy service. This may bring injectables back into the mix under drug costs for many insurers and employers. Either way, the utilization of biologics need to be given a lot of thought; pharmacoeconomic information is becoming of greater interest in this area as more biologics come to market, formulations change, and indications expand. For many drug categories, formulary decisions need to be all inclusive and involve more than the pharmacy department.

Formulary decisions may be much more effective under the following conditions: 1) P & T committee members represent all departments and institutions involved in the pharmacy care process; 2) pharmacoeconomic studies are planned with respect to the needs of various providers in the integrated healthcare system; 3) care providers have a vested interest in collecting and storing clinical data for pharmacoeconomic studies; and 4) performance measures are used to evaluate the cost-effectiveness of services and quality of care.

Providers across departments can be directly involved in the planning stages for pharmacoeconomic studies. Plan managers can determine the providers' roles and responsibilities in system planning. Communication channels should be established to allow information exchange and to work through any initial glitches that arise from the implementation of new study plans. Each department shares responsibility for monitoring progress in the implementation stages as well as determining when key endpoints are reached.

The main driver for decompartmentalization has been the need to collect and manage clinical data. As managed healthcare systems continue to grow, more emphasis is placed on the ability of providers to collect pharmacoeconomic data internally and to use these data to support or refute information obtained externally through national and international data sources. Decision analytic models, structural equation models, and other economic models are necessary tools to help providers condense information and package it into meaningful segments. Information systems and electronic medical records have great potential to address some of these issues and to integrate patient information across healthcare systems. Professionals who can resolve conflict and help managers establish norms for information use and exchange, and who can create opportunities for trust formation through goal development will be vital as providers consolidate resources for the sake of efficiency.

REINTEGRATING PHARMACY OUTCOMES WITH MEDICAL OUTCOMES

After members understand how pharmacoeconomic data can be integrated and used to achieve desired outcomes and measure performance, action can be taken to ensure that pharmacy care processes are linked to medical outcomes. To analyze the relationship between process and outcome, pharmacy care processes or intermediate pharmacy outcomes must be evaluated to determine if they contribute to medical outcomes. A focus on pharmacy and medical outcomes provides the foundation for improving patient care processes and reported outcomes. Patient reported outcomes (PROs) may include patient loyalty, quality of life, satisfaction, compliance, value, and quality. PROs work in conjunction with system measures that convey information about the efficiency, effectiveness, success, and quality of medical services. These topics are discussed in the next section.

PATIENT REPORTED OUTCOMES

Patient reported outcomes are the measurement of a patient's health status that is reported directly from the patient. PROs do not include any outside interpretation by a physician, healthcare worker, or anyone else. PROs are not only used in research but also are included in clinical trials. In these trials, PRO information may be used to evaluate the impact of an intervention on one or more aspects of patients' health status. The patient's health status may be reported as purely symptomatic, for example a headache, or more complex, such as the capacity to perform life's daily activities. Even more complex outcomes that may be reported include the humanistic outcome of quality of life, patient satisfaction, and preferences from the aspect of physical, psychological, and social perspectives.

PRO instruments provide a means for measuring treatment benefits by capturing concepts related to how a patient feels or functions with respect to his or her health or condition. The concepts, events, behaviors, or feelings measured by PRO instruments can be either readily observed or verified (e.g., walking) or can be non-observable, that is, known only to the patient and not easily verified (e.g., feeling depressed).

Including PRO instruments enhances clinical information in the evaluation of new medical products because:

- Some treatment effects are known only to the patient.
- The desire to know the patient's perspective about the effectiveness of a treatment.
- Systematic assessment of the patient's perspective may provide valuable information.
- Without PROs, the patient's opinion is filtered through a clinician's evaluation of the patient's response to clinical interview questions.[65]

Wilke et al.[66] measured the treatment impact and concluded that, although quite variable as a class of study endpoints, PROs have a significant role in the development and evaluation of new medicines. Also, their study concluded that additional formal guidance from the FDA about use of such measures along with continued collaboration by PRO researchers to develop and disseminate standards will enhance the appropriate use of PROs in future drug development and labeling.[67]

To ensure that patients' needs are satisfied, providers must have a sufficient number of individuals ready to answer questions, take care of complaints, represent patients, and provide quality medical services. Healthcare professionals should focus efforts on building long-lasting relationships with patients to ensure that healthcare resources are used efficiently. Integrated data systems will allow physicians, pharmacists, and nurses to store current information regarding patients, thus allowing professionals to anticipate patients' medical problems before they occur. Providers must ensure that the concentration of personnel is large enough to have a significant impact on service delivery.

Patient reported outcome measures are used extensively in many service-related industries. Opportunities to collect data pertaining to patient satisfaction, quality of life, and compliance are equally promising for healthcare providers in hospitals and MCOs. In fact, the need to evaluate patients will become more important as managed care continues to pervade all aspects of healthcare delivery. To meet these needs, new departments will begin to evolve with the sole function of patient evaluation and assessment. Employees of these departments will dedicate their time to survey instrument development in the areas of patient satisfaction, compliance, and quality of life. These instruments will be used to measure quality across providers, over time, and for comparison within a specific MCO or provider group. Consumer coalitions such as the Foundation for Accountability are developing performance standards based on criteria established by the National Committee for Quality Assurance (NCQA). The NCQA developed the Health Plan Employer Data and Information Set, a set of standardized measures used to compare the performance of managed care organizations in various clinical, administrative, and financial areas.[68] Pressures to integrate health standards in MCOs will continue to grow as patients seek value from the healthcare system and manufacturers seek accountability from providers regarding the management of healthcare resources.

SYSTEM PERFORMANCE

Shareholders seek to optimize equity value. Common measurements of equity value include revenue growth, economic profit, cash flow, and key strategic accomplishments. Responsibilities for the accomplishment of these goals can be allocated more efficiently when management units are decompartmentalized. Using this strategy, each department must develop and determine performance standards as they relate to patient care. Financial indicators will become the major determinants of value, particularly when questioning whether service delivery was valued according to performance standards.

In addition to being measured internally, value can be assessed externally through the analysis of customer satisfaction (e.g., customer survey results, opportunities to provide service input, number of complaints), success (e.g., referrals, morbidity, and mortality), and quality (e.g., timely services, waiting periods, technology, trained personnel). When patients stay with one healthcare provider, their care is easier to manage and the system is more cost-efficient because future needs for medical resources can be anticipated and managed.

SOURCES OF DATA

A number of data sources are available for conducting pharmacoeconomic research and the choice is based on the pharmacoeconomic question in hand. For example, during early drug development process (e.g., phase two), there may be an interest in determining the overall economic impact of the disease to a healthcare system (e.g., HMO) and therefore a role the new drug may have in lessening the burden (e.g., cost of illness study). Large databases containing clinical and economic outcomes maintained by HMOs (e.g., Kaiser Permanente) do lend themselves to answering questions like estimation of cost-effectiveness and investigations of risk predictions in populations. Pharmacoeconomic modeling (e.g., cost-effectiveness analysis [CEA]) generally is carried out prior to a drug launch, alongside clinical trials to demonstrate the clinical and economic benefits of the drug over the current status quo. In conjunction with clinical outcomes, data on resource use are collected to calculate CEA ratios. One of the primary concerns of collecting such resource use data in a clinical trial is the issue of protocol driven costs.[68] Therefore, it is recommended that such modeling studies be based on data within clinical trials in combination with observational data representing more typical resource use. Pharmacoeconomic studies conducted post-launch (also known as Phase IV studies) rely on singly or a combination of clinical trial data, literature (e.g., meta-analysis), and/or observational or sometimes also known as retrospective databases. When little or no published information is available in a particular area, expert opinions are obtained via a Delphi panel.[69] Delphi studies are research exercises conducted by a panel of experts. It involves surveying experts in two to four stages of data collection to obtain convergence of opinion in a particular area. There is no face-to-face contact between the respondents, and the respondents do not know who else is serving on the panel. A 2003 pharmacoeconomic study evaluated the cost-effectiveness of adding up to 20 weeks of becaplermin, a genetically-engineered growth factor in a hydro-gel vehicle in healing chronic foot ulcers of patients with adequate vasculature receiving best clinical care, compared to the standard care.[70] A one-year decision-analytic model was developed using clinical data from published clinical trial study and resource utilization from an expert panel using a Delphi approach.

Repositories containing "real-world" or observational data may be broadly classified into private and public databases. Private databases may be further categorized into those that are primarily built for insurance billing purposes (e.g., claims database), or for tracking quality of care and improving patient care (e.g., General Electric's Logician database). Specific examples of applications of such databases are numerous. For example, a claims database from a particular MCO used to conduct a retrospective analysis to determine physician prescribing behavior for hypertension patients may include frequency of physician visits, medications filled, procedures performed, and hospitalizations.

Public sector data are available from the Department of Health and Human Services and from state Medicaid programs. A state Medicaid database contains prescriptions and medical claims for respective Medicaid recipients. The prescription claims dataset may include patient demographics and prescription data (e.g., strength, quantity, national drug code identifier number, and amount of reimbursement). The Medicaid medical claims dataset usually includes diagnostic and procedure codes for outpatients and inpatients. In a 1998 study of healthcare utilization, researchers used the Idaho State Medicaid database to profile a resource use pattern of Medicaid patients with migraines.[71] Some of the readily available federal databases include: Behavioral Risk Factor Surveillance System (BRFSS), National Health and Nutrition Examination Survey (NHANES), National Health Interview Survey (NHIS), Medical Expenditure Panel Survey (MEPS), National Ambulatory Medical Care Survey (NAMCS), National Hospital Discharge Survey (NHDS), Nationwide Inpatient Sample (NIS), Surveillance, Epidemiology, End Results (SEER), the Department of Defense (DoD), and the Veterans Administration (VA). Purpose, unit of observation, method of data collection, the timeframe, and sample size of each of these databases vary. The advantages of using such sources are the national representation of the sample and the longitudinal follow-up, which requires sophisticated analytic techniques (i.e., accounting for sampling weights) to conduct a valid pharmacoeconomic study. Finally, financial data such as the average wholesale prices on drugs and costs of various resources are available from sources such as the *Red Book* (Thompson Reuters) and the Center for Medicare and Medicaid Services (CMS).

All of these data sources can be used to conduct pharmacoeconomic studies that analyze current trends and practice patterns across various healthcare providers. Pharmacoeconomic studies utilizing these data sources are useful in determining the role of new products in the marketplace. The results of these studies may be analyzed to improve the delivery of healthcare across various healthcare settings. Thus, database management has and continues to enter into areas involving home therapy, diagnostics, dialysis clinics, chemotherapy, biologicals, and innovative delivery systems. Pharmaceutical manufacturers will work with healthcare organizations in these areas to develop databases that use a prospective and proactive format for data collection.

OPPORTUNITIES FOR PHARMACISTS IN PHARMACOECONOMIC RESEARCH AND APPLICATIONS

The Health Economics Leaders Study showed very encouraging results for the field of pharmacoeconomics and health economics research.[72] An ISPOR organized task force evaluated how pharmacoeconomic studies are used by decision makers.[73] The study results identified 16 different surveys of decision makers and 15 published guidelines for the use of economic evaluations. The conclusion of the task force study raised awareness that there might be the need for more requirements of the pharmacoeconomic studies, that decision makers may need more education in economic evaluation, as well as the possible need for more evaluation of the healthcare decision-making process. Although the marketplace for health economics research continues to develop, many respondents were satisfied with the health economics–related research that they evaluated. Furthermore, most of these decision makers wanted to see a lot more of this type of research. In fact, many of the MCOs wanted to partner with pharmaceutical companies as well as other related organizations to conduct sound and relevant research. With new pharmaceutical products rapidly entering the marketplace, it is necessary for the MCOs to have the results from pharmacoeconomics and health economics research available to make formulary decisions. There is a high demand for healthcare professionals to design and conduct this type of research as well as evaluate the results of these studies.

Sources of these pharmacoeconomic data will continue to evolve. The FDA will continue to struggle with the inclusions of pharmacoeconomic data in drug approval decisions. Because of this, pharmaceutical companies will continue to be reluctant to compromise FDA approval by collecting data targeted to the payor. At the same time, the demand for pharmacoeconomic information from the payor continues to increase, with consistent formats supporting the collection and dissemination of such information. Although pharmaceutical companies have clearly recognized this demand and hired post-graduate trained pharmacists and other scientists, there remains a bit of skepticism to studies done exclusively by the industry. Therefore, many academic centers are involved in industry sponsored pharmacoeconomic research to bring additional collaborations into the work and a sense of academic credibility. Most pharmaceutical companies now have separate departments that concentrate solely on pharmacoeconomics and health outcomes research. These departments design and monitor studies that support the development and marketing of their company's product portfolio, analyzing and reporting the data collected from the studies and disseminating the results of their research to different healthcare organizations. However, the department also may focus on activities that are not directly linked to a specific product. Some of these activities consist of disease management initiatives, evaluations of healthcare delivery systems, and different practice patterns throughout the country. Pharmacists have the specialized training and the ability to interact with researchers and medical personnel on a scientific level. These unique qualities make them an invaluable resource within this field and allow them to work on pharmacoeconomics-related research within the pharmaceutical industry, managed care, and academia. Pharmacists' understanding of drug therapies and the healthcare market allows them to grasp the complexities of new drug therapies, health policies, procedures, and the ever changing marketplace. These qualities enable pharmacists to contribute greatly to pharmacoeconomics and health economics research.

CONCLUSION

Pharmacoeconomics is becoming increasingly important and influential in drug development and utilization. Pharmaceutical manufacturers are using pharmacoeconomics to define drug value and support strategic marketing plans. There are numerous uses of pharmacoeconomic information in the healthcare industry. P & T committees of MCOs are using pharmacoeconomic data to consider drug value, rather than cost alone, when selecting drug products for formularies. The growing importance of pharmacoeconomic information presents many opportunities for pharmacists involved in managed care to make pharmacotherapy decisions to pursue both cost and quality of care objectives.

Acknowledgment
The authors would like to acknowledge the significant contributions of Barbara Roper, PharmD candidate 2009 to the finessing of content, editing, and formatting of the final document.

REFERENCES

1. Gabel J., Claxton G., Gil I., et al., Health benefits in 2005: premium increases slow down, coverage continues to erode. Health Tracking Trends. *Health Affairs*. 2005; 24(5): 1273-1280.
2. Kaiser Family Foundation, *Health Insurance Coverage in America, 2003 Data Update*, November 2004, Table 1, p. 28. Available at http://www.kff.org/uninsured/7153.cfm. Accessed 27 June 2008.
3. Boston Consulting Group, The Contribution of Pharmaceutical Companies: What's at Stake for America. *Ann NY Acad Sci* 1994; 729(1): 111–126.
4. Racine E., Justifying high-cost anticoagulant therapy, *Am J Health Syst Pharm*. 2002; 59(20 Suppl 6): S18-S20.
5. Legg R.F., Sclar D., Nemec N.L., et al., Cost-effectiveness of sumatriptan in a managed care population. *Am J Manag Care*. 1997; 3(1): 117-122.
6. Legg R.F., Sclar D., Nemec N.L., et al., Cost benefit of sumatriptan to an employer. *J Occup Environ Med*. 1997; 39(7): 652-657.
7. Joish V.N., Donaldson G., Stockdale W., et al., The economic impact of GERD and PUD: examination of direct and indirect costs using a large integrated employer claims database. *Curr Med Res Opin*. 2005; 21(4): 535-544.
8. Drummond M.F., Stoddart G.L., O'Brien B.J., Torrance G.W., *Methods for Economic Evaluation of Health Care Programmes*. Oxford: Oxford University Press; 1997.
9. Howard K.B., Blumenschein K., Rapp R.P., Azithromycin versus erythromycin for community-acquired pneumonia: a cost-minimization analysis. *Am J Health Syst Pharm*. 1999; 56(15): 1521-1524.
10. Newby D., Hill S., Use of pharmacoeconomics in prescribing research. Part 2: cost-minimization analysis—when are two therapies equal? *J Clin Pharmacy Therapeut*. 2003; 28: 145-150.
11. Brixner D.I., Outcomes research, pharmacoeconomics and the pharmaceutical industry, *J Manag Care Pharm*. 1996; 2(1): 48-52.
12. Donaldson C., Shackley P., Does 'process utility' exist? A case study of willingness to pay for laparoscopic cholecystectomy. *Social Sci Med*. 1997; 44: 699-707.
13. Bootman J.L., Townsent R.J., McGhan W.F., *Principles of Pharmacoeconomics*, 3rd Ed. Cincinnati, OH: Harvey Whitney Books Co.; 2004.
14. Ettinger B., Pressman A., Schein J., et al., Alendronate use among 812 women: prevalence of gastrointestinal complaints, noncompliance with patient instructions, and discontinuation. *J Manag Care Pharm* 1998; 4(5): 488-492.
15. Rich P., et al., Onychomycosis: symptoms and quality of life associated with this medical condition. Abstract presented at the 56th Annual Meeting of the American College of Foot and Ankle Surgeons, Orlando, FL, February 1998.
16. The GUSTO Investigators, An international randomized trial comparing four thrombolytic strategies for acute myocardial infarction. *N Engl J Med*. 1993; 329(10): 673-682.
17. Neumann P.J. Zinner D.E., Paltiel A.D., The FDA and regulation of cost-effectiveness claims. *Health Affairs*. 1996; 15(3): 54-71.
18. Mark D.B., Hlatky M.A., Califf R.M., et al., Cost effectiveness of thrombolytic therapy with tissue plasminogen activator as compared with streptokinase for acute myocardial infarction. *N Engl J Med*. 1995; 332(21): 1418-1424. Erratum *N Engl J Med*. 1995; 333(4): 267.
19. Huybrechts K.F., Caro J.J., Wilson D.A., O'Brian J.A., Health and economic consequences of sevelamer use for hyperphosphatemia in patients on hemodialysis. *Value Health*. 2005; 8(5): 549-561.
20. Pashos C.L. Klein E.G., Wanke L.A., eds., *ISPOR Lexicon*. Princeton, NJ: International Society for Pharmacoeconomics and Outcomes Research; 1998.
21. Marchetti A., Piech C.T., McGhan W.F., et al., Pharmacoeconomic analysis of oral therapies for onychomycosis: a US model. *Clin Ther*. 1996; 18(4): 757-778.
22. Motheral B.R. and Fairman K.A., The use of claims databases for outcomes research: rationale, challenges, and strategies, *Clin Ther*. 1997; 19(2): 346-366.
23. Patsy B.M., Heckbert S.R., Koepsell T.D., et al., The risk of myocardial infarction associated with antihypertensive drug therapies. *JAMA*. 1995; 274(8): 620-625. Comments in *J Hum Hypertens*. 2006; 20(6): 465-466; *JAMA*. 1995; 274(8): 654-655.

24. Cheng J.W. and Behar L., Calcium channel blockers: association with myocardial infarction, mortality and cancer. *Clin Ther.* 1997; 19(60): 1255-1268.

25. Motheral B., Brooks J., Clark M.A., et al., A checklist for retrospective database studies–report of the ISPOR Task Force on Retrospective Databases. *Value Health.* 2003; 6(2): 90-97.

26. Brixner D.I., Said Q, Corey-Lisle P.K., et al., Real world impact of second generation antipsychotics on weight gain. *Ann Pharmacother.* 2006; 40: 626-632

27. Gianfrancesco F., Pesa J., Wang R.-H., Comparison of mental health resources used by patients with bipolar disorder treated with risperidone, olanzapine, or quetiapine. *J Manag Care Pharm.* 2005; 11(3): 220-230.

28. Hay J.W., Appropriate econometric methods for pharmacoeconometric studies of retrospective claims data: an introductory guide. *J Manag Care Pharm.* 2005; 11(4): 344-348.

29. Lyman G.H., Berndt E.R., Kallich J.D., et al., The economic burden of anemia in cancer patients receiving chemotherapy. *Value Health.* 2005; 8(2): 149-156.

30. Amato M.P., Pharmacoeconomic considerations of multiple sclerosis therapy with the new disease modifying agents. *Exp Opin Pharm.* 2004; 5: 2115-2126.

31. Erkan D., Physician treatment preferences in rheumatoid arthritis of differing severity and activity: the impact of cost on first-line therapy. *Arthritis Care Res.* 2002; 47: 285-290.

32. Summers K.H. and Szeinbach S.L., Formularies: the role of pharmacy and therapeutics (P&T) committees. *Clin Ther.* 1993; 15(2): 433-441.

33. American Society of Health-System Pharmacists, *Survey of Managed Care and Ambulatory Care Pharmacy Practice.* Washington, DC: ASHSP; 1997.

34. Roberts M.J. and Summerfield M.R., Formulary management to reduce cost: P&T committee strategies, *Hosp Formul.* 1986; 21(4): 481-483, 488-492.

35. Carlson J.A., Antimicrobial formulary management: meeting the challenge in a health maintenance organization. *Pharmacotherapy.* 1991; 11: 32S-35S.

36. Standish R.C., Evans P.J., Bell J.E., Preparing the P&T committee agenda for new drug requests. *Hosp Formul.* 1984; 19: 792-800.

37. National Institute of Standards and Technology, *Malcolm Baldridge National Quality Award: 1998 Criteria for Performance Excellence.* Gaithersburg, MD: Malcolm Baldridge National Quality Program; 1997.

38. Summers K.H., et al., The use of economic models in managed care pharmacy decisions. *J Manag Care Pharm.* 1998; 4(1): 42-50.

39. Hoffmann R.P., Perspectives on the hospital formulary system. *Hosp Pharm.* 1984; 19: 359-364.

40. Rasccati K.L., Survey of formulary system policies and procedures. *Am J Hosp Pharm.* 1992; 49: 100-103.

41. Huskamp H.A., Managing psychotropic drug costs: will formularies work? *Health Aff (Millwood).* 2003; 22(5): 84-96.

42. Gottlieb D., Dubin W.R., Ning A., Gardiner G.C., Improving psychiatric drug benefit management: IV. Experiences of a pharmacy advisory committee. *Psychiatr Serv.* 2004; 55(11): 1210-1212.

43. Cave D., Personal communication, phone conversation. September, 1998, St. Louis, MO.

44. Neumann P.J., Evidence-based and value-based formulary guidelines. *Health Aff.* 2004; 23(1): 124-134.

45. Van Den Bos J., Watkins J., Reed K., Shreve J., The formulary decision process: what are they doing in there and can actuaries help? *Health Section News.* 2005; 9: 18, 20-25.

46. Balu S., O'Connor P., Vogenberg R., Contemporary issues affecting P&T committees part 2: Beyond managed care. *P&T.* 2004; 29(12): 780-783.

47. Sullivan P.W., Valuck R., Brixner D.I., Armstrong E.P., Managed care's response to a pharmacoeconomic model of serotonin reuptake inhibitors. *P&T.* 2005; 30(3): 178-182.

48. Todd C., What makes health economics research useful to decision makers? *Pharmacoeconomics & Outcomes News Weekly.* 1998; 170: 3-4.

49. Suh D.C., Okpara I.R., Agnese W.B., Toscani M., Application of pharmacoeconomics to formulary decision making in managed care organizations. *Am J Manag Care.* 2002; 8(2): 161-169.

50. Avorn J., Balancing the cost and value of medications: the dilemma facing clinicians. *Pharmacoeconomics.* 2002; 20(Suppl 3): 67-72.

51. Rucker T.D. and Schiff G., Drug Formularies: Myths-in-Formation. *Med Care.* 1990; 28: 928-942.

52. Rich D.D., Experience with a two-tiered therapeutic interchange policy. *Am J Hosp Pharm.* 1989; 46: 1792-1798.

53. Green E.R., Chrymako M.M., Rozek S.L., Kitrenos J.G., Clinical considerations and costs associated with formulary conversion from tobramycin to gentamicin. *Am J Hosp Pharm.* 1989; 46: 714-719.

54. Bailey M. and Ferro K., Innovative drug formulary management through computer assisted protocols. *J Manag Care Pharm.* 1998; 4(3): 246-252.

55. Bull S., Shoheiber O, Bailey M., Utilization of pharmacy claims data to evaluate therapeutic interchange programs. *J Manag Care Pharm.*

56. Horn S.D., Unintended consequences of drug formularies. *Am J Health-Syst Pharm* 1996; 53: 2204-2206.

57. Curtiss F.R., Drug formularies provide a path to best care. *Am J Health-Syst Pharm.* 1996; 53: 2201-2203.

58. Kravitz R.L. and Romano P.S., Managed care cost containment and the law of unintended consequences. *Am J Manag Care.* 1996; 2: 232-234.

59. Cranor C.W., Christensen D.B., The Asheville Project: long-term clinical and economic outcomes of a community pharmacy diabetes care program. *J Am Pharm Assoc (Wash).* 2003; 43(2): 173-184.

60. Goldberg K.B., Managing the pharmacy benefit: the formulary system. *J Manag Care Pharm.* 1997; 3(5): 565-573.

61. Navarro R.P., *Trends and Forecasts.* CibaGeneva Pharmacy Benefit Report. Summit, NJ: Ciba-Geneva; 1996.

62. Rascati K.L., Drummond M.F., Annemans L., Davey P.G., Education in pharmacoeconomics: an international multidisciplinary view. *Pharmacoeconomics.* 2004; 22(3): 139-147.

63. Gunter M.J., Worley A.V., Carter S., et al., Impact of a seizure disorder disease management program on patient-reported quality of life. *Dis Manage* 2004; 7(4): 333-347.

64. Trost L.F. III, Wender R.C., Suter C.C., et al., Diagnosis and management of epilepsy in adults: an algorithm-based approach for primary care. *Postgrad Med.* 2005; 116(6): 22-26.

65. *Guidance for Industry Patient Reported Outcomes Measures: Use in Medical Product Development to Support Labeling Claims.* February 2006. Available at http://www.fda.gov/cder/guidance/5460dft.pdf. Accessed 28 June 2008.

66. Willke R.J., Burke L.B., Erickson P., Measuring treatment impact: a review of patient-reported outcomes and other efficacy endpoints in approved product labels. *Control Clin Trials.* 2004; 25(6): 535-552.

67. Knight W., "Quality of Care," in *Managed Care: What It Is and How It Works.* Gaithersburg, MD: Aspen Publishers, Inc.; 1998.

68. Coyle D., Lee K.M., The problem of protocol driven costs in pharmacoeconomic analysis. *Pharmacoeconomics.* 1998; 14(4): 357-363.

69. Kennedy H.P. Enhancing Delphi research: methods and results. *J Adv Nurs.* 2004; 45(5): 504-511.

70. Sibbald R.G., Torrance G., Hux M., et al., Cost-effectiveness of becaplermin for nonhealing neuropathic diabetic foot ulcers. *Ostomy Wound Manage.* 2003; 49(11): 76-84.

71. Joish V.N., Cady P.S., Shaw J.W., Health care utilization by migraine patients: a 1998 Medicaid population study. *Clin Ther* 2000; 22(11): 1346-1356.

72. Fellowship Program, Program Guide for "Future Pharmacy Leaders: Building the New Foundation." East Hanover, NJ: Bimark Healthcare Communications; 1998.

73. Drummond M., Brown R., Fendrick M., et al., Use of pharmacoeconomics information: report of the ISPOR Task Force on use of pharmacoeconomic/health economic information in healthcare decision making. *Value Health.* 2003; 6(4): 407-416.

chapter 13

PHARMACY & THERAPEUTICS COMMITTEES IN MANAGED CARE ORGANIZATIONS

ROBERT P. NAVARRO

DANIEL C. MALONE

ELAINE MANIERI

RAULO S. FREAR

TIMOTHY S. REGAN

PAUL N. URICK

T. JEFFREY WHITE

INTRODUCTION

Drug product evaluations and selections have been made as long as drug choices have been available. In open and unmanaged systems, the prescriber makes the medication choice after considering pharmacological properties of alternative drugs, the unique patient care needs, and patient cost. Within organized healthcare delivery systems, such as hospitals or managed care organizations, Pharmacy & Therapeutics (P & T) Committees are authorized by the organization to conduct drug reviews and analyses, and make population-level drug formulary decisions. The formulary is then provided to participating physicians to select agents when making patient-level prescribing decisions. However, the responsibilities of the P & T Committee transcend simply compiling a list of recommended drugs. According to the American Society of Health-System Pharmacists (ASHP) *Statement on the Pharmacy and Therapeutics Committee*, the Committee ". . . evaluates the clinical use of drugs, develops policies for managing drug use and drug administration, and manages the formulary system . . . is a policy-recommending body to the medical staff and the administration of the organization on matters related to the therapeutic use of drugs."[1] The Committee must consider how drugs will be distributed, administered, monitored, and managed, as well as the cost impact to all stakeholders, and must also attempt to determine if outcomes suggested by clinical trial efficacy data will be borne out in real world practice, given the myriad of benefit design structures that may influence drug use and adherence.

The responsibilities of the P & T Committee have far-reaching implications for all healthcare professionals, plan sponsors, patient members, and indeed the health care organization itself. Appropriate selection and use of a pharmaceutical is often the most cost-effective form of prevention or therapy for many medical conditions. It is the responsibility of the P & T Committees, using a standardized drug evaluation process, to make pharmacotherapy recommendations for all healthcare professionals and members of the organization as well as consider and expeditiously process patient-specific exceptions.

This chapter describes the genesis of managed care Pharmacy & Therapeutics Committees, their role and structure, the drug evaluation and review process, and how Committee decisions become manifested in the organization's drug formulary.

GENESIS OF P & T COMMITTEES IN MANAGED CARE

Organized healthcare delivery systems, such as hospitals and managed care organizations (MCOs), have empowered a group of knowledgeable healthcare professionals, usually physicians and pharmacists, with the authority and responsibility to make pharmacotherapy evaluations and recommendations on behalf of the entire hospital or system. This group is now generally termed a *Pharmacy & Therapeutics Committee* or *Drug Formulary Committee*. The Committee's decisions are driven by organizational philosophy, goals, and objectives, and serve as the basis for drug therapy decisions made by all healthcare professionals within the system. The Committee communicates their decisions to professionals via the publication of a compendium of drugs approved by the Committee.

This compendium was initially termed a *pharmacopeia* in the United States in the late 18th century,[1] and today it is often called a *drug formulary*. In the 1920s, U.S. hospitals began creating drug formularies to eliminate therapeutic duplication.[2] By the 1960s, virtually every hospital in the United States had established a formulary system, largely influenced by the publication of the American Hospital Formulary Service by the American Society of Hospital Pharmacists (ASHP) in 1959.[3] In addition to the identification of a drug compendium or drug formulary for the health system or hospital, the P & T Committees became involved in drug storage, administration, monitoring, outcomes research, physician and patient drug use education, and other activities that would promote the appropriate use of formulary medications, guidelines for use of non-formulary medications, and procedures for procurement and use of investigational drugs.

The use of formularies has spread beyond the institutional setting. As described in Chapters 1 and 2, by the 1970s, health maintenance organizations (HMOs) began to flourish in several regions of the United States. As these HMOs expanded their benefits beyond medical and hospital, and added pharmacy benefits, they naturally hired pharmacists to manage the pharmacy benefit. Many early managed care pharmacy directors came out of hospital practice, and they logically applied the practices and principles of drug formulary development and management they learned in hospitals to the managed care practice environment. HMOs began developing drug formularies, and to provide the independent, critical evaluation of available drugs, they began forming their own Pharmacy & Therapeutics Committees fashioned after the hospital model. In fact, the principles of drug review are quite similar, although the type of drugs reviewed, administration and utilization parameters (i.e., controlled in-patient vs. uncontrolled out-patient environments), and organizational goals and objectives are quite different.

HMOs began developing P & T Committees and publishing their own drug formulary (formularies are discussed in depth in Chapter 9). The use of a P & T Committee, comprised largely of independent community-based physicians and pharmacists lends clinical credibility to the decisions. An HMO making its own drug decisions would be accused of selecting drugs based upon parsimony rather than outcomes. One current MCO published *Drug Formularies: Myths and Facts*, and defends its formulary decision process as follows[5]:

> **Myth #4:** Bean counters determine which drug appears on any formulary.
>
> The fact is, a formulary is established by a clinical committee of doctors and pharmacists. This committee compares each drug's safety, side effects, effectiveness, and relative costs. Based on research and discussion, the clinical committee decides which ones are best for the formulary. In addition, our doctors and pharmacists stay current on the newest nationwide developments in medicine, and update our formulary based on the latest research.

To emphasize the focus on quality of care, many P & T Committees will consider a drug's cost or contract impact only after they make a favorable formulary decision based upon clinical and safety data.

P & T Committees are now *de rigueur* within MCOs, and are largely accepted by public and private plan sponsors, physician providers, or individual members. Often there are two layers of P & T Committees in formulary decisions. Pharmacy benefit managers (PBMs) (see Chapter 4) have their own P & T Committee, and often their MCO customers also have their own P & T Committee. Large employer groups are becoming more sophisticated in managing its employee's health. One way that employers are taking an active part in taking care of their employees is by employing physicians, nurses, and pharmacists. Large employer groups may form their own P & T Committee or become an active participant in their MCO's P & T Committee. Although the vast majority of MCOs use a PBM for some or most pharmacy benefit management services (see Chapters 2 and 4), approximately 80% of MCOs who use a PBM also make their own formulary decisions with their own P & T Committee.[6] They evaluate the PBM recommendations and may take advantage of PBM contracting but ultimately use their own P & T Committee for plan formulary decisions.

MCO and PBM P & T Committees are evolving. In 2003, the Medicare Modernization Act (MMA) provided for the development of Medicare Part D pharmacy benefit. Participating Medicare Advantage–Prescription Drug (MA-PDs) plans and prescription drug plans (PDPs) were required to make drug formulary decisions for members through a P & T Committee. MMA legislation required that the Committee include at least one pharmacist and physician member with expertise in the care of geriatric patients, and those members be free of conflicts of interest. Additional language specified the frequency of P & T Committee meetings, the types of formulary management and utilization management activities for which the committee was responsible, and also specified that drugs and drug classes should be reviewed in a regular and timely manner. The increasing use of specialty pharmaceuticals will require the P & T Committees to include or regularly consult with specialists who commonly use such injectable biologicals and other specialty medications to make certain this class of medications is fairly and appropriately evaluated. Due to the extremely high cost of specialty pharmaceuticals, which in many cases will extend the life of a patient only by a few months, P & T Committees are increasingly adding or consulting with ethicists to consider the ethical issues involved on these drug selection additions.

ROLE OF THE MANAGED CARE P & T COMMITTEE

Members of any organization's P & T Committee have the opportunity and responsibility to offer what their experience and analysis shows to be the best drugs available to patient members of their organization. Their decisions will affect patient care and clinical outcomes, have a significant financial impact on the MCOs and customers, and may even influence the lives of many individuals with medication therapy needs. However, the Committee's first responsibility is to the patient, and to select the safest and most cost-effective drugs available for formulary inclusion.

In 1999, a coalition of several organizations convened to discuss the principles of a sound drug formulary system. The Coalition Working Group participants met to identify the principles of a sound drug formulary system (**Table 13-1**). The Working Group succinctly emphasized that the responsibilities of the P & T Committee go beyond creating the formulary, and include promoting the *effective use* of formulary products through the following statement[7]:

TABLE 13-1   Principles of a Sound Drug Formulary System Coalition Working Group Members

- Academy of Managed Care Pharmacy (AAMC)
- American Medical Association (AMA)
- American Society of Health-System Pharmacists (ASHP)
- Department of Veterans Affairs (VA)
- National Business Coalition on Health (NBCH)
- U. S. Pharmacopoeia (USP)
- American Association of Retired Persons (AARP; observer)

Source: AMCP. *Principles of a Sound Drug Formulary.* Alexandria, VA: Academy of Managed Care Pharmacy, October 2000. Available at http://www.amcp.org/data/nav_content/drugformulary.pdf. Accessed 19 Aug 2008.

"The Pharmacy and Therapeutics (P & T) Committee . . . is the mechanism for administering the formulary system, which includes developing and maintaining the formulary and *establishing and implementing policies on the use* of drug products" (emphasis added).

Recommendations of the Working Group Coalition for P & T Committee activities are found in **Table 13-2.**

The Academy of Managed Care Pharmacy published the *Formulary Management* concept paper that also emphasizes the broad responsibility of the Pharmacy & Therapeutics Committee to include the following[8]:

"A formulary system is much more than a list of medications that are approved for use by a managed healthcare organization . . . Policies and procedures for the procuring, dispensing, and administering of the medications are also included in the system. Formularies often contain additional prescribing guidelines and clinical information which assists healthcare professionals to promote high quality, affordable care for patients. Finally, for quality assurance purposes, managed healthcare systems that use formularies have policies in place to give physicians and patients access to non-formulary drugs where medically necessary."

Clearly, when a P & T Committee evaluates a drug for formulary consideration, the members also must determine how the organization can ensure that the product is effectively managed, accurately monitored, and optimally used.

When a P & T Committee evaluates a drug for formulary consideration, the members must determine how the physicians and pharmacists of the organization will prescribe, dispense, monitor, and ensure appropriate utilization. P&T Committees also review and evaluate clinical programs and utilization management strategies. These P & T

TABLE 13-2 Working Group Coalition Recommendations for P & T Committee Activities

- Objectively appraises, evaluates, and selects drugs for the formulary.
- Meets as frequently as is necessary to review and update the appropriateness of the formulary system in light of new drugs and new indications, uses, or warnings affecting existing drugs.
- Establishes policies and procedures to educate and inform healthcare providers about drug products, usage, and committee decisions.
- Oversees quality improvement programs that employ drug use evaluation.
- Implements generic substitution and therapeutic interchange programs that authorize exchange of therapeutic alternatives based upon written guidelines or protocols within a formulary system. (Note: Therapeutic substitution, the dispensing of therapeutic alternates without the prescriber's approval, is illegal and should not be allowed.)
- Develops protocols and procedures for the use of and access to non-formulary drug products.

Source: AMCP. *Principles of a Sound Drug Formulary.* Alexandria, VA: Academy of Managed Care Pharmacy, October 2000. Available at http://www.amcp.org/data/nav_content/drugformulary.pdf. Accessed 19 Aug 2008.

Committee decisions touch all participating providers and members, and have far-reaching implications on health and economic outcomes. Decisions made by the P & T Committee may be challenged or appealed. In some situations, a Committee may reconsider and/or reverse a decision. For this reason, many Committees have a consumer member whose role is to represent the interests of patients. However, the Committee operates independently and decisively in the best interest of the patient, and ideally is uninfluenced by any other internal or external special interest person or group.

AN ILLUSTRATIVE EXAMPLE OF A P & T COMMITTEE STRUCTURE

Pharmacy and Therapeutics Committees are generally similar in their structure, size, authority, and the process they observe, allowing for differences in model type (e.g., open or closed, and product line: HMO, PPO, POS), and membership (e.g., commercial, Medicaid, Medicare). The reader is advised that while we discuss the P & T Committee of a typical mid-size health plan to illustrate an example, organizations are different. Organizational by-laws as well as the state-filed Certificate of Coverage provide the authority and responsibility for the formation and function of a "formulary decision entity," (e.g., a P & T Committee) to make drug product selection decisions for the organization. The Committee consists of healthcare professionals, usually physicians and pharmacists, although nurses, quality assurance directors, ethicists, or economists may be committee members of some larger organizations. In very select instances, MCOs have begun including plan members in the role of patient advocates as members of P&T Committees. At the time of this writing, it is unclear as to whether this practice will become more widespread. The Committee members are predominantly independent practitioners not employed by the sponsoring MCO or PBM, but generally are participating plan providers. Staff or group model plans may use physicians employed by the health system or the exclusively contracted medical group. Some organizations may include faculty members from medical and/or pharmacy schools.

While this committee often is named the Pharmacy & Therapeutics Committee, it may be termed the Drug Formulary Committee or a similarly named group. The Committee size varies among organizations, and some large MCOs or PBMs may have therapeutic subcommittees of the National P & T Committee. In general, a typical medium size MCO has a P & T Committee consisting of 10 to 15 members, although some have up to 20 members. The largest group represented is comprised of physician members who generally represent the specialties who are experts in the most commonly used therapeutic categories, including family practice, general internal medicine, oncology, pulmonology, cardiology, obstetrics and gynecology, or pediatrics. Committees often invite additional specialists to attend a specific meeting to discuss certain therapeutic categories if the Committee does not believe the members have adequate expertise or experience (e.g., endocrinology, infectious diseases, neurology, psychiatry, gastroenterology, or other specialties). Due to the growing number of elderly and individuals with special needs with drug benefits covered under Medicare Part D, many P&T Committees include physicians and pharmacists who specialize in geriatrics in order to consider the unique needs of these subgroups.

In addition to clinical expertise, ideal committee members understand managed care business principles, the organization's pharmacy benefit management philosophy, and the plan sponsor base. They also must appreciate and consider the impact of their decisions on participating physicians, pharmacists, case managers, quality assurance directors, and most importantly, patients. Committee members agree to serve often for a staggered one or two year term, so that the committee continuously evolves yet maintains continuity.

A typical mid-sized open-model health plan P & T Committee may consist of the following members, usually with equal voting authority:

- Committee Chair (independent community-based participating physician or the plan medical director)
- Nine to fourteen additional independent community-based participating physicians
- Health plan medical director (if not the Committee chair)
- Health plan pharmacy director
- Geriatrician for Medicare Part D programs

In addition, the pharmacy department clinical pharmacists and the pharmaceutical contract manager often attend Committee meetings as non-voting staff members to present and discuss clinical and financial impact or contract information. Plans may differ. Larger health plans and PBMs may have broader Committees that may include an economist, an ethicist, quality assurance representatives, or a non-clinical lay plan member. Organizations may also use therapeutic category subcommittees that have the responsibility to review and render expert opinion recommendations to the full P & T Committee on specific therapeutic categories. Multi-state MCOs and PBMs may have a corporate or national P & T Committee that constructs a primary organizational formulary (or National Formulary for organizations with a national presence) that is "customized" at a state or regional plan level, for large self-insured plan sponsors, or by MCO clients of PBMs that have their own P & T Committee. Some organizations separate discussions of drug cost or pharmaceutical manufacturer contract terms from clinical discussions, and only review the contracts or the financial impact after a drug has received a positive review (e.g., a "may add" or a "must add" decision) from the P & T Committee. Typically, medications given "do not add" designation by the P & T Committee are not listed or added to formularies irrespective of financial considerations.

Frequently, subcommittees are formed to conduct reviews of highly sophisticated or unique therapies generally limited to specialists. For example, large organizations may have oncology, neurology, rheumatology, or hemophilia subcommittees to review emerging biotechnology agents often distributed through specialty pharmacies. Subcommittees also are useful to perform emergency reviews between full committee meetings, such as the release of a new break-through therapy, black box safety warnings, or the publication of post-marketing drug research with important results.

It is important to note that new drugs are not reviewed in isolation, but are compared with other existing or soon-to-be-launched pharmacotherapy options, regardless of their therapeutic category. This is key difference between the functions of the Committee and the role of the FDA. The FDA only evaluates one entity at a time in terms of effectiveness and safety. Whereas the P & T committee will consider all viable alternative treatments, including those treatments that may not be pharmacological, or the off-label use of existing medications.

PHARMACY DEPARTMENT ROLE IN NEW DRUG EVALUATION

As discussed in previous chapters, MCO or PBM pharmacy departments have the responsibility to design and administer an effective pharmacy benefit for organization clients. A dynamic drug formulary, developed by the P & T Committee and executed by the pharmacy department, is a seminal requirement for an effective pharmacy benefit designed to optimize clinical and economic outcomes.

Connection between the P & T Committee and the MCO or PBM is maintained to the sponsoring organization through the medical director of pharmacy staff members on the P & T Committee. The organization's pharmacy department generally coordinates and supports the P & T Committee meetings and activities by orchestrating and scheduling meetings, providing drug review material and summaries to Committee members, recording and distributing Committee meeting minutes, and putting Committee decisions into action (e.g., changing claim adjudication drug file, publishing formulary changes to providers and members). **Figure 13-1** illustrates the flow of information among the pharmacy department groups, the P & T Committee, and health plan providers.

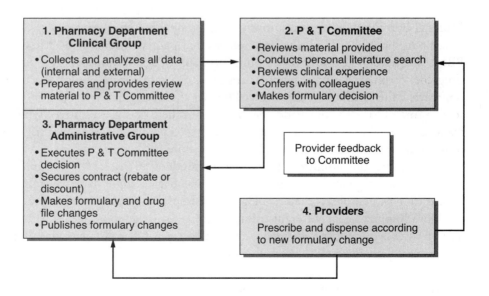

FIGURE 13-1   Information Flow among Pharmacy Departments, P & T Committee, and Providers.

There are three basic pharmacy department activities involved in supporting and executing the P & T Committee decisions:

1. *Clinical Pharmacy Activities.* The clinical pharmacists manage the data and information collection and analysis process, prepare and disseminate P & T Committee meeting materials, interface with Committee members and consultants, and coordinate the P & T Committee agenda.
2. *Pharmaceutical Relations and Contract Management.* The contract manager will review P & T Committee decisions and complete negotiations as appropriate related to pharmaceutical manufacturer discount or rebate contracts.
3. *Pharmacy Benefit Program Management.* Formulary changes must be reflected in drug file and claims adjudication processes, and executed in accordance with pharmacy benefit design contracts; this includes coordination of printing member and provider formularies as well as developing a Web site application.

CLINICAL PHARMACY RESPONSIBILITIES

Clinical pharmacists play a central role in the drug review and drug formulary management processes, and are an important conduit through which critically analyzed new drug information reaches the members of the P & T Committee. For each evaluation of a new drug product by the Committee, clinical pharmacists gather a broad array of new drug and related clinical data. They will review, analyze, and organize, and then transform the information into a cogent summary, usually termed a *new drug monograph*, of evidence-based information for further review by the P & T Committee members. The information sources consulted by clinical pharmacists when conducting a drug review and analysis are discussed later in this chapter. Clinical pharmacists review cost and utilization data of relevance within their own organization, and often model the utilization and cost impact of potential formulary changes.

Physician and other healthcare professional P & T Committee members have additional sources of information upon which they will make their formulary decision, including personal clinical and research experience, recommendations of key opinion leaders, their own review of published peer-reviewed literature, scientific meetings and abstracts, continuing education programs, and pharmaceutical company scientific and marketing material.

PHARMACEUTICAL RELATIONS AND CONTRACT MANAGEMENT

A pharmacist generally will lead the work group responsible for managing the business and contract relationships between the MCO or PBM and pharmaceutical companies. Discount and rebate contracts with pharmaceutical companies are important to pharmacy benefit management, as the rebate income reduces the net cost of contracted products (see Chapters 14 and 15). Although cost remains secondary to clinical and safety considerations in P & T Committee decisions, a lower net cost may influence drug formulary positioning (see Chapter 9) when the therapeutic outcomes expected from comparable medications are considered to be equal or very similar. MCOs may operate under the pharmaceutical contracts of their PBM, or maintain their own contractual relationships with drug companies.

Net drug cost is an important consideration in drug comparisons and formulary positioning when comparative drugs are therapeutically undifferentiated. The MCO or PBM pharmaceutical relations and contract management group has the responsibility of pursuing rebate contracts (or discount contracts when organizations, such as group or staff model plans or PBMs with mail service, take possession of drugs) and assessing the financial impact on forecast drug utilization.

While the net cost of reviewed drugs is important, various MCOs and PBMs introduce the financial data at different times in the drug review process. Traditionally, the pharmacy department contract manager would pursue a contract offering from a pharmaceutical company prior to the P & T Committee meeting, so that the drug cost and a drug cost impact assessment can be presented to the Committee when formulary addition and positioning are considered. Contract details are usually not shared, but the pharmacy department considers the contract rebate level, the pharmacy reimbursement level, the likely copayment, and uses the estimated net cost in pharmacy budget impact analysis models.

However, some MCOs and PBMs do not share cost or contract information with the P & T Committee to make certain formulary decisions are made solely on efficacy and safety data. Cost is not considered until after the drug under review offers clinical value. In this latter situation, a contract is pursued only after the P & T Committee determines the drug receives a positive review. If the Committee renders a "must add" or "may add" decision, the pharmacy contract manager pursues a contract offering so that a pharmacy budget impact model may be constructed to reflect anticipated cost to the organization. Based upon the contract obtained, net cost, and anticipated budget impact, the pharmacy department will determine the appropriate formulary position based upon guidance provided by the P & T Committee.

PHARMACY BENEFIT PROGRAM MANAGEMENT

Once a Committee's decision has been made, changes in the drug files used for pharmacy claims adjudication must be made as soon as possible to allow accurate reimbursement of formulary products. Although a rather detailed and often tedious process, pharmacists working with customer account managers make certain formulary additions or deletions are consistent with customer benefit designs and formularies. As drug formulary changes, it is important to incorporate this new information into client formularies in accordance with their benefit design requirements and specific formulary expectations. Many purchasers and employers dislike frequent formulary changes that disrupt member prescription benefit expectations and utilization patterns. Some states require that formulary changes be made only at specific times in the year, and require plan sponsor approval to delete a formulary product. In order to minimize patient disruption, organizations have established policies to ensure formulary changes are made, at the most, no more frequently than four times yearly.

CMS is very specific with respect to the timing and frequency of formulary changes in Medicare Part D programs. In general, most pharmacy benefit management companies will evaluate medications throughout the year for addition to the formulary, with deletions from the formulary made only at the beginning of the plan or calendar year.

DRUG EVALUATION AND REVIEW PROCESS IN MANAGED CARE

Although P & T Committee schedules vary among organizations, many health plans convene their committee on a quarterly basis, others more frequently, such as monthly. The Committee meeting agenda is usually set 60 to 90 days in advance of the meeting to make certain the health plan pharmacy department has adequate time to complete their drug information collection, analysis, and evaluation, and prepare and distribute materials for the P & T Committee members well in advance of the meeting. Some organizations also schedule an annual review of all important therapeutic categories on a staggered schedule.

NEW DRUG REVIEW WAITING PERIOD

New drugs are often reviewed by a P & T Committee prior to the drug's anticipated launch so that on the first day the drug may be dispensed, complete reimbursement data are provided to participating pharmacies via the online claims adjudication system. When presented a prescription, participating pharmacies must know if the new drug is eligible for reimbursement, the level of reimbursement, the copayment or coinsurance to collect, and if there are any step-care or other limitations on dispensing. Without providing the dispensing pharmacists complete reimbursement information, the MCO or PBM customer and provider services departments are flooded with reimbursement inquiries from frustrated and confused patients, physicians, and pharmacists.

The initial P & T Committee review of a new drug often results in a provisional decision regarding reimbursement when launched. This preliminary decision is usually effective for six months, and new drugs are often placed in a non-preferred formulary tier (e.g., the highest consumer cost-sharing amount, such as the 3rd tier in a three copayment system). MCOs and PBMs are reluctant to provide full approval for a new product without months of real-world prescribing and utilization history. Adverse effects may not be fully expressed in controlled clinical trials and fully realized only after months of real-world experience. Many high-profile medication withdrawals in recent years have served to add credibility to this "wait-and-see" evaluation process. Thus, many MCOs and PBMs generally review products approximately six months after a new drug launch to assess their utilization experience and review contemporary literature and adverse event reports, and only then will the P & T Committee render a final decision on formulary placement and reimbursement.

Many MCOs and PBMs require manufacturers of new drug products to submit clinical and economic data and information in a standard format, such as that adopted by the Academy of Managed Care Pharmacy (see Chapters 9 and 11). This comprehensive dossier of information about the efficacy, safety, and pharmacoeconomic qualities of a new drug product is often not available until many months after a medication's approval, further delaying a full formulary evaluation.

Developing and managing a dynamic drug formulary requires a continual process and work cycle. **Figure 13-2** illustrates a typical process flow of drug review and formulary management activities culminating in a P & T Committee formulary decision. The pharmacy department is continuously engaged in various phases of formulary management. Harvesting of new drug information and review of clinical data is constantly ongoing, and drugs review are continuously being prepared and updated with new information.

As indicated above, an additional tool used to manage formularies is the scheduled review, typically on an annual basis, of all therapeutic classes of drugs. These reviews are an important part of the maintenance of a cost-effective, clinically sound formulary in that they facilitate the gathering and reporting of new, relevant information about the medications listed on the MCO or PBM formulary. In addition to scheduled reviews, the introduction of a new drug to a therapy class or significant newly-published information about the safety or efficacy of existing medications will trigger a therapeutic class review by the P & T Committee.

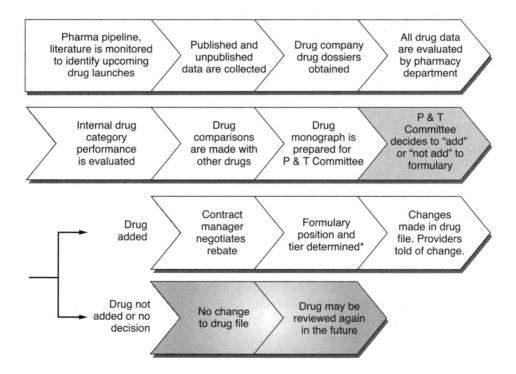

FIGURE 13-2 Drug Evaluation and Formulary Decision Process.

NEW DRUG REVIEW INFORMATION SOURCES AND ANALYSIS

The review of a specific drug commences within the pharmacy department many months before the Committee meeting at which the drug is reviewed. The submission of a New Drug Application (NDA), to the FDA is a common trigger for the pharmacy department to begin the process of collecting relevant information about the new medication that may come to market in the United States. MCO and PBM pharmacists within follow the U.S. drug development pipeline by monitoring a variety of sources, including the following:

- U.S. FDA Center for Drug Evaluation and Research[9]
- Commercial publications, such as *Next Generation Pharmaceutical*[10] and *Pipeline Drugs: Drugs in Clinical Trials*[11]
- Investment company research (e.g., brokerage and investment firm pharmaceutical industry reports)[12]
- Pharmaceutical company Web sites
- Meetings with scientific liaisons from the pharmaceutical industry
- Scientific literature and meetings

Months before a drug's anticipated launch and continuing post-launch, MCO and PBM pharmacy departments aggressively collect data and information from a variety of sources as they build, and embellish, their new drug information cache from which they will develop the new drug monograph for the P & T Committee meeting. Large organizations may have a drug information department that continually monitors a variety of medical and pharmaceutical sources for the most updated drug information. In addition to the pipeline sources listed above, clinical pharmacists collect information from a broad array of resources that may include the following (some may be available only after the drug launch but before the P & T Committee review):

- P & T Community[13] and Formulary[14] publications and Web sites
- Agency for Healthcare Research and Quality's evidence-based practice reports
- *Cochrane Reviews*[15]
- The *FDA Approved Drug Products with Therapeutic Equivalence Evaluations* ("Orange Book")[16]
- Drug information and clinical research Web sites
- PBM publications, such as Caremark *TrendsRx Drug Pipeline & News*[17]
- International drug review and regulatory agencies, such as the United Kingdom's National Institute for Health and Clinical Excellence[18] or the Canadian Coordinating Office for Health Technology Assessment[19]
- Scientific meetings and abstracts
- Global peer reviewed medical and pharmaceutical publications
- P & T Society resource material[20]
- Internal pharmacy and medical claims data analysis
- Economic models, either developed internally or by pharmaceutical companies

- Pharmaceutical company new drug dossiers that generally observe the *AMCP Format* (see Chapter 11)
- Recommendations from key physician opinion leaders

MCO or PBM clinical pharmacists prepare and distribute the new drug monograph with supporting literature reprints to each P & T Committee member to review well in advance of the meeting. Some organizations publish the drug monographs on a secure Web site for P & T Committee members to review. Clinical pharmacists then present the previously distributed clinical information during the P & T Committee meeting and encourage a vigorous dialogue and debate as well as requests for further information.

P & T COMMITTEE MEETING DECISION PROCESS

As discussed above, the P & T Committee members receive and review new drug monographs prior to the meeting. At the meeting, a clinical pharmacist often presents the new drug to be reviewed, presents utilization data of existing class therapeutic drugs, forecasts the new drug's potential role and impact on the class, summarizes the drug monograph findings, and makes a recommendation for formulary positioning. Many plans present cost, contract, and net cost information. Several organizations do not share any cost or contract information with the Committee, and contracts are pursued only after a positive review is rendered by the Committee.

The P & T Committee members consider a broad array of clinical (efficacy and safety), administrative, financial, economic, and quality of life issues when considering a new drug for formulary inclusion. The weight of the type of information depends upon the characteristics of the drug being considered. For example, with a new drug offering imperceptible clinical differentiation in an already crowded therapeutic class (e.g., angiotensin blocking drugs, statins, and beta blockers), the net price and potential utilization rate may be the most influential factors. When a highly unique new drug is launched for a life-threatening condition (e.g., oncology), clinical efficacy and safety will be the most important factors, regardless of price. **Table 13-3** illustrates the relative importance of nine formulary decision criteria. In general, efficacy and safety are universally the two most important decision criteria. Price is an important tertiary criterion, but exerts more relative weight when new drugs are largely undifferentiated from existing products in efficacy and safety.

Pharmacy departments make recommendations that are "evidence based," which weigh the strength of evidence available regarding the efficacy and safety of a new drug product. The P & T Committee then evaluates this evidence to make a decision.

Following a deliberation by Committee members, the Committee chairman calls for a formulary inclusion or exclusion motion and then the members will vote. Committee decisions usually result in one of the following general conclusions.

1. The drug is determined to offer significant clinical value, and should be added to the formulary.

2. The drug is found to possibly offer some clinical value and may be added if the price is acceptable.

3. The drug is not found to offer any clinical value, and will not be added to the formulary. The drug may be reviewed in the future should additional clinical information be available.

4. The drug review is inconclusive. The pharmacy department is requested to collect additional information for a future formulary review.

In all cases when a drug is added to the formulary, the exact formulary position (e.g., tier and copayment or coinsurance, the application of limitations or restrictions, that is, quantity limits, step care, prior authorization) will depend on the price, the new product's clinical differentiation from other drugs currently on formulary, any existing contract conflicts, and anticipated level of utilization. Drugs are not added simply because they are inexpensive. They must offer a clinical and or safety advantage compared with alternative medications. Addition of a new product may result in existing products being deleted from the formulary or repositioned. Large PBMs will also share their P & T Committee decisions with their health plan and employer group clients. The PBM MCO clients with their own P & T Committees will conduct their decision process and make formulary decisions. While the MCO's decisions are often similar to that of their PBM, they are free to make their own decisions based upon regional clinical practices, state laws or pharmacy, or benefit philosophy.

The organizations that do not share financial information with the P & T Committee follow this practice to separate drug clinical value from drug cost, to remove any suggestion that drug costs influence formulary decisions. In such organizations, the pharmacy department contract manager will pursue a rebate contract only after a favorable P & T

TABLE 13-3 Relative Importance of Drug Formulary Decision Criteria

Rank	Formulary Decision Criterion	Importance Rating*
1	Efficacy	4.9
2	Safety	4.8
3	Pharmacy budget impact (net of copays and rebates)	4.6
4	Labeled indications	4.5
5	Included in national guideline	4.3
6	Physician specialist recommendation	3.6
7	Economic data and models	3.0
8	Physician demand	2.8
9	Quality of life	2.6

*Rating scale: 5 = very important; 1 = very unimportant.

Committee decision is rendered, and a separate committee of the pharmacy department may determine formulary position based upon guidance from the P & T Committee. Rebate contracts are discussed in Chapter 15.

At any time during the year, plan participating physicians and pharmacist often communicate comments regarding P & T Committee decisions back to the Committee in the form of phone calls, letters, or emails to the pharmacy department, the medical director, or P & T Committee chairman. Such communications are documented, logged, and discussed at subsequent Committee meetings to determine if a formulary amendment or change is required.

DRUG FORMULARY CHANGE EXECUTION

Following a P & T Committee decision to change the drug formulary (e.g., drug addition, deletion, formulary tier change, addition of a limitation or restriction), the MCO or PBM pharmacy department must immediately make changes in the organization's drug file used by participating pharmacies (including retain, mail, specialty) to adjudicate claims. First Data Bank[21] is an example of a third party provider of a pharmaceutical drug product pricing file used by MCOs and PBMs. The pharmacy department must make immediate reimbursement changes in their drug file so that participating pharmacies may adjudicate claims accurately.

Formulary changes also may require implementation of change of a pharmacy dispensing adjudication edit. For example, the P & T Committee may apply a prior authorization requirement, step-edit, or other limitation to a formulary drug. The pharmacy department must develop and execute the adjudication edit process according to the guidance of the P & T Committee.

Pharmacists within MCOs and PBMs must apply the formulary changes appropriately to the pharmacy benefit designs purchased by the customers (other MCOs [for PBMs], employer groups, of government-sponsored plans). For example, a P & T Committee decision to delete a drug or change formulary position of a drug must be executed in accordance with plan sponsor-specific benefit design requirements.

Many organizations have a written policy to inform members or employers of formulary changes before the change is made, especially if it is a negative formulary change such as "drug not covered" or moving a drug to a higher copayment tier. The notification can be in written or electronic form and can be sent to either all or selected members or employee groups. Online formularies have the benefit of being updated quickly. In addition, some organizations still print a drug formulary or drug list that is updated two to four times annually.

CONCLUSION

Pharmacy & Therapeutics Committees represent a broad array of pharmacy and medical specialty interests that are necessary to develop, maintain, and manage a dynamic and cost-effective drug formulary. The P & T Committee works closely with, and is dependent upon, a highly effective pharmacy department that helps provide the Committee with a complete suite of data and information for new drug analysis as well as to promptly and accurately execute P & T Committee decisions.

Pharmaceuticals are a cost-effective approach to improve and/or maintain health. The P & T Committee has the opportunity and responsibility to develop a highly effective formulary system to yield optimal clinical, economic, and humanistic outcomes.

REFERENCES

1. American Society of Health-System Pharmacists. *ASHP Statement on the Pharmacy and Therapeutics Committee*. Available at http://www.ashp.org/s_ashp/bin.asp?CID=6&DID=5391&DOC=FILE.PDF. Accessed 1 July 2008.

2. Iglehart J., Health Policy Report: the American health care system—expenditures. *N Engl J Med.* 1999; 340(1): 75.

3. Zellmer W.A., "Overview of the history of hospital pharmacy in the United States," in *Handbook Institutional Pharmacy Practice*, 4th ed, Brown T.R., Ed. Bethesda, MD: American Society of Health-System Pharmacists; 2006: 19-32.

4. American Society of Health-System Pharmacists homepage. Available at http://www.ashp.org/s_ashp/index.asp. Accessed 1 July 2008.

5. *Drug Formularies: Myths and Facts*. Coventry Health Care. Available at http://www.healthamerica.cvty.com/content/items/14322/FormularyMyths.pdf. Accessed 1 July 2008.

6. Navarro R.P., unpublished data, various research projects 2005–2007.

7. Consensus document. *Principles of a Sound Drug Formulary*. Alexandria, VA: Academy of Managed Care Pharmacy, October 2000. Available at http://www.amcp.org/data/nav_content/drugformulary.pdf. Accessed 19 Aug 2008.

8. The Academy of Managed Care Pharmacy Concepts in Managed Care Pharmacy. Available at http://www.amcp.org/. Accessed 1 July 2008.

9. U.S. FDA Center for Drug Evaluation and Research. Available at http://www.fda.gov/cder/. Accessed 1 July 2008.

10. Next Generation Pharmaceutical homepage. Available at http://www.ngpharma.com/pastissue/article.asp?art=26442&issue=159. Accessed 1 July 2008.

11. Pipeline Drugs: Drugs in Clinical Trials, *Drugs at the Clinical Stage—In the Pipeline*. Available at http://www.pipelinedrugs.com/. Accessed 1 July 2008.

12. Lawler, B. Know your drug stock ABCs: part 3. The Motley Fool Web site. 2007. Available at http://www.fool.com/investing/high-growth/2007/03/05/know-your-drug-stock-abcs-part-3.aspx. Accessed 19 August 2008.

13. P & T Community homepage. Available at http://www.pharmscope.com. Accessed 7 August 2008.

14. Modern Medicine Network, *Formulary Journal*, "Formulary FDA pipeline preview, November 2007." Available at http://www.formularyjournal.com/formulary/In+the+Pipeline/FDA-pipeline-preview-November-2007/ArticleStandard/Article/detail/476079. Accessed 1 July 2008.

15. The Cochrane Collaboration. An introduction to Cochrane reviews and the Cochrane library. Available at http://www.cochrane.org/reviews/clibintro.htm. Accessed 19 August 2008.

16. FDA, Department of Health and Human Services, *Electronic Orange Book: Approved Drug Products with Therapeutic Equivalence Evaluations*. Available at http://www.fda.gov/cder/ob/. Accessed 1 July 2008.

17. Caremark. *TrendsRx Drug Pipeline & News*. Available at https://www.caremark.com/portal/asset/DPN_Mar_2007.pdf. Accessed 1 July 2008.

18. National Institute for Health and Clinical Excellence. Available at http://www.nice.org.uk/. Accessed 1 July 2008.

19. Health Canada, *Drugs and Health Products*. Available at http://www.hc-sc.gc.ca/dhp-mps/index_e.html. Accessed 1 July 2008.

20. P & T Society. Available at http://www.pandtsociety.org/pages/home.php. Accessed 1 July 2008.

21. First Data Bank homepage. Available at http://www.firstdatabank.com/. Accessed 1 July 2008.

SUGGESTED READING

Rucker T.D. and Schiff G., Drug formularies: myths-in-formation. *Medical Care*. 1990; 28(10): 928-942.

Plumridge R.J., Stoelwinder J.U., Rucker T.D., Drug and therapeutics committees: the relationship among structure, function, and effectiveness. *Hosp Pharm*. 1993; 28(6): 492-493, 496-498, 508.

Simon G.E., Psaty B.M., Hrachovec J.B., Mora M., Principles for evidence-based drug formulary policy. *J Gen Intern Med*. 2005; 20(10): 964-968.

Shih Y.C. and Sleath B.L., Health care provider knowledge of drug formulary status in ambulatory care settings. *Am J Health-Syst Pharm*. 2004; 61: 2657-2663.

Chapter 14

ROLE OF THE PHARMACEUTICAL COMPANY IN MANAGED CARE

KEVIN J. MCDERMOTT

ELIZABETH TAYLOR HOLLAND

ROBERT P. NAVARRO

INTRODUCTION

Managed care and the pharmaceutical industry theoretically should have a natural symbiotic relationship. As described in previous chapters, the pharmacy benefit is a critical component of comprehensive health care, and over 80% of all prescriptions dispensed in the United States are reimbursed, at least in part, by a private or public (e.g., Medicaid, Medicare) third party entity. Pharmacists with managed care organizations (MCOs) are the focal point for interaction with pharmaceutical companies due to the director's responsibility in managing all aspects of prescription drug benefits, from designing the benefit, developing the formulary, negotiating contracts with the pharmaceutical industry, conducting drug use research projects, and implementing clinical and medication therapy management programs to optimize drug use outcomes. Pharmaceutical manufacturers have a mission to develop and market pharmaceuticals, and to do so in a managed markets environment, they must also meet the needs of their plan sponsors and, ultimately, patient-members. Truly engaged manufacturers can provide support to help MCO and pharmacy benefit manager (PBM) pharmacy departments accomplish their program outcome objectives. In turn, pharmacists developing and managing pharmacy benefit programs can influence physician access and utilization of pharmaceuticals. This affects drugs sales and pharmaceutical company profitability. For many medical conditions, the appropriate use of the proper pharmaceutical is the most cost-effective therapy available. Cost minimization will always be a component of managed care. However, if managed care pharmacy directors and pharmaceutical companies can demonstrate clinical, economic, and humanistic outcomes with formulary drugs, plan sponsors and health care policymakers may better understand the value of pharmaceuticals within a managed prescription drug benefit. It is at the intersection of the MCOs' pursuit of cost-effective drug programs and the pharmaceutical manufacturers' commitment to the appropriate use of the drugs that they bring to market where the congruence of interests occur.

MANAGED CARE RELATIONSHIP WITH THE PHARMACEUTICAL INDUSTRY

Through private commercial insurance, Medicaid, Medicare, TRICARE, and other governmental programs (e.g., Indian Health Service), more than 250 million citizens have access to prescription drugs provided by the pharmaceutical industry. Pharmaceutical companies (PCs) are business enterprises seeking to recoup revenue from the discoveries they have brought to market as well as to fund future drug discovery, and understandably have a high interest in having their drugs used whenever appropriate. Prior to the development of managed care, PCs primarily marketed products to physicians through various professional promotional strategies. However, over the past two decades, MCOs and PBMs have increased power and influence over drug product reimbursement as well as physician prescribing behavior. As a result of this shift or sharing of drug prescribing and utilization control with managed care, PCs have developed their own internal managed care marketing expertise. The pharmaceutical industry often prefers the term *managed markets* rather than *managed care* to reflect the breadth of healthcare delivery systems adopting managed care pharmacy program policies (see Chapters 1 and 2) as well as to reflect the business aspect of drug distribution. Also, the pharmaceutical industry often dissects the broad marketplace into generally distinct but interactive market distribution "channels" such as the hospital channel, the health plan channel, the PBM channel, the specialty pharmacy channel, the Medicare channel, Medicaid channel, Veterans Affairs (VA), Department of Defense (DoD), etc. The health plan, PBM, and even Medicare channel may be combined. Health plans and PBMs are logically similar in that they both offer commercial managed care programs, and very often the same health plans and PBMs also offer Medicare Part D pharmacy benefits. It's this segmentation that drives the designs of the account management teams and marketing programs.

Pharmaceutical companies have different structural organizations, but in general, most have dedicated internal teams or business units that mirror their target market channels and correspond with their current and future product portfolio. For example, a pharmaceutical company that markets drugs into the hospital channel will have institutional sales and marketing teams. Most PCs that distribute non-specialty drugs to the outpatient market have a trade sales and marketing team that focuses on drug wholesaler and retail pharmacy relationships. A state government sales and marketing team concentrates on State Medicaid programs, VA, and the DoD, and the managed markets team will generally develop sales and marketing programs targeted at commercial managed care and Medicare Part D programs (as very often the same organizations offer commercial programs and Medicare Part D benefits). The primary role of all of these groups is to develop materials to properly position the PC's products with managed care but also to create materials for the PC's sales forces to promote their portfolio's reimbursement status to community-based physicians. **Figure 14-1** illustrates how a pharmaceutical company may develop internal teams to mirror the distribution channels most important to their product portfolio. Of course, all PCs are different and use different names and organizational structures, yet all are similar in that they develop expertise in sales and marketing strategies to most effectively and appropriately promote their products to meet the needs of their target physician and market channel.

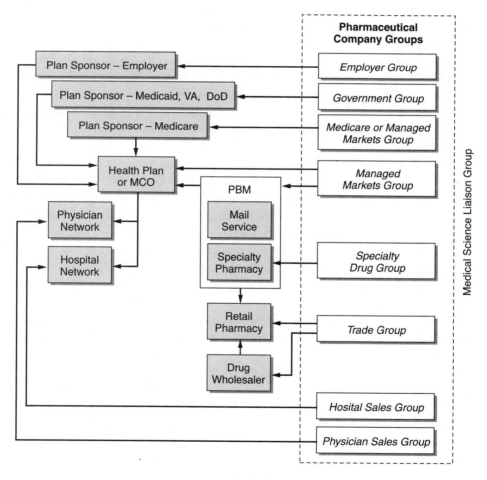

FIGURE 14-1 Pharmaceutical Company Groups that Interact with Managed Markets' Components. Drug wholesalers and community pharmacies are independent entities, not internal components of a managed care organization, but are important entities in the distribution of pharmaceuticals within the system.

MANAGED MARKETS' GROUP ROLE WITHIN PHARMACEUTICAL COMPANIES

The pharmaceutical industry has learned over the past twenty years that managed care is a powerful gatekeeper and market shaper with the ability to influence physician prescribing, pharmacist dispensing, and member utilization of pharmaceuticals. PCs vary widely in their commitment to work with managed care based on their internal assessment of their ability to successful sell into targeted markets. It is almost a linear relationship between the amount of effort and resources put into managed care directly correlated with the complexity and control of managed care in the PC's key therapeutic areas. The largest PCs with broad portfolios have had managed markets departments for almost twenty years, and dedicate enormous resources to sustain large managed markets sales and marketing activities. Smaller, emerging companies may have no one specifically designated as a managed markets specialist, but this responsibility is added to the other job responsibilities such as someone on a brand team or within the sales organization.

The importance given to managed care sales and marketing activities within a pharmaceutical company is often dependent upon the size of the pharmaceutical company, and the breadth and uniqueness of the drug portfolio subject to managed care reimbursement and coverage influence. While the first criterion is highly variable, it is common to find a drug with reimbursement heavily influenced by managed care. Exceptions in the past have been injectable products for severe, debilitating diseases, such as multiple sclerosis, rheumatoid arthritis, or cancer. Today even such unique products with a limited and highly individualized patient population are subject to coverage and reimbursement limitations. This trend has been driven, in part, by the MCO's vigilance over spending trends. If a category begins to expand, systems and tools are now more commonly available to managed care to identify this movement and model the impact. Also, as discussed in previous chapters, the vast majority of all drug use is touched by the control philosophy and policies of managed care. In essence, the greater the chance for managed care "interference" into the marketing plans of a brand, the greater the likelihood for a large, structured, and diverse managed markets team within a PC.

The managed markets group interacts with and supports many other teams within the pharmaceutical company, including sales (including primary, specialty and institutional sales groups if present), marketing, finance, medical services, market research, clinical development, and health outcomes. As over 80% of all outpatient prescriptions are influenced or reimbursed by an MCO or PBM, the managed markets group must provide managed care expertise throughout the company by providing education and training, and supporting the strategy development and tactical programs of other groups. Regardless of where they are organizationally, they must interact and liaise with many other internal functional units, including the sales and marketing team. Customer and market trend information is required to keep medical services, brand teams, health outcomes, market research, finance (contract administration), legal, clinical development, disease management, and others on top of the issues that challenge sales.

ORGANIZATION STRUCTURE OF MANAGED MARKETS TEAMS

Managed markets groups within pharmaceutical companies are structured to meet short- and long-term organizational needs, and may have various reporting responsibilities in organizational charts. The managed markets group may report into the highest echelon of U.S. commercial operations in pharmaceutical companies highly dependent upon managed care access. Often the managed markets group is found under the corporate sales or marketing business units. The managed markets group mission is typically twofold: 1) support the managed care knowledge of other internal teams, and 2) achieve appropriate access at targeted managed care customers.

Account managers often have defining titles that indicate the type of managed care customer on which they call, although titles vary among pharmaceutical companies. Regional account managers (RAMs) are responsible for regional health plans or PBMs. *National account managers (NAMs)* may call on health plans or PBMs with a national presence. Some pharmaceutical companies call their NAMs *corporate account managers* denoting a closer connection between the account managers and headquarter functions. NAMs and RAMs must coordinate their activities when dealing with a national insurer's regional affiliates or the local accounts that use a national PBM. In some instances the account managers may have a direct or a dotted-line relationship with the regional sales unit. **Figures 14-2 and 14-3** illustrate two of many organizational structures of a pharmaceutical

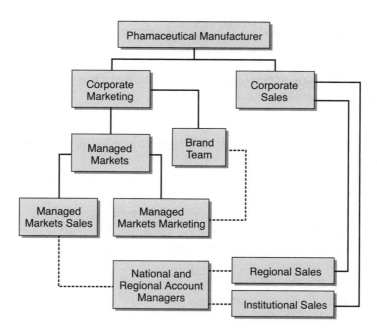

FIGURE 14-2   Example of Managed Markets' Group Reporting into Corporate Marketing with Indirect Sales Responsibility (Dotted Line to Sales).

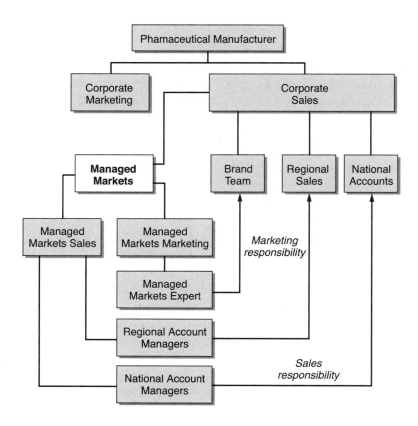

FIGURE 14-3   Example of Managed Markets' Group Reporting into Corporate Sales with Direct Sales Responsibility.

company managed markets group and the interaction of a RAM or NAM with sales and marketing activities.

A newer addition to some managed market teams is the hybrid organizational structure that includes a *regional marketing manager (RMM)*. This team member works in tandem with a RAM for a specific geographic area of the country (i.e., Southeast). In this structure, the RAM is solely responsible for obtaining formulary access through contracting and/or negotiations, and the RMM acts as the liaison between the account managers and the field, with job responsibilities to include pull-through and push-through initiatives, promotional fund disbursement to promote wins, training, managed care messaging, and answering field questions that arise regarding the managed care terrain in a geographic area. The RMM position can be an asset in the view of some pharmacy directors, as this has positive implications on market share increase for preferred products.

INTERACTION WITH THE PRODUCT BRAND TEAM

A pharmaceutical company brand manager is responsible for orchestrating promotional messages and marketing activities on behalf of their assigned brand(s). As a result of the enormous influence on drug access and reimbursement on brand performance, it is imperative that the brand team include involvement of the managed markets team to provide market intelligence, education on benefit designs and reimbursement trends, and to assist in development of the various activities targeted to solidify a brand's value to managed markets customers. This includes sales and marketing campaigns, product value messaging, physician promotional marketing, formulary dossier and economic model distribution, phase IV studies, health outcomes research, product pull-through programs, and disease management product support.

Managed markets team members must interact with brand teams to recommend managed markets-focused sales and marketing strategies and tactics to help increase access and utilization of key brand products, and serve as a communication conduit between the brand team and the managed markets group. Ideally, the managed markets team should be integrated into the core brand team to advise on development of a managed care marketing strategy and message, product promotion to managed care customers, development of the managed care dossier (see Chapter 11), customer contracting, product pull-through programs, and health outcomes research. Many companies have a fully dedicated team of marketers who specialize in managed markets marketing, allowing the core brand team to concentrate on physician-directed marketing. The source of personnel for these managed markets marketing managers is many times experienced RAMs or NAMs who have shown a strong ability and affinity to this area and understand the needs of the managed market customer.

Companies may have one or a limited number of people on the managed markets team as permanent members of the brand team and usually have those people's time split between managed markets and more traditional physician marketing responsibilities. Other companies that invest in a managed markets operation that "carves out" managed care activities to a separate team typically have assessed that the demands are large enough to warrant that type of overhead. In return for that investment, the managed markets marketing functions are often asked to take on a greater role with the brand, such as developing and managing rep-driven programs like coupons and compliance and persistency offers. It's difficult to say which model a company uses is correct because most are responding to the market conditions with which they have been challenged. Successful companies anticipate the requirements in advance so that the managed markets marketing team can assist in market development activities prior to a product's launch to help the company understand the potential for a new agent. In this case, the managed markets team may actually have relationships with new product planning versus what is called in-line brand marketing.

SUMMARY OF INTERACTIONS WITH OTHER INTERNAL PHARMACEUTICAL COMPANY TEAMS

Other teams within the pharmaceutical company the managed markets group may interact with include the following:

- *Marketing team.* Advises on product, portfolio, and corporate marketing and branding strategies that will be meaningful to managed care customers.
- *New product planning.* Advises on requirements of the market and current treatment patterns that would have to be acknowledged when evaluating a new product's probability of success in the market.
- *Sales team.* Secures preferred formulary access to support physician promotion and advises the sales team (corporate, regional, and local) on strategies for physician promotion with formulary disadvantaged products.
- *Market research group.* Advises on effective market research that captures the broad managed care market trends, channel trends, and unique customer cohort differences, to produce more actionable research findings.
- *Health outcomes and outcomes research group.* Advises on designing economic study methodologies to produce data outputs that will be meaningful to managed care customers, and recommends methods to develop a meaningful economic model to accompany the new drug product dossier.
- *Business development group.* Provides forecasted reimbursement information data that may influence valuation of product development, in-licensing opportunities, pivotal trial study design, and future product launch forecasts.
- *Pricing.* Advises on quantitative and qualitative pricing sensitivity research that considers the impact of managed care formulary tiers and member copayments.
- *Contract administration.* Recommends reasonable and performance-oriented rebate and discount contracts for various managed care customer types.
- *Legal department.* Secures a balance of risk management and compliance adherence with market competitiveness into rebate and discount strategy.
- *Institutional, trade, and specialty pharmacy teams.* If appropriate, these are based upon the product line, if there will be interaction among hospitals, retail pharmacies, or specialty pharmacies that may be influenced by managed care formulary policies.
- *Supply chain/manufacturing.* Assures special packaging that allows for a more efficient distribution of a product(s).
- *Medical science liaisons* to partner the business side of the equation (managed care) with the corporate clinical expertise in order to achieve a true value proposition offering.

ROLE OF THE MANAGED MARKETS ACCOUNT MANAGER WITHIN MANAGED CARE CUSTOMERS

Managed markets managers function as the primary point of contact of the pharmaceutical company with the managed care customer. As discussed above, specialized managed markets account managers from various teams call on commercial, Medicaid,

Medicare, TRICARE, VA, and other managed care customer channels through a variety of organizational structures among various pharmaceutical companies. For purposes of this discussion, we focus on the managed markets account managers (regional or national) who call on commercial health plans or PBMs serving commercial and Medicare Part D customers.

The account manager is the primary representative of the pharmaceutical company to his or her managed care customer. At the first meeting, the account manager must have a thorough understanding of the topics listed on **Table 14-1** before he or she meets the customer pharmacy director for the first time (i.e., visiting the plan's Web site at the very minimum). Pharmacy directors are willing to educate the account manager on plan-specific information but no longer have time to provide a basic managed care education. Because the average tenure of an account manager has lessened due to high levels of restructuring among pharmaceutical manufacturers in the mid-2000s, pharmacy departments have grown a bit weary of breaking in new account managers. Over time, an effective account manager will harvest customer-specific intelligence (**Table 14-2**) that will assist him or her, and the pharmaceutical company, to more effectively penetrate the organization's formulary and increase appropriate product utilization.

The account manager must be versed on all points of interaction between the pharmaceutical company and assigned managed care customer accounts. The ideal account manager can detail a company's products as well as any top representative *(rep)* but has the wisdom to present the features and benefits that really matter to a pharmacy department. The primary basis of the relationship between the account manager and the pharmacy director is to satisfy each others' needs. The pharmacy director desires to select the most cost-effective products for the organization's drug formulary, and to obtain desired program support resources. The account manager should never underestimate the effectiveness of being passionate about the product and disease state he/she represents. If that is visibly

---

TABLE 14-1   Minimum General Managed Care Knowledge Base Requirements for Pharmaceutical Company Managed Markets' Account Managers

• Managed care business objectives	• Pharmacy network reimbursement
• General managed care benefit management policies and practices	• Pharmacy & Therapeutics Committee operations
• Commercial, Medicare, and Medicaid benefit design options and policies	• New drug data collection and review process
• Managed care use of drug price metrics (e.g., WAC, AWP, MAC)	• Specialty pharmacy distribution (if applicable for product portfolio)
• Drug formulary development and management strategies and tactics	• Rebate contracting, therapeutic category, and benefit design management objectives
• Consumer directed programs	• HEDIS and other quality measures
• Copayment and coinsurance operations	• Fundamental knowledge of use of outcomes studies, and evidence-based medicine

TABLE 14-2 Customer-Specific Knowledge Necessary for Effective Pharmaceutical Company Managed Markets' Account Managers

- Customer-specific business objectives

- Financial stability and success (medical and pharmacy loss ratios)
- Customer base and product offerings
- Benefit design
- Formulary management style (e.g., open, closed, amount and type of edits, PAs)
- Customer loss or renewal rate
- Identification of important decision-makers (e.g., pharmacy director, medical director, quality director, marketing director)
- Demographics and population of patient types for promoted product(s)
- Federal, state, and local regulations that may affect discussions on disease state management programs
- Business challenges of employers, unions, and other major payers serviced by customer
- Interest in customer to pursue health outcomes research or consider health outcomes in formulary decisions
- Physician reimbursement mechanism (e.g., capitation, discounted fee-for-service) and if physicians are at-risk for drug costs

- Pharmacy distribution network (e.g., retail, mail, specialty [if applicable]) and level of pharmacy reimbursement
- Pharmacy & Therapeutics Committee process, schedule, and members
- Level of competition in customer's market
- Future marketing plans of customer
- Importance of quality assurance (NCQA accreditation; HEDIS scores)

- Customer creativity and willingness to innovate
- Level of customer disease management program offerings

- Disease state priorities

- Regulations of federal and state funded programs customer may participate in

- Business performance of customer, especially if publicly traded
- Epidemiologic data for disease states in customer service areas

strong, the pharmacy director has a solid insight into the caliber and quality of the account manager's sales force's expertise as clinical knowledge and account management have not traditionally been strongly correlated. The pharmacy director expects the account manager to provide complete clinical and economic drug product data and information and an aggressive rebate contract offer with or without external help. Combined, the clinical, economic, and contract information assist the Pharmacy & Therapeutics (P & T) Committee in determining the value of the account manager product portfolio and drug formulary position (see Chapters 9, 12, 13, and 20). Essentially, value is a product of the perceived clinical outcomes and net product cost (net of copayment and rebate) when compared with competing formulary products. Secondarily, and only if the product is accepted for the drug formulary, the pharmacy director may be interested in certain support resources, such as promotional messaging, number of rep details relative to the competitive agents, patient education, advancement of the therapeutic area through landmark trials, or disease management program resources offered regardless of contractual relationship.

The account manager's needs in this relationship are perhaps a bit more limited but of equal importance back to the manufacturer. He or she desires to obtain the best possible drug formulary position for the lowest possible (or no) rebate contract to satisfy internal pressures. Secondarily, the account manager desires to satisfy any other needs expressed by the pharmacy director, or someone else within the organization, because relationships are key in this very close environment or "small world" that comprises the U.S. managed care market. Of course, this is a simplistic analysis of a complex relationship, but the time-tested truths of effective account management include trust, responsiveness, respect, honesty, and performance (as one promised in the negotiation phase of an agreement) as the basis for a positive managed care business relationship. If any of these components are missing, the relationship between the account manager and the pharmacy director will be superficial and easily discarded once a better value proposition comes along. It may seem that the account manager is being required to exert far more effort into the relationship than the pharmacy director, but good account managers know that his/her customers always have choices especially because there are very few exclusive markets anymore. It truly is easier to get it right from the start than to have to react to competitive services/offers without the benefit of a solid relationship.

Eventually, the account manager should earn the respect of the pharmacy director and seek references to others in the managed care company who influence access and reimbursement decisions. The goal here (with positions such as the medical director) is to solidify the awareness of one's product(s) attributes across multiple departments that may benefit from the product profile. It is highly advisable and generally mandatory to inform the pharmacy director of all interactions with other departments, especially the medical director. The pharmacy director may report to the medical director, who then is ultimately responsible for medical services (essentially everything other than pharmacy) in addition to pharmacy services. Alternatively, the medical director may not be responsible for pharmacy, and may report on a parallel track with the pharmacy director to a higher echelon. However, as drug use is inextricably linked with the prevention and treatment of most medical conditions, the medical director and pharmacy director generally function as a team, and both have a mutual concern over the pharmacy benefit management and drug formulary product selection. The medical director may be the chairman, and most certainly is a member—along with the pharmacy director—of the organization's P & T Committee.

Contact with other individuals within the health plan or PBM generally is orchestrated by the pharmacy director, and depends on whether the organization has identified resource needs from which they are willing to seek external support and have decided that pharmaceutical companies are a valid and unbiased source of such support or resources. **Table 14-3** provides a list of other individuals within the health plan outside of the pharmacy department with whom the account manager may interact. Typically, other resources produced by the pharmaceutical company (often termed *value added resources*) are in

TABLE 14-3 Other Managed Care Positions that May Interact with Pharmaceutical Company Account Managers, and the Purpose of Such Interactions

MCO and PBM Contacts*	Purpose of Interaction
Medical director	• May be responsible for pharmacy benefits • Is a member of the Pharmacy & Therapeutics Committee • May champion drug economic value
Quality director	• May utilize company resources to support organizational quality initiatives (e.g., HEDIS measures)
Case or care management director	• Company resources may support case or disease management initiatives
Health outcomes research department	• Health outcomes research support to show value of pharmaceutical company's drug
Training department	• Pharmaceutical company may offer educational modules or support resources
Marketing department	• Pharmaceutical company may offer program or benefit support to plan sponsors
Mail service pharmacy	• Company products may be appropriate for mail distribution and adherence programs
PBM Clinical Program (CP) management	• CP manager may include pharmaceutical manufacturer resources in programs with PBM customers

* Beyond the pharmacy department director; not all MCOs and PBMs include all departments.

response to a well researched and typical challenge faced by a majority of MCOs. It is important to note that the offering of such services be completely separated from discussions on a company's access status because the linking of such requires specific acknowledgment in federal pricing reporting. Ideally, these support resources should be intended to advance the care of any patient suffering from a condition that the pharmaceutical company engages in, not just those on a company's products.

The pharmacy director is generally the primary contact within a health plan. In large health plans and PBMs, the account manager will interact with various healthcare professionals, who are mostly pharmacists. In national insurance companies and PBMs, these individuals often reside throughout the country and may be called on by various account managers within a pharmaceutical company. This causes communication and coordination challenges for the national insurer or PBM as well as the pharmaceutical company. The ideal national account relationship has the NAM (or CAM) quarterback the overall plans by regional account so that a consistent and coordinated strategy is executed at a national account. Without that collaboration and coordination, many customer headquarters often refuse to support a company's request for a national program, because the regional efforts to drive demand "boxed in" corporate to make a decision and any negative decision would tarnish regional/headquarter relationships. **Table 14-4** lists some of the individuals within a pharmacy department with whom an account manager may interact, and the purpose for the interactions.

PHARMACY DIRECTOR'S EXPECTATIONS OF A PHARMACEUTICAL COMPANY ACCOUNT MANAGER

The managed care pharmacy director is under enormous pressure to develop and administer a pharmacy benefit that provides for all clinical needs of covered members and also satisfies the financial expectations of the parent organization, plan sponsors, and plan members. The pharmacy director expects that the pharmaceutical company account manager will bring all the resources of his or her company to help the pharmacy director achieve business objectives, including high value drugs with a competitive price, an aggressive contract, and other desired resources. In exchange, the pharmacy director offers the account manager an opportunity for a favorable drug formulary position for the cost-effective pharmaceuticals. Once on a formulary, the account manager informs her or his sales colleagues, who can then launch a physician promotional campaign describing the favorable formulary position of their product on the plan's drug formulary.

The pharmacy director expects the account manager to be a conduit for all pharmaceutical company resources, and to know how to access desired resources on behalf of her or his managed care customers. The pharmacy director also expects the account manager to effectively communicate the drug formulary status and reimbursement policy of his or her company's drugs to all relevant sales professionals within the pharmaceutical company, so that

TABLE 14-4 Managed Care Pharmacy Department Contacts for Pharmaceutical Company Managed Markets' Account Managers

Pharmacy Department Contact*	Purpose for Interaction
Pharmacy director	• General pharmacy department operations
	• Discuss corporate-level programs between the MCO or PBM and the pharmaceutical company
Clinical pharmacist	• Drug product clinical and economic presentations
	• Present drug dossier and economic model
	• Discuss Pharmacy & Therapeutics Committee agenda and data needs
MTM pharmacist and/or DUR pharmacist**	• Discuss disease management, MTM, and adherence program resources
Contract administrator	• Present and negotiate rebate contract
	• Monitor rebate contract performance
Health outcomes researcher	• Research endeavors and support

* Positions in large MCOs and PBMs may be at the vice president level.
** See Chapters 8 and 21.

physicians are provided accurate drug coverage information that is consistent with the reimbursement information provided to the health plan. The effective account manager will meet with and educate local sales representatives about the managed care customer formulary status of their products, reimbursement policies, and of any other coverage information relevant to physician promotion. The account manager may bring his or her regional director or RMM into the managed care customer especially if both organizations are pursuing a drug formulary switch or product pull-through campaign that benefits both entities.

The pharmacy director also expects his or her account manager to present an aggressive rebate contract for drugs desired by the health plan. Account managers often are given the discretion for negotiation with established ranges, but ultimately contracts must be approved by the headquarters' finance contract administration department. Account managers must understand the market potential, the level of contract necessary to obtain a preferred formulary position, and know if the health plan or PBM has the benefit designs necessary to achieve the expected utilization benchmarks. An account manager must not only "sell" his or her company/products to the plan but must "sell" the MCO to his or her contracting committee to secure the highest rebate possible for that MCO within an acceptable range. Any information that a pharmacy director can provide that gives the account manager further insight into the MCO's level of control, future increases in membership, or preferred brand initiatives that might encourage market share growth can help the account manager better "sell" the MCO to upper management.

Beyond the specific performance expectations, the pharmacy director expects the account manager will act honestly and professionally, understand the local managed care environment and market trends, and deliver the promised services in a timely manner. In summary, the pharmacy director expects the account manager to be a business partner as well as to act as the interface to all other departments and resources within the pharmaceutical company. The account manager may not know all of the answers him- or herself, but can quickly obtain the desired information. **Table 14-5** lists some of the expectations pharmacy directors may have of pharmaceutical companies' managed markets account managers.

TABLE 14-5 Pharmacy Director Expectations of Pharmaceutical Company Managed Markets Account Managers

• Understand managed care, the regional market and trends, and specific customer business operations	• Provide an aggressive contract for formulary products
• Provide requested product clinical, economic, and other marketing data and information	• Provide effective communication with the regional sales representatives regarding managed care customer policies
• Deliver the new drug dossier and economic model	• Effectively support and coordinate joint pull-through and adherence initiatives
• Be an effective conduit to other pharmaceutical company resources	• Recommend useful pharmaceutical company resources when appropriate (e.g., research support, disease management resources)

REBATE CONTRACTING

Many pharmaceutical companies offer rebate contracts to managed care customers to improve access position and improve the relative cost-effectiveness ratio of key drug products within and across therapeutic alternatives. As discussed in greater detail in Chapters 9, 13, and 15, clinical efficacy and safety data are of paramount importance when considering a drug for formulary addition, and price is of tertiary importance. However, in the absence of significant clinical differentiation among competitive products, the net price (net of WAC, rebates, and copayments) becomes an extremely influential decision criterion. It is important to emphasize that clinical value trumps net price, and many large MCOs and PBMs make formulary decisions based upon a drug's clinical value before a contract is pursued.

Managed care customers often evaluate their account manager's contracting knowledge and effectiveness on a continuum of low to high.[1] Because price and rebate contracting are so central to the business relationship, managed care customers judge their account managers very quickly based on their handling of this specific area. Commonly, the account manager who is only capable of quoting their product's AWP and WAC pricing is considered to have a low skill level. Account managers who discuss the financial impact in terms of unit cost or daily therapy cost, or even cost per course of therapy are considered to have higher level of understanding. Account managers who can discuss the net cost to the plan as well as that of the competitor(s) and who offer cost-impact modeling based upon various utilization scenarios are most helpful and are considered to have the highest level of contracting understanding.

The types of financial models described above are created by account managers in a format where the plan can actually input their own utilization, pharmacy discounts, dispensing fees, and rebates for each product. They then are able to speculate about the financial impact of the potential addition of a product. The plan's analytics department can check for integrity of formulae and this type of tool saves the plan the time and money of creating its own. Financial models are met with a receptivity that pharmacoeconomic models are not, as pharmacoeconomic models are seen as marketing contrived and not pure like the financial model described above.

The decision for a pharmaceutical company to contract is driven by the brand forecast, competitive net price, and expected utilization rate (sales). Managed markets and the brand team, with input from market research, will determine the net profit contribution likely in various formulary positions, with and without different rebate levels, within various managed care key customers types. The expected contract return on investment (ROI) is based on the ability of various contract offerings to secure preferred formulary access, or prevent a disadvantaged position or restricted reimbursement at key customers. Chapter 15 discusses contracting in greater depth. Recently, due to benefit design changes, an additional rationale

---

[1] Mark Newton of GTx Inc., contributed to this discussion of rating the contracting skill level of account managers.

for contracting has emerged that is especially related to chronic conditions. In these disease states, long-term adherence and compliance to therapy has been shown to be challenged by the amount of copay the patient has to outlay per prescription. Copays, coinsurance, and consumer-driven benefit designs have put out-of-pocket expenses at the top of the list in the patient's mind of whether to take a medication. If the out-of-pocket exceeds the patient's willingness to pay, then adherence begins a significant and, in most cases, dramatically steep decline. This dynamic has driven many pharmaceutical companies to deploy strategies that don't just get preferred access, but access that will translate into adherence to their chronic medications. This could involve contracting or direct to patient programs should the benefit designs net out of pocket exceed the patient's willingness to pay.

Once a contract is in place, many companies are required to drive market share for the financial agreement to work for both parties. In those instances, additional relationships are executed to assure that success is achieved. Formulary conformance programs (i.e., *pull-through programs*) that increase the use of preferred formulary medications within a specific therapeutic category or for a targeted medical condition are a large part of an account manager's accountability to his/her company and the contracted client. In many such programs, the MCO or PBM and the pharmaceutical company initiate communicate and incentive programs to encourage (or require) physicians and members to use preferred (and usually contracted) formulary products when clinically appropriate. These initiatives, often termed pull-through programs, benefit both parties by increasing the use of cost-effective formulary drugs from the partnership pharmaceutical company.

MANAGED CARE AND PHARMACEUTICAL COMPANY JOINT PROGRAMS

Separate and distinct from the contractual relationship is the condition where a pharmaceutical manufacturer recognizes the additive role a MCO or PBM could play in disease education by studying the effects of the pharmaceutical company's product on a population from an economic perspective or helping to drive adherence. This capability of the managed care company leads many pharmaceutical companies to pursue service relationships with customers. Such programs include the following:

- Disease and care management programs often are developed and executed by the MCO or PBM using resources of a pharmaceutical company partner. Several pharmaceutical companies have excellent program and patient educational resources for some of the high-prevalence and high-cost medical conditions (e.g., various cardiovascular diseases, depression, asthma, COPD) that are unbranded and non-promotional.
- Drug adherence programs target non-adherence members and result in sustained prescription use of targeted products.
- Clinical and economic research support may be provided through unrestricted financial grants, or by retaining a reputable third-party research consultancy or university to conduct the research.

These programs—often mislabeled as *value added programs*—are indeed true service offerings and should be treated as such by both parties. Many MCOs and PBMs are reluctant to accept any non-financial support to avoid any suggestion of impropriety. It's important that both parties establish the fair market value of the service offering(s) and account for that in the reporting required to government agencies. Many excellent unbranded programs exist in the market that have addressed appropriate legal and regulatory guidelines for managed care–pharmaceutical company relationships and benefit MCOs and PBM members today.

PHARMACEUTICAL COMPANY ACCOUNT MANAGER EXPECTATIONS OF A PHARMACY DIRECTOR

A successful managed care–pharmaceutical company business relationship requires that both parties are treated with respect, have open and frequent communications, and concentrate on both the short- and longer-term aspects of each other's business models. Just as pharmacy directors have expectations of account managers and of pharmaceutical companies, so do account managers have expectations of the pharmacy director. Primary expectations are that the pharmacy director be trustworthy, responsive, honest, and open to hearing about the research a company performs on its drugs. Ultimately, the best pharmacy director delivers on promises, especially in contractual relationships.

If the pharmacy director is to be effective for the account manager, he or she (or properly trained and empowered staff members) must be available to provide requested information to the account manager in a timely manner. Some of the important information critical to the account manager includes the following:

- Complete and accurate description of the organizational structure, business model and objectives, product offerings, membership, growth expectations, benefit design, and trends.
- Explanation of the drug formulary, tier and copayment or coinsurance structure, P & T Committee process and schedule, new drug review data and information collection process, expected timing of data needs from the account manager, and interest in the account manager bringing in company clinicians or economists for in-house presentations.
- Description of the rebate negotiation schedule and process. In the case of the account having their pharmacy benefit managed by a PBM, this includes what that relationship looks like and how the account manager should communicate local needs back to the PBM.
- Understanding of the MCO or PBM interest in pharmaceutical company resources.
- Interest in joint programs (described above).
- Understanding of customer drug formulary and benefit design philosophy, objectives, therapeutic category management priorities, and having possession of accurate customer utilization data.

The account manager can be an effective representative of the pharmaceutical company only if the pharmacy director takes the time to periodically update the account manager on any organizational activity and anticipated change(s) that may influence the use of drugs or program resources available from the pharmaceutical company. The reason this mutual respect and commitment to communication is necessary is that staff from all other internal pharmaceutical company departments mentioned previously that are touched by a managed care company depend on information to do their jobs. Managed care has asked (sometimes even demanded) that the pharmacy department be the gatekeeper for the managed care/pharmaceutical company relationship. If that "gate" is never opened, then the account's reputation is many times tarnished inside the pharmaceutical company as not being a true partner. Whether that title is deserved or not, the fact is that resourceful managed care companies are always looking for an edge to tackle the business challenges they face. By closing the door on the vast disease-specific and market development skills that the pharmaceutical industry has developed, an MCO limits its own ability to compete in the marketplace.

MEASURING THE PERFORMANCE OF THE MANAGED MARKETS GROUP WITHIN A PHARMACEUTICAL COMPANY

Pharmaceutical companies also have key performance indicators and expectations of their managed markets group. The managed market group's performance metrics among pharmaceutical companies are highly variable based upon the importance of managed care to the company's product portfolio, the relative size and sophistication of the pharmaceutical company in managed markets, and the managed market group's ability to directly influence sales. Specific performance metrics used to measure the success of the managed markets group as well as individual account managers may include the following:

- The number of covered lives (and prescription utilization data) for which account managers have been able to gain unlimited (without edits or prior authorization) or preferred formulary access for the company's key products.
- Product utilization (sales) compared with national and regional market share, new prescriptions, and total prescription growth trends are the typical measures.
- Product profitability after rebates. Some account managers have a profit-and-loss accountability for their assigned accounts.
- Success in helping regional sales representatives sell their products when in a disadvantaged formulary status (e.g., Tier III).
- Ability to use alternatives to rebates to obtain unlimited or preferred formulary access without using rebates. Alternative approaches include member coupons, loyalty cards, and other methods to offset a Tier III copayment. Coupons may be distributed by sales representatives directly to physician offices or may be applied online by the pharmacist using the pharmacy point-of-service claims adjudication system (not used for Medicaid or Medicare Part D beneficiary prescriptions).
- Managed markets team effectiveness in supporting other internal pharmaceutical company groups (e.g., new product development, brand teams, sales representative training, or disease management teams).

- Ability to accomplish other assignments, such as market-based initiatives (e.g., develop an employer marketing initiative) or customer-specific programs (e.g., joint pull-through program, disease management program support).
- Recognition by their customers for outstanding service. There are many national surveys that seek out that information for pharmaceutical companies; the results of those surveys matter when the criteria used for a "best" nomination are the elements that the pharmacy department (or medical and quality) need most in a pharmaceutical company relationship.
- Success in establishing regular and effective communications and interactions with key departments and individuals within customer accounts.

The ultimate recognition that can come to a pharmaceutical company's managed care group is the elevation of the function to its own group with direct ties to the very top of a company's management structure. An independent (yet cross-functionally aware) seat at the biggest decision-making tables is really in the best interests of the managed care accounts as well. When this level of recognition is achieved, managed care companies should feel confident that their relationship will be given the highest review and regard in strategic planning and business development. The first step towards achieving that for the managed care department is by making the account manager/pharmacy director relationship a truly great business venture that delivers results for both parties.

CONCLUSION

MCOs, PBMs, and pharmaceutical companies have forged a relationship anchored by the important role pharmacotherapy plays as one of the most cost-effective forms of preventive, acute, and chronic care for most medical conditions. The appropriate and adherent use of cost-effective pharmaceuticals benefits all stakeholders in the healthcare delivery system. Cost-effective drugs will continue to be developed by pharmaceutical companies in order to be selected and preferentially used. The responsibility of the pharmaceutical company is also to back up these advances with sound support resources and programs, the most important of which is a well trained and respected account manager. Companies that commit to this equation should flourish in this highly managed environment.

SUGGESTED READING

Appleby C., Making the case to managed care. *Biotechnology Healthcare*. December 2004. Available at http://www.biotechnologyhealthcare.com/journal/fulltext/1/6/BH0106016.pdf. Accessed 6 July 2008.

Moran D.W., Prescription drugs and managed care: can 'free market détente' hold? *Health Affairs.* 2000; March/April: 63-77. Available at http://content.healthaffairs.org/cgi/reprint/19/2/63.pdf. Accessed 6 July 2008.

Smith M.C., Kolassa E.M., Perkins G., Sieker B. (eds), Pharmaceutical Marketing Drugs in the 21st Century. Binghampton, NY: Haworth Press; 2001.

Wertheimer A.I., Smith M.I., Fincham J. (eds.), Pharmacy and the U.S. Health Care System, 3rd Ed. Binghamton, NY: Haworth Press; 2005.

Chapter 15

MANAGED CARE CONTRACTS WITH PHARMACEUTICAL MANUFACTURERS

ROBERT P. NAVARRO

JAMES T. KENNEY

RUSTY HAILEY

DALE KRAMER

PAUL N. URICK

INTRODUCTION

Managed care organizations (MCOs) and pharmacy benefit managers (PBMs) must develop and manage pharmacy benefits to satisfy both the clinical needs as well as the financial expectations of plan sponsors and members. Clinical outcomes and patient care considerations are always paramount in pharmacy benefit management. However, in this highly competitive environment, pharmacy program and prescription drug costs are important decision criteria second only to clinical considerations to both plan sponsors and members. The pursuit of cost-effective decisions must not compromise quality of care.

In previous chapters, we have discussed the importance of a responsive and dynamic drug formulary within a comprehensive pharmacy benefit design to help satisfy clinical and financial needs of plan sponsors and members. The MCO and PBM clinical pharmacy departments and their Pharmacy & Therapeutic (P & T) Committees select the most cost-effective drug options based upon scientific evidence. The pharmacy program benefit design, utilization review activities, and disease and case management departments help assure formulary drugs are optimally utilized. Although many resources are available to maximize the clinical quality numerator component of the value equation, the responsibility to minimize the drug product cost denominator rests with the pharmacy department pharmaceutical contracting group and the pharmaceutical manufacturer.

This chapter discusses the discount and rebate contracts offered by pharmaceutical manufacturers to MCOs and PBMs that help decrease the cost of select formulary medications, and ultimately the cost of pharmacy benefits to plan sponsors and members. Contracts are highly confidential and proprietary, and the topic will be discussed in general terms to illustrate how contracts are structured, the responsibilities of interested parties, and how contracts may influence formulary positioning, drug utilization, and total pharmacy program costs.

Pharmaceutical companies consider their innovative contracting offerings to be highly proprietary and an important business strategy to differentiate their company from competitors. Some contracts are quite standard, while others are highly creative and may include clinical performance guarantees. To avoid compromising any company's proprietary contracting approaches, we are specifically not including a co-author from the pharmaceutical industry. Thus, this chapter solely expresses the perspective and opinions of managed care pharmacy directors with extensive experience in contracting, with over 100 years of combined experience in contracting with pharmaceutical manufacturers.

OVERVIEW

Pharmaceutical manufacturers offer drug discounts or rebates to MCOs and PBMs through contracts. Legally, contract components generally include: 1) an offer; 2) an acceptance; and 3) consideration, or an exchange of value. In exchange for an offer of net price reduction, manufacturers expect their contracted products will receive a more favorable formulary and copayment positioning that will result in increased sales and utilization.

DISCOUNT AND REBATE CONTRACTS

Discount and rebate contracts are the two different types of offers from pharmaceutical manufacturers to MCOs or PBMs. *Discount contracts* offer up-front invoice price reductions at the time of purchase, and are generally reserved for MCOs or PBMs that take possession of products (e.g., MCO with owned pharmacies or PBM with mail service pharmacy).

Rebates are the best known and most widely used contracts for any pharmacy program using a third party community pharmacy network. Rebates are paid by the manufacturer usually quarterly to MCOs and PBMs *after* drug utilization has been reported and validated. Similar to a mail-in rebate coupon when a consumer retail product is purchased, the rebate is paid after product purchase evidence is demonstrated to the manufacturer.

Both discounts and rebates have the ultimate impact of reducing the net price of contracted products. Hundreds of formulary drugs are subject to either discounts or rebates, which has the effect of reducing the cost of pharmacy benefit premiums and copayments to plan sponsors and members as a result of the pharmacy department contracts with manufacturers.

DISCOUNT CONTRACTS

Discount contracts consist of a purchase agreement that typically offers a discount percentage off of the wholesale acquisition cost (WAC) or other published price for each drug by National Drug Code (NDC). The amount of the discount often increases as the purchase volume increases over a given time period, provided that the volume increase is consistent with an increase in market share or level of formulary control and the discount is taken up front when a product is purchased and before the drug is utilized. Discounts are offered to those organizations that take possession of a drug product, such as staff or group model plans with owned pharmacies, integrated systems with hospitals, or PBM mail service pharmacies. Discount contracts are restricted to hospitals and staff/group model health maintenance organizations (HMOs) due to their ability to take possession and control distribution of contracted products for their "own use." A U.S. Supreme Court ruling from 1976 related to the Robinson-Patman Act is often used as a basis to defend discounts for hospitals "own use."[1]

Drugs are most often purchased through drug wholesalers (some drugs may be purchased directly from pharmaceutical companies), but the discount is always negotiated with the drug company, which reimburses the drug wholesaler the amount of the discount through a chargeback payment. The flow of dollars in a discount contract is shown in **Figure 15-1**.

The discount is applied by the wholesaler when a contracted drug is purchased by the MCO. The wholesaler then invoices the manufacturer the difference between their purchase

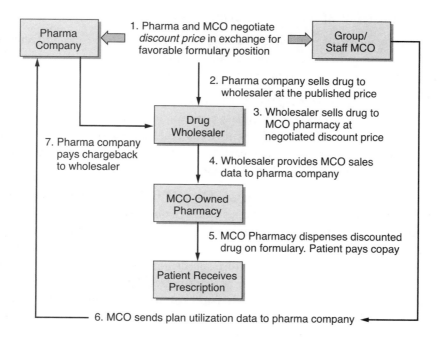

FIGURE 15-1 Schematic of the Flow of Product and Dollars in a Managed Care Discount Contract.

price and the discount purchase price paid by the MCO. This price difference reimbursement paid by the manufacturer to the drug wholesaler is termed a *chargeback*.

REBATE CONTRACTS

One of this chapter's co-authors (R.N.) was involved in 1984 at United HealthCare, when the first rebate contract was developed as a novel method by which independent practice associations (IPAs) and network model HMOs could compete on a pharmacy program cost basis with group and staff model HMOs. IPA and network model HMOs used community pharmacy networks and were not eligible for traditional discounts. Their contracted community pharmacies served members of many different HMOs as well as cash-paying patients, so "own use" could not be guaranteed. Community pharmacies purchase the drugs for all participating third party programs as well as cash customers. MCOs and PBMs reimburse the pharmacy at contracted rates on behalf of plan members. The key distinction between discount and rebate contracts is that rebates are paid retrospectively, usually quarterly, based upon reported drug utilization, whereas the discount is applied at the time of drug purchase by the manufacturer through the dispensing entity (e.g., owned MCO pharmacy or PBM mail service pharmacy). The flow of rebate dollars in a rebate contract is shown in **Figure 15-2**.

REBATE ACCESS AND PERFORMANCE COMPONENTS

Rebates are paid retrospectively based upon reported utilization of contracted products, and after the drugs have been dispensed and paid by the MCO or PBM. Rebate contracts often contain both access and performance components:

1. The access rebate is generally a flat or fixed percent off of the WAC awarded for adding a drug to a specific formulary position (e.g., Tier II).
2. The performance rebate component is a variable percent off of the WAC based upon achieving specific performance parameters specified in the contract. Performance is typically based on market share increases.

Rebate contracts require participating MCOs and PBMs to submit utilization reports, per contract terms, to pharmaceutical companies on a quarterly basis. Most rebate submission requests are provided to manufacturers within 30 to 60 days after the end of the reporting quarter, and most payments are received by the MCO or PBM within 60 days. Any rebates received within 60 days of invoice submission can be booked as assets on the balance sheet of health plans (per newer accounting regulations) and this places additional pressure on manufacturers to turn the rebates around more quickly. Most companies are paying faster, with select manufacturers making partial payments early and reconciling at the end of the quarter after the data are fully analyzed.

Rebate contracts may provide for an audit of rebate submission reports that should include detailed Health Insurance Portability and Accountability Act (HIPAA)-compliant member level prescription utilization reports or even an in-pharmacy "bench" audit to verify the claimed utilization rate of a contracted drug.

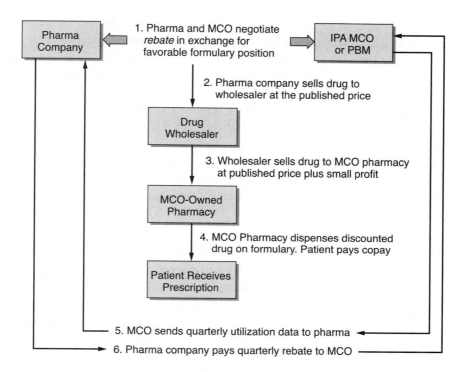

FIGURE 15-2 Schematic of the Flow of Product and Dollars in a Managed Care Rebate Contract.

Rebate Performance Components   Original rebate contracts consisted of only flat access components. Performance components were added to rebate contracts in the late 1980s to offer incentives for managed care plans to implement effective formulary steerage strategies (e.g., formulary tiers) to encourage the use of contracted (preferred) products if clinically appropriate. Increased utilization of contracted products supported contract goals for both parties.

Market share performance parameters may be based upon achieving a certain percent over national market share (with a defined market basket), or an intra-plan market share. It is important that both parties agree on the drug products included in the market basket, and that they are competitive products. For example, a performance market share rebate contract may include all brand drugs within a given therapeutic category, such as all branded proton pump inhibitors. Generic drugs are most often a less expensive option to any brand drug, and philosophically most MCOs and PBMs prefer generic alternatives be used when medically appropriate; therefore, generic drugs are generally excluded from the performance contract market basket to avoid a conflict between the philosophy to prefer generic drugs and the desire to increase the use of contracted brand products.

Performance tiers often require the increase in market share to be a certain percent (e.g., 5% or more) over national market share. The pharmaceutical company reasonably expects to pay only for performance over what would normally occur as a result of their marketing activities. However, the percent requirement over the national share must be realistic. Many plans prefer a local or regional market share parameter, as drug use may often exhibit regional variances. **Tables 15-1** and **15-2** illustrate two examples of performance rebate contracts (market share and volume). All rebates are paid as a percent of the drug's WAC.

Both parties benefit from a clinically appropriate increased use of contracted products that does not compromise generic drug utilization. MCOs and PBMs as well as manufacturers consider the ability of the other party to contribute to contract performance. MCOs

TABLE 15-1   Rebate Contract Example: Performance Rebate Agreement Based upon Percent Utilization Within Defined Therapeutic Category Market Basket

Access Rebate Potential	Additional Performance Rebate Potential Based Upon Achieving the Following Performance Benchmarks		
	Performance Level I	Performance Level II	Performance Level III
Access Rebate Component	National Market Share plus 5%	National Market Share plus 8%	National Market Share plus 10%
5% for Tier II position	Additional 3%	Additional 3%	Additional 4%
Total Rebate Income = 5%	Total Rebate Income = 8%	Total Rebate Income = 11%	Total Rebate Income = 15%

TABLE 15-2   Rebate Contract Example: Performance Rebate Agreement Based Upon In-Plan Year-Over-Year Volume Increases

Access Rebate Potential	Additional Performance Rebate Potential Based Upon Achieving the Following Performance Benchmarks		
Access Rebate Component	5% greater Rx volume over same quarter last year	10% greater Rx volume over same quarter last year	15% greater Rx volume over same quarter last year
5% for Tier II position	Additional 3%	Additional 5%	Additional 8%
Total Rebate Income = 5%	Total Rebate Income = 8%	Total Rebate Income = 13%	Total Rebate Income = 21%

and PBMs may consider the professional promotional and marketing power of a pharmaceutical company to increase physician awareness and use of contracted products. Pharmaceutical companies will consider MCO and PBM benefit design and the ability of the formulary to influence physician and member behavior to select and utilize contracted formulary products.

ROLE OF THE PBM IN REBATE CONTRACTING

As discussed in Chapter 4, many MCOs use PBMs to administer all or part of the pharmacy benefit. PBMs offer their MCO clients an opportunity to be included in the PBM rebate contract. This is a convenient way for the MCO to gain access to a large number of contracted products and manufacturers. The flow of utilization data and rebate dollars in different plan sponsor, MCO, and PBM relationships are illustrated in **Figures 15-3** through **15-5**. In Figure 15-3, an MCO administers a pharmacy program without a PBM and contracts directly with pharmaceutical manufacturers. In Figure 15-4, an MCO uses a PBM to administer the pharmacy benefit and the MCO is covered under the PBM contracts. Figure 15-5 illustrates a situation where a self-funded plan sponsor (e.g., large employer group) contracts directly with a PBM for pharmacy benefits, and contracts separately with an MCO for medical benefits.

However, the role and importance of membership volume must be put into perspective. The key word to describe the driver of the most successful discount and rebate

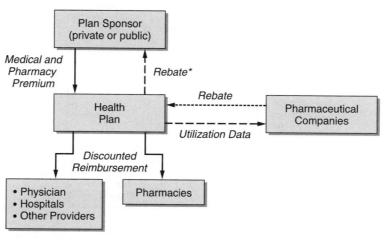

*Allocation of rebate value to plan sponsor is contract dependent.

FIGURE 15-3   MCO Contracts Directly with Pharmaceutical Manufacturer without a PBM.

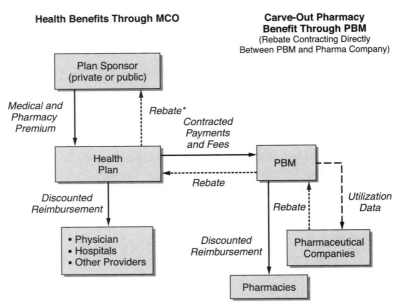

*Allocation of rebate value to plan sponsor is contract dependent.

FIGURE 15-4 PBM Contracts with Pharmaceutical Manufacturer on Behalf of MCO.

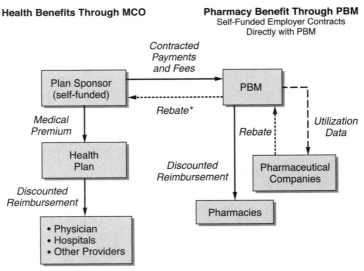

*Allocation of rebate value to plan sponsor is contract dependent.

FIGURE 15-5 Self-Funded Employer Contracts Directly with PBM for Pharmacy Benefit and Contracts with MCO for Health Benefits.

* Allocation of rebate value to plan sponsor is contract dependent.

contracts is *control*. PBMs enjoy selling the concept of volume of combined customer membership to negotiate greater rebates. However, most MCO clients of PBMs have their own P & T Committee and manage their own formulary. As a result, the ultimate control of the formulary and rebate contract performance is managed by the MCO at the plan level. A flat rebate may be paid for preferred access; however, the greatest rebates are realized when control is demonstrated and market share movement occurs that favors manufacturers' contracted products.

MEDICARE PART D REBATE CONTRACTS

Contemporary commercial rebate contracts contain both flat access and performance components for preferred Tier II brand products. Although highly variable, the flat access typically represented 30% to 50% of the total rebate, while performance generated 50% to 70% of the total potential rebate. It should be noted that Medicare Part D contracts remain separate and distinct from any commercial contracts.

In 2006 when Medicare Part D began, no one could anticipate the level of drug use, due to the complex benefit design and the unknown impact of the coverage gap ("donut hole"). Additionally, early Medicare Advantage Prescription Drug program (MAPD) plans and prescription drug programs (PDPs; see Chapter 19) offered multiple benefit and formulary options to satisfy member desire for choice and to sell the products as rich in benefits. A 2007 study of Part D PDP plans in California found formularies had multiple tiers and included an average of 2,452 drugs, with a range of 987 drugs to 3,763 drugs.[2] To help mitigate the uncertainty of Part D performance rebate contracts, initial Medicare Part D contracts were more often flat access rebate contracts rather than performance based. However, now with two years of experience, contracts may now have added performance components. Successful contracts are dependent on formulary structure, benefit design, and the level of benefit controls utilized by the plan administrator.

REBATE CONTRACT TRENDS

As a result of increased benefit controls, some MCOs and PBMs are transitioning more of their commercial contracts back to flat access rebate contracts. Others organizations continue to prefer performance components, especially in competitive therapeutic categories (e.g., statins, angiotensin II receptor blockers, proton pump inhibitors) where performance is a key contract condition. Additionally, those Tier III products previously not contracted are now being rebated because the less advantaged (more disadvantaged) formulary position of Tier III reduces access to products. In addition, benefit designs of Tier IV or higher products and benefit restrictions (e.g., step edit or prior authorization), along with reimbursements at a coinsurance rate or non-coverage in a closed formulary design, encourage contracting by the manufacturers.

Flat access contracts are easier to administer and it is easier to predict potential rebate income, as it is not dependent upon achieving a specific market share (although rebate income increases in parallel with drug utilization). Understandably, most MCOs and PBMs would prefer flat access contracts, whereas typically pharmaceutical manufacturers prefer performance contracts that inspire and require the MCO or PBM to aggressively increase the market share of contracted formulary products to maximize their rebate income.

PERFORMANCE REBATE CONTRACTS

Clinical performance contracts have been explored for over a decade but remain quite uncommon due to difficulty in administration. Such contracts offer to link a financial payment to drug clinical performance (e.g., achieving a clinical outcome) or safety (e.g., payment for the cost of adverse events over a specific rate). Three examples are offered:

1. A manufacturer may offer payment to the health plan for patients demonstrating a defined adherence level of a contracted drug who do not achieve a specific objective clinical endpoint (e.g., HbA1c for an insulin; blood pressure for an antihypertensive) within a specific timeframe.
2. A manufacturer of a contracted product with a potential safety concern may reimburse a health plan for the frequency and treatment costs of confirmed and defined adverse drug events over a specific baseline rate.
3. Manufacturers also are known to offer financial experience controls for new, expensive drugs. For example, if a health plan is concerned about potential overuse of a new drug, the manufacturer may offer to "cap" the plan's drug expenditures over a specific utilization level. That is, any drug use over a pre-defined level would be reimbursed back to the plan in the form of a rebate.

Performance components complicate the relatively simple rebate contracts. Although clinical performance contracts appropriately shift the focus from drug cost to drug clinical value, such contracts are difficult to implement, eligible outcomes may be disputed, the ability to merge medical and pharmacy claims can be challenging (primarily due to the delay and inaccuracy of some medical claims), contract management is laborious, and the financial outcomes are unpredictable. As a result, such clinical performance contracts remain relatively uncommon.

IMPACT OF PHARMACEUTICAL MANUFACTURER CONTRACTS

The P & T Committees of MCOs and PBMs develop and manage drug formularies to help them achieve the clinical and financial objectives of their plan sponsor customers. Clinical outcomes are of paramount concern, but cost is a crucial secondary consideration. Pharmacy benefit costs are a product of drug cost times the utilization rate. Quite simply, pharmaceutical contracts reduce the net cost of clinically desirable drug products. As a drug's price declines, its economic value increases either in a cost-minimization analysis or a cost-effectiveness analysis, and as the drug's value rises, it is often promoted to a position of preference on the drug formulary.

Decision makers balance clinical value and cost of a new drug, but also consider it in comparison with therapeutic competitors. Assuming equivalent clinical value with competitors, a discount or rebate may reduce a drug's net cost and improve the cost-effectiveness ratio. This interaction of clinical value and net cost is illustrated simply in **Figures 15-6A** and **15-6B**. The most desirable drug is shown in quadrant I, with higher clinical value at a lower cost (compared with competitors). Quadrant IV displays a higher cost, clinically inferior drug (least desirable of the four choices). Quadrant II includes a drug with higher clinical value but

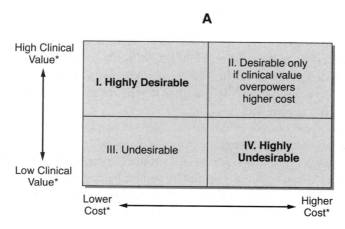

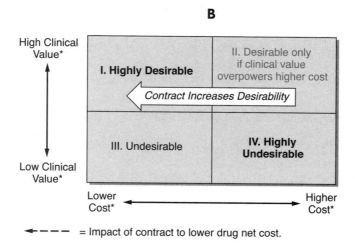

FIGURE 15-6 **(A) Interaction of Drug Price and Drug Clinical Value in Drug Desirability. (B) Interaction of Drug Price and Drug Clinical Value in Drug Desirability: Impact of a Lower Net Drug Price in Drug Desirability.**

Source: Adapted from the concepts of Lowry A. and Hood P., *The Power of the 2 × 2 Matrix: Using 2 × 2 Thinking to Solve Business Problems and Make Better Decisions.* Jossey Bass, imprint of John Wiley Publisher, Hoboken, NJ, 2008.

at a higher cost. The arrow in Figure 15-6B joining quadrants I and II illustrates the impact of a lower net cost (arrow from quadrant II to quadrant I). This lower net cost results in increased desirability (drug value from quadrant II to quadrant I).

Tables 15-3 through **15-5** demonstrate the potential power of rebates and copayments to reduce drug and pharmacy program costs. The savings will not be realized unless the contracted products are actually dispensed. This requires an effective pharmacy benefit and drug formulary to assure that physicians prescribe, pharmacies dispense, and members utilize formulary drugs, as described in Chapter 9. If non-preferred, non-contracted drugs are used in place of the preferred, contracted products, the potential programs savings will not be realized. Interestingly, on occasion the higher copay of a non-preferred drug may result in a lower net cost for a specific prescription; however, plans and sponsors encourage the use of preferred drugs with various formulary incentives to avoid this occurrence.

To support these objectives, MCOs and PBMs employ the formulary copayment tier system to provide financial incentives to use generics and preferred (contracted) products, rather than non-preferred (non-contracted) products, which are normally found in higher copayment tiers. When building a formulary and evaluating pharmaceutical contracts, pharmacy directors consider the effectiveness of the pharmaceutical manufacturer to promote contracted products to physicians as well as any other formulary or contract conflicts that may result in poor contract performance.

TABLE 15-3   Calculation of Drug Net Cost for Drug A without Rebate

Step		Drug A
1	Drug AWP	**$ 120.00**
2	Drug WAC	$ 96.00
3	Pharmacy Reimbursement (AWP − 16%)	$ 100.80
4	Pharmacy Dispensing Fee	$ 1.50
5a	Patient Tier II Copayment (−$30.00)	$ (30.00)
5b	Patient Tier III Copayment (−$50.00)	
6	*MCO/PBM Pharmacy Reimbursement*	*$ 69.30*
7	Pharmaceutical Rebate Percent	0%
8	Rebate Amount	$ —
9	**Net Drug Price to MCO/PBM**	**$ 69.30**

TABLE 15-4   Calculation of Drug Net Cost for Drug A and Drug B with Rebate

Step		Drug A	Drug B
1	Drug AWP	$ 120.00	$120.00
2	Drug WAC	$ 96.00	$ 96.00
3	Pharmacy Reimbursement (AWP – 16%)	$ 100.80	$100.80
4	Pharmacy Dispensing Fee	$ 1.50	$ 1.50
5a	Patient Tier II Copayment (–$30.00)	$ (30.00)	$(30.00)
5b	Patient Tier III Copayment (–$50.00)		
6	*MCO/PBM Pharmacy Reimbursement*	$ 69.30	$ 69.30
7	Pharmaceutical Rebate Percent	0%	20%
8	Rebate Amount	$ —	$(19.20)
9	**Net Drug Price to MCO/PBM**	**$ 69.30**	**$ 50.10**

TABLE 15-5   Calculation of Drug Net Cost: Impact of Rebate and Copayment

Step		Drug A	Drug B	Drug C
1	Drug AWP	$ 120.00	$ 120.00	$ 144.00
2	Drug WAC	$ 96.00	$ 96.00	$ 115.2
3	Pharmacy Reimbursement (AWP – 16%)	$ 100.80	$ 100.80	$ 120.96
4	Pharmacy Dispensing Fee	$ 1.50	$ 1.50	$ 1.50
5a	Patient Tier II Copayment (–$30.00)	$ (30.00)	$ (30.00)	
5b	Patient Tier III Copayment (–$50.00)			$ (50.00)
6	*MCO/PBM Pharmacy Reimbursement*	$ 69.30	$ 69.30	$ 69.46
7	Pharmaceutical Rebate Percent	0%	20%	0%
8	Rebate Amount	$ —	$ (19.20)	$ —
9	**Net Drug Price to MCO/PBM**	**$ 69.30**	**$ 50.10**	**$ 69.46**

REBATE IMPACT ON DRUG NET COST

Rebates reduce the net cost of clinically desirable contracted drugs to make them more attractive to MCOs and PBMs. Pharmacy directors consider a variety of drug price metrics when evaluating the financial impact of formulary alternatives, including wholesale acquisition cost (WAC), and average wholesale price (AWP). However, the most important considerations are the drug's net price and the expected utilization rate to forecast the drug's overall financial impact. The drug net price is calculated by subtracting the formulary tier copayment and rebate amount from the pharmacy reimbursement obligation.

The net cost calculation is shown for Drug A in Table 15-3. The pharmacy director approaches this calculation sequentially:

1. Steps 1 and 2: Obtain the published WAC and AWP.
2. Step 3: Subtract the pharmacy reimbursement rate (AWP − 16% in this case).
3. Step 4: Add the pharmacy dispensing fee ($1.50 in this example).
4. Step 5a: Subtract the member copayment ($30.00 for Tier II in this case).
5. Step 6: This is the reimbursement due to the pharmacy from the MCO or PBM. If there is no rebate, the calculation ceases and this becomes the drug net price.

The net price calculation for Drug A shows the discounted pharmacy reimbursement rate and the copayment reduce the drug price by 31%. This demonstrates the "baseline" net price available without a rebate.

Table 15-4 illustrates the power of the rebate in reducing the net price. Drugs A and B have identical AWPs and WACs, and are both on Tier II with the same $30.00 member copayment. However, a 20% rebate on Drug B reduces the net price by $19.20 (illustrated in steps 7 and 8 in Table 15-2). There is no rebate for Drug A.

If the two drugs are clinically equivalent, Drug B would logically be preferred as a result of the 20% lower net price. The rebate causes Drug B to be more cost-effective than Drug A. As suggested in Chapter 9, if there is no need to maintain Drug A on Tier II; it may be placed on Tier III. The rebate satisfies two contract considerations:

1. The pharmaceutical company's contracted drug is awarded a preferred formulary position and presumably enjoys higher utilization as a result.
2. The MCO or PBM reduces their pharmacy benefit costs, which lowers the pharmacy premium for their customers.

Table 15-5 summarizes and compares the effects of a copayment and rebate. Drugs A and B have identical AWPs and WACs, while the AWP and WAC of Drug C are 20% higher than Drugs A and B. Assuming all three drugs are clinically equivalent, Drug C is placed on non-preferred Tier III due to the higher price. However, the higher Tier III member copayment reduces the net price of Drug C to essentially equal the net price of Drug A, and it is 39% higher than Drug B, as preferred in Tier II.

The total value of pharmaceutical contracts increases as more expensive and heavily utilized drugs are under contract. Large MCOs and PBMs may have 200 rebate contracts in force that cover hundreds of drug products. The total impact on pharmacy program costs may vary depending on the health plan model type, formulary style and conformance level, and number of drugs under contract. Aggressive pharmaceutical contracts typically reduce overall pharmacy program costs by up to 25%.

REBATE AND DISCOUNT CONTRACTING PROCESS

Pharmaceutical discount and rebate contracts provide potential benefits for both parties. MCOs or PBMs are offered a price discount or rebate on selected drug products and agree to place the contracted products in a more favorable formulary position. However, to achieve contract performance, both parties also must effectively participate in pre-contract information gathering, contract negotiations, and contract management. As most of the considerations apply to both rebate and discount contracts, both types of arrangements will be implied with the word "contract" unless specified.

PRE-NEGOTIATION ACTIVITIES

Both parties must clearly understand the potential benefit as well as their responsibilities associated with contract participation. As described in Chapter 14, pharmaceutical manufacturers may offer a variety of resources to MCOs and PBMs depending upon the size of the company and their drug portfolio. Larger companies generally offer a broader array of desirable drug products. Larger companies also may offer additional "value added" resources, such as disease management, patient education, patient registries, physician education, professional sales staff for contract pull-through, and other support.

These non-contract "value added" resources are not considered in the formulary decision process, and are considered only after a contract is executed. Some MCOs and PBMs may be interested in non-contract resources but will only discuss non-contract related resources after a contract is executed. Many MCOs and PBMs will not accept any non-contract resources from pharmaceutical companies to prevent any suggestion of bias in drug formulary decisions.

MCOs and PBMs select a drug for formulary inclusion based first on clinical value (defined by the elements of efficacy, safety, and tolerability), and second, on the cost impact (enhanced with a contract). If a drug must be prescribed for a member, MCOs and PBMs prefer it to be a formulary drug. MCOs and PBMs employ a variety of activities to increase formulary conformance, including closed formularies, tiered formularies, point-of-sale pharmacy edits, and physician and patient communications. MCOs and PBMs also expect their pharmaceutical company partners to offer resources to increase the use of formulary drugs. This is obviously in the interest of pharmaceutical companies as well. Therefore, MCOs and PBMs consider the ability of a pharmaceutical company to support contract "pull-through." Some resources used by pharmaceutical companies include physician professional sales and marketing activities and patient education or marketing campaigns. It neither benefits the MCO or PBM customer nor the pharmaceutical company if a non-contracted product is used in place of a contracted product.

Tables 15-6 and **15-7** provide examples of factors MCOs or PBMs and pharmaceutical companies may consider about each other when evaluating contracting opportunities. In general, MCOs and PBMs want to know if the contract savings potential will be realized, and the pharmaceutical company wants to be certain they will experience an incremental increase in sales of contracted drugs greater than sales without a contract.

Before commencing contract negotiations, each party must complete their due diligence and completely understand the potential business opportunities, the ability of the contract partner to satisfy their responsibilities, and the likelihood of actually achieving contract potential.

TABLE 15-6   Factors Considered by Pharmaceutical Companies When Evaluating Contracting Opportunities with MCO and PBM Customers

MCO or PBM Evaluation Factors	Examples of Factors to Consider
Corporate and business considerations	• MCO or PBM financial stability and model (e.g., profit or non-profit) • Market dominance and reputation • Business focus (e.g., low cost vs. high quality of care)
Type of health or pharmacy benefit products	• Commercial, Medicaid, Medicare (PDP or MA-PD) • Membership and growth potential of each product • Type of customers (e.g., government programs, self-funded companies)
Formulary type and level of control	• Number of members covered by each formulary type (e.g., closed, open, tiered formularies; edits and limitations) • Source of formulary decisions (e.g., role of MCO and PBM in formulary decisions) • Ability to influence drug product selection and utilization by physicians, pharmacists, and patients
Contracting history and relationships with pharmaceutical manufacturers	• Honesty in contracting (e.g., willingness to avoid conflicting contracts) • Behavior in contract disputes • Willingness to honor contracts • Interest in partnership on other programs (e.g., disease management)

TABLE 15-7 Factors Considered by MCOs and PBMs When Evaluating Contracting Opportunities with Pharmaceutical Companies

Pharmaceutical Manufacturer Evaluation Factors	Examples of Factors to Consider
Corporate and business considerations	• Pharmaceutical company financial stability (likeliness to remain independent or be purchased)
	• Business focus (e.g., research-based company, breadth of pipeline)
Portfolio and contracting offerings	• Number of drugs
	• Therapeutic category of drugs
	• Clinical value of drugs
	• Rebate value and potential to realize rebate value
Contracting history and relationships with pharmaceutical companies	• Honesty in contracting
	• Behavior in contract disputes
	• Willingness to honor contracts
	• Interest in partnership on other programs (e.g., disease management)

CONTRACT NEGOTIATIONS

Only after each party completes their due diligence should contract negotiations commence. Discount and rebate contract execution often involves protracted negotiations. After the offer is presented, MCOs and PBMs will consider the contract's potential value, weigh the requested formulary changes in relation to other drugs and other potential contract offers, and consider the contract parameters (e.g., formulary exclusivity, performance benchmarks) as well as reporting requirements.

Negotiation of the initial contract between parties may take several months. Subsequent contracts or contract renewals, especially when the contract performance for both parties has been satisfactory, is generally swift and efficient. While the pharmaceutical company account manager and the MCO or PBM contract manager may find the essential contract terms, responsibilities, and opportunities quite sensible and fair, it is often legal department issues behind the scenes at each organization that causes the negotiations to become tedious marathons.

MCO and PBM contract managers appreciate an account manager who has reasonable ability to negotiate, rather than to have to send all contract changes and requests back to headquarters resulting in significant delays. Many customer contract managers pursue contract opportunities prior to a Pharmacy & Therapeutics (P & T) Committee meeting so that the net price potential as a result of the contract offer may be considered during the drug evaluation. In Chapter 13 we discussed that some MCOs and PBMs will not present contract offers or discuss price at their P & T Committee meetings to make certain the formulary decision is based solely on efficacy and safety considerations. In these organizations, a contract offer is pursued only after the P & T Committee determines the drug should or may be added to the formulary. The contract offer ultimately may determine the formulary position of the product.

Contract offers and negotiations are confidential. Pharmaceutical account managers will not divulge contract discussions with competitors of MCOs or PBMs, and customer contract managers will not reveal any contract offers to other account managers from competing companies to influence a contract offer. Exact contract terms are generally not shared with the P & T Committee. Rather, net price impact models are prepared for the P & T Committee to illustrate the relative financial impact of any committee decisions. Confidentiality and credibility are very important to both parties in building future relationships.

IMPACT OF THE "BEST PRICE" PROVISIONS

The Omnibus Budget Reconciliation Act of 1990 (OBRA '90) requires that pharmaceutical manufacturers offer State Medicaid pharmacy programs their "best price." That is, if a pharmaceutical manufacturer offers a discount or rebate to a commercial health plan or PBM, the company is legally required to offer State Medicaid programs the same price. Therefore, the greatest rebate given to any private MCO or PBM is considered the "best price" and must be offered to State Medicaid programs. Medicaid rebating is complicated, often including mandatory supplemental rebates, but generally the minimum rebate offered is 15.1% (see Chapter 17). Therefore, pharmaceutical companies often considered 15.1% as their "best" rebate or ceiling rebate. If this is exceeded, the higher rebate must automatically be offered to State Medicaid programs, significantly increasing the rebate payment liability of the drug company. Pharmaceutical companies claim this "best price" limit as a reason why their commercial contracts may be limited to a maximum 15.1%, benefit. The OBRA '90 "best price" limitation does not apply to Medicare Part D pharmaceutical contracts and certain exempt organizations.

There are exceptions for "nominally priced" products. Nominal prices are defined by the Center for Medicare and Medicaid Services (CMS) to be less than 10% of the average manufacturer's price, but today approximately 2% of all contracted drugs are nominally priced. Nominal pricing is intended for government and other non-profit entities.

In addition to the mandatory 15.1% rebate requirement, any price increases on products greater than the Consumer Price Index (CPI) for pharmaceuticals on an annual basis also affect best price. The delta between CPI and the price increase per product is added to the best price and carries forward on an annual basis. For example, if the CPI increase for each of five years was 3% and the manufacturer of a product increased their prices 8% each year, the additional 5% times five years, or 25%, gets added to the best price, which becomes 40.1%. In addition, a manufacturer may choose to contract at a rate in excess of 15.1% for certain customers. This percent is confidential and is not something that can easily be leveraged during a contract discussion. If 50% of contracts are in excess of 15.1%, then most companies are discounting at higher rates. Exemptions from best price include the federal supply schedule and any Medicare part D contracting. **Table 15-8** includes some common pricing terminology used in rebate contracting.

TABLE 15-8 Definition of Various Pricing Terms Used in Contracting

Pricing Term	Description
Average Manufacturer Price (AMP)	The average price paid to a manufacturer by wholesalers for distributing to retail pharmacies. AMP was a benchmark created by Congress in 1990 in calculating Medicaid rebates and is not publicly available. FSS and 340B prices, as well as prices associated with direct sales to HMOs and hospitals, are excluded from AMP under the rebate program. The Congressional Budget Office estimates AMP to be about 20% less than AWP for more than 200 drug products frequently purchased by Medicaid recipients.
Average Sales Price (ASP)	A new system created by Federal and State government prosecutors in settlements with pharmaceutical manufacturers TAP and Bayer to ensure more accurate price reporting. ASP is the weighted average of all non-Federal sales to wholesalers and is net of chargebacks, discounts, rebates, and other benefits tied to the purchase of the drug product, whether it is paid to the wholesaler or the retailer.
Average Wholesale Price (AWP)	A national average of list prices charged by wholesalers to pharmacies. AWP is sometimes referred to as a *sticker price* because it is not the actual price that larger purchasers normally pay. Actual acquisition cost at the pharmacy level is often in the AWP less 18% range. Discounts for HMOs and other large purchasers can be even greater. AWP information is publicly available.
Best Price (BP)	The lowest price available to any wholesaler, retailer, provider, health maintenance organization (HMO), nonprofit entity, or the government. BP *excludes* prices to the Indian Health Service (IHS), Department of Veterans Affairs (DVA), Department of Defense (DoD), the Public Health Service (PHS), 340B covered entities, Federal Supply Schedule (FSS) and State pharmaceutical assistance programs, depot prices, and nominal pricing. BP *includes* cash discounts, free goods that are contingent upon purchase, volume discounts, and rebates.
Maximum Allowable Cost (MAC)	The maximum reimbursement amount paid by an MCO or CMS to a participating communicating pharmacy. MACs are often established on highly price competitive, multi-source generic products that are bioequivalent with the brand drug equivalent. The MCO, PBM, or CMS establishes a MAC on the generic chemical entity. The MAC is the highest level of reimbursement regardless of whether the pharmacy dispenses the brand or generic version. A physician "dispense as written" order may override the MAC reimbursement depending upon the pharmacy benefit design contract.

(continues)

TABLE 15-8 (continued)

Pricing Term	Description
Medicaid Best Price	The lowest price paid to a manufacturer for a brand name drug, taking into account rebates, chargebacks, discounts or other pricing adjustments, excluding nominal prices. Best price is a variable used in the Medicaid rebate statute to calculate manufacturer rebates owed to State Medicaid agencies. Prices charged to certain governmental purchasers are statutorily excluded from best price, including prices charged to the VA, DoD, Indian tribes, FSS, State pharmacy assistance programs, Medicaid, and 340B covered entities. Best price data are not publicly available.
Medicaid Rebate Net Price	The effective price paid for covered outpatient drugs by State Medicaid programs taking into account the manufacturer rebates received by States. The basic rebate for brand name drugs is the greater of 15.1% of the AMP, or the difference between AMP and Medicaid best price. Rebates for generic drugs are 11% of the AMP. Manufacturers must pay a supplemental rebate on brand name drugs for which the AMP increases faster than the rate of inflation, based on the consumer price index. Information on rebate amounts is publicly available; AMP and best price are not.
Wholesale Acquisition Cost (WAC)	The drug price published by a pharmaceutical manufacturer and paid by a drug wholesaler for drugs purchased from the wholesaler's supplier, typically the manufacturer of the drug. On financial statements, the total of these amounts equals the wholesaler's cost of goods sold. Publicly disclosed or listed WAC amounts may not reflect all available discounts. Wholesalers typically add a small percentage (< 2%) to the WAC when selling the drug product to pharmacies.

Source: Adapted by R.P. Navarro using definitions provided by the U.S. Department of Health and Human Services, Health Resources and Services Administration, Pharmacy Affairs and 340B Pharmacy Pricing Program Glossary of Terms. Available at http://www.hrsa.gov/opa/glossary.htm. Accessed 7 July 2008. The definition of "MAC" is sourced solely to R.P. Navarro, 2008.

It is common for a manufacturer to offer a discount on a new to market product in excess of 15.1% to secure preferred formulary placement. A new product has no Medicaid liability early in its life cycle and a manufacturer can build the discount into the drugs finances for years to come. It is more difficult for an established product to exceed best price long after launch because an immediate Medicaid rebate liability is incurred in the quarter impacted by the new price.

CONTRACT COMPONENTS AND PROVISIONS

One co-author (J.K.) describes pharmaceutical contracts as having four basic components: 1) boilerplate terms, 2) specific terms, 2) legislative terms, and 4) special contract provisions.[3] Each component is further described below.

BOILERPLATE CONTRACT TERMS

Every contract is first a legal document that is written in, and contains, standard legal language and components, including the following:

1. Identification of contracting parties
2. General business statements
3. Definitions of contract terms
4. Contract term and termination process
5. Governing State/Federal law
6. Confidentiality of contract terms among the parties
7. Right of first refusal (right of contracting parties to respond to competing offers)
8. Indemnification
9. Assignment in the event either party is acquired or sold to another entity
10. Use of company name or trademarks
11. Settlement of disputes (e.g., arbitration terms)
12. Audit rights of each party
13. Notices
14. Signatures

SPECIFIC CONTRACT TERMS

Every contract also contains specific terms pertaining to the specific customer and contracted drugs that define the potential contract value for each party.

1. Obligations of manufacturer
2. Obligations of health plan
3. Formulary requirements
4. Market share or volume requirements
5. Pricing (including rebates or discounts)
6. Reporting requirements
7. Amendments
8. Appendices
9. Membership changes
10. Plan changes
11. Decision to sell or distribute a product

LEGISLATIVE CONTRACT TERMS

1. "Own Use" (e.g., assurances that the health plan will not claim discounts or rebates of contracted products beyond covered membership)
2. OBRA '90 (Medicaid best price considerations, described below)
3. Medicare exclusion
4. Medicaid exclusion
5. Maine unitary pricing (example of a state specific legislative requirement)

SPECIAL CONTRACT PROVISIONS

Some contracts may contain additional specific obligations and considerations that may influence contract performance.

1. Temporary clauses
   a. Guarantee a specific discount for an interim period
   b. Provisional rebate pending a formulary review (rebate offered to newly launched products during a waiting period before a formal P & T Committee review)
   c. Ramp up period (rebates available as market share builds)
2. Co-promotion activities (e.g., plan therapeutic interchange program)
3. Value added programs (e.g., disease management, patient education, adherence programs, or other consideration offered by the pharmaceutical company)

Contracts are legal instruments and must be well crafted and thorough when negotiated and executed to avoid subjective interpretation and ambiguity if contract management or payment questions and disputes arise that threaten the contractual relationship.

CONTRACT DURATION

MCOs and PBMs attempt to offer a stable drug formulary to minimize member therapy disruptions caused by changing preferred products in response to new offers from competing manufacturers. Contracts often have two-year durations but may have a life of up to five years or longer. It often takes about six months to see the impact of formulary changes as a result of a new contract, which leaves about 18 months to realize the contract impact in a typical two-year agreement. Many contracts offer an automatic renewal provision option, however the actual rebate amounts are frequently renegotiated to reflect price increases, market changes, and other competitive issues.

CONTRACT RENEWALS

It is common for a contract to be extended for an additional term if there are no changes anticipated in the therapeutic category and the contract is performing well for both parties. Contract renewal/renegotiation discussions generally commence three-to-six months prior to contract termination, depending upon the level of substantive changes anticipated. Some contracts allow for automatic renewal unless one party objects, although the level of contract discounts or rebates may be updated periodically based upon market changes, price changes, or competitive issues. In situations where both parties desire to extend a contract, but negotiations may require lengthy discussions, the parties may execute a letter of intent to renew the contract so that the contract may remain effectively in force beyond the contract termination date or simply extend the current agreement by an additional quarter to allow time for the renegotiation process to be completed.

CONTRACT DISPUTE RESOLUTION

Managed care desires stable yet dynamic formularies. A stable formulary encourages physicians to learn and follow drug formularies, and minimizes disruptions in chronic drug use for patients. A dynamic formulary allows managed care to make formulary changes in response to new drug launches or the publication of new clinical data. Contracts generally allow managed care to modify their formularies—and possibly obtain a variance from an in-force contract—for the following legitimate reasons:

- A new competing drug is launched with data demonstrating clinical superiority or safety compared with contracted products. Managed care has the responsibility to offer their members the "best" available products as determined by their P & T Committees.
- Newly published peer-reviewed scientific evidence that may reveal new safety or clinical effectiveness data regarding formulary drugs.
- Drug recalls that may remove a contracted product from the market (e.g., Vioxx®)

Both managed care and the pharmaceutical industry dislike premature contract terminations. Most MCOs and PBMs take pride in never (or rarely) terminating a contract. Rather, pharmacy directors attempt to anticipate potential conflicts (e.g., launch of a competitor or a generic), include contract provisions for such occurrences, and attempt to renegotiate contract disputes rather than terminate contracts. Pharmacy directors of large MCOs and PBMs may have up to 200 contracts in place with 80 to 100 different pharmaceutical companies. One drug may have three separate contracts for commercial, Medicaid, and Medicare Part D. Contract negotiation, implementation, and management consume significant time, and contract termination may be quite disruptive for physicians and members. Therefore, managed care attempts to amicably resolve contract disputes through renegotiation and only reluctantly terminates at the most one or two contracts a years as a result of unsolvable situations.

Launch of a Generic Competitor   The launch of a generic form of a contracted product or a competitor to a contracted product may produce controversy if not specifically addressed in the contract. Managed care desires to use the least expensive, clinically appropriate drug product within a therapeutic category. A generic introduction is usually accepted without any need to change the contract unless the generic product is an AB-rated interchange for the branded product under contract. If a significantly lower priced AB-rated generic form of the contracted version becomes available, managed care logically would encourage the use of the generic and possibly apply a Maximum Allowable

Cost (MAC) reimbursement limit that would virtually eliminate use of the contracted brand product. In fact, the manufacturer will terminate any rebate for a MAC-brand product. This situation illustrates the desire of managed care to encourage the use of the lowest net cost equivalent form of the drug (the generic) rather than promoting the more expensive brand drug and collect a rebate.

Mid-term contract changes may occur when a new branded agent launches in the same competitive market that includes the same therapeutic class of products. Also, the launch of a new generic may lead to a decision to implement a step edit or prior authorization on a contracted product. Typically this would void the existing contract agreement.

In addition to evaluating the net price (factoring in the copay and rebate), managed care philosophically supports generics when possible, but to promote a brand drug when a generic is available is incongruent with this "generic first" benefit design philosophy, and presents an inconsistent message to physicians and members. In this case, the contracted product is eliminated from the agreement and other products on the contract would normally continue without any changes. Managed care pharmacy directors closely monitor the anticipated patent loss of important brand drugs, and will execute contracts that specifically provide for generic preference, should they be launched prior to contract expiration.

SUMMARY

The managed care contracting process with pharmaceutical manufacturers is complex and involves many aspects of the pharmacy benefit process. Critical requirements include drugs with strong efficacy and safety profiles and demand from physician and patients populations. In addition, the financial benefit of a contract must integrate with the formulary design of the specific plan and provide value in the form of a return on the investment in the contract process. Although many plans defer the contracting program to a PBM, it is effective for health plans to manage the contracts on their own. The critical factor in the success of a pharmaceutical contract program is the element of control. The greater the degree of formulary control that a plan can deliver will yield greater opportunities for aggressive contracts from manufacturers. In addition to control, the health plan must provide an increase in market share as appropriate for each drug in a specific therapeutic basket of competing products. Although volume would appear to be a logical driver of contract discounts, control and market share are essential requirements to a successful contracting program. Volume is important for purchase agreements involving generic drugs that are purchased as commodities; however, volume does not drive branded product contracts. Many departments and committees also provide critical input and support to the contracting process including the P & T Committee, legal department, case management, and many others. A successful pharmacy contracting program will incorporate the needs of many internal and external customers with the ultimate goal of providing efficacious, high quality, safe, and cost-effective pharmaceutical products for all patients. In the end, the patient should be the ultimate driver of the process.

REFERENCES

1. Greenberg, R.B., Portland Retail Druggists Association vs. Abbott Laboratories et al, part 1. *Am J Hosp Pharm.* 1976; 33(6): 572-573. Available at http://www.ajhp.org/cgi/content/abstract/33/6/572. Also, Greenberg R.B., Mandl F.L., Portland Retail Druggists Association vs. Abbott Laboratories et al, part 2. *Am J Hosp Pharm.* 1976; 33(7): 648-651. Available at http://www.ncbi.nlm.nih.gov/pubmed/941919. Accessed 7 July 2008.

2. Avalere Health Care, LLC. The Medicare Drug Benefit in California, Facts and Figures, July 2007. Available at http://www.chcf.org/documents/insurance/MedicareDrugBenefitFactsAndFigures 2007.pdf. Accessed 7 July 2008.

3. Kenney J., Personal Communication, March 18, 2008.

SUGGESTED READING

Murninghan J.K., *Bargaining Games: A New Approach to Strategic Thinking in Negotiations.* New York: William Morrow; 1992.

Ury W., *Getting Past No.* New York: Bantam Books; 1993.

Fisher R. and Ury W., *Getting to Yes.* New York: Penguin Books; 1991.

Waitley D. *The Double Win (Success Is a 2-Way Street).* Westwood, NJ: Fleming H. Revell Co.; 1985.

Shell G.R., *Bargaining for Advantage.* New York: Penguin Books; 2006.

Cohen H., *Negotiate This.* New York: Warner Business Books; 2003.

IMPACT OF MANAGED CARE ON PHARMACY PRACTICE

KENNETH W. SCHAFERMEYER

![ruled divider]

INTRODUCTION

One of the greatest challenges facing managed care organizations (MCOs) today is the rapid increase in expenditures for prescription drugs. From 2003 to 2004, the average annual expenditure per member increased by 8.4% (from $336.26 to $364.65).[1, p48] Although drug costs comprise less than 15% of total healthcare expenditures, they are increasing more rapidly than other healthcare expenditures and are a major concern of employer groups and health insurers. Consequently, MCOs and pharmacy benefit managers (PBMs) are intensifying their efforts to control prescription drug utilization and expenditures, which, in turn, are having a significant influence on the way pharmacies are providing and being reimbursed for services.

Changes in managed care prescription programs present both threats and opportunities to pharmacy practice today. While managed care prescription plans have contributed to declining pharmacy margins, they also have influenced pharmacy managers to become more efficient and to explore new services and opportunities.

While most chapters in this book address topics from the perspective of the MCO or PBM, this chapter presents the perspective of community pharmacies that participate in managed care prescription programs. It is important for managed care pharmacists to understand this perspective in order to effectively collaborate with their network pharmacies for the benefit of all parties concerned. Specifically, this chapter describes the impact of managed health care on pharmacy practice today and outlines measures that pharmacies and MCOs have applied to constrain increases in prescription expenditures without compromising quality.

ADMINISTRATION OF MANAGED CARE PRESCRIPTION CONTRACTS

NETWORKS

Because the administration of managed care pharmacy programs is complex and requires a large prescription volume to be conducted efficiently, MCOs often carve out prescription benefits and arrange to have them managed by PBMs. In 2004, 96.3% of health maintenance organizations (HMOs) used PBMs to administer pharmacy services, an increase from 93.7% in 2003.[1 p38] Using PBMs helps MCOs to isolate cost centers and concentrate a workforce of prescription benefit experts to manage the prescription program. PBMs provide two basic functions: 1) they serve as brokers for prescription benefits by arranging services between payers and providers, and 2) they use databases and various tools to influence the cost and quality of healthcare services. As brokers and managers of data, costs and quality, the administrative services provided by PBMs include:

- Combining existing pharmacies into large networks
- Communicating with both patients and providers to explain and update administrative policies
- Providing reports to plan sponsors
- Identifying eligible beneficiaries
- Processing claims submitted by pharmacies
- Reimbursing network pharmacies
- Creating and maintaining formulary systems
- Performing disease-management programs
- Conducting drug utilization review
- Educating providers
- Auditing pharmacies

Many of these functions are defined and described in a participating pharmacy agreement, which is a contract that stipulates the pharmacy services that will be provided in exchange for a specified, discounted reimbursement. Typically, PBMs contract with existing community pharmacies to create a large network of pharmacies from which patients can receive prescriptions. The network may be an *open panel* in which all community pharmacies are invited to sign participating pharmacy agreements, or it may be a *closed panel* in which only selected or "preferred" pharmacies may participate. In selecting a network, PBMs consider such factors as the pharmacy's:

- location
- willingness to accept the PBM's reimbursement terms, and
- ability to perform services specified in the participating provider agreement.

Carried to an extreme, the closed network could contract with a very limited number of pharmacies (sometimes only one chain) and become what is known as an *exclusive provider organization (EPO)*. Being excluded from participating in a PBM's network can aversely affect a pharmacy. When faced with the possibility of losing a major portion of their clientele, many pharmacies see no option but to agree to a contract and accept low reimbursement.

Some HMOs develop a network of pharmacies that they own and operate. Twenty-nine percent of HMO prescriptions were dispensed through on-site pharmacies in 2004, down from 32.5% in 2003. This strategy is employed more commonly by staff model HMOs; 77% of them had an in-house pharmacy in 2004.[1] p37

MAIL ORDER

Participation of community pharmacies in managed care plans also can be limited by the use of mail-order pharmacies. Due to large prescription volumes, most PBMs offer mail-service pharmacies as part of their service and negotiate discounts on product costs in an effort to reduce dispensing costs. PBMs may require members to use only a mail-service pharmacy for certain prescriptions—usually maintenance medications for chronic conditions—or they may give incentives, such as discounted copayments, to encourage members to use the mail-service pharmacy. Even when made mandatory, utilization of the mail service benefit by enrollees, however, was modest; HMO plans dispensed an average of only 36% of their prescriptions through mandatory mail service, and 12% when use was voluntary.[2] p25 When a prescription benefit plan makes the mail-service program optional, community pharmacies are wise to make their patients aware of their advantages regarding accessibility and the value of face-to-face interaction between pharmacist and patient.

REIMBURSEMENT FOR MANAGED CARE PRESCRIPTIONS

As illustrated in **Figure 16-1**, three factors influence the costs incurred in fee-for-service prescription plans: 1) unit costs, 2) utilization rate, and 3) program administration costs. Each of these components is described below.

UNIT COSTS

Unit costs, the average amount paid by the MCO to the pharmacy for each prescription, consist of two components: 1) the cost of drug ingredients, plus 2) a professional dispensing fee. This sum is reduced by any amount that the patient is required to pay out-of-pocket (i.e., patient cost sharing). The first component, drug ingredient costs, represents

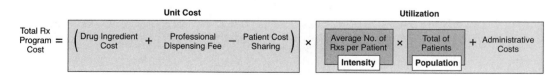

FIGURE 16-1　Components of Fee-for-Service Prescription Costs.
Source: Copyright © Foundation for Managed Care Pharmacy.

between 75% and 80% of the prescription price. **Figure 16-2** illustrates the unit cost for a fee-for-service prescription program in more detail.

Drug Ingredient Costs   Traditionally, pharmacy reimbursement for drug ingredient costs has been based on the average wholesale price (AWP), which is a list price established by the manufacturer. Because AWP does not closely represent actual acquisition cost (AAC), it is being replaced by a new metric known as average manufacturer's price (AMP). The difference between the pharmacy's AAC and the amount paid by the PBM is known as the *earned discount*. These discounts are very important because they decrease the pharmacy's acquisition cost, resulting in a higher *gross margin (GM)* (i.e., the difference between the selling price and the cost to the pharmacy for the product that was sold). By supplementing low dispensing fees, earned discounts have allowed pharmacies to participate in managed care plans that would otherwise have been unprofitable.

Managed care plans usually limit reimbursement for multiple-source drugs to the price for a selected generic equivalent, referred to as the *maximum allowable cost (MAC)*. Each managed care plan creates its own MAC list. On those occasions when a physician requires the brand-name product, some managed care plans allow full reimbursement for the higher-cost product if the pharmacist indicates that the prescription was a *dispense as written (DAW)* order.

Dispensing Fee   The second component of unit costs illustrated in Figure 16-2, the professional dispensing fee, is designed to cover the pharmacy's overhead expenses (also known as the cost of dispensing) plus a reasonable net profit. The easiest and most common way to lower costs has been to restrict pharmacy dispensing fees, which decreased from $2.05 in 2003 to $1.95 in 2004.[2 p4] However, dispensing fees represent a very small percentage of prescription costs and the potential savings to be achieved by controlling drug ingredient costs and prescription drug utilization rates are much greater.

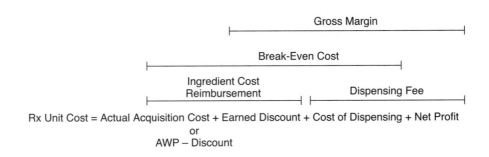

FIGURE 16-2 Unit Cost Components for a Fee-for-Service Prescription.
Source: Copyright © Foundation for Managed Care Pharmacy.

Usual and Customary Prices   PBMs will not reimburse pharmacies more than their usual and customary price (i.e., the amount charged to cash customers for prescriptions). Pharmacy computers should transmit the correct usual and customary price when required by the PBM. *Usual and customary* has different definitions, but basically it is translated as the cash price normally charged to patients who do not have prescription insurance coverage. This is an attempt by the PBM to assure that they are not getting charged more than the current "market" prices for medications.

Patient Cost Sharing   Managed care organizations commonly require beneficiaries to pay a portion of the cost of their prescriptions. This patient cost sharing is designed to control utilization of health services by discouraging patients from seeking care for insignificant problems, while not impeding them from obtaining care for problems that are significant.[3 p54]

Plans without any patient cost sharing have "first-dollar coverage." Although first-dollar coverage was once common, most plans use patient cost sharing as a financial incentive to avoid using unnecessary healthcare services. To be effective, however, patient cost-sharing provisions should not be so high as to discourage use of necessary health services.

Patient cost sharing takes one of three forms: copayments, deductibles, and coinsurance. Copayment, the most common form of patient cost sharing for prescription benefits, requires patients to pay a specified dollar amount for every prescription received (e.g., $10.00 per prescription).

Deductibles require patients to pay for all of their prescription expenses until a specified dollar amount has been paid out-of-pocket during a given period of time, usually a year. For example, the prescription plan may cover prescriptions only after the patient has paid the first $1000 of prescription expenses. With the expansion of online computerized claims processing, more programs are including deductibles because the pharmacist is informed by the computer of the amount of cost-sharing the patient must pay. The use of deductibles as a way to manage costs has increased by approximately 50% since 2000. Almost 16% of employers reported deductible use in 2004 compared with 8% in 2000. Deductible amounts increased by two-thirds since 2000.[2 p20]

Coinsurance requires patients to pay a specified percentage (usually 20%) of the prescription cost while the payer covers the remainder. The percentage of employers using coinsurance increased from 22% in 2001 to 32% in 2004.[2 p19] Although most employers who use coinsurance generally use it for all drug categories, some employers use coinsurance only for certain non-preferred drug categories. This approach allows plans more flexibility to ensure that patients pay a consistent portion of the benefit cost, while providing an additional incentive to use generic drugs.[2 p19]

The pharmacy is supposed to collect the patient's share of the prescription cost at the time the prescription is dispensed; this amount is then deducted from the PBM's reimbursement. Patient cost sharing, therefore, serves multiple functions: it decreases the PBM's unit cost, helps control utilization, and channels patients and providers toward using less expensive products.

UTILIZATION

The second component of managed care prescription costs is utilization. As shown in Figure 16-1, *utilization* is the product of intensity (i.e., the average number of prescriptions per patient) multiplied by the population (i.e., the total number of patients enrolled in the program). The utilization rate multiplied by the average unit cost is the total program reimbursement for prescription drugs. Program intensity is an important benchmark used to compare managed care prescription plans. Prescription intensity was 8.5 prescriptions per person per year in 2004, up from 8.2 prescriptions in 2003.[1 p34] Prescription utilization rates have grown because of the aging of the population, an increase in the number of members enrolled in managed care that now have a more affordable prescription drug benefit, the growing availability of unique drug products, and the influence of direct-to-consumer advertising of prescription drugs.

Administrative Costs   The third component of managed care prescription costs is the administrative costs incurred in managing the prescription benefit. MCOs incur costs in contracting with pharmacies, communicating with patients and providers, maintaining pricing files, processing claims, making payments, maintaining formularies, operating drug utilization review (DUR) programs, and performing other functions. To reduce costs, PBMs can look at any of the three components listed in Figure 16-1. Because dispensing fees are less than one-fourth of total costs, the additional amount of savings that can be achieved by further decreasing fees is limited. Greater savings can be earned by increasing patient cost sharing or by decreasing drug ingredient costs through the use of generics and formularies.

IMPACT OF MANAGED CARE PROGRAMS ON PHARMACY

The growth of managed care prescriptions has changed the economics of the retail pharmacy marketplace. For private-pay prescriptions, retail prices have traditionally been set by the pharmacy in response to the competitive market. Managed care prescription plans, however, are able to demand significant discounts from regular retail prescription prices through their contractual arrangements with pharmacies. While decreasing reimbursement, managed care prescriptions also can increase the work required for prior authorization, online prospective DUR, formulary compliance, and answering patients' questions about their prescription benefit plan.

During the last decade, usual and customary prescription charges have increased significantly while dispensing fees for managed care prescriptions have decreased. This, along with other competitive forces, has contributed to a shrinkage of the average pharmacy's gross margin from 26.3% of sales in 1996 to 23.6% of sales in 2005, a drop of 2.7% (**Table 16-1**).[4 p8] For those pharmacies that have survived, the average net profit has consistently remained at 3.0% of sales or higher. Pharmacies that have remained in business have succeeded at least in part by decreasing expenses and becoming more efficient,

TABLE 16-1 Changes in Pharmacy Operations, 1996–2005*

	1996 (%)	2005 (%)	Change (%)
Sales	100	100	0
Cost of goods sold	73.7	76.4	+2.7
Gross margin	26.3	23.6	-2.7
Expenses	23.3	19.9	-3.4
Net profit	3.0	3.7	+0.7

* Expressed as a percentage of sales.

Source: Adapted from West D. (ed.), *2006 NCPA-Pfizer Digest.* Alexandria, VA: National Community Pharmacists Association; 2006: 8.

primarily through computerization and the use of pharmacy technicians. It also appears that pharmacies need to maintain a net profit above 3% percent in order to stay in business, otherwise the business' resources could be put to more profitable use elsewhere.

There is evidence that pharmacies with high managed care prescription volumes (greater than 75% of their total) have significantly lower gross margins, lower proprietors' incomes and lower net profits as a percentage of sales than do pharmacies with low managed care prescription volumes (less than 50%). (**Table 16-2**).[4] [p54] Although the number of pharmacies is increasing (from 51,579 in 1996 to 58,665 in 2005),[4] [p6] the average number of hours of operation per pharmacy has increased as well. This suggests that pharmacists may work longer hours to compensate for declining gross margins.

Although many community pharmacy managers may believe that dispensing fees are too low, there is little pressure on PBMs to increase fees as long as there is an adequate network of participating pharmacies. It is often assumed that if fees were inadequate, pharmacies would not accept them. In fact, MCOs could interpret some pharmacies' willingness to accept fees from other PBMs that are even lower than theirs as evidence that fees may actually be higher than necessary.

TABLE 16-2 Effect of Managed Care Prescriptions on Pharmacy Operations, 2005*

	Pharmacies with Low Managed Care Activity (%)**	Pharmacies with High Managed Care Activity (%)***
Sales	100	100
Cost of goods sold	76.1	78.1
Gross margin	23.9	21.9
Expenses	19.2	19.7
Net profit	4.6	2.2

* Expressed as a percentage of sales.
** Low managed care activity defined as less than 50% of prescriptions paid by managed care programs.
*** High managed care activity defined as at least 75% of prescriptions paid by managed care programs.

Source: Adapted from West D. (ed.), *2006 NCPA-Pfizer Digest.* Alexandria, VA: National Community Pharmacists Association; 2006: 54.

Why then do pharmacies participate in managed care plans while claiming that reimbursement is inadequate? The answer is not simple and varies from pharmacy to pharmacy:

1. Pharmacists do not want to lose long-term customers and want to do what they can to continue providing services to these patients.

2. Many pharmacy managers have not quantified the effect that managed care plans have on their profitability and, consequently, do not have adequate information to make an informed business decision.

3. Even if pharmacy managers know that some plans are unprofitable, they may be willing to accept these losses provided that the plans are relatively small.

4. Businesspeople know they can take small losses on certain lines of business and still meet overall financial objectives as long as they can earn sufficient above-average profits from other lines of business. Therefore, some managers may claim that losses from low managed care reimbursement can be absorbed by pharmacies that can make additional profits from either: 1) non-prescription sales or 2) prescription sales to cash customers. These "cost-shifting" strategies worked for some pharmacies when managed care prescriptions represented a relatively small percentage of prescriptions. Because the majority of prescriptions are now covered by managed care plans, cost shifting is no longer a viable strategy for most pharmacies.

5. Pharmacies have fixed costs (i.e., rent, utilities, insurance, payroll, etc.) that will be incurred whether or not they participate in a given managed care plan. Pharmacy owners and managers know that any revenue received in excess of their variable costs (i.e., those costs that increase with each unit sold, such as ingredient costs and prescription vials and labels) will help cover these fixed costs. Without this additional revenue to help defray the fixed costs, pharmacies may lose even more by not participating. As difficult as it may seem, deciding upon whether or not to sign some managed care contracts may present a choice between losing a little money or a lot of money.

Pharmacy owners or chain pharmacies' managed care departments must evaluate whether they can afford to participate in each program. To do so, they must know the impact of accepting or rejecting any given contract. Pharmacy owners and managers must understand that low reimbursement rates require that the pharmacy department be run efficiently and economically in order for the pharmacy to prosper.

The following sections of this chapter describe some strategies that pharmacy owners and managers can use to work effectively with managed care prescription programs.

STRATEGIES FOR WORKING WITH MANAGED CARE PLANS

To succeed in the current managed care environment, it is essential that pharmacy personnel are able to:

- properly identify and control overhead costs,
- document services that enhance patient outcomes, and
- understand the needs of payers.

IDENTIFYING AND CONTROLLING COSTS

To remain profitable, pharmacies must earn revenues that exceed expenses. Because prescription reimbursement rates are fixed by managed care plans, it is cost—not retail price—that is the primary target for control.

Two types of costs can be controlled. The first is the cost of drug ingredients, also known as the *cost of goods sold (COGS)*.

Pharmacy managers must reduce cost of goods sold by purchasing inventory as efficiently as possible, usually by earning discounts and using generics as much as possible. Community pharmacies often participate in buying groups to obtain volume discounts. Other discounts available to pharmacies from manufacturers are cash discounts (for paying early) and trade discounts (special deals and promotions). These discounts are very important because they decrease the pharmacies' acquisition costs, which will increase gross margins. By supplementing low dispensing fees, earned discounts have allowed pharmacies to participate in managed care plans that would otherwise have been unprofitable.

Pharmacies also can decrease their COGS by:

- Purchasing efficiently and earning volume discounts from suppliers
- Increasing the inventory turnover rate
- Returning out-dated merchandise in a timely manner

If pharmacies can purchase efficiently by earning discounts from suppliers, then they may be able to purchase inventory at prices slightly less than the cost that is estimated by the MCO. Therefore, purchasing the right products from the right suppliers at the right price is a critical function for pharmacy departments.

One of the most important measures of pharmacy department efficiency is the *inventory turnover rate*. This is measured by dividing COGS for a period of time by the average inventory on hand during the same period. This calculation shows how many times the inventory has been sold and replaced during the year and is a key indicator of efficiency.

$$\text{Inventory Turnover Rate} = \frac{\text{Cost of Goods Sold}}{\text{Average Inventory}}$$

In general, a higher inventory turnover rate indicates greater efficiency. According to the *NCPA-Pfizer Digest*, the average pharmacy turns its inventory over 10.4 times per year.[4 p14]

The second is overhead costs for dispensing prescriptions, also known as the *cost of dispensing (COD)*.

The economic viability of an effective pharmacy depends upon its revenues exceeding associated expenses. Developing an understanding of a firm's cost of doing business is among the most basic and vital business functions. The cost of doing business should be assessed and used for pricing prescriptions as well as in contract negotiations, cost management, and other decisions.

In order to price prescriptions competitively and yet realize a fair profit, prescription pricing decisions and decisions regarding participation in managed care contracts must be based on accurate measurements of costs. Because pharmacies make thousands of transactions, each having a relatively small dollar value, minor miscalculations in deciding price relative to cost is multiplied thousands of times in the course of a year.

Restating a concept explained previously, the components of a retail prescription drug price include the cost of drugs, COD prescriptions, and a reasonable return on investment. The COD is calculated by totaling all prescription department expenses over a given period and dividing by the number of prescriptions dispensed during that time. The average COD in 2005 was $10.53.[4 p48]

$$\text{Cost of Dispensing} = \frac{\text{Total Rx Dep't Costs}}{\text{Number of Prescriptions}}$$

A COD analysis can be as simple or detailed as needed. The simplest approach would be to classify all expenses into two categories: 1) direct costs, and 2) indirect costs. *Direct costs* are those incurred only by the prescription department and include:

- Licenses required for the pharmacy to operate
- Pharmacy computer expenses
- Salaries for pharmacists, technicians and clerks
- Employee benefit expenses (medical, dental, etc.)
- Prescription vials and labels

Indirect costs are those shared with the rest of the store or other departments and include:

- Rent
- Utilities
- Advertising

Direct costs would be applied 100% to the prescription department while indirect costs could be allocated in proportion to the percentage of total store sales generated from the prescription department. Further refinements may be made to satisfy the internal management needs of the firm conducting a COD analysis. (Two examples are allocating *fixed costs*—those costs that do not increase because of increases in sales—in proportion to the amount of store area occupied by the prescription department and allocating personnel costs in proportion to the percentage of each employee's time spent working in the prescription department.)

Although it may be important to apply the same cost-accounting procedures to all pharmacies participating in industry-wide COD surveys, this uniformity is not necessary or even desirable for individual companies that are interested in analyzing their own costs. Because it is possible that expenses that are variable in one pharmacy may be fixed in another, it would be best if costs could be assigned by someone familiar with each particular pharmacy's operation.

The potential profitability of a particular managed care contract depends in part on the proportion of beneficiaries that are new customers versus the proportion who were private-pay customers but converted to the plan. A well-known accounting text states that "present business should be charged with all present costs [in other words the cost of dispensing], and additional business should be charged only with incremental or differential costs [in other words, only variable costs—those costs that will increase with an increase sales]."[5] [p899] Therefore, for current patients who are converted from private pay to the managed care plan, the pharmacy will make a profit only if the gross margin from the plan exceeds the pharmacy's cost of dispensing. For new patients, the gross margin earned from the plan must exceed only the variable costs of dispensing the new prescriptions, of course, provided there are a sufficient number of other prescriptions with reimbursement sufficient to cover the pharmacy's fixed costs.

Pharmacies face the difficult task of trying to reduce overhead costs as much as possible, while at the same time maintaining good quality services. Two ways to help accomplish these tasks are: 1) minimizing the pharmacists' role in drug distribution by delegating non-clinical functions to technicians, and 2) using automation and technology to create additional efficiencies.

In many cases today, delegating dispensing functions to technicians requires that pharmacies alter their workflow. Sometimes this will require remodeling and restructuring the pharmacy department to allow technicians to:

- Receive prescriptions
- Facilitate data entry to produce labels
- Count, pour, and package medications
- Set-up prescriptions for final pharmacist check

An efficient workflow enables pharmacists to work closer to the "out window" and be free to:

- Check the final prescription before dispensing
- Counsel patients
- Monitor drug therapy and interact with patients

MODIFYING PHARMACY WORKFLOW

Pharmacies in today's healthcare marketplace face the difficult task of trying to reduce overhead costs to the extent possible while at the same time increasing their level of pharmaceutical care services. To accomplish these seemingly opposing objectives, pharmacies must: 1) minimize pharmacists' roles in drug distribution by delegating these functions to technicians, and 2) use automation and technology to create additional efficiencies.

Delegating dispensing functions to technicians requires that pharmacies alter their workflow so that pharmacists are free to counsel patients, monitor drug therapy, and intervene with patients when necessary. In turn, this modified workflow may require some remodeling of the pharmacy so that technicians receive prescriptions, type labels, and count or pour medications while pharmacists work closer to the "out window" to check prescriptions processed by the technicians, review computerized patient records, and interact with patients. A counseling area that offers patients privacy should be close to the pharmacist's workstation.

Increasing productivity, that is, the effectiveness of workers' efforts, is another way to decrease overhead costs. Optimum productivity is the result of efficiently controlling payroll expenses while maximizing results, or sales. Employee productivity is sometimes measured by "sales per employee." However, sales per employee have remained relatively stable from $398,449 in 2004 to $393,560 in 2005 despite increasing use of technology.[4 p12] Increased costs to administer complex managed care prescription programs and preparation for the implementation of Medicare Part D are possible explanations for the stagnation.[4 p12] Pharmacies have been relatively successful decreasing overhead costs, but increasing financial pressures requires a continuing commitment to creating additional efficiencies.

DOCUMENTING PATIENT OUTCOMES

Pharmacists must demonstrate that pharmaceutical care services have value. For example, patient counseling can improve patient compliance, which hopefully will result in more favorable patient outcomes: cure, alleviation of symptoms, or decreased use and expense for other healthcare services such as physician office visits, lab tests, hospitalization, and nursing home admissions.

Pharmacists' future survival and prosperity depends in part on the ability to demonstrate value of their services and to get reimbursed accordingly. The steps involved in developing a reimbursement strategy for cognitive services include: 1) identifying key participants in the reimbursement decision, 2) demonstrating patient need for the service, 3) marketing to establish payer demand, 4) documenting the link between services provided and patient outcomes, and 5) setting prices to reflect value to the payer.[6] Reimbursement will not be easy to achieve as MCOs will pay for these services only if they are convinced that doing so is in their best interest. Several pharmacy organizations, computer companies, and managed care programs have been working for over a decade to develop standardized methods to pay for pharmacy interventions.

Providing cognitive services requires that pharmacists excel at counseling patients, monitoring therapy, conducting utilization review, assuring compliance, and maximizing therapeutic outcomes. The most commonly offered services are blood pressure monitoring, comprehensive medication reviews, diabetes training/management, anticoagulation therapy monitoring, dyslipidemia monitoring/management, and influenza immunizations.

The number of pharmacists billing for their services increased in 2005,[4 pp28,29] including cash fees charged directly to the patient as well as those billed to managed care plans for services provided. Future opportunities may include mental health, nutrition, oncology, geriatrics, pediatrics, hypertension, depression, gastric disorders, digestive diseases, and respiratory, cardiac and circulatory problems. It is evident that community pharmacists are providing a range of patient care services and are setting up structure and processes in their pharmacies to offer high-quality care.[4 p29]

PROCEDURES FOR WORKING WITH MANAGED CARE ORGANIZATIONS

The previous discussion on pharmacy workflow and medication therapy management (MTM) services underscores the need for pharmacists to delegate many managed care functions to well-trained pharmacy technicians. This section discusses procedures that can be employed to optimize the use of pharmacy personnel, reduce costs, reduce the number of rejected or delayed claims payments, and maximize opportunities provided by managed care plans.

ELIGIBILITY

The participating pharmacy agreement specifies how covered employees and dependents will be identified. Some plans' identification cards list the names of the cardholder and all dependents eligible to receive prescriptions. Other plans do not list eligible family members; instead, they define eligibility coverage. For example, dependent children may be covered up to age 18 or, in other cases, they may be covered up to age 23 or 24 (depending on the specific plan) if they are full-time students, etc. Even though PBMs issue identification cards, pharmacy personnel should still verify patient eligibility through an online point-of-service (POS) verification system that also indicates the portion of the cost of the prescription the patient must pay (i.e., the amount of patient cost sharing).

By linking pharmacies to PBMs at the time a prescription is dispensed, POS claims' adjudication systems help pharmacies to:

- Verify that the patient is eligible for coverage
- Determine whether the prescribed medication is covered
- Determine the maximum quantity that may be dispensed
- Conduct online prospective drug utilization review
- Confirm the amount the pharmacy will be paid
- Determine the patient's copayment
- Submit the claim for payment

Pharmacies can reduce the possibility of rejected claims by making sure that all patient information submitted is accurate. Patient birth date is a required element relating to eligibility, benefit design, and DUR messaging, so it must be recorded accurately. The patient's relationship to the cardholder has a code that will determine coverage limits. Pharmacy personnel need to be familiar with each PBM's use of dependent codes. In some cases, college students are covered and in other cases they are not. Although the primary card holder (the person in whose name the prescription coverage is listed) is designated by the person code "00" by some PBMs, others use the code "01."

CLAIMS

Data Collection and Documentation   The participating pharmacy agreement specifies how claims will be submitted and paid. Many of these requirements can be met by ensuring that all necessary information is gathered accurately and documented in the correct place either in the pharmacy's computer system or on the hard copy of the prescription.

Information that must be collected from the patient to process a claim includes, but is not limited to:

- Name
- Date of birth
- Gender
- Address
- Phone number
- Medication allergies
- Chronic medical conditions
- Insurance identification numbers

It is also helpful to obtain the prescriber's name, address, phone number, and identification number.

This information generally is collected and maintained in the pharmacy's computer system and is transmitted to the PBM to adjudicate a prescription claim. Although most participating pharmacy agreements do not mandate that this information be documented in either the computer or on the hard copy prescription itself, it is beneficial to document this information in the event that it is needed for a possible future audit.

Package Size and NDC Number   To avoid lost revenue and possible audit problems, pharmacy personnel must be careful when entering claims data to ensure that the proper patient codes and national drug codes (NDC) are used.

The pharmacy must make sure that the actual drug dispensed matches with what was billed. Purchasing a drug in 500 size or 1000 size and billing under the NDC for the 100 size will lead to audit problems. Many federal and state regulations place responsibilities on pharmacists to bill correct NDC numbers. The best solution is to record the NDC numbers for the prescription claim directly off of the manufacturer's package. This is important not only on the original fill, but also on prescription refills. Audit problems caused by using the wrong NDC numbers on claims can be quite substantial, especially if the pharmacy's computer software doesn't actually accommodate and historically track NDC changes on refills.

Quantity Billed versus Quantity Dispensed   When entering a prescription, special attention is necessary to correctly record the quantity that is billed to the PBM. Each insurance plan will have specific quantity limits that are allowed for the members covered under that plan. If a higher quantity is entered than the allowable amount, a rejection message will be returned to the pharmacy's computer.

Dispensing and billing the prescription for the quantity prescribed by the physician averts many problems. Some pharmacies get into trouble by dispensing quantities other than what is written on the prescription, even if the number of refills and maximum days supply under health plan coverage permits it. This can be especially tough as some patients are well educated about their plan maximums and sometimes insist on receiving a larger quantity. In those cases, the physician should be contacted to write a new prescription for the quantity actually dispensed.

The quantity that is actually dispensed to the patient must also match the quantity of the medication that is billed to the PBM. This may seem obvious, but there are some cases where there is a gray area that must be interpreted. The most common of these is dealing with partially filled prescriptions. There are times when the pharmacy does not have the entire amount of medication that a prescription is written for. In this case, if the patient decides to take the amount of medication on hand and return for the remainder later, it is important that the pharmacy does not overcharge for the prescription.

PBMs will want to assure that if the remainder of the medication is not picked up by the patient, the PBM is charged only for the amount dispensed. The PBM also wants to ensure that only one dispensing fee is paid for the full prescription. Many pharmacies sign a Corporate Integrity Agreement (CIA) in which they agree that they will only bill for medication that is actually received by patients.

Each pharmacy will have a slightly different method for handling partially filled prescriptions. It is important that the amount of medication dispensed to a patient is the same as the amount that is billed to the PBM. Partial filling may be viewed by the plan as fraud or abuse. The best method is to only bill the claim when the completed prescription is dispensed.

Days Supply   The maximum allowable quantity that a PBM will allow is based upon the number of days that the prescription will last. The allowable quantity that each PBM will pay for varies by the individual plan. Many will pay for a one-month supply (usually 30 to 34 days). Accurate calculation of days supply can be difficult for certain types of medications such as topical creams/ointments, inhalants, and injectables. Days supply for inhalants, like albuterol and nasal steroids, can be determined because each of these will contain a set number of doses (sprays/puffs) that can be divided by the number of doses per day. For example, an albuterol inhaler prescription (total doses per inhaler = 200) written with directions of two puffs four times daily will have a 25-day supply ($200 \div 8$). Injectable medications, like insulin, can be handled much the same way with the total amount per vial divided by the total dose per day. Days supply is more difficult to determine for topical medications and may require some judgment.

There are instances that require information be written directly on the prescription itself regardless of the documentation entered into the pharmacy computer system. One case where this is appropriate is when a prescription is written with directions of "use as directed." Because there is a quantity written but no directions for use, it is impossible for the pharmacy to accurately determine the number of days supply to dispense as required by the PBM. The pharmacist may have to call the prescriber's office to determine either the correct directions for use or how long the prescriber anticipates the quantity written will last. In the latter case, the days supply must be documented on the hard copy in case of a future audit. It is also a good idea to document any information needed to justify a prior authorization.

Claims Rejections When a claim is submitted, a PBM will either accept the claim as submitted or send back a response indicating why the claim was not accepted. These responses are often in the form of a uniform set of "reject codes" established by National Council for Prescription Drug Programs (NCPDP). Depending on the computer software the pharmacy uses, it may either see the code or it will be translated into an explanation. Not all codes are uniformly adopted by all payers and various pharmacy computer systems translate the codes differently. If a resubmitted claim is still rejected, the pharmacy may need to contact the PBM's help desk for information needed to resolve the rejection and obtain payment for the claim.

FORMULARIES

Restrictions Formulary systems not only provide a list of preferred drug products but also may create other types of restrictions such as: 1) limits on the number of refills; 2) limits on the number of dosage units dispensed (e.g., a maximum of a one-month supply); 3) restrictions on use according to age and gender; and 4) limits on prescribing specified medications to physicians practicing in certain specialties. The latter are usually very expensive medications that require a high level of expertise. For example, the use of growth hormone may be restricted to endocrinologists and prescribing intravenous chemotherapy may be limited to oncologists.

NDC blocks are sometimes used to prevent non-formulary drugs from being covered but more often are used to exclude entire therapeutic categories. For example, PBMs may exclude drug categories such as fertility agents, appetite suppressants, and over-the-counter medications. They also may establish a lifetime limit for some drug products, such as one course of nicotine patches.

Generic Preference Each managed care plan creates its own MAC list. On those occasions when a physician requires a brand-name product, some managed care plans allow full reimbursement for the higher-cost product if the pharmacist indicates that the prescription was a dispense as written (DAW) order.

The NCPDP has developed nine DAW codes designed to communicate the circumstances for which a certain multiple-source drug product was used or not used (**Exhibit 16-1**). Most plans recognize only a few of these codes and strictly limit their use. The inappropriate use of DAW codes can result in inaccurate payments to the pharmacy and trigger an audit.

DAW codes reflect the preference of the physician or patient regarding substitution of equivalent generic products for more expensive brand-name medications. Because DAW

EXHIBIT 16-1   DAW CODE VALUES.

0 = No Product Selection Indicated

This is the field default value that is appropriately used for prescriptions where product selection is not an issue. Examples include prescriptions written for single source brand products and prescriptions written using the generic name and a generic product is dispensed.

1 = Substitution Not Allowed by Prescriber

This value is used when the prescriber indicates, in a manner specified by prevailing law, that the product is to be Dispensed As Written.

2 = Substitution Allowed - Patient Requested Product Dispensed

This value is used when the prescriber has indicated, in a manner specified by prevailing law, that generic substitution is permitted and the patient requests the brand product. This situation can occur when the prescriber writes the prescription using either the brand or generic name and the product is available from multiple sources.

3 = Substitution Allowed - Pharmacist Selected Product Dispensed

This value is used when the prescriber has indicated, in a manner specified by prevailing law, that generic substitution is permitted and the pharmacist determines that the brand product should be dispensed. This can occur when the prescriber writes the prescription using either the brand or generic name and the product is available from multiple sources.

4 = Substitution Allowed - Generic Drug Not in Stock

This value is used when the prescriber has indicated, in a manner specified by prevailing law, that generic substitution is permitted and the brand product is dispensed since a currently marketed generic is not stocked in the pharmacy. This situation exists due to the buying habits of the pharmacist, not because of the unavailability of the generic product in the marketplace.

5 = Substitution Allowed - Brand Drug Dispensed as a Generic

This value is used when the prescriber has indicated, in a manner specified by prevailing law, that generic substitution is permitted and the pharmacist is utilizing the brand product as the generic entity.

6 = Override

This value is used by various claims processors in very specific instances as defined by that claims processor and/or its client(s).

7 = Substitution Not Allowed - Brand Drug Mandated by Law

This value is used when the prescriber has indicated, in a manner specified by prevailing law, that generic substitution is permitted, but prevailing law or regulation prohibits the substitution of a brand product even though generic versions of the product may be available in the marketplace.

8 = Substitution Allowed - Generic Drug Not Available in Marketplace

This value is used when the prescriber has indicated, in a manner specified by prevailing law, that generic substitution is permitted and the brand product is dispensed since the generic is not currently manufactured, distributed, or is temporarily unavailable.

9 = Other

This value is reserved and currently not in use. NCPDP does not recommend use of this value at the present time. Please contact NCPDP if you intend to use this value and document how it will be utilized by your organization.

Source: Materials reproduced with the consent of © National Council for Prescription Drug Programs, Inc. 2008 NCPDP.

codes can affect the amounts of payments and patient copayments, it is important that the pharmacy uses the correct code for each claim. The particular reason for using the DAW code should be recorded also.

The need for documentation is important to justify the use of DAW codes. For example, to transmit a DAW-1 code, a written prescription must have the prescriber's signature on the DAW line or there must be a check mark in the DAW box (depending on state requirements). In the event of a telephoned prescription, the pharmacist must record the nature of the DAW request on the hard copy of the prescription along with the name of prescriber's agent who authorized the DAW. If the patient has stated that the brand-name version is preferred to a generic version (by authorizing "substitution permitted"), this request must be documented on the hard copy of the prescription by pharmacy staff. The pharmacy could lose a large sum of money if an audit cannot find the documentation supporting the use of these codes.

PREFERRED DRUGS AND TIERED COPAYMENTS

Formularies can be categorized as being *open* (i.e., most prescription products are covered), *incented* (i.e., patients pay lower copayments for preferred products), or *closed* (i.e., reimbursement is limited to selected drug products within each therapeutic class). Most PBMs have migrated from open to incented formularies to the use of tiered copayments. In a three-tier copayment plan, generics will require a relatively low copayment (e.g., $10) from the patient; preferred brand-name drugs will have a higher copayment (e.g., $25), and non-preferred brand-name drugs will have the highest copayment (e.g., $50). Some plans have a fourth tier for so-called *lifestyle drugs* such as those for erectile dysfunction.

Retail copayments increased across all tiers from 2003 to 2004; they increased by 6% for the first tier; increased by 8% for the second tier; and increased by 7% for the third tier.[2] p15 Tiered copayments are sometimes confusing to patients, so pharmacy personnel must be prepared to explain why copayments vary from one prescription to another. To sensitize patients to actual drug therapy costs, some plans utilize coinsurance in which the patient pays a percentage of the total cost (e.g., 20%, 30%, or 50%) in lieu of copayments.

Prior Authorization   Formulary guidelines specify policies that determine the specific situations in which certain high-cost drugs may be used. Usually the prescriber must explain why a particular drug product is considered superior to a preferred formulary product and obtain authorization from the PBM before the pharmacy may dispense the drug and obtain reimbursement. Pharmacies receiving a prescription for a drug restricted by a prior authorization (PA) program may have to contact the physician and/or the PBM to make sure the proper authorization is obtained before the drug can be dispensed. Although this may be inconvenient for the patient, pharmacist, and physician, it does reduce expenditures without unnecessarily denying access to medications when they are needed. Although 92% of HMOs use prior authorization,[1] p35 the administrative expenses associated with operating PA programs usually requires that PBMs apply this restriction to relatively few drug products.

Prior authorizations are often required for specific products such as high-cost injectables. Some plans require that certain low-cost or low-risk alternatives be tried first before a non-formulary drug will be approved. Some examples of drugs or situations requiring prior approval are:

- Certain injectable medications, such as Lupron® or growth hormone.
- The use of a drug for a purpose other than what was approved by the FDA. For example, prescribing Viagra® for a female patient, or prescribing oral contraceptives for a male.
- Drugs in a therapeutic class that has been excluded, such as drugs used for cosmetic purposes. For example, some plans will not pay for Retin-A® for use by patients over the age of 25 unless the prescriber obtains prior approval.
- Brand-name multi-source drugs that are deemed to be medically necessary. These products can sometimes be approved with a PA even though the PBM does not allow routine DAW overrides for the product.
- Non-formulary brand-name products.

In some cases, a prescriber will contact the PBM or health plan medical director to explain the reason for prescribing a non-formulary product. In most cases, a prescriber does not know when a PA is needed for a particular product. The pharmacy submitting a claim will receive a rejection notice and will need to call the PBM help desk to determine the reason for the rejection. The help desk will tell the pharmacy the process that the PBM requires for prior approval. The pharmacy ultimately informs the prescriber of the need for obtaining a PA and the process to follow for approval.

Some plans specify that pharmacies must telephone the PBM to receive approval before they are allowed to dispense certain prescriptions. If the plan authorizes the prescription, the pharmacy is given a code that is used to document the approval. Authorization may be given for one prescription, several refills, or a year's worth of refills for a patient. In any case, the pharmacy must follow the PBM's specific procedures for obtaining authorization.

The PA process will vary from one PBM to another. Some PBMs will accept prior authorization requests through their Web sites; in most cases, though, the pharmacy needs to contact the PBM help desk, and follow the plan's procedures.

Some PBMs, after approving a prior authorization request, will adjust their processing computers to accept the prescription the pharmacy submits. Some PBMs may require the prescriber to include a prior approval number on the prescription, and require the pharmacy to submit that number along with the claim. Other PBMs may require the pharmacy to call the PBM help desk to obtain the authorization number to submit with the claim. There are other methods a PBM may use for approving a prior authorization. Whatever the process, once approval is obtained, the prescription can then be submitted for online adjudication.

Some plans require that *Treatment Authorization Requests (TAR)* be filed to receive a prior authorization for a medication. This request is usually a form for which the pharmacy will input various data regarding the patient, pharmacy, physician, medication, and justification, and fax in to the PBM for review and authorization.

There may be instances where a plan will not approve a PA request. If this is the case, the patient needs to be advised that the prior authorization request was denied by the plan. The pharmacy can call the prescriber to obtain a different prescription or explain to the patient that he or she has the option of paying cash for the prescription as originally written.

DISEASE STATE MANAGEMENT

Disease management programs are designed to promote rational drug utilization, especially for patients with certain common, high-cost diseases. For pharmacists, this means not only dispensing drugs but also educating patients, encouraging compliance, monitoring patient progress, and intervening when necessary to assure positive outcomes.

These types of services generally require specialty training in a particular area, as well as the use of diagnostic devices and supplies. The number of pharmacists billing for their services increased in 2005,[4] p28 indicating that managed care is becoming more comfortable with providing a separate "cognitive" skills fee reimbursement to pharmacists for their involvement.

With the recognition of MTM services through Medicare Part D, it is expected there will be more opportunities for pharmacists to become more involved as pharmacotherapy managers and get reimbursed for these services.

DRUG UTILIZATION REVIEW

One of the primary tools used by PBMs to control utilization is DUR. DUR is a very important tool that has a significant impact on community pharmacy practice. Traditional DUR programs have attempted to control unnecessary utilization by avoiding duplication of therapy and reducing drug abuse and misuse. All reporting HMOs had DUR programs in 2004.[1] p33

Controlling program utilization can save more money than restricting expenditures for drug ingredients or dispensing fees. For example, patients who continue taking a proton pump inhibitor beyond the time recommended for acute treatment of ulcers cause significant and unnecessary costs for the program. By limiting medication use to the recommended dosage and duration, the MCO can save hundreds of dollars for just one patient.

DUR may be prospective or retrospective. Retrospective DUR involves the review of prescription claims databases well after the prescriptions have been dispensed. Because these programs are primarily educational, the focus is on alerting physicians and pharmacists to prescribing habits with the hope that they will be able to improve patients' outcomes using less costly medications.

Prospective DUR, on the other hand, occurs before the prescription is dispensed and results in alert messages being sent to the pharmacy's computer when problems are detected. When this occurs, pharmacists must review the alert message and take appropriate action that may require a phone call to the physician, a discussion with the patient, or a call to the PBM to resolve the problem. These alerts also may result in a prescription being changed or not filled, if that is determined to be in the patient's best interests.

There are two types of information that are reviewed in the DUR process:

1. *Non-clinical (administrative):* Messages involve evaluating the prescription claim for compliance with the insurance plan for each patient's prescription. Administrative messages focus on issues such as patient and dependent eligibility, drug exclusions and limitations, and formulary requirements.
2. *Clinical:* Messages that focus on issues relating to patient safety and enhancing the appropriate use of medications with the patient. Examples include review for potential:

   - Drug interactions
   - Duplication of therapy
   - Inappropriate dosage
   - Inappropriate duration of therapy
   - Contraindications

While prospective DUR messages about clinical issues (i.e., drug interactions) often duplicate information generated by the pharmacy's own computer system, sometimes they can provide information that wouldn't otherwise be available for patients who use more than one pharmacy.

CLAIMS RECONCILIATION

When PBMs reimburse pharmacies for prescription claims, the check is usually accompanied by a "remittance advice," "claims detail," or other document that shows the amount paid for each claim, the copayment amount, and other messages that help explain how each claim is paid. This remittance advice is used to reconcile prescription claims with payments.

Because of the difficulty in determining the accuracy of a payment response at the time of filling, many pharmacies have developed systems that allow them to properly handle claims and collect payments. Claims management systems record claims transactions, create receivables files (what the pharmacy expects to be paid), and reconcile payments against claims. This helps to identify differences between expected payments and actual payments. A claims management system will also help pharmacy personnel to determine:

- *Was the adjudicated claim paid at all?* During prescription processing, the PBM sends a response indicating what they will pay for a particular claim. Once the information has been processed by the PBM and the pharmacy dispenses the prescription, the claim is then labeled as *adjudicated*. Sometimes an adjudicated claim does not make it onto a payment voucher. Pharmacy personnel need to check each claim against payment registers to be sure the claim was paid.

- *Was the claim paid at the rate indicated by the adjudication response?* The adjudicated response is what the PBM says it will pay. Payments may sometimes be adjusted by the PBM through its internal claim review process. If payment does not agree with the adjudicated response, pharmacy personnel should check to find the reason and, if necessary, contact the PBM's help desk to determine the reason for the discrepancy.

- *Was the claim paid at the correct contract rate?* This is very difficult to determine unless the pharmacy can determine the plan in which the patient was enrolled. Some PBMs provide information on their remittance advice. In these cases, pharmacy personnel can compare the payment with the contracted rate.

- *Was the claim paid in full?* If the claim was paid in an amount other than the amount anticipated, the pharmacy should determine the payment differential and determine why the claim payment varied from the anticipated payment. Payment variances can occur from MAC pricing, incorrect NDC numbers, incorrect quantities, or incorrect copayments.

When payment is delayed, the pharmacy should attempt first to determine the cause of the unresolved claim. If the problem claim resulted from an incorrect billing entry at the store, it may be possible to correct and re-bill the claim. If the pharmacy dispensed a brand-name drug in place of a generic product and was paid at MAC, there may be no way to recover the outstanding payment. If this problem occurs, it would be a good idea to establish a procedure for dispensing generics and make sure all pharmacy personnel know the importance of following this procedure.

CLAIM ADJUSTMENTS

Even though a claim is paid, it may not have been paid in accordance with the plan schedule. It also may not have been paid in accordance with the amount returned by the PBM's adjudication response. Most PBMs have the ability to audit adjudicated claims for reasonableness prior to sending payment. If a claim seems to be unreasonable, such as 100 vials of insulin (rather than 100 units of insulin), and this was not adjusted during the dispensing process, the PBM may review and adjust the claim.

Among the most frequent reasons for claims adjustments are:

- *Error in package size.* If the NDC submitted for an asthma inhaler refers to a package size of 22.5 mL and the pharmacy submitted a quantity of 2.25 mL, a payment reduction will occur.

- *Error in metric quantity.* Some PBMs require the billing of injectable products as number of vials while others may require the number of milliliters or the number of packages. For example, a drug with a package size of 7.5 mL may need to be entered as 7.5 mL rather than as "1" unit. The incorrect billing unit will result in a payment different than is anticipated.

- *Invalid DAW code.* DAW codes help the payer to understand why a generic product was or was not dispensed. If the pharmacist dispensed a brand-name product instead of a generic, because the physician instructed the prescription to be DAW and did not indicate the proper DAW code, the claim amount billed will be adjusted down as if the generic product had been dispensed.

- *Paid from MAC list.* This is the maximum allowable cost for a multiple-source drug. This indicates that the plan pays only for generics even if a brand-name drug was dispensed. If a brand-name drug was dispensed, that is money lost that cannot be recovered.
- *Change in drug acquisition cost.* Because payers and pharmacies may use different data sources and update their files at different times, the cost information used by the pharmacy to calculate reimbursement may differ from that used by the payer.
- *Incorrect fee.* Dispensing fees vary by plan and are subject to change. The pharmacy may anticipate reimbursement at one rate and be paid another.
- *Claim subject to usual and customary pricing.* Some plans require the pharmacy to submit its usual and customary price along with the prescription claim. These plans will pay the contract price or the usual and customary price, whichever is lower.

Pharmacies should have an individual—perhaps a technician—who has the responsibility for researching and resolving those claims that are paid incorrectly. When payments differ from the expected payments, the person responsible for reconciling billings with payments should create reports comparing anticipated payments with the actual payment and include all of the claim and payment data elements.

Whatever the reason for a variance, it is important to document the findings. The more documentation the pharmacy has, the greater the likelihood of determining the cause of the variance and recovering any under-payments by following the specific procedures. If, for example, a product that had been multi-source no longer has a generic counterpart but the PBM continues to pay at the generic rate, the pharmacy's documentation will help in resolving the payment.

Not all variances are recoverable. If the pharmacy is unable to recover further payment from the PBM, it will need to account for the loss by decreasing the amount of sales recorded in its financial records or show the loss as an expense (i.e., "bad debts"). Each pharmacy has its own procedures for handling these adjustments.

CHARGEBACKS

Occasionally, a PBM may assert that it has overpaid a claim in error, or paid a claim incorrectly and will charge back to the pharmacy the amount in question. Whenever receiving a chargeback, the pharmacy should review the original claim, the adjudication response, and the payment response to determine the facts involved in the chargeback request. If the chargeback is appropriate, the pharmacy will need to make appropriate financial adjustments in accordance with its financial procedures. If the chargeback is determined to be inappropriate, the pharmacy should gather all appropriate documentation and call the PBM's help desk.

CLAIM REVERSALS

Because pharmacy systems record a billing upon dispensing a prescription, there may be circumstances where an adjudicated prescription needs to be reversed or "unbilled." This happens when a patient does not pick up their prescription within a reasonable period of time.

Prescriptions may not be picked up by patients for a variety of reasons: the patient no longer needs the medication, the physician has changed the medication, the patient decides to get the prescription at another pharmacy, the patient forgot to pick it up, or the patient no longer wants the prescription. Each pharmacy should have appropriate procedures to address prescriptions that are not picked up.

AUDITS

Because of the increasing cost of health care, managed care plans want assurances that all steps outlined within the participating pharmacy agreement are being followed. This holds true for all sectors of health care from hospitals, physicians, and pharmacies. As a way to address this concern, most PBMs audit prescription claims. Audits come in many different forms that range from automated reviews of electronic claims (desk audits) to on-site audits in a community pharmacy (*field audits*).

Audit programs have three primary goals:

1. *Identify overpayments.* Insurance companies are legally bound to do this by a fiduciary responsibility to their clients.
2. *Provide a significant deterrent to abuse.* It is perceived that people who are aware of audit activity are more likely to follow plan guidelines.
3. *Encourage compliance.* Audits can help healthcare providers learn (sometimes the hard way) to understand and follow program guidelines.

The best way to prepare for an audit is to develop day-to-day policies that will address many of the areas that will trigger an audit and stick to them. By being proactive and employing effective procedures, a pharmacy can avert expensive problems later.

EFFECT OF MANAGED CARE ON HOSPITAL PHARMACIES

BACKGROUND

The rapid rise in hospital costs during the last several decades has been fueled by an oversupply of hospital beds, lack of price competition among hospitals, and generous reimbursement methods. With the passage of the Hill-Burton Act in 1946, the federal government provided money to build new hospitals in many communities throughout the country. The number of hospital beds, admissions, and average length of stay increased significantly. Hospitals also were reimbursed on a "cost plus" basis that created few incentives to contain costs. As a result of this generous fee-for-service reimbursement, it was not necessary for hospitals to compete on price. Instead, hospitals competed with each other to attract physicians who could fill the beds. The most effective way of attract-ing physicians was to provide the latest medical technology, which is a very costly but effective strategy.

Effective restraints on hospital costs were finally introduced in 1983 with prospec-tive reimbursement methods known as *diagnosis-related groups (DRGs)* and capitation. Under DRGs, hospitals were paid a specified amount for each admission based on patient diagnosis. This new reimbursement method encouraged hospitals to become more efficient and to improve effectiveness of treatment to reduce patient length of stay. In 2004, 10.7% of contracted hospitals were reimbursed using DRGs, continuing an annual increase since 2001.[1 p86]

While DRGs are still used by some MCOs, many MCOs continue to negotiate with hospitals to establish *per diem* or capitation, rates. Although 76.3% of contracted hospi-tals accepted *per-diem* payments in 2004, the popularity of this method has also been declining.[1 p86] One reason may be that hospital pharmacies can control their own pro-duction efficiency but have little control over the prescribing habits of the physicians. Therefore, a pharmacy can provide services and prescriptions very efficiently but still may lose financially if physicians prescribe many and/or expensive products.[7]

IMPLICATIONS FOR HOSPITAL PHARMACIES

Through prospective reimbursement systems, MCOs have profoundly changed the way hospitals operate. Hospitals now have strong incentives to eliminate unnecessary services and to promote efficiency. Some hospitals have closed, and others have eliminated some of their licensed beds. Most hospitals have either consolidated into large hospital corpora-tions or developed affiliations with other hospitals to benefit from economies of scale in their purchasing, advertising, and central administration.

The advent of prospective reimbursement transformed hospital pharmacies from profit centers into cost centers and created incentives to eliminate unnecessary services and promote efficiency. The primary cost-cutting targets for hospital pharmacies have been the two areas that contribute the most to costs: 1) inventory and 2) personnel. Almost all hospital pharmacies have reduced inventory costs by working with the medical staff to adopt extensive formulary systems. They also reduced the cost of goods by joining with other hospitals to form volume purchasing groups that solicit competitive bids from pharmaceutical manufacturers.

Personnel costs have been reduced by delegating routine functions to pharmacy tech-nicians and by automating dispensing procedures. Automated dispensing machines and robots reduce personnel time and enhance accountability by delivering medications to the nursing staff on demand. Many hospital pharmacy departments have increased the extent of their on-the-job training programs, and some have encouraged or required pharmacy technicians to enhance their knowledge and skills by passing a certification exam. Automation and extended use of pharmacy technicians, however, have not always reduced pharmacy staff. In many cases, these efficiencies have allowed pharmacists to become more involved with patient-focused care, dosage recommendations, discharge counseling, and case management. By working with the medical staff to achieve positive patient outcomes, hospital pharmacists can help reduce patients' length of stay and, consequently, minimize overall hospital costs.

CONCLUSION

The impact of managed care prescriptions on pharmacy margins and workload is readily recognized by pharmacists. These changes, though, are a natural progression of a medical industry that is in the advanced stages of evolving from a cottage industry to a post-industrial revolution industry with a focus on efficiencies, economies of scale, consolidation, and continuous quality improvement.

Until recently, healthcare services were *financed* but not *managed*. Historically, government and private employers sponsoring health insurance programs demanded cost controls but showed relatively little interest in improving quality or ensuring positive outcomes, which are ordinary management functions for most businesses. More attention is now being devoted to analyzing claims databases to assess and improve the quality of healthcare services in an effort to control costs and enhance patient outcomes.

Pharmacy practice and pharmacy education have no choice but to adapt and change in order to fit into the evolving managed care environment. Successful pharmacists now need to be more than good practitioners; they need to understand business, technology, marketing, and how to improve patient outcomes.

Pharmacists will continue to play a greater role in managed care. All pharmacists—staff or management, community or institutional—are affected by the problems and opportunities presented by managed care prescription programs. The extent to which pharmacists use their skills to minimize problems and take advantage of opportunities will determine to a large extent the profession's future success.

REFERENCES

1. *Managed Care Digest Series: 2005.* Bridgewater, NJ: Aventis Pharmaceuticals Corporation; 2005.
2. *The Prescription Drug Benefit Cost and Plan Design Survey Report: 2005 Edition.* Lincolnshire, IL: Takeda Pharmaceuticals North America, Inc.; 2005.
3. Brian E.W. and Gibbens S.F., California's Medi-Cal co-payment experiment. *Med Care.* 1974; 12(Suppl 12): 1–303.
4. West D., (ed.), *2006 NCPA-Pfizer Digest.* Alexandria, VA: National Community Pharmacists Association: 2006.
5. Pyle W.W. and Larson K.D., *Fundamental Accounting Principles,* 9th Ed. Homewood, IL: Richard D. Irwin, Inc.; 1981.
6. Rupp M.D., Strategies for reimbursement. *Am Pharm.* 1992; NS32: 79-85.
7. Larson L.N., Financing Health Care in the United States, Chapt 2, in Smith M.I., et al. (eds.): *Pharmacy and the U.S. Health Care System,* 3rd Ed. Binghamton, NY: The Haworth Press, Inc., 2005.

Chapter 17

FUNDAMENTALS OF HEALTHCARE BENEFITS FROM THE EMPLOYER PLAN SPONSOR'S PERSPECTIVE

CRAIG S. STERN

PART I — **FUNDAMENTALS OF HEALTHCARE BENEFITS FROM THE EMPLOYER PLAN SPONSOR'S PERSPECTIVE**

INTRODUCTION

Healthcare benefits are designed to meet the needs of beneficiaries. Benefits must rest on the foundation of the organization's needs and expectations. As such, a benefit is not defined until there are analyses of demographics, utilization, and the current and future requirements of the beneficiary population. Then the healthcare resources, costs and financial projections are analyzed to determine the infrastructure that will be required to deliver the benefits. This chapter focuses on the elements of healthcare benefits.

WHAT IS THE NEED FOR HEALTH INSURANCE?

Individuals at different age levels must ascertain their need for healthcare services. The uncertainty of one's health and the expense of requiring hospitalization, physician care, or other health resources lead many to consider purchasing health insurance. As an economic and cultural decision, some purchase monthly benefits, while others choose only catastrophic care for unintended problems requiring hospitalization.

WHAT ARE THE TYPES OF HEALTH INSURANCE?

Individuals (*beneficiaries*) may receive health insurance protection through several vehicles. They may be covered under federal and state government sponsored plans like Medicare and Medicaid, Blue Cross/Blue Shield service organizations, or health maintenance organizations (HMOs) and preferred provider organizations (PPOs). They also may participate in group insurance plans offered by their employers, or purchase individual insurance through mass purchasing groups (e.g., credit unions, or professional or trade associations).

The decision for purchasing individual or group healthcare insurance is based on "insurability." To purchase individual insurance, a person must fill out a health questionnaire and complete a medical examination. Insurability is based on the applicant's personal health, medical history, age, habits, and income. Group health plans, on the other hand, are governed by the Health Insurance Portability and Accountability Act of 1996 (HIPAA). Under HIPAA an applicant does not have to take a medical examination. Group health is based on the *law of large numbers* such that the impact of individual health risks is mitigated by insuring a large number of individuals. Group health plans must find a balance between the number of healthy versus sick people in order to mitigate the impact of high cost and utilization in the population insured.

The most popular type of health insurance in the United States is employer-sponsored group coverage. As of 2003, 159.2 million people were covered by employment-based plans, according to the Employee Benefit Research Institute. This includes non-elderly full time employees (people under age 65 who work more than 34 hours per week), and part-time employees (people who work between 21 and 34 hours per week). As of 2006, 62.2 percent of the non-elderly population had employment-based health insurance, according to EBRI reports. This compares with 62.7 percent in 2005.

WHAT IS GROUP HEALTH INSURANCE?

Group health insurance includes medical, dental, vision, prescription drug, mental health, and long-term care coverage. Beneficiaries receive full or partial reimbursement for their various expenses, which usually include hospital and surgical expenses, diagnostic x-rays, tests, and physician visits. Coverage is defined in a master contract issued to the group and relayed to beneficiaries through the Summary Plan Description (SPD).

Group health is commonly purchased by employers for their employees and retirees. Because insurance is governed by the *law of larger numbers*, large employers can purchase their own health insurance at favorable rates, or pool resources and purchase jointly as coalitions. Small employers can use similar methods by pooling their employee lives into joint purchasing groups or coalitions.

Unions commonly receive healthcare benefits through collective bargaining with employers. Typically they offer group health insurance to their members through a *trust*. The trust, or Taft-Hartley Plan, is jointly managed by the union and employers. The trust purchases the group health policy for members who are employed by the same company, or for union members employed by different companies.

Insurance also is offered by professional, trade, retail, and chamber of commerce organizations. These groups commonly offer insurance that is specific to their business, for example, malpractice insurance. If membership in the organization is based on employment, the groups are known as multiple employer welfare arrangements (MEWA), or multiple employer trusts (MET). If they offer health insurance, they are known as Association Health Plans (AHPs). In AHPs, the groups purchase the insurance policy and offer it to their members for a fee.

States and cities also can sponsor coalitions of small employers called *health insurance purchasing coalitions*, or *cooperatives*. These coalitions are formed to improve the purchasing power of their members. Their intent is to make healthcare insurance more available and affordable, where individuals are offered multiple health plans to choose from, but the employers pay only one bill. Examples of these groups are the Pac Advantage in California and HealthPass in New York City. There is an opportunity for multiple state cooperatives to join together and jointly purchase health insurance. By pooling their resources, they receive lower costs and can promote value-based purchasing through requirements on quality or quality incentives for better care. This is commonly known as *pay for performance (P4P)*.

HOW DO COMPANIES BUY HEALTH INSURANCE?

The diversity and complexity of the various health insurance options available in the marketplace is usually beyond the scope of employers, including the larger ones. Therefore, most companies use intermediaries to help them develop a plan, research their options, and negotiate competitive bids. These intermediaries may be insurance agents (who represent insurance companies), *brokers* (who represent employers), health benefit consultants, or third party administrators (TPAs). These intermediaries work with the *underwriters* at insurance companies to define the employer's or group's acceptability for insurance based on risk. *Risk* in insurance terms is the chance that the claims will exceed the expected level. Underwriters evaluate companies by developing risk profiles that consider the composition of the employer or group according to age, sex, prior claim experience, and the plan design. The risk will define the premium level that will be paid.

WHY AND UNDER WHAT CIRCUMSTANCES WOULD AN EMPLOYER SELF-FUND GROUP HEALTH INSURANCE?

Some large employers decide that funding their own health insurance is less expensive than purchasing it from an insurance company. As well, the employer may determine that the benefit plan that they desire is not available at a reasonable cost or that the risk for loss is less than that determined by the insurance company's underwriter. Whether for cost or breadth of benefit offering, an employer or group that decides to self-fund must make several critical decisions. A self-funded program avoids the overhead costs of an insurance company, but they must decide whether to pay claims internally or outsource this function. Typically, self-funded programs contract with a TPA or insurance company to handle the benefit administrative functions. These functions are directed to the payment of claims in an expeditious manner, to managing the resolution of claims problems and reporting on benefit utilization.

WHO REGULATES HEALTH INSURANCE?

Benefits provided under insurance contracts are governed by state laws as defined by the McCarran-Ferguson Act of 1948. Health plans are covered under the rules and regulations of the Department of Insurance (DOI) for the state in which the employer is licensed. The DOI publishes a *Health & Safety Code* that lists rules and regulations. Self-funded health plans, that is, employers that fund health plans themselves, are covered under ERISA that preempts state laws (see next section).

WHAT IS ERISA AND HOW DOES IT APPLY TO GROUP HEALTH INSURANCE?

Federal law does not require employers to provide medical coverage for their employees. However, once a health plan is established, there are federal laws that regulate the entities. These include: the Employee Retirement Income Security Act of 1974 (ERISA); the Health Insurance Portability and Accountability Act of 1996 (HIPAA); the Mental Health Parity Act of 1996 (MPHA); the Newborn's and Mothers' Health Protection Act of 1996 (NMPHA); Consolidated Omnibus Budget Reconciliation Act of 1985 (COBRA); the Pregnancy Discrimination Act (PDA; 1987 amendment to the Civil Rights Act of 1964); the Age Discrimination in Employment Act of 1967 (ADEA); Omnibus Budget Reconciliation Act of 1993 (OBRA '93); the Women's Health and Cancer Rights Act of 1998 (WHCRA); and Family and Medical Leave Act of 1993 (FMLA).

ERISA was written to protect employee pensions, not medical insurance plans. The law includes a definition of "welfare plans" that broadly includes health plans within its scope. ERISA requires that plans must meet certain requirements:

- Plans must have a written document defining the plan.
- Plans must be administered according to the document.
- The document must be understandable to the average employee, and copies of the plan (the SPD) must be given to employees.
- The document must describe covered benefits, and clearly define the conditions for denying coverage of a service.
- The document must indicate who administers the plan and how the benefit is funded.
- Annual financial reports must be provided to the government, and summaries (*summary annual reports [SARs]*) must be given to participants.

COBRA is another piece of legislation that implicates medical insurance. COBRA requires coverage under the employer's medical plan after termination of employment provided that the employee pays the full cost of the coverage.

WHAT ARE BLUE CROSS/BLUE SHIELD PLANS AND HOW DO THEY DIFFER FROM PRIVATE INSURERS?

Blue Cross associations were established in the 1930s under the auspices of the American Hospital Association. Blue Shield associations were established in the 1940s under the auspices of the American Medical Association. Blue Cross organizations guaranteed payment in full to hospitals for services, while Blue Shield organizations provided a similar guarantee to physicians. The close association between hospitals and physicians with the Blues prompted the providers to offer discounts on fees. Later, many Blue Cross and Blue Shield organizations associated to form Blue Cross/Blue Shield (*the Blues*) associations.

Blues plans contract directly with physicians, hospitals, and other healthcare providers to establish the charges for services to their members. When a member goes to a healthcare provider, the bill for charges is sent to the Blues for payment. The Blues offer health plans similar to private insurers but often at deeper discounted prices. Typically, the Blues offer base medical plans with supplemental major medical plans if employers wish to purchase more coverage. They also offer many types of managed care plans, for example, HMO, PPO, or point-of-service plan (POS).

Private insurers offer supplemental insurance to the plans offered by the Blues. As for-profit organizations, they pay premium taxes (about 2.5%) to the state. In contrast, many of the Blues are still non-profit organizations and pay no premium tax to the state. As a non-profit organization, the Blues (many are now for-profit) receive exclusive rights to hospital discounts granted by the state; however, in return for these rights, the Blues allow state regulation of their rates and eligibility criteria for individual contracts. As a result, many of the Blues have experienced higher costs without being able to raise premium rates or to deny coverage for certain pre-existing conditions similar to private health plans. Their response has been to raise group health premiums for employers to cover the short-fall in individual contracts. This has lead employers to seek alternative options to lower costs consistent with their actual cost trend (or inflation).

HOW DO EMPLOYERS DESIGN HEALTHCARE PLANS?

Employers use group health insurance as employee benefits, or even as a competitive strategy to hire desired employees. The economic climate often determines the level of benefits that employers can afford. They may also consider their corporate culture, and the demographics of their employee population. Given these baseline fundamentals, employers frequently follow one of five general strategies for health benefit design:

- *Managed Competition:* Employees are offered choices between multiple health plans with the goal of driving employees to the most cost-effective plan.
- *Total Compensation:* Employee benefits are negotiated as a single package together with base salary and incentive pay with the goal of driving employees to consider their total take-home compensation. The result is to drive employees to consumer-

driven health plans (CDHPs) that shift more costs to employees by requiring them to make value judgments about the most cost-effective plan for them.

- *Paternalistic:* Employees are fully covered, or require a modest employee contribution with the goal of making the employee the dependent of the employer. The employer utilizes PPOs to control costs.
- *Flexible/Market Driven:* The most common of strategies where employees are offered several options of PPO, HMO, and CDHP with the goal of allowing employers to maintain a competitive hiring and employee retention position in the marketplace by responding to employee needs.
- *Consumer Driven:* These strategies (i.e., CDHPs) move more of the benefit expense to the employee with the goal of making them a more informed consumer supported by financial incentives, information, and comparisons between available options.

WHAT TYPES OF HEALTH PLANS ARE AVAILABLE?

Group health plans fall into the two broad categories of traditional or managed care. Traditional group health is a basic medical plus major medical plan (also known as *base-plus* or *first-dollar* plan), or a comprehensive medical plan (also known as *comprehensive*).

The base-plus plan is a two-part health insurance plan composed of basic medical coverage (hospitalization, surgery, physicians' visits, diagnostic laboratory tests, and X-rays) and major medical, which covers other expenses. The base-plus has limits on the services, e.g., number of hospital days covered, but there are no deductibles or coinsurance for the employee to pay. Employees are compensated for the total expense from the first-dollar of expenses.

The major medical is broader and, as a result, while there are fewer limits, the employee is required to pay more of the expense through deductibles and coinsurance until a maximum out-of-pocket (MOOP) expense is reached. After that threshold is reached, the employer reimburses expenses in full.

A comprehensive plan provides coverage for most healthcare expenses using a standard reimbursement formula based on a deductible and a coinsurance paid by the employee for all covered expenses until a MOOP is reached, after which the employer pays all expenses in full.

Managed care is a healthcare delivery system where the plan or insurer influences the type of medical care delivered. Managed care actively "manages" both the medical and financial aspects of patient care by providing comprehensive plans for predetermined prices. The onus is on the plan to determine the most cost-effective and efficient methods to deliver the required care.

WHAT TYPES OF SERVICES ARE COVERED BY HEALTH PLANS?

Covered expenses are eligible for payment under group health plans, although employees may be required to pay whole or part of the expense. Covered expenses vary by plan, but usually include professional services of physicians and osteopaths, hospital charges for semiprivate rooms, surgical charges and anesthesia, nursing services, home health care, diagnostic x-ray or radium treatments, blood transfusions, oxygen, prescription drugs, ambulance services, durable medical equipment (DME), artificial limbs and prostheses, casts, and wheelchairs. Outpatient services are covered for emergency treatment, surgery, and services rendered in outpatient labs or x-ray departments. Mental health may be included or insured separately (*carve out*) with a separate premium. Hospice care is covered by Medicare Part A but may not be covered by traditional plans because this type of care does not cure illness. Traditional plans must cover palliative care to include hospice coverage for their beneficiaries. More controversial are alternative therapies (i.e., herbal remedies, acupuncture, etc.), which are covered by only some plans. A common criterion for coverage for acute, outpatient, and emergency treatment is that they are all regulated by applicable licensing agencies so that there is oversight of safety and compliance with state laws.

Experimental treatments have traditionally not been a covered benefit. The problem lies in the definition of "experimental" used in the benefit language. Where does treatment become non-experimental? How is a treatment tested to determine if it has any value and if it is safe? These questions lie at the root of the problem, and have lead to the difficulty in covering experimental treatments.

WHAT ARE THE ELEMENTS OF CONSUMER-DRIVEN HEALTH PLANS?

Traditional health plans are based on providing *defined benefits* (DB) for employees. These benefits are listed in the SPD given to employees to define what is covered on their health plan. When services are rendered, the employee receives an *Explanation of Benefits (EOB)* to define which services are covered in their plan, and a rationale for the cost share that is the employee's responsibility. With the rising cost of healthcare services, emphasis has shifted from providing defined benefits, to making a *defined contribution* (DC) to the employee. The defined contribution shifts the responsibility for payment and selection of healthcare services from the employer to the employee, according to the Employee Benefit Research Institute. DC assumes that an employee will spend their own money more wisely than if they are spending their employer's money. DC forces employees to shop for healthcare the same as they do for other goods and services.

There are several types of DC benefit plans; namely, health reimbursement accounts (HRAs), medical savings accounts (MSAs), health savings accounts (HSAs), and consumer-driven dental care. An HRA is paid solely by the employer, where the employee is reimbursed for medical expenses up to a maximum dollar amount for a defined period of time. Any unused portion is carried forward to the next period to increase the maximum dollar amount in that period. In an MSA, the employer gives a fixed dollar amount and the employee sets up their own account. Medical expenses are drawn from the MSA and any balances can build over time. An HSA is a tax-exempt trust that is established for the exclusive purpose of paying qualified medical expenses for the beneficiary. An individual may establish an HSA as long as the health plan includes a high-deductible feature (usually $1,000 annual MOOP for an individual). In DC, the employee decides which type of plan is best for his/her needs. The selection of the DC plan is based on one of at least three models:

- The employer gives the employee a fixed dollar amount (*voucher*) that the employee may use to buy whichever health plan they choose.
- The employer identifies a group of health plans with varying services and costs for which the employer has pledged to pay a fixed premium amount. Any surpluses are paid to the employee and any balance of payment must be borne by the employee.
- The employer can construct a medical savings account with a financial entity or an HMO, which then tracks the utilization and pays cost from the account.

CONCLUSION

The subject of medical insurance is complex and Part I of this chapter only scratches the surface. It is not sufficient to define the needs of a population and contract a provider network. Regulatory, legislative, tax, and financial implications must be considered as well. The dynamic nature of insurance as populations change, and the role of different financial and delivery models as design experiments is at the heart of the issue. The employer-based group health model is one such experiment that is now undergoing radical change to consumer-based models. The marketplace will eventually decide which of these models will remain.

PART 2   MEASURING HEALTH PLAN PERFORMANCE

INTRODUCTION

Managed care is based on aligning insurance models and delivery systems to provide medical care that meets the expectations of patients and payers. The alignment of the various stakeholders in the medical system requires that there be methods to test performance, financial controls, and fiscal intermediaries (e.g., TPAs, pharmacy benefit managers [PBMs]) to ensure compliance with benefit designs. This section focuses on the use of audits, contracts, and market intelligence to provide oversight and management of these systems.

AUDITS

All organizations are obligated to establish financial controls on their operations to protect the interests of their owners, shareholders, and employees. They also are obligated to ensure that when they contract services to outside vendors, their benefits and health plan objectives are administered in a fashion that is consistent with their plan obligations. A contract defines the obligations of both parties when an outsourced vendor is used.

How do we test compliance with contracts, contractors, and internal control systems? Are claims administration policies sufficient to ensure a high level of accuracy in claims payments? When should we audit? What do we audit?

Audits are the standard approach for testing systems and validating the results when the systems are applied. Their purpose is to provide accountability for managers and officials to their governing boards. All managers and officials that are entrusted with the handling of public or corporate resources "are responsible for applying those resources efficiently, economically, and effectively to achieve the purposes for which the resources were furnished" (Government Auditing Standards, 1.13.b). As a result, the term *audit* refers to both financial and performance audits. *Financial audits* provide independent reports directed to an entity's financial performance. They identify if the financial information is presented fairly and if its internal controls comply with laws and regulations. *Performance audits* provide an assessment of the performance of organizations, programs, activities, or functions of an entity. They improve accountability, oversight, and are used as a basis for decision-making or corrective actions.

FINANCIAL AUDITS

Financial audits include financial statements (balance sheets, income statements, cash flow) as defined by a strict accounting perspective. These audits include determinations of: 1) whether the information is presented in accordance with established criteria; 2) whether the entity has adhered to financial compliance requirements; and 3) whether the internal controls over financial reporting and safeguarding of assets is suitably designed and implemented to achieve the objectives. These criteria are detailed in financial audit criteria established by the American Institute of Certified Public Accountants (AICPA).

Audits that are commonly performed in healthcare systems fall under the *attestation standards* developed by the AICPA in the AT Section of the *Statements on Standards for Attestation Engagements*. Attestation standards focus on contract compliance and reviews of systems to determine if they meet adequate standards. Opinions are given on the adequacy of these controls.

Attestation audits (also called *engagements*) require a standard for comparison. For example, the methods for paying incurred services (e.g., pharmacy claims) needs to be clarified and codified. The pharmacy vendor or fiscal intermediary has standards for payment. The goal of the engagement is to achieve clarity such that all concerns are addressed. This may include re-pricing of claims, testing of eligibility for benefits, and validation of prior authorization controls for payment of non-benefit claims. The role of the auditor in this regard is to provide an independent opinion of the veracity of claim administration and to push for more clarity and transparency of systems.

PERFORMANCE AUDITS

Performance audits are "objective and systematic examinations of evidence for the purpose of providing an independent assessment of performance" of an organization, program, activity, or function (Government Auditing Standards). The goal of these audits is to provide accountability and to assist decision makers with the information that they need for oversight of their operations. Performance audits have three elements: economy, efficiency, and program audits.

Economy and *efficiency* in this context include determinations of: 1) the appropriate use of resources (people, funds); 2) the causes of any inefficient processes; and 3) compliance with rules and regulations. *Program audits* apply to determinations of: 1) the extent to which the desired results of programs, functions, or activities are achieved; 2) the effectiveness of organizations and their programs; and 3) compliance with rules or standards relating to specific programs, functions, or activities.

Ultimately, the goal of performance audits is to provide information. Managed care organizations and their many contractors have both regulatory and business requirements for oversight. Performance audits provide the information necessary for effective oversight.

ELEMENTS OF A VENDOR CONTRACT

Because attestation audits focus on contract compliance, it is often necessary to define a model contract. How can an entity be sure that critical elements are included in contracts? As with any vendor contract, there are specific elements that must be included to ensure that the entity is receiving the services and pricing that are consistent with their business requirements. A PBM, TPA, or fiscal intermediary (FI) contract is no different. Provider contracts are frequently boilerplate and allow for minimal customization. The entity, as the client, must decide which elements are important and how to measure the performance of the vendor.

What elements should be considered in any contract? A contract with an intermediary (used collectively for all PBMs, TPAs and FIs that administer pharmacy benefits) must consider the fundamental service portfolio that is offered and how it fits with desired service requirements. Intermediary service portfolios can be distilled into the following:

- Pharmacy and specialty injectable claim administration
- Pharmacy benefit administration
- Pharmacy network contracting and oversight, including mail service, internet, and specialty providers
- Formulary construction and management (drug utilization review), and prior authorization support
- Rebate collection and management
- Data and reporting
- Value-added programs (e.g., disease management)

To administer a contract, the intermediary must have their incentives aligned with those of their client. Of particular concern is that pricing methodologies are well defined and transparent, services are delivered on a timely basis for both members and administrative issues, and that the network of providers is delivering optimal services as defined in the contract.

As the fiduciary, the managed care entity or employer defines the benefit. The intermediary administers the benefit in compliance with all applicable rules and regulations. To ensure compliance with the benefit, the intermediary contract includes measurable parameters for all critical performance elements. All service and chargeable elements have performance and service guarantees, as well as financial penalties for non-performance to ensure contract compliance.

MARKET INTELLIGENCE: ELEMENTS OF A REQUEST FOR INFORMATION OR A REQUEST FOR PROPOSAL

The process of assessing the performance of current benefits and providers requires an evaluation of the current marketplace. This type of market intelligence ensures that contracts and pricing reflect current market realities. Market intelligence also allows payers and employers to benchmark their benefits and contracts with other similar entities. There are several methods for assessing the market, two of which are request for information (RFI) and request for proposal (RFP).

The RFI is an informal request for information. The payor or employer is trying to determine market benchmarks for pricing, access, contracts, vendor performance, or the competitive elements of various value-added programs. The answers to an RFI are non-binding and are not used as a basis for contracting.

An RFP is a formal request to determine the current marketplace for access, service, and price. In a competitive market the vendors offer their best pricing and service as well as an offer that is consistent with the RFP questions. All benefit elements and service needs should be considered for inclusion in an RFP. There are also standard elements that should be included, namely:

- Short description of the vendor, their business model, and disclosure of any conflicts of interest with the client or their customers
- Service portfolio required with guarantees and penalties
- Benefit design and member eligibility requirements
- Reporting and data requirements
- Pricing guarantees required on a pass through claim basis to validate manufacturer pricing
- Value-add programs of interest, including performance measurement and return on investment (ROI)

The critical element is that the RFP must clearly define and guarantee the member access, service requirements (member and administrative), and pricing that are non-negotiable. Negotiable services can be added based on interest, discretion, and perceived value; however, the value must be clearly defined.

CONCLUSION

The process of auditing and evaluating the effectiveness of managed care systems is frequently mundane, but critical. The public, patients, payors, employers, and others who use and pay for medical care expect a high degree of efficiency and consideration for their needs. Expectations are high for both payors and providers that they are engaged in ethical conduct, and that the systems for implementing the provisions of medical insurance are constantly improved. To achieve exemplary outcomes, systems must constantly be re-evaluated and motivated to greater achievements. In this context, everyone is an auditor.

SUGGESTED READING

American Institute of Certified Public Accountants, Statements on Standards for Attestation Engagements, 2002. Available at http://www.aicpa.org/Professional+Resources/Accounting+and+Auditing/Authoritative+Standards/attestation_standards.htm. Accessed 26 September 2008.

Barcia S.M., Requests for proposals: do we really need them? *Health Manag Technol.* 1999; 20(8): 24-25.

Broekemeier R.L., Brewer P.E., Johnson M.K., Audit mechanism for hospital drug distribution., *Am J Hosp Pharm.* 1980; 37(1): 85-88.

California Health Decisions, Drug Formularies, A Consumer Tool. Available at http://www.calpers.ca.gov/eip-docs/member/health/edu/pharm-kit-07.pdf. Accessed 10 July 2008.

Corchnoy B., Pharmacists as fiscal auditors save hospital millions of dollars. *Hosp Pharm.* 1987; 22(11): 1101-1104.

Cornelis W.A., Audit criteria for drug-use review. *Am J Hosp Pharm.* 1986; 43(7): 1685-1686.

Daniels N., Teagarden J.R., Sabin J.E., An ethical template for pharmacy benefits. *Health Aff.* 2003; 22(1): 125-137.

Department of Human Services, Med-Quest Division, Kapolei, HI, Request for proposals. June 2002, No. RFP-MQD-2002-007

Edlin M., Cost and utilization correlations force plans to study their drug benefits. *Manag Healthcare Exec* 2004; 14(10): 46-48.

Enright S.M., Developing the request for proposal. *Top Hosp Pharm Manage.* 1989; 9(3): 1-8.

Garner J. C., *The Health Care Answer Book,* 7th Ed. New York: Wolters Kluwer/Aspen Publisher; 2007.

Ghotbi L., Managing pharmaceutical trend: a California perspective. 20th Annual Research Meeting, The premier forum for health services research, Nashville, TN, June 27-29, 2003.

Gilderman A., Trends in Effective Formulary Development, July, 2004; Clinical Services, Prescription Solutions.

Habeger H.E., Hardy D.L., Auditing function for staff pharmacists. *Am J Hosp Pharm.* 1985; 42(5): 1038, 1040.

Hoffmann R.G., Auditing hospital pharmacies. *Osteopath Hosp Leadersh.* 1987; 31(4): 20-21.

Huber S.L., Patry R.A., Hudson H.D., Godwin H.N., Strengthening the formulary system by implementing a drug usage guidelines program. *Hosp Formul.* 1984; 19(8): 664-668.

Josephs A., UR/Quality and Compliance Collaboration, Corporate Compliance Hillcrest Health System, Texas Medical Foundation; 2004 (provider meeting).

Kamal-Bahl S, Briesacher B., How do incentive-based formularies influence drug selection and spending for hypertension? Health Aff. 2004; 23(1): 227-236.

Keys P.W., Giudici R.A., Hirsh D.R., Gonzales S.M., Pharmacy audit: an aid to continuing education. *Am J Hosp Pharm.* 1976; 33(1): 52-55.

Landon B.E., Reschovsky J.D., Blumenthal D. *Physicians' views of formularies: implications for medi-*

care drug benefit design. Health Aff. 2004; 23(1): 218-226.

Malkin J.D., Goldman D.P., Joyce G.F., The changing face of pharmacy benefit design. *Health Aff.* 2004; 23(1): 194-199.

McGovern E.M., Campbell A., Lindsay H., et al., Quality improvement in community pharmacy practice. *Int J Pharm Pract.* 2002;10(suppl):R8.

Miller L.L., Miller J.E., Designing your health benefit plan. *Empl Benefits J.* 2003; 28(1): 41-46.

Neal T., Developing the request for proposal. *Am J Hosp Pharm.* 1982; 39(3): 475-480.

Neubrecht F., Third party pharmacy audits: can they be improved? *J Am Pharm Assoc* (Wash). 2000; 40(5): 666-669.

Neumann P.J., Evidence-based and value-based formulary guidelines. Health Aff 2004; 23(1): 124-134.

Nitkin D., Brooks L.J., Sustainability auditing and reporting: the Canadian experience. J Bus Ethic. 1998; 17(13): 1499-1507.

Parmenter E.M., Health care benefit crisis: cost drivers and strategic solutions. Journal of Financial Service Professionals. 2004; 58(4): 63-79.

Pharmacists meet monthly to discuss findings of QA audits. Hospitals. 1980; 54(23) 39-40.

Pietrusko R.G., Seaman J.J., Professional practice audit. *Am Pharm.* 1980; NS20(9): 49-50.

Principles of a Sound Drug Formulary System, 2000, Coalition Working Group.

Roberts M.B. and Keith M.R., Implementing a performance evaluation system in a correctional managed care pharmacy. *Am J Health-Syst Pharm.* 2002; 59(11): 1097-1104.

Schneider P.J., Brier K.L., Caryer K.E, Administrative audits of professional services: effective residency

training experience. *Am J Hosp Pharm.* 1981; 38(3): 339-342.

Specialty Pharmaceutical Management Strategies for Health Plans and Employers. Two-day national conference, March 16–17, 2004, Chicago, IL; presented by International Quality & Productivity Center.

Stern C.S., Evaluating the pharmacy benefit. Empl Benefit Plan Rev. 1994; 49(6): 22-25.

Stern C.S., How to evaluate pharmacy benefit offerings. Empl Benefit Plan Rev. 1995; 50(6): 27-30.

The Commonwealth Fund, Project HOPE/The People to People Health Foundation Inc. Jan/Feb 2004. Available at http://www.commonwealthfund. org/grants/grants_list.htm?grantee_organization= Project%20HOPE%2FThe%20People-to-People %20Health%20Foundation%2C%20Inc. Accessed 10 July 2008.

Tripodi M., Avoiding pharmacy fraud through automation and audit. *Manag Care Interface.* 1998; 11(12): 97-100.

Troy T.N., Growing PBMs face tough challenge in a 'highly undifferentiated' niche. *Manag Healthcare.* 1998; 8(5): 30-31.0.

United States Government Accountability Office, Federal Government Audit Standards, July 2007 Revision. Available at www.gao.gov/cgi-bin/getrpt?rptno= GAO-07-731G. Accessed 26 September 2008.

West J. and Glickman S., Developing an RFP for outstanding investment management, health financial management. July 1997.

Zoloth A., Yon J.L., Woolf R., Effective decision-making in a changing healthcare environment: a P & T Committee interview. *Hosp Formul.* 1989; 24(2): 85-87, 90, 93.

Chapter 18

MEDICAID PHARMACY BENEFIT MANAGEMENT

MARY KAY OWENS

INTRODUCTION

Medicaid was established as a federally mandated and state-operated program to provide health care and related benefits to Americans unable to afford such benefits. In 2006, Medicaid provided health coverage and long-term care assistance to more than 55 million people. This included the provision of Medicaid services to 41 million people in low-income families and nearly 14 million elderly people and persons with disabilities.[1] Most states have allowed some recipients to obtain Medicaid benefits through private or state-run managed care organizations (MCOs) in an attempt to contain rapidly rising program costs. Medicaid benefit requirements and membership demographics create special management challenges in traditional managed care programs. This chapter discusses how managed Medicaid prescription drug benefit design differs from that of commercial programs and how managed care pharmacy directors can operate Medicaid programs to optimize cost and quality of care objectives.

LEGISLATIVE HISTORY

The Federal Social Security Act was amended in 1965 to add Title XIX, which created the general public assistance program known as *Medicaid*. This national program of medical assistance for low-income individuals and families is funded by federal and state governments. Medicaid is the primary source of healthcare coverage to America's poor and disabled and accounts for a significant portion of U.S. health expenditures, yet Medicaid cost projections are once again declining, reflecting slower Medicaid spending growth in recent years.[2]

The federal government establishes regulations, guidelines, and policy interpretations that define the broad scope within which each state operates individual programs. Each state's Medicaid agency determines its own operational and administrative procedures and provider reimbursement policies in accordance with legislative directives and annual budget appropriations. Many states have had a relatively long history of applying managed care delivery methods and strategies to Medicaid populations. States may apply for a waiver from the Centers for Medicare and Medicaid Services (CMS) to experiment with novel financing and healthcare delivery mechanisms, including managed care. As a result, in 2006, there were nearly 30 million Medicaid members enrolled in managed care plans, representing 65% of the total Medicaid membership.[3] By contrast, nearly 48% of Medicaid beneficiaries were enrolled in managed care plans in 1997. **Figure 18-1** illustrates the growing percentage of total Medicaid enrollees covered by managed care.

ADMINISTRATION OF MEDICAID BENEFITS

At the federal level, oversight of the Medicaid program is provided by the CMS under the Department of Health and Human Services (DHHS). Individual states usually assign administrative responsibility for Medicaid to a specific governmental department or

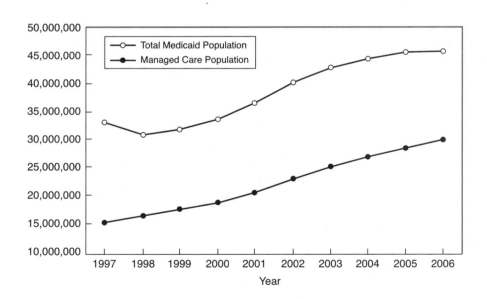

FIGURE 18-1   Total Medicaid Enrollment and Medicaid Enrollment in Managed Care.

These statistics represent point-in-time enrollment as of June 30 for each reporting year.

Source: Medicaid Managed Care Enrollment Report as of June 30, 2006, Centers for Medicare and Medicaid Services. Available at http://www.cms.hhs.gov/MedicaidDataSourcesGenInfo/Downloads/mmcer06.pdf. Accessed 13 July 2008.

agency, often designated as the department of public health and welfare or health care administration. States must designate a medical assistance office that is responsible for developing, analyzing, and evaluating the Medicaid program. Operational activities for administering each state Medicaid program include provider and recipient enrollment, reimbursement policy implementation, claims processing within the Medicaid Management Information System (MMIS), compliance auditing, and quality of service assessment. Each state is responsible for the following activities:

- Establishing recipient eligibility criteria
- Determining the type, amount, duration, and scope of services
- Setting reimbursement rates for each provider service
- Defining the administrative and organizational program structure

FUNDING MEDICAID BENEFITS

All state Medicaid services, including pharmacy services, are funded through a combination of state and federal dollars. The specific ratio of funding from each source varies in each state according to the federal match percentage for each state, known as the *Federal Medical Assistance Percentages (FMAP)*. The proportion of federal funds states receive range from 50% to 83%.[4] Wealthier states with the highest per capita incomes receive less federal funding and those with the lowest per capita income receive more federal funding.

MEDICAID ELIGIBILITY

Medical services are provided to recipients who are eligible to receive cash payments under one of the existing welfare programs established by the federal Social Security Act. There are two categories of recipients: 1) those for whom health coverage is mandated at the federal level and 2) those for whom coverage is determined by the state. In order to receive Title XIX funding from the federal government, states must provide benefits to certain "categorically needy" persons, including: those receiving financial assistance primarily through the Temporary Assistance for Needy Families (TANF) program for adults, children, and pregnant women; and the Supplemental Security Income (SSI) program for the elderly and disabled.

Other groups that are categorically needy and therefore eligible for Medicaid are infants born to Medicaid-eligible women, some low-income Medicare beneficiaries, recipients of adoption assistance or foster care, and children under age six whose family income is below 133% of the federal poverty level (FPL). Most states also provide optional coverage to other groups not subject to mandatory coverage. For example, these groups may include individuals that are "medically needy" and have excessive medical expenses even though they do not qualify for Medicaid due to low-income criteria.

IMPACT OF THE MEDICARE MODERNIZATION ACT ON STATES

The Medicare Modernization Act (MMA) of 2003 created a significant expansion of the Medicare program by establishing the new Medicare prescription drug benefit (Part D). The new coverage has major implications for states' Medicaid programs because, for the first time ever, beneficiaries who are eligible for both Medicare and Medicaid (dual eligibles) now receive prescription drug benefits not from Medicaid but from Medicare.

States provided drug coverage through Medicaid for the roughly 6.4 million low-income seniors and people with disabilities enrolled in both Medicaid and Medicare.[5] These 6.4 million individuals are often referred to as "dual eligibles" and represent approximately 50% of total Medicaid drug spending. As of January 1, 2006, the MMA ended Medicaid drug coverage for dual eligibles and required that they instead secure their medications through private Medicare drug plans known as prescription drug plans (PDPs) under Medicare Part D (**Figure 18-2**). Though states no longer provide drug coverage to dual eligibles through Medicaid, states have had a major role to play in assisting them make the transition to new Medicare PDPs.

The MMA impacts the Medicaid program by carving out the coverage of drugs for dual eligibles and transferring this responsibility to the Medicare program. States are expected to send "clawback" payments to the federal government on a monthly basis to fund 90% of the Medicare Part D benefit. States face new administrative expenses and responsibilities as many assist Medicare beneficiaries with the application and qualification process for low-income subsidies available under Part D.

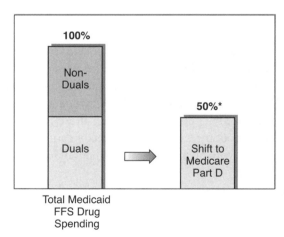

FIGURE 18-2   Percentage of Medicaid Fee-for-Service Drug Spending Shifted to Medicare Part D, January 2006.

Source: Southeastern Consultants, Inc., 2007. Adapted from the 2004 Expenditure Report, National Association of State Budget Officers. Available at http://www.nasbo.org/Publications/PDFs/2004ExpendReport.pdf. Accessed 13 July 2008.

Additionally, states are assessing the impact of MMA on Medicaid cost containment initiatives and other programs such as disease management, drug utilization review (DUR), Medicare subsidies, and managed care benefit structures. While these requirements are finalized and will not likely be changed, states do have a number of opportunities to influence the effectiveness of the new Part D program and re-evaluate future Medicaid policy and program design decisions.[6] Examples of state initiatives related to MMA may include decisions as to:

- Cover non-Part D drugs, non-formulary drugs, and/or copayments for dual eligibles
- Create incentives or mandate pharmacies to waive copayments for dual eligibles that cannot pay
- Establish a dedicated unit for education and assistance for dual eligibles related to plan selection, benefit use, and appeals
- Re-evaluate existing and planned cost containment policies, such as preferred drug lists
- Re-evaluate current DUR program structures and objectives
- Re-evaluate disease and care management program structures and vendor contracts
- Review current managed care program structure and benefit design
- Review current and proposed long-term care programs and alternative structures

MEDICAID SERVICES

Title XIX mandates that states provide certain basic services to all categorically needy persons to obtain federal matching funding. These mandatory services include:

- inpatient and outpatient hospital services
- physician services
- prenatal care
- vaccines for children
- nursing facility services for persons aged 21 and older
- family planning services and supplies
- rural health clinic services
- home health care for persons eligible for skilled nursing services
- lab and x-ray services
- nurse-midwife services and pediatric and family nurse practitioner services
- federally qualified ambulatory and health center services

It is of interest to note that pharmacy benefits are not a federally mandated program. However, states also may receive federal matching funds for providing certain optional services. Those most commonly provided by states include:

- diagnostic services
- clinic services
- intermediate care facilities for the mentally retarded (ICFMR)
- prescribed drugs

- prosthetic devices
- optometrist services and eyeglasses
- nursing facility services for children under age 21
- transportation services
- rehabilitation and physical therapy services
- home- and community-based care to persons with chronic diseases

Currently, all states include prescribed drugs as a covered service even though it is listed as an optional service. States have appropriately realized that pharmaceuticals help prevent disease progression, morbidity, and mortality in a cost-effective manner.

MEDICAID BENEFIT DESIGN

Under Title XIX of the Social Security Act, states are required to ensure that four basic criteria are met in the overall Medicaid benefit design:

1. Amount, duration, and scope of covered services
2. Comparability of benefits
3. Uniform geographic distribution and access
4. Freedom of choice

States are required to ensure that each covered service is sufficient in amount, duration, and scope to achieve its purpose. Additionally, a state may not arbitrarily place limits on benefits that discriminate among beneficiaries based on medical diagnosis or condition. States are required to make available equal services to all categorically needy individuals and are required to offer the state's plan to all geographic areas in each state. Finally, the freedom of choice provision mandates that states allow Medicaid recipients to obtain services from any enrolled participating provider, institution, or pharmacy.

MEDICAID REFORM AND DEFICIT REDUCTION ACT

Over the past five years, states began to grapple with increasing healthcare costs in the traditional fee-for-service Medicaid reimbursement system. States became interested in pursuing a managed care model often utilizing a capitation-based reimbursement fee structure. It is important to note that not all managed care programs use the capitation-type fee structure used by MCOs. Some "managed care" plans still operate on a fee-for-service basis but offer care management or assignment of a gatekeeper physician as the "managed care" component of the plan.

The Deficit Reduction Act of 2005 (DRA) reduces federal and state Medicaid spending and also changes healthcare access and coverage for low-income beneficiaries. It allows families with disabled children to buy into Medicaid, different benefits to be tied to each eligibility group, and now allows some waiver groups to be eligible without a waiver. The DRA also establishes a five-year look-back period for transfer of assets and requires new applicants as well as most current beneficiaries at re-determinations, to document their citizenship. Under the DRA, states may require premiums to be paid by those over 150% of the federal poverty level. The DRA includes net savings of $4.9 billion and $11.5 billion in gross savings over the next five years.[7]

MEDICAID DEMOGRAPHIC CHALLENGES

The Medicaid population poses some unique challenges that merit a brief discussion. The Medicaid population uses healthcare services more intensively than the general population. The elderly and disabled Medicaid population (13 million people) account for 23% of beneficiaries and 68% of expenditures (**Figure 18-3**).[8] Annual average drug expenditures for elderly and disabled patients are five to seven times the average adult's drug expenditures and ten to thirteen times those of a child (**Figure 18-4**).

Prior to January 1, 2006, the highest prescription drug utilizers represented primarily the elderly patients with compromised health and complex, multi-system diseases. Many of these patients were residing in long-term care facilities or were over the age of 65 and thus not usually enrolled in a Medicaid managed care plan. Even most elderly, ambulatory

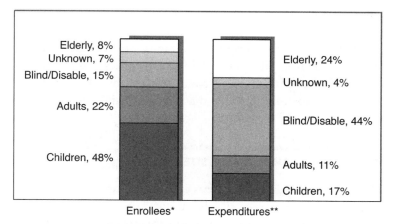

Elderly/Blind/Disabled = 23% of Enrollees and 68% of Expenditures

*Enrollees are recipients of actual services.
**Total expenditures exclude administrative expenses.

FIGURE 18-3 Percent Enrollees and Expenditures by Enrollment Group.
Source: Southeastern Consultants, Inc., 2007. CMS, MSIS 2003 data, Table 9. Available at http://www.cms.hhs.gov/ MedicaidDataSourcesGenInfo/Downloads/MSISTables2003.pdf. Accessed 13 July 2008.

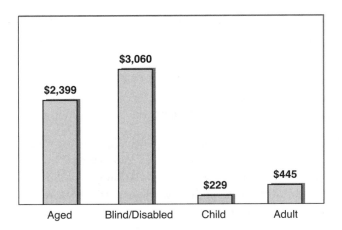

FIGURE 18-4 Average Annual Medicaid Drug Spending per Medicaid Prescription Drug User.
Source: CRS Report for Congress, Prescription Drug Coverage Under Medicaid, Updated February 21, 2006. (Data are extracted from MSIS 2003 Data.) Available at http://www.cms.hhs.gov/MedicaidDataSourcesGenInfo/Downloads/MSISTables2003.pdf. Accessed 13 July 2008.

patients had been on Medicaid for many years, and had advanced medical problems such as diabetes, congestive heart failure, emphysema, and other chronic diseases. Often these patients did not receive preventative or coordinated care for many years and suffered from declining health status with much co-morbidity. Following the Medicare Part D implementation, the remaining majority of Medicaid patients with high drug utilization represent patients with chronic disease and co-morbidity who are not Medicare eligible.

In Federal Fiscal Year (FFY) 2001, 96% of enrollees had annual spending less than $25,000, and represented 51% of all costs. Conversely, approximately 4% of enrollees had average annual spending greater than $25,000 and represented 49% of all costs (**Figure 18-5**).[9]

DEVELOPMENTAL AND CULTURAL ISSUES

Patients often become Medicaid eligible as a result of existing mental and physical developmental disabilities. This can pose significant challenges in the areas of patient education and compliance. However, there is often a primary caregiver assigned to these patients who can be educated and encouraged to take an active part in the health maintenance of the patient. In these cases, providers must be innovative in their approach to the delivery of services and willing to facilitate the caregiver's role to achieve desirable outcomes.

Medicaid programs in states such as Florida, New York, Texas, and California have large, culturally diverse patient populations that can further challenge the delivery mechanisms and efficiency of services. Some cultural and social factors can compromise patient care by discouraging patients from seeking appropriate care. Specifically, the fields of infectious disease and psychiatry are often associated with a stigmatism in our own culture

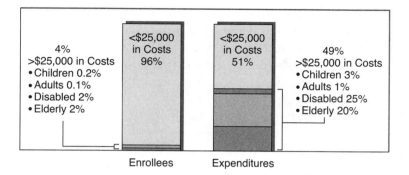

FIGURE 18-5 Small Share of Medicaid Population Accounts for Large Share of Expenditures. *Source:* Medicaid's High Cost Enrollees: How Much Do They Drive Program Spending? Kaiser Commission on Medicaid and the Uninsured, March 2006. Available at http://www.kff.org/medicaid/upload/7490.pdf. Accessed 13 July 2008. This information was reprinted with permission from the Henry J. Kaiser Foundation. The Kaiser Family Foundation, based in Menlo Park, California, is a nonprofit, private operating foundation focusing on the major healthcare issues facing the nation and is not associated with the Kaiser Permanente or Kaiser Industries.

and more intensely in other cultures. For this reason, those who often have the most serious illnesses will not seek treatment at all or will only allow a local, primary care physician to provide care. Also, racial and ethnic groups can have different physiological responses to drugs (e.g., differences in metabolism, clinical effectiveness and side-effect profiles) as well as different psychosocial views of disease and the medications used to treat them.

Cultural diversity also may serve as a challenge to the successful delivery of medical and pharmaceutical educational services. For example, printed materials are often very useful to physicians and pharmacists in performing patient education and encouraging proper use and adherence to drug therapy. However, these materials are usually not available in languages such as Haitian Creole or Vietnamese. Many state Medicaid programs have recognized this, yet translated materials continue to represent a significant challenge from a resource perspective to budget for the development of tracts in multiple languages targeted at these groups. Culture is a known driver that encourages patients to reside in like ethnic communities and consequently seek medical care in those areas. It is important to realize that treating healthcare providers also reside in these same communities and are often of similar cultural and ethnic backgrounds. This offers advantages for patients because these providers usually speak the language and are culturally sensitive to many patient issues.

MANAGED CARE WAIVERS

In order to pursue managed care as an alternative payment system, states had to obtain a waiver from the federal government's CMS. The purpose of this waiver is to allow states to "waive" the legal requirements outlined in the original plan and apply for exemptions to those four requirements as previously discussed. The process of applying for and obtaining a waiver from CMS is very labor intensive and takes, on average, over a year to complete and implement. In order for states to move Medicaid recipients from a traditional fee-for-service plan into a managed care plan, more than one type of waiver is required. For example, a Section 1915(b), two-year waiver allows states to restrict the providers from whom a recipient receives services, implement care management, and mandate recipient enrollment into a managed care plan.

Another waiver that states usually seek from CMS to establish managed care programs is the Section 1115 waiver is known as a *research and demonstration waiver*. These waivers are used by states to test special projects that target specific populations and provide flexibility to design new healthcare delivery systems that focus on appropriate healthcare service utilization. A Section 1115 waiver is usually granted for a five-year period; however, states like Arizona have operated under this waiver for over fifteen years. Currently, 28 states have active Section 1915(b) waivers and 11 states have obtained a Section 1115 research and demonstration waiver to test new and innovative Medicaid program concepts and to expand coverage for populations such as the uninsured.[10]

In 2001, the Secretary of Health and Human Services released new waiver guidelines, called the Health Insurance Flexibility and Accountability (HIFA) initiative, which encouraged states to look to Section 1115 waivers as a way to expand coverage within "current-level" resources.

Recently, waivers have been promoted as a way to expand the number of people covered within existing resources and cites as a model for Medicaid reform. Some waivers have included coverage expansions, but increasingly, states are implementing waivers as a way to reduce state costs.[11] Several states have filed new or expanded Section 1115 waivers to completely change the current Medicaid delivery system and reduce the rate of expenditure growth in their Medicaid programs. This new initiative known as *Medicaid Reform* is being promoted by the states and complemented by a national Medicaid reform effort in Congress. Florida, California, South Carolina, Georgia, Tennessee, Vermont, and Ohio are leading the way with state-based reform efforts, some of which include a private sector approach to contracting and delivery of services, consumer choice, integrated care models, and patient incentive programs for achieving better health status.

The basic reform model allows states to receive a block grant of federal dollars to fund the Medicaid program for a period of several years. The goal is for states to have flexibility in how to structure benefit packages and payments for those packages based on patient-specific determined need rather than be held to the current federal mandates, which require the same amount, scope, and duration of benefits be offered to all mandatory enrolled patients. The reform plans generally require payments be provided under a managed care capitation arrangement where premiums are paid directly to the managed care plan selected by the patient. Patient advocates are most concerned with the increased patient cost sharing provisions that the reform plans are proposing for all healthcare services provided. It is too early to tell whether the states will be successful with this new approach to Medicaid service delivery and cost containment.

MEDICAID MANAGED CARE CONTRACTS

Most states have chosen to contract with MCOs on a capitation fee basis. The Medicaid managed care population has grown from nearly 21 million patients in 2001 to nearly 30 million as of 2006, according to CMS.[3] The patients in 2006 enrolled in a managed care plan was approximately 52% of the total U.S. Medicaid population, with approximately 48% enrolled in a non-comprehensive risk managed care plan and 48% enrolled in a comprehensive risk managed care plan (**Figure 18-6**).

It is important to note that most state Medicaid managed care programs historically have concentrated on moving only those recipients who qualify under the Temporary Assistance for Needy Families (TANF) regulation. This group includes predominately young and healthy female patients with small children and excludes from managed care plans those patients who are elderly, disabled, chronically ill, or residing in a long-term care facility. However, in an emerging trend, states are applying for special reform waivers to extend access to managed care programs for the more costly elderly and chronically ill population.

Under the current structure, an MCO must cover the cost of providing all medical services to a patient with the capitated monthly fee paid by the state. The monthly fees are set by the state based on a level usually equal to between 92% and 95% of the regular fee-for-service rates paid for the total medical services of comparable sets of patients. These rates are calculated from claims histories and vary depending on specific factors such as demographics, geographic regions, eligibility category, and provider service type, and can be adjusted periodically as necessary. Most managed care contracts require that the same scope and type services be provided to patients in a managed care plan as are required in the traditional fee-for-service system. In addition, all services deemed to be medically necessary,

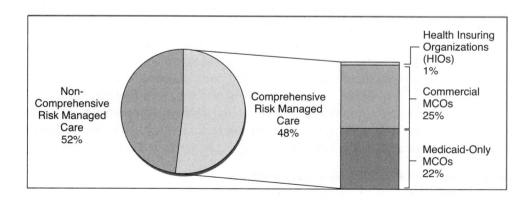

FIGURE 18-6   Medicaid Enrollment in Managed Care.
Source: Southeastern Consultants, Inc., 2007. (Data are extracted from CMS Medicaid Managed Care Enrollment Report Summary Statistics.) Available at http://www.cms.hhs.gov/MedicaidDataSourcesGenInfo/Downloads/mmcer06.pdf. Accessed 13 June 2006.

appropriate, and which conform to professionally accepted standards of care are usually covered by the managed care plan. These requirements are likely to change as Medicaid reform efforts are allowed to proceed based on waiver approval by the federal government.

PERFORMANCE MEASURES AND MEMBER SATISFACTION

Managed care organizations contracting with state Medicaid programs are required to establish a system to receive and monitor patient grievances within the managed care plan. Many states report that as a part of their quality care management, the plans are required to submit grievance and beneficiary complaints to the state Department of Insurance or the Medicaid agency. States also have set up toll-free numbers that direct patients to state offices and officials who can assist and answer questions for plan-related problems and enrollee complaints.

Continuous monitoring of managed care plan practices, quality of care, and access-related issues is a key concern for Medicaid officials. Most states have a review process in place to ensure that minimum standards are being achieved, process measures are in place, and that care is provided appropriately. However, early in the process some states sanctioned and fined managed care plans for not meeting the minimum standards. A few states have enacted legislation that require all participating plans to meet national accreditation standards such as those set by the National Committee for Quality Assurance (NCQA). According to surveys, most patients are pleased with the care they receive through managed care plans and desire to remain enrolled in those plans.

MEDICAID PHARMACY BENEFIT DESIGN

Most state managed care Medicaid plans include pharmacy benefits as part of their contracting, comprehensive medical capitation rates, as is the case in commercial managed care plans. Some states "carve out" the pharmacy benefit from the capitation rate and reimburse for drugs on a separate fee-for-service arrangement. State Medicaid managed care contracts usually make provisions regarding drug coverage and formulary status that require coverage of similar therapeutic products that are covered under the state's fee-for-service formulary. In many states that would include selected non-prescription (over-the-counter [OTC]) medications and prescription drug products. States that have more stringent guidelines on their fee-for-service formulary, such as prior authorization procedures and refill or quantity limitations, often allow managed care plans to apply similar policies and restrictions.

OVER-THE-COUNTER PRODUCT COVERAGE

Medicaid fee-for-service plans are now covering more OTC products, including smoking cessation, cough and cold, antihistamine, vitamin, and acid suppression products. Because Medicaid managed care plans must often allow coverage for the same or similar drugs covered under the fee-for-service plan, many patients now have access to these OTC products.

Though states vary substantially, state Medicaid programs are more likely to cover OTC drugs than are private plans.[13] According to a recent compilation by the National Pharmaceutical Council titled *Pharmaceutical Benefits Under State Medical Assistance Programs*, all 50 states offer some classes of OTC products such as allergy/asthma/sinus, analgesics, cough and cold, smoking deterrents, digestive products, feminine products, and topical products.[12] The policy to cover OTC products is primarily driven by the recent movement of many products from prescription to OTC status. It is possible that the utilization of OTC products may increase as more Medicaid patients move into managed care. Traditionally, the Medicaid population has not sought to self-medicate with OTC products. Instead, they generally have chosen to seek unnecessary urgent care services such as costly physician or hospital emergency department visits. Managed care plans strive to teach patients to utilize phone triage services and other mechanisms to prevent patients from seeking unnecessary and expensive visits for the treatment of minor ailments. Pharmacists are often an underutilized resource who should be recognized and compensated by managed care for their ability to assist patients with selection of OTC medications in the treatment of minor illnesses and thus perform a great cost containment service.

Additionally, managed care plans must be careful to ensure that patients have an incentive to use OTC products. If patients are required to pay five dollars for a physician office visit and the cost of an OTC medication is ten dollars, the patient may seek the services of a physician instead of purchasing the OTC product. It is imperative for health plans to view policy reimbursement in the context of the total medical expenditures and not make shortsighted departmental budget decisions.

MEDICAID PRESCRIPTION COPAYMENTS

Most states have small copayments for pharmacy services in the Medicaid program. These copayments vary from state to state per prescription and may be dependent on whether a generic or brand name drug is dispensed or whether a preferred or non-preferred drug is dispensed. It is widely recognized that even a small copayment can act as a significant barrier to patient drug therapy adherence in low-income populations. For this reason alone, some states have eliminated the copayment requirement as they do not wish the copayment to be a barrier that prevents the member from obtaining a necessary prescription. Federal Medicaid law prevents a pharmacy from withholding treatment based on a Medicaid patient's inability to pay the copayment. Some state pharmacy associations and pharmacists have successfully lobbied their state legislatures to rescind the policy of instituting and enforcing copayments for Medicaid patients. The pharmacies viewed the policy as financially burdensome because they were required to forgive the copayment if the patient could not afford to pay. However, this trend could change significantly with the implementation of Medicaid reform efforts by states and the federal Deficit Reduction Act (DRA) of 2005.

New provisions under the DRA allow states the option of imposing cost sharing up to 5% of a beneficiary's income. Under the new provisions of the DRA, copayments are now "enforceable," meaning that providers or pharmacists can deny services or access to drugs if a beneficiary cannot pay the cost sharing amount at the point of service. However, states are prohibited from imposing premiums and cost sharing for services and preferred drugs on certain groups, such as for persons in institutions, categorically needy persons enrolled in MCOs, pregnant women, foster children, hospice patients, and women in the breast or cervical cancer program. States also are prohibited from imposing cost sharing for emergency services and mandatory and preventative children's services.

SPECIAL OPTIONAL COST SHARING PROVISIONS FOR PRESCRIPTIONS UNDER DRA

Increases to prescription cost sharing rules may now occur via state plan amendment and no longer require a waiver, but may require legislative approval in a specific state. Prescription cost sharing is counted as part of the aggregate cost sharing limits of 5% of monthly or quarterly family income. Cost sharing can be excluded or waived for specific drugs and/or drug classes as well as for preferred drugs. Cost sharing amounts can be waived also for non-preferred drugs and reduced to preferred amounts based on a prior authorization process where a preferred drug is deemed ineffective for a patient.

DISPENSING FEES

Dispensing fees are fees that are part of the overall formula for prescription reimbursement and are paid to the pharmacy for the act of performing administrative tasks related to the processing and filling of a prescription. For example, a typical Medicaid reimbursement formula would be as follows:

Drug Ingredient Fee + Dispensing Fee − Patient Copayment = Total Prescription Reimbursement

These dispensing fees encompass a wide range from approximately $0.50 to $2.00 in a Medicaid managed care plan, or $1.75 to $11.46 per prescription in a traditional Medicaid fee-for-service plan.[13] Each state sets the Medicaid fee-for-service dispensing fee under state administrative law; however, each participating state managed care plan is not bound by state law and can set the fees at any level. All participating pharmacies must accept that managed care rate of reimbursement even if it is significantly lower than the Medicaid fee-for-service rates. Managed care plans generally reduce the dispensing fees and provide much lower drug ingredient cost reimbursement to pharmacies as part of a cost containment mechanism in the pharmacy services budget.

PHARMACEUTICAL MANUFACTURER REBATES

A preferred drug list (PDL) is a list of selected drugs that healthcare providers are permitted to prescribe without prior authorization. Before any non-PDL drug can be dispensed, providers must obtain prior authorization from the state Medicaid agency or its contractor.

A PDL is most often administered in conjunction with a supplemental manufacturer rebate program in which states collect rebates in addition to the required federal CMS base rebates.

Preferred drug lists primarily achieve cost savings on drugs used to treat chronic illnesses, which are refilled on a regular basis. These include drugs for diabetes, gastrointestinal conditions, high blood pressure, heart disease, arthritis, asthma, epilepsy, cancer, mental illness, and high cholesterol. Elderly and disabled patients are more greatly impacted by a PDL because they suffer from more chronic illnesses than younger and non-disabled patients.

As of the beginning of 2007, at least 44 Medicaid programs had a PDL in operation or pending in law.[14] The Medicare Modernization Act shifts responsibility of prescription drug benefits for dual eligible patients from Medicaid to Medicare Part D, thereby reducing the volume of prescriptions available for supplemental rebate savings through a PDL program. Therefore states will need to conduct a cost benefit analysis of PDL programs following the implementation of the Medicare Part D program to determine if enough savings exist that warrant the continuation of the PDL program.

Traditional fee-for-service Medicaid receives a minimum 15.1% rebate on brand drug products from the manufacturers as mandated by the DHHS and federal law. These dollars are paid back to the states each quarter based on invoices submitted by the states to each manufacturer detailing specific drug product claims and utilization. Medicaid managed care plans do not receive separate, additional rebates on their Medicaid enrollees, but do collect rebates as they would for all their commercially enrolled patients. Managed care plans typically receive rebates direct from the manufacturers on a quarterly basis, as do most other health plans. Prescription rebates are often used as a tool to assist health plans with offsetting the increasing drug budget expenses, primarily due to increased utilization driven by an aging population with accelerating rates of chronic disease.

Following the implementation of a PDL with supplemental rebate requirements, states have been able to increase their average rebates on brand drugs to approximately 30%. This has prompted some states to shift the coverage for drugs provided under Medicaid managed care plans back into the fee-for-service drug program to achieve greater total rebates not available to managed care plans. However, the practice of separating payment of the drug benefit from the medical care benefit causes fragmentation of care, which is considered contrary to the original concept of "managed" care.

CHALLENGES AND OPPORTUNITIES IN MEDICAID PHARMACY BENEFIT MANAGEMENT

Recently, health plans have reported increasing expenses in the pharmacy services budget. Medicaid pharmacy expenditures also have been growing at an increasing rate. Because the rate of growth has not been constant each year, it is particularly challenging to project the annual pharmacy budget. State Medicaid programs have begun to explore various methods to identify inappropriate utilization and implement intervention strategies to address these issues for both fee-for-service and managed care patients. It is important to recognize the many challenges that confront state Medicaid programs and how these impact various components of the overall plan operations. Conversely, there are many excellent opportunities in the Medicaid pharmacy benefit area to enhance patient care while ensuring cost effectiveness through a combination of targeted provider education initiatives and integrated disease and care management programs.

TRADITIONAL FEE-FOR-SERVICE MEDICAID BENEFIT MANAGEMENT CHALLENGES

Numerous challenges exist in managing pharmacy benefits for the Medicaid population. Some are systems and legal related, while others observed in this population result from patient-specific factors, such as demographic and health characteristics. Most pharmacy utilization in the Medicaid population is confined to patients with chronic and/or complex multi-system disorders. A significant percentage of these patients with chronic and serious illness are dual eligibles who, prior to January 2006, received their pharmacy benefits through the Medicaid program and their medical benefits through the Medicare program. Following the transition of these dual eligible patients into the Medicare Part D drug program, a number of states realized that their elderly and chronic disease populations had been dramatically reduced and therefore began to enroll the remaining chronic disease patients into managed care plans. Medicaid MCO plans traditionally have not enrolled chronically and severely ill patients with complex multi-system disorders, so they will need to prepare for the many challenges that arise from managing this complex population.

FREEDOM OF CHOICE LAWS

Traditional fee-for-service Medicaid programs face many system and legal challenges to providing integrated patient care. The system encourages lack of coordinated care by permitting patients to seek care from multiple physician and pharmacy providers. Often patients do not remain under the care of one primary care physician or clinic and during a month's time period they may have sought care from several different physicians and pharmacies. Under federal Medicaid law, patients are entitled to "freedom of choice," meaning that they are permitted to seek care from any enrolled Medicaid provider for any covered services. Many states have implemented a primary care case management (PCCM) program to encourage patients to seek care through a gatekeeper physician. However, these programs do not necessarily prohibit patients from accessing any provider they choose. Federal law does allow "lock-in" programs; however, states most often use a provider referral process to enroll patients into these programs and states do not necessarily enforce the provisions of these lock-in programs. Surveys show that most states only have a small number of patients enrolled in these programs and states are not aggressively mining the claims data to identify patients for lock-in program enrollment. The result is that many thousands of patients are not being appropriately enrolled who could benefit from increased coordination of care where a gatekeeper physician authorizes and coordinates all of their services. In this manner, the system does not ensure the coordination of pharmacy and medical care or promote cost effective utilization of services. Many provisions proposed under comprehensive Medicaid reform waivers address these inefficiencies in the current system and seek to provide better coordination of care.

UTILIZATION PATTERNS

A small percentage of patients do over-utilize pharmacy services; however, of equal concern is the fact that under-utilization of prescribed drugs used to treat chronic conditions has been substantially documented in many states. The recent move towards disease management and implementation of national medical practice guidelines has stimulated states to mine and analyze data from their claims systems. Results demonstrate that many patients are not receiving pharmaceutical services according to recommended guidelines and are not being properly monitored by one physician to coordinate their care. In many diseases, such as HIV, diabetes, and asthma, it is known that the appropriate use of cost-effective drugs according to best medical practice standards can significantly reduce unnecessary hospitalizations and promote improved clinical outcomes and quality of life.

Recent analyses conducted using states' claim level data sets reveal the need for better coordination of care. Patients were screened for patterns of uncoordinated care, such as utilizing excessive numbers of prescriptions, therapeutically duplicative drugs, frequently changing drug therapies, using multiple prescribers and multiple pharmacies concurrently and in random patterns, accessing the ER frequently and for non-emergent care, and numerous other access patterns often indicative of uncoordinated care.

The state analyses findings showed that uncoordinated care patients had significantly increased average annual prescription and medical costs compared to the coordinated care group (**Figure 18-7**). Even when patients are matched by disease, demographic, and severity of illness profiles, there are significant cost differences between the groups. In addition, these uncoordinated care patients comprised about 10% of Medicaid-Only patients (excluding dual eligibles and long-term care) but accounted for about 45% of total prescriptions, 46% of prescription costs, and 36% of total medical and drug costs combined.[15]

Further analyses reveal that there is a direct and linear relationship between the number of prescribers and markedly increased average annual drug and other medical costs (**Figure 18-8**). Tremendous cost savings can be achieved by reducing the number of prescribers involved in treatment with enhanced coordination of care through case and disease management activities and the use of health information technology.

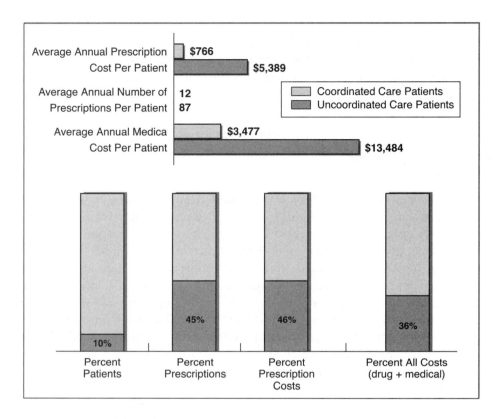

FIGURE 18-7 Utilization and Cost Comparison for a Selected State.
Source: Southeastern Consultants, Inc., 2007. Adapted from independent state claims analysis conducted for the Ohio Commission to Reform Medicaid, 2005.

MEDICAID FRAUD AND ABUSE

Providers and patients are able to abuse and misuse the Medicaid system where there is a lack of internal controls. This has resulted in a significant amount of fraud and abuse in the system. State Medicaid programs recently have begun to dedicate resources to implement and design expensive system edits and computer software enhancements that can identify aberrant provider and patient behaviors through sophisticated claims analysis. As part of the federally-required Medicaid retrospective DUR process, it has been documented that some pharmacies have inappropriately filled prescriptions that were medically unnecessary. Unscrupulous physician and laboratory providers also have been the subjects of abusive billing practices encouraged by the fee-for-service payment system. These are issues that warrant tightly targeted utilization review and

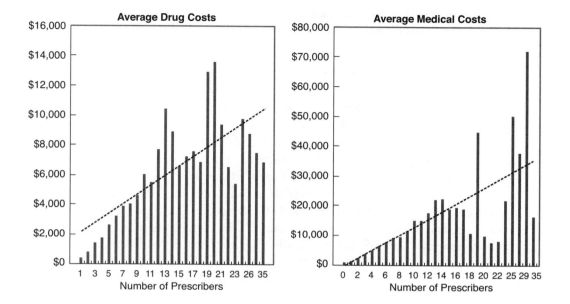

FIGURE 18-8   Average Annual per Patient Cost by Number of Prescribers for Selected State.
Source: Southeastern Consultants, Inc., 2007. Adapted from independent state claims analysis conducted for the Ohio Commission to Reform Medicaid, 2005.

audit programs to efficiently and appropriately manage pharmacy and medical benefits. Many third party plans and now more state Medicaid plans invest in system enhancements and targeted provider auditing that can identify and reduce these inappropriate expenditures.

MEDICAID ELIGIBILITY CRITERIA

Other system and legal challenges result from the Medicaid criteria that determines a patient's eligibility to receive services based on income and health status. Those who are at or below the determined poverty level or have serious health problems are deemed eligible to participate and remain eligible for services. It has been argued that this type of system criteria creates a negative incentive for patients to become healthy and obtain employment because doing so would disqualify them from Medicaid coverage. Many federal and state reform initiatives have been directed at this component of the system to allow low income workers to qualify for and retain Medicaid eligibility, which has increased Medicaid enrollment significantly, while reducing the uninsured population.

MEDICAID REIMBURSEMENT POLICIES

An often unrecognized challenge results from differences in Medicaid fee-for-service reimbursement policies versus other third party plans. Physician specialists typically do not enroll as Medicaid providers as often as they enroll in other health plans due to a lower service fee structure. There is a noted incentive for physicians not to order tests and procedures as often due to the differences in fees paid on those services or a lack of coverage for specific services, the results of which could contribute to decreased patient lab ordering for appropriate prescription monitoring and a decrease in overall prescribing. Conversely, most pharmacies have always enrolled Medicaid providers due to the high reimbursement fee structure for prescription services. Medicaid pays the highest dispensing fees and ingredient remuneration of any third party health plan. This can act as a patient benefit in that pharmacies have a financial incentive to encourage refills and prescription compliance and persistence. Under the provisions of the federal Deficit Reduction Act, there are new reductions in the drug product reimbursement rates paid to pharmacies for specific drugs and new requirements for reporting and calculating these prices. The DRA requires that a federal upper limit (FUL) price be set for all multi-source (generic) drugs at 250% of the average manufacturer's price (AMP; which is the average price paid by drug wholesalers for products distributed in the retail class of trade). In addition, the AMP is further defined to exclude prompt pay discounts to wholesalers, and manufacturers are required to report these wholesaler discounts, the AMP, and the best price for each product at the end of each rebate quarter. The DRA also requires the AMP be calculated monthly for both multi-source (generic) and single-source (brand) drugs.

MANAGED CARE CHALLENGES IN PROVIDING MEDICAID BENEFITS

Medicaid management provides challenges to managed care that are difficult to control due to the complexities of federal and state management, lack of information system infrastructure, benefit mandates, and member turnover.

INFORMATION SYSTEMS

Medicaid managed care faces different challenges than traditional fee-for-service plans in both medical and pharmacy benefit management. The federal waiver process has provided states with some enhanced flexibility in lifting the "freedom of choice" provision for selection of provider services. This in effect allows managed care plans to place the patient under a "gate keeper" physician who is responsible for primary medical management and coordination of their total care. Theoretically, this physician should act as the primary provider and authorize all medical services and specialty referrals. The goal is to ensure continuity of care and cost effectiveness. This works well as long as there are appropriate edits in the system and the managed care plan has an integrated computer network among various clinic and provider sites. Unfortunately, many managed care plans do not have networked medical records or system edits that actively track patient encounter data, thus compromising the concept of managing patient care.

Another significant challenge to pharmacy benefit management is the lack of specific medical encounter data. This makes conducting drug and medical utilization review very difficult versus the traditional Medicaid plan where all data are present, integrated, and accessible from one database. In a capitated reimbursement structure, a monthly fee is paid to the MCO for all patient healthcare services; therefore, there is little financial incentive for the plan to track and report each patient encounter because there is no payment received for individual medical services. Pharmacy services are billed individually to the health plan by the provider pharmacy. Many MCOs use a pharmacy benefit manager (PBM) to process prescription claims, conduct DUR, and enforce specific formulary restrictions. Another widely recognized challenge to managing the pharmacy benefit and conducting comprehensive DUR is the lack of integration between the PBM pharmacy claims data and the MCO medical diagnoses codes and encounter data.

OPEN FORMULARY PROVISIONS

Managed care plans are challenged significantly with managing prescription benefits in Medicaid populations due to mandates that states must have formulary coverage that is at least as comprehensive as the fee-for-service program. Some states specify the managed care plans must allow patient access to any drug product that is covered under the traditional fee-for-service plan. This eliminates the formulary cost containment mechanism that MCOs rely on heavily for their commercial patients. This lack of formulary cost containment has prompted some states to take back the drug benefit from the managed care plans so that the state may realize larger rebates. States receive greater federally required base rebates and supplemental rebates under the fee-for-service PDL programs than are available to Medicaid managed care plans.

ENROLLMENT TURNOVER RATES

Managed care plans are most effective when patients stay enrolled in one health plan for at least a year, preferably more. This is known as a plan "lock-in" provision, which ensures that the MCO has a chance to properly diagnose and stabilize a patient as well as provide preventive care services for a reasonable time period. The original waivers granted to states to implement managed care programs did not allow for plan specific "lock-in" provisions, such as for a 12-month period. This has created serious challenges for managed care plans and negates the entire process of providing continuity of care. Medicaid managed care plans have experienced excessive turnover rates in enrollment that has been detrimental to both the MCOs and the Medicaid program in general.

The managed care TANF patients are, by system eligibility determining factors, a very fluid population. The movement of patients due to frequent changes in eligibility status as well as the absence of a plan-specific "lock-in" provision simply compounds the turnover rate. The administrative burdens and expense of processing and reprocessing enrollment for thousands of patients each month have wreaked havoc on all parties. In some states, this issue was a contributing factor for some Medicaid MCOs filing for bankruptcy. Consequently, the excessive enrollment turnover between plans severely limits the success of managing the pharmacy benefit. Many states have requested and received CMS authorization for a reasonable plan-specific "lock-in" period for managed care patients. The federal government is permitting states to use plan-specific lock-in mechanisms but has stated that extensive choice counseling should be offered to patients prior to the patient's voluntary selection and enrollment in a specific managed care plan. This choice counseling must include a thorough comparison of each health plan in the patient's geographic area and in-depth discussion of the different types of medical and pharmacy services offered among the various health plans. Once a patient selects a specific MCO, they are required to remain in that plan for a one-year period unless extenuating circumstances can be cited.

PHARMACY BENEFIT MANAGEMENT OPPORTUNITIES

The management strategies managed care has applied to the commercial populations can be applied, with limitations, to the Medicaid population. Therefore, managed care has an increased ability to manage Medicaid successfully to achieve both cost management and quality of care objectives.

PROVIDER SELECTION

Managed care organizations participating in Medicaid programs are permitted to require that patients use only designated plan providers including certain pharmacies. For example, a managed care plan can contract exclusively with a limited number of pharmacies to provide all the prescription services to their patients. This is a vital cost containment mechanism for MCOs in that they can negotiate substantial discounts and reduced fees for pharmacy services for all their patients.

PROVIDER PROFILING

Managed care plans have typically recognized the importance of provider profiling to track and analyze patterns of prescribing among physicians. This is a powerful tool for identifying those providers that are prescribing inappropriately and targeting them for educational programs, academic detailing, and comparison reporting. Managed care groups have been successful at providing peer comparisons or "report cards" to physicians to stimulate individual prescribing behavior changes. Physicians are generally more receptive to this from an MCO because they have an economic incentive to hold down costs and prescribe appropriately. Managed care plans also have a distinct advantage in eliciting physician cooperation for academic and educational programs due to the more integrated provider infrastructure. Additionally, these physicians are often very receptive to the implementation of best practice guidelines that enhance the pharmacy benefit management process and improve patient outcomes.

DISEASE MANAGEMENT

Many states have decided to take the high risk, elderly, and chronically ill patients and implement disease management programs incorporating some "managed care" practices into the traditional fee-for-service Medicaid system. Disease management programs are underway in most states addressing various diseases and conditions. The challenge many states face in designing and implementing these programs centers on the issue of data mining. Medicaid programs have not previously needed to categorically analyze disease-specific related expenditures and utilization data. The complex and time consuming process of extracting the claims data using diagnosis codes, procedure codes, and drug code querying must be accurately completed prior to determining the disease management focus and program structure. For example, Florida Medicaid has determined the need to concentrate efforts on HIV, asthma, congestive heart failure, and diabetes disease areas first. They prioritized these based on a thorough retrospective claims analysis of the database. However, another state such as Texas or Louisiana may find upon analysis that they should focus on a different set of diseases. Over the past several years, states have realized that co-morbidity is very significant in this population and therefore a single disease approach is not effective when delivering disease management interventions. In response, many of the vendor companies have consolidated and developed an integrated approach to manage multiple chronic diseases. It is apparent that many states now recognize the value of disease management and will continue expanding initiatives in disease management (**Table 18-1**).

PROVIDER AND PATIENT EDUCATION

One important prerequisite to successful disease management is an updated knowledge base of the prescribing and treating healthcare providers. Providers are overwhelmed with the pace of medical advancement and the proliferation of drug therapy options in the marketplace. Health plan organizations are finding that they must develop internal mechanisms to facilitate the exchange of medical information and treatment guidelines to their providers. The most efficacious manner of accomplishing this is to teach providers to use technology such as the Internet to promote continuous quality improvement in medical education and the application of national treatment guidelines for best medical practices. Other effective resources for physicians are face to face consults with other physicians and the use of clinical pharmacists in their decision support processes. It takes the appropriate balance of different resources and training methods to accomplish these educational objectives.

Patient education is an equally significant factor in determining the success of disease management and appropriate drug therapy utilization. Consequently, it must be approached from two perspectives: the patient and the provider. Providers such as physicians, nurses, and pharmacists have a vital role to play in communicating with patients regarding the importance of proper medication usage, behavior modification, and personal

TABLE 18-1   State Medicaid Disease Management Program History

Medical Condition	States
Asthma	Alabama, Colorado, Florida, Georgia, Illinois, Indiana, Maryland, Mississippi, Missouri, Montana, New Hampshire, New Jersey, North Carolina, Ohio, Oklahoma, Oregon, South Carolina, Texas, Virginia, and Washington
Cancer	Colorado and Montana
Congestive Heart Failure	Florida, Indiana, Missouri, Montana, New Hampshire, New Jersey, North Carolina, Oregon, Texas, and Washington
Diabetes	Colorado, Florida, Illinois, Indiana, Maine, Maryland, Minnesota, Mississippi, Missouri, Montana, New Hampshire, New Jersey, North Carolina, Ohio, Oregon, South Carolina, Texas, Vermont, Virginia, Washington, and West Virginia
End-Stage Renal Disease	Florida, New Hampshire, and Washington
Hemophilia	Florida and Utah
High-Risk Pregnancy (and High-Risk Neonates)	Arkansas, Colorado, and Maryland
HIV/AIDS	Florida and Indiana
Hypertension/Coronary Artery Disease	Florida, Indiana, Maine, Mississippi, New Hampshire, South Carolina, Texas, and Virginia
Mental Health/Depression/Schizophrenia	Colorado, Florida, Missouri, New Hampshire, Texas, and Virginia
Sickle Cell	Florida
Other (including Pain Management and Immunizations)	Maine and Montana

Source: Southeastern Consultants, Inc., 2007. Based upon data available at National Pharmaceutical Council, http://www.npcnow.org; Medicaid Disease Management Programs; Gillespie and Rossiter, *Dis Manage Health Outcomes* 2003; 11(6): 345-361, available at http://www.npcnow.org/resources/PDFs/DM_HO.pdf; and National Conference of State Legislatures, State Disease Management Program Descriptions, available at http://www.ncsl.org/programs/health/StateDiseaseMgmt1.htm, updated July 2007. Accessed 13 July 2008.

health responsibility. Conversely, patients must take an active role in their own health care for disease management programs to be successful and mutually beneficial to the patient and the health plan.

FUTURE TRENDS

Medicaid membership in managed care will continue to expand based on the various Medicaid reform models being proposed and implemented by states. Those MCOs that understand the unique healthcare requirements of the Medicaid population and are able to manage risk will be in the best position to achieve acceptable financial performance while providing necessary care for Medicaid members.

ADVANCED TECHNOLOGY APPLICATIONS

Other future trends include the continued development and implementation of interactive technology-based provider and patient education programs via the Internet. These programs will be used to expose providers and patients to national treatment guidelines and will function as a vital component of an integrated disease management approach to care. Many states are developing and testing various types of advanced technology tools. Examples include Web-based provider access to electronic medical records and utilization profiles as well as the implementation of electronic prescribing, both of which will significantly enhance physician prescribing and treatment decision-making at the point of care. As more patients and providers recognize the role of the Internet in disease management, services will be designed to assist them in achieving their goals in patient assessment, monitoring, education, and treatment adherence. Attaining each of these goals is equally important and vital in ensuring optimal medical and pharmacy patient outcomes.

According to the DHHS *Federal Register*, more than 3 billion prescriptions are written in the United States, and prescription medications are used by 65% of the U.S. public in a given year.[16] A provision of the Medicare Modernization Act will reduce medication errors due to bad handwriting or other errors with electronic prescribing. This system will allow doctors to write a prescription via a hand-held device and electronically transmit that prescription to the patient's pharmacist. Because each prescription can be electronically checked at the time of prescribing for dosage, interactions with other medications, and therapeutic duplication, e-prescribing potentially could improve quality, efficiency, and reduce costs substantially. The integration of electronic prescribing with other advanced features such as clinical decision support tools and two-way electronic communications between the health plan and providers will further enhance the quality and efficiency of care. Recent studies report that approximately 22% of physicians indicated that information technology was available in their practices to allow electronic prescribing.[17] The Secretary of HHS released the final uniform standards for electronic prescribing in the April 7, 2008 *Federal Register*[18], which goes into effect in 2009.

Florida initiated a pilot project in 2001 that provided electronic prescribing hand-held devices to physicians that displayed the Medicaid preferred drug list to test whether physicians found it easier to prescribe a medication from the approved list. In 2002, the project was expanded to provide clinical information about prescription drugs in order to alert physicians to adverse drug interactions and to allow for the inclusion of patient medical histories, so that physicians would be aware of patient drug allergies and could detect therapeutic duplication with other prescribers. Cost savings for the project have been documented at $700 per enrolled physician per month.

NEW APPROACHES IN DRUG UTILIZATION REVIEW

Other specific trends directly impacting pharmacy benefit management programs include the integration of medical and pharmacy utilization databases for in-depth DUR analysis and targeted disease management. This integration will facilitate new approaches to conducting DURs for many state Medicaid programs and other health plans. If state Medicaid and other health plans intend to effectively use the DUR process as an integral component to successful disease management, they must shift from the traditional product-centered approach to a complete patient-centered approach.

Current DUR procedures in most health plans focus on product specific utilization trends. For example, the highest ranking drug products in terms of dollars spent and total units dispensed are often targeted for utilization management and provider educational intervention even if the product is being used appropriately in most patients. Often criteria such as continued use of a drug for an extended period of time may be the only drug use patterns used to generate a DUR alert and intervention. It is common for products in the gastrointestinal and narcotic therapeutic classes to be subject to this type of "exceeds time duration or quantity dispensed" criteria. For example, a profile of a patient who has been receiving a proton pump inhibitor for several months is flagged by the computer for DUR review and intervention based on the "exceeds appropriate duration of use" criteria edit. This product-centered approach does not cross-match to the diagnosis or procedural claims codes present that indicate a history of severe erosive esophagitis or gastric surgery. In most cases, the drug is being used appropriately; however, the DUR reviewer is forced into a specific drug product-based review that does not take into account the complete clinical status or history of that patient. The results of this approach are numerous, including unwarranted physician inquiries and interventions that are strictly drug product utilization-based and not clinically relevant (**Figure 18-9**).

Shifting to a patient-centered DUR approach involves identifying populations of individuals at high-risk or with a history of adverse events due to inappropriate drug and medical service utilization. Inappropriate utilization can involve over- or under-utilization of drugs, contraindicated adjunctive drug therapy, or concomitant disease presence that

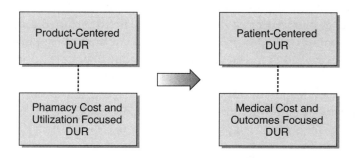

FIGURE 18-9 Shift to Patient-Centered Drug Utilization Review (DUR).
Source: Southeastern Consultants, Inc., 2007.

predisposes patients to increased risk. These adverse events may have been documented in the claims data or may be events that are anticipated to occur immediately or that may occur in the near or distant future. A broader definition of the term *adverse event* should be applied to include any preventable progression of disease or development of a related co-morbidity (**Table 18-2**).

Furthermore, DUR criteria should be defined in the context of the subpopulation that is being targeted for review and then applied only to that specific group. The defined subset of the health plan population could have specific DUR criteria developed that focus on an area of known concern regarding drug use. For example, elderly patients at high risk or with a prior history of falls and resulting bone fractures could be screened for use of drugs that potentially cause additional falls and fractures. This may include excessive dosages or improper selection of drugs in the therapeutic categories of benzodiazepines and sedatives. Other DUR criteria may involve identifying patients with a specific disease (e.g., diabetes or congestive heart failure) to determine whether there is appropriate selection and prescribing of drugs, in the right combinations and dosages, based on established medical guidelines (**Table 18-3**).

TABLE 18-2 Drug Utilization Review Criteria Compared

Product-Centered DUR Criteria	Patient-Centered DUR Criteria
Use of gastrointestinal (GI) agent for more than 8 weeks	Use of GI agent with absence of GI diagnosis or concurrent nonsteroidal anti-inflammatory (NSAID)drug use
Therapeutic duplication of two selective serotonin reductase inhibitors (SSRIs)	Uncoordinated care + presence of multiple prescribers, new inpatient mental health visits, or increased office visits
Excessive refills of inhaled beta-agonist	Absence of inhaled corticosteroids + presence of emergency department visits

Source: Southeastern Consultants, Inc., 2007.

TABLE 18-3 Diagnosis Criteria for Patient Identification

Population Segment	Service Categories	Criteria
Age greater than 70 and a nursing home resident	Inpatient hospital, physician office/clinic, and pharmacy	Diagnosis code with fall or fracture + use of benzodiazepine or sleep agent in past six months
Female 14 to 45 years old	Physician office/clinic, and pharmacy	Diagnosis code of pregnancy or related diagnosis + use of any specific teratogenic drugs by generic or therapeutic class codes

Source: Southeastern Consultants, Inc., 2007.

Software programming for this type of patient-centered DUR is more complex and should include criteria for predefined diagnosis and procedure codes in addition to therapeutic drug code criteria parameters. The programming also should accommodate input variables for demographic criteria such as age, race, and gender. Following the criteria selection and input, all the criteria are then matched against the claims data to target those selected high-risk, high utilization, and/or high cost patients. Interventions can then be performed with the providers caring for those patients in an effort to prevent significantly probable untoward events and enhance the overall disease management process.

MANAGED CARE EXPANSION

Legislation was passed—the Federal Balanced Budget Act (BBA) of 1997—that made significant changes to the Medicaid program by providing states more opportunities to enroll patients in managed care without undergoing the burdensome process of obtaining waivers. Under the new provisions of the BBA, states have been able to mandate enrollment of patients into managed care or primary care management without a waiver. The BBA guidelines provide assurances of access and quality of care as well as address marketing of managed care plans and enrollment requirements.

Medicaid managed care will continue to evolve and expand as states embrace reform in the next few years and implement provisions of the Deficit Reduction Act of 2005 (DRA). The expanded enrollment to include long-term care, the chronically ill, and the medically complex populations will further necessitate the implementation of an integrated and comprehensive disease and care management model.

REFERENCES

1. Smith V., Gifford K., Ellis E., et al., Kaiser Commission on Medicaid and the Uninsured, Low Medicaid Spending Growth Amid Rebounding State Revenues, October 2006. Available at http://www.kff.org/medicaid/upload/7569.pdf. Accessed 11 July 2008.
2. CMS Office of Public Affairs. "Medicaid Spending Projections Down Again, Reflecting Effective Federal and State Steps to Slow Spending Growth," CMS Fact Sheet, July 11, 2006. Available at http://www.cms.hhs.gov/apps/media/press/release.asp?Counter=1895. Accessed 11 July 2008.
3. Finance Systems and Budget Group, of the Centers for Medicare and Medicaid Services, 2006 Medicaid Managed Care Enrollment Report as of June 30, 2006. Available at http://www.cms.hhs.gov/MedicaidDataSourcesGenInfo/Downloads/mmcer06.pdf. Accessed 11 July 2008.
4. Department of Health and Human Services, Centers for Medicare & Medicaid Services, GPO Access, The *Federal Register* Main Page; 2007; 72(16). Available at http://www.gpoaccess.gov/fr/index.html. Accessed 11 July 2008.
5. Smith V., Gifford K., Kramer S., Kaiser Commission on Medicaid and the Uninsured, Implications of the Medicare Modernization Act for States: Observations from a Focus Group Discussion with Medicaid Directors. January 2005. Available at http://www.kff.org/medicaid/upload/Implications-of-the-Medicare-Modernization-Act-for-States-Observations-from-a-Focus-Group-Discussion-with-Medicaid-Director-Report.pdf. Accessed 11 July 2008.
6. Schofield L. and Owens M.K., *The Impact on States of the Medicare Drug Benefit*. National

Pharmaceutical Council, April 2005. Available at http://www.npcnow.org/resources/PDFs/Medicare_Admin.pdf. Accessed 11 July 2008.

7. Rudowicz R. and Schneider A., Kaiser Commission on Medicaid and the Uninsured, The Nuts and Bolts of Making Medicaid Policy Changes: An Overview and a Look at the Deficit Reduction Act, August 2006. Available at http://www.kff.org/medicaid/upload/7550.pdf. Accessed 11 July 2008.

8. Owens M.K., State Medicaid Resource Kit: Maintaining Quality and Patient Access to Innovative Pharmaceuticals in Challenging Economic Times. National Pharmaceutical Council, December 2006. Available at http://www.npcnow.org/resources/PDFs/MedicaidKit.pdf. Accessed 11 July 2008.

9. Sommers A. and Cohen M., Kaiser Commission on Medicaid and the Uninsured, Medicaid's High Cost Enrollees: How Much Do They Drive Program Spending? March 2006. Available at http://www.kff.org/medicaid/upload/7490.pdf. Accessed 11 July 2008.

10. HHS.gov Web site homepage. A Map of State Waiver Programs and Demonstrations. Centers for Medicare and Medicaid Services. http://www.cms.hhs.gov/medicaid/waivers/waivermap.asp. Accessed 11 July 2008.

11. Artiga S. and Mann C., Kaiser Commission on Medicaid and the Uninsured, Coverage Gains under Recent Section 1115 Waiver: A Data Update, August 2005. Available at http://www.kff.org/medicaid/upload/Coverage-Gains-Under-Recent-Section-1115-Waivers-A-Data-Update-Issue-Paper.pdf. Accessed 11 July 2008.

12. National Pharmaceutical Council, Pharmaceutical Benefits under State Medical Assistance Programs, 2005-2006. Table: Coverage of Over-the-Counter Medications: 4-45, 46. Available at http://www.npcnow.org/resources/PharmBenefitsMedicaid.asp. Accessed 11 July 2008.

13. Pharmaceutical Benefits under State Medical Assistance Programs, 2005-2006. National Pharmaceutical Council, Table: Pharmacy Payment and Patient Cost Sharing: 4-56. Available at http://www.npcnow.org/resources/PharmBenefitsMedicaid.asp. Accessed 11 July 2008.

14. Crowley J.S., Ashner D, Elam L., Kaiser Commission on Medicaid and the Uninsured, State Medicaid Outpatient Prescription Drug Policies: Findings from a National Survey, 2005 Update. October 2005. Available at http://www.kff.org/medicaid/upload/State-Medicaid-Outpatient-Prescription-Drug-Policies-Findings-from-a-National-Survey-2005-Update-report.pdf. Accessed 11 July 2008. State Medicaid Web sites accessed 13 July 2008.

State	Medicaid Web site
Alabama	http://www.medicaid.state.al.us
Alaska	http://www.hss.state.ak.us/dhcs
Arkansas	http://www.medicaid.state.ar.us/
California	http://www.dhs.ca.gov/mcs
Colorado	http://www.chcpf.state.co.us
Connecticut	https://www.ctdssmap.com/ctportal/
Delaware	http://www.dhss.delaware.gov/dhss/dph/index.html
District of Columbia	http://www.dchealth.dc.gov
Florida	http://www.fdhc.state.fl.us/Medicaid/index.shtml
Georgia	http://www.communityhealth.state.ga.us
Hawaii	https://hiweb.statemedicaid.us/Home.asp
Idaho	http://www.healthandwelfare.idaho.gov/Default.aspx
Illinois	http://www.hfs.illinois.gov/pharmacy/
Indiana	http://www.indianamedicaid.com/ihcp/index.asp
Iowa	http://www.ime.state.ia.us/index.html
Kansas	http://www.khpa.ks.gov/MedicalAssistanceProgram/default.html
Kentucky	http://chfs.ky.gov/dms/
Louisiana	http://www.dhh.state.la.us/offices/?ID=92
Maine	http://www.maine.gov/dhhs/bms/
Maryland	http://www.dhmh.state.md.us/mma/mmahome.html
Massachusetts	http://www.state.ma.us/dma
Michigan	http://www.mdch.state.mi.us/msa/mdch_msa/msahome.HTM
Minnesota	http://www.dhs.state.mn.us/healthcare/

Mississippi	http://www.dom.state.ms.us
Missouri	http://www.dss.mo.gov/mhd/index.htm
Montana	http://www.dphhs.mt.gov/PHSD/
Nevada	http://dhcfp.state.nv.us/
New Hampshire	http://www.dhhs.state.nh.us/DHHS/DHHS_SITE/default.htm
New Mexico	http://www.hsd.state.nm.us/mad/index.html
New York	http://www.health.state.ny.us/health_care/medicaid/index.htm
Ohio	http://jfs.ohio.gov/ohp/index.stm
Oklahoma	http://www.ohca.state.ok.us/
Oregon	http://www.oregon.gov/DHS/healthplan/index.shtml
Pennsylvania	http://www.dpw.state.pa.us/omap/dpwomap.asp
Rhode Island	http://www.dhs.state.ri.us/dhs/dheacre.htm
South Carolina	http://www.dhhs.state.sc.us/dhhsnew/index.asp
Tennessee	http://www.state.tn.us/tenncare/
Texas	http://www.hhsc.state.tx.us/Medicaid/
Vermont	http://ovha.vermont.gov/
Virginia	http://www.dss.virginia.gov/
Washington	http://fortress.wa.gov/dshs/maa/
West Virginia	http://www.wvdhhr.org/bms/
Wisconsin	http://www.dhfs.state.wi.us/medicaid/
Wyoming	http://wdh.state.wy.us/

15. Ohio Medicaid Prescription Utilization Analysis: Final Findings and Recommendations. Southeastern Consultants, Inc., report to The Ohio Commission to Reform Medicaid, June 2005. Available at http://sec-rx.com/Ohio%20Final%20Findings%20and%20Recommendations.pdf. Accessed 13 July 2008.

16. Department of Health and Human Services, Centers for Medicare and Medicaid Services, Federal Register, 42 CFR Part 423, Final Regulation, Medicare Program. *E-Prescribing and the Prescription Drug Program*, November 7, 2005. Available at http://www.cms.hhs.gov/EPrescribing/. Accessed 13 July 2008.

17. Grossman JM, Gerland A, Reed MD, Fahlman C., Physicians' experiences using commercial e-prescribing systems. *Health Aff.* 2007; 26(3): w393-w404.

18. Department of Health and Human Services, GPO Access, *Federal Register*, 2008; vol 73. Available at http://frwebgate.access.gpo.gov (key word search: Standards for e-prescribing under Medicare Part D.) Accessed 11 July 2008.

SUGGESTED READING

Commission on Medicaid and the Uninsured, *Low Medicaid Spending Growth Amid Rebounding State Revenues: Results From a 50-State Medicaid Budget Survey State Fiscal Years 2006 and 2007.* October 2006. Available at http://www.kff.org/medicaid/upload/7569.pdf. Accessed 13 July 2008.

Deficit Reduction Act of 2005, S. 1932, Congressional Budget Office, January 27, 2006. Available at http://www.cbo.gov/ftpdocs/70xx/doc7028/s1932conf.pdf. Accessed 13 July 2008.

Headen A. and Masia N. Exploring the potential link between medicaid access restrictions, physician location, and health disparities. *Am J Manag Care.* 2005; 11: SP21-SP26.

Holahan J., Weil A., Wiener J.M., eds., *Federalism and Health Policy.* Washington, DC: Urban Institute Press; 2003.

Kaiser Commission on Medicaid and the Uninsured, *Medicaid: A Primer.* March 2007. Available at http://www.kff.org/medicaid/upload/Medicaid-A-Primer-pdf. Accessed 13 July 2008.

Kaiser Commission on Medicaid and Uninsured, *State Medicaid Outpatient Prescription Drug Policies: Findings from a National Survey, 2005 Update.* October 2005. Available at http://www.kff.org/medicaid/upload/State-Medicaid-Outpatient-Prescription-Drug-Policies-Findings-from-a-National-Survey-2005-Update-report.pdf. Accessed 13 July 2008.

Kaiser Commission on Medicaid and the Uninsured, *The Medicaid Program at a Glance.* March 2007. Available at http://www.kff.org/medicaid/upload/7235-02.pdf. Accessed 13 July 2008.

Kaiser Commission on Medicaid and the Uninsured, *The Medicaid Resource Book.* July 2002. Available at http://www.kff.org/medicaid/2236-index.cfm. Accessed 13 July 2008.

Lichtenberg F.R., The effect of access restrictions on the vintage of drugs used by Medicaid enrollees. *Am J Manag Care.* 2005; 11: SP7-SP13.

Murawski M.M. and Abdelgawad T., Exploration of the impact of preferred drug lists on hospital and physician visits and the costs to Medicaid. *Am J Manag Care.* 2005; 11: SP35-SP42.

National Pharmaceutical Council, Resources and Publications, *Pharmaceutical Benefits Under State Medical Assistance Programs.* Available at http://www.npcnow.org/resources/PharmBenefitsMedicaid.asp. Accessed 13 July 2008.

Owens M.K. and Schofield L., State Medicaid Program Issues: Preferred Drug Lists (Conducting a Cost Benefit Analysis). National Pharmaceutical Council, July 2004. Available from the author at mowens@sec-rx.com.

Owens, M.K., *State Medicaid Resource Kit: Maintaining Quality and Patient Access to Innovative Phar-maceuticals in Challenging Economic Times.* National Pharmaceutical Council, December 2006. Available at http://www.npcnow.org/resources/PDFs/MedicaidKit.pdf. Accessed 13 July 2008.

Owens M.K. and Schofield L., *The Impact on States of the Medicare Drug Benefit.* National Pharmaceutical Council, April 2005. Available at http://www.npcnow.org/resources/PDFs/Medicare_Admin.pdf. Accessed 13 July 2008.

Virabhak S. and Shinogle J.A., Physicians' prescribing responses to a restricted formulary: the impact of Medicaid preferred drug lists in Illinois and Louisiana. *Am J Manag Care.* 2005; 11: SP14-SP20.

Wilson J., Axelsen K., Tang S., Medicaid prescription drug access restrictions: exploring the effect on patient persistence with hypertension medications. *Am J Manag Care.* 2005; 11: SP27-SP34.

MEDICARE PHARMACY BENEFITS

DEBI REISSMAN

INTRODUCTION

In the 2006 American Community Survey, the U.S. Census Bureau reported that over 37 million (12%) of the 299 million people in the United States were over the age of 65.[1] As the baby boomer generation begins to reach retirement age in the year 2010, this percentage will begin to dramatically increase. By 2030, it is estimated that almost 20% of the U.S. population or one in every five Americans will be over 65.[2] Not only is the number of older Americans increasing; Americans are living longer, making older Americans one of the fastest growing segments of the U.S. population. Additionally, the U.S. Census Bureau estimates that by the year 2050, the number of elderly (over age 65) will exceed 86 million, more than double the number of U.S. elderly today with as many as 48 million of these (56%), being 75 years or older.[3]

Despite representing only 12% of the population, the elderly used a disproportionate amount of healthcare services and purchased almost 20 percent of the nearly $1.4 trillion U.S. health care dollars spent in 2004.[3] These consumption patterns are expected to increase as the elderly grow to constitute an increasingly greater proportion of the population. To add to the growing cost, during the 2003 legislative year, landmark legislation was passed that, for the first time, brought Medicare beneficiaries a comprehensive prescription drug benefit, expanding the Medicare program (as initially estimated by the Congressional Budget Office [CBO]) by $400 billion over the following 10 years. This chapter describes the history of Medicare and the opportunities and challenges involved in managing a prescription drug program for Medicare beneficiaries.

HISTORY OF MEDICARE

Since the passage of Title XVIII of the Social Security Act in 1965 entitled, "Health Insurance for the Aged," a substantial portion of the medical costs for elderly Americans has been paid by the Centers for Medicare and Medicaid Services (CMS; previously known as the Health Care Financing Administration [HCFA]) through two programs: *Medicare* for physician and hospital care and *Medicaid* for long-term care. Americans under age 65 who have long-term disabilities or end-stage renal disease also receive reimbursement from Medicare; however, more than 85% of Medicare enrollees are over 65. Upon implementation in 1966 more than 19 million Americans were enrolled in Medicare.[3] In 2005, more than 42 million Americans (approximately 36 million elderly and 7 million disabled) received medical insurance through Medicare.[3] Beneficiaries are predominantly white (79%) and female (56%) and more than half have at least two chronic medical conditions.[2,3] In 2004, Medicare benefit payments totaled $295 billion, with Medicare paying 30% of the nation's hospital costs and 32% of home healthcare expenses, but only 2% of prescription drug costs.[3] **Figure 19-1** shows the number of Medicare beneficiaries from 1970 through 2030.

Passed in 1982, the Tax Equity and Fiscal Responsibility Act (TEFRA) was one of the first solutions to curb spending in Medicare. TEFRA gave Medicare beneficiaries the

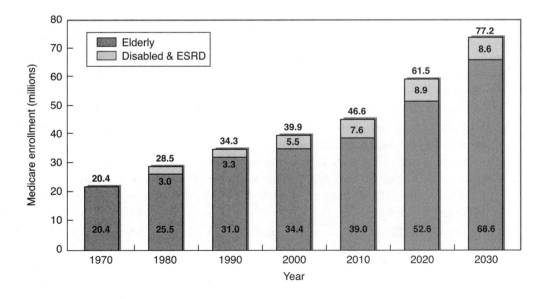

FIGURE 19-1   Number of Medicare Beneficiaries, CY 1970–2030.
Source: Health Care Financing Administration. *Medicare 2000: 35 Years of Improving Americans' Health and Security.* July 2000. Available at http://www.cms.hhs.gov/TheChartSeries/downloads/35chartbk.pdf. Accessed 25 September 2008.

option of enrolling in managed care plans and introduced a true option in medical care to Medicare enrollees. Following TEFRA, the Balanced Budget Act of 1997 included extensive changes to the program and established Part C of the Medicare program, *Medicare + Choice*, creating an array of new managed care and other health plan choices for beneficiaries including private fee-for-service plans (PFFS), health maintenance organization (HMO), and preferred provider organization (PPO) plan options. The Medicare Prescription Drug, Improvement, and Modernization Act (MMA) was signed into law in 2003, creating Medicare Part D (an outpatient drug program), new regional PPO options, and renaming Medicare + Choice as *Medicare Advantage*. In 2005, approximately 4.9 million Medicare beneficiaries (13%) were enrolled in a Medicare Advantage plan with the majority (95%) being enrolled in an HMO and less than 5% in a PFFS or PPO plan.[3] The Department of Health and Human Services (DHHS) estimates that 30% of Medicare beneficiaries will be enrolled in a Medicare Advantage plan by 2013.[3]

COMPONENTS OF MEDICARE

Medicare medical benefits are now broken into four major components: Hospital Insurance (HI; also known as Part A), Supplemental Medical Insurance (SMI; also known as Part B), Medicare Advantage health plan options (previously called Medicare + Choice, also known as Part C), and Prescription Drug Coverage (also known as Part D).

MEDICARE PARTS A AND B

Medicare Part A covers the costs of inpatient hospital services as well as some nursing home, some home healthcare costs, and hospice. Individuals over age 65 who are eligible for Social Security are automatically entitled to this coverage. Costs for the program are paid out of the Social Security payroll deductions taken from employees and employers for individuals with more than 40 quarters of Medicare covered employment. For those with less than 40 quarters of employment, a monthly premium applies.

Part B covers physician services, outpatient hospital services, home health services that are not covered in part A, and other services such as durable medical equipment and ambulance services. To receive part B benefits, enrollees must enroll and pay a monthly premium. Part B premiums adjust based on income level starting in the year 2007. In 2008, seniors with annual incomes that are *less than or equal to* $82,000 for singles and *less than or equal to* $164,000 for couples pay $96.40 monthly. Seniors with higher incomes pay a greater Part B monthly premium.[4]

Both Part A and Part B of Medicare are subject to enrollee deductibles and coinsurance for services received in addition to the premiums paid. For example, in 2008, under part A, enrollees pay the first $1,024 of each hospitalization (deductible). Additionally, they pay a portion of the costs (coinsurance) for hospital stays past 60 days and nursing home stays between 21 and 100 days. In 2008, the Part B deductible was $135 per year for outpatient expenses, with a coinsurance of 20% for most services at the time each service is rendered.[4]

MEDICARE PART C

Medicare Advantage (i.e., Part C), allows Medicare beneficiaries to enroll in a PFFS plan, HMO or PPO rather than using the traditional Medicare system. These plans must offer the same basic coverage as the traditional Medicare program and may offer additional "non-covered" benefits such as eyeglasses, hearing aids, or health club membership, or a reduced monthly premium, and also may charge premiums and copayments for extra benefits provided.

MEDICARE PART D

In 2004, outpatient prescription drugs were offered to enrollees for the first time since Medicare's inception through Medicare Part D. Initially, in June 2004, a drug discount card program became available that continued through May 2006. The comprehensive prescription drug benefit program began on January 1, 2006.

Initial budget estimates suggested that this benefit would cost $400 billion over the coming 10 years. More recent estimates place the cost at closer to $243 billion due to the slowing of drug cost trends, lower estimates of plan spending, and higher rebates from drug manufacturers.[5] The program costs will be offset through member premiums, copayments, and government subsidies. See **Figure 19-2** for the projected cost of the Medicare prescription drug benefit, in billions.

SUPPLEMENTAL INSURANCE COVERAGE

Medicare has limited long-term care benefits, does not cover eyeglasses, hearing aids, or dental care, and until 2006 did not pay for outpatient prescription drugs. In 2002, bene-

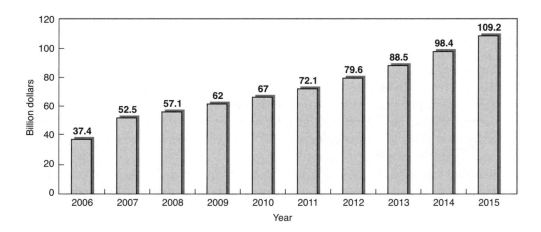

FIGURE 19-2 Projected Cost of the Medicare Prescription Drug Benefit, in Billions.
Source: Rxperts Inc, 2007. Adapted from the President's FY 2006 Budget Proposal: Overview and Briefing charts. Available at http://www.kff.org/uninsured/7294.cfm. Accessed 23 October 2008.

ficiaries paid on average $2,223 (19%) of their healthcare expenses. In 2005, the average out-of-pocket cost for prescription drugs alone was estimated to be $1,139.[3]

Most Medicare beneficiaries have some type of supplemental insurance coverage to help pay for services not covered by Medicare and to cover Medicare's cost-sharing requirements (deductibles and coinsurance). Supplemental insurance may be obtained through an employer sponsored retiree benefit, Medicare Advantage plan, individually purchased Medi-gap policy, or Medicaid for low-income beneficiaries.[3]

HOW MEDICARE RECIPIENTS HISTORICALLY HAVE OBTAINED PRESCRIPTION MEDICATION

Although Medicare Part A and Part B currently cover medications administered while in the hospital or the physicians' office, they cover relatively few medications for chronic outpatient use, such as those used to treat diabetes, hypertension, arthritis, congestive heart failure, lipid disorders, or even Alzheimer's disease. As a result, until 2006, many Medicare beneficiaries ran the risk of having no form of outpatient prescription drug coverage or assistance.

Less than 50% of Medicare beneficiaries had some form of prescription drug coverage in 2002, although over 90% of beneficiaries were taking at least one prescription medication.[3] Of those with drug coverage, 34% of beneficiaries had coverage through an employer-sponsored retiree program, 12% through a Medicare + Choice (now Medicare Advantage) plan and 14% having coverage under dual eligibility with Medicaid.[3] Many of these enrollees may have had only limited coverage. **Figure 19-3** shows the percentages of Medicare beneficiaries with drug coverage in 1999 versus 2006.

While in 2003 79% of Medicare beneficiaries had access to a Medicare + Choice plan, fewer had access to a plan that offered at least some prescription drug coverage. By 2004, due to plan closures and benefit cut-backs, only about one-third of beneficiaries had prescription drug coverage through a Medicare + Choice plan. Of those enrollees, 28% had only coverage for generic therapies, and anther 19% had prescription coverage for only up to $750 annually.[6] Since 2006, the majority of Medicare recipients with limited coverage or without current coverage receive drug coverage through the Part D benefit.

MEDICATION COVERAGE UNDER MEDICARE PART B

Part B covers physician services, outpatient hospital services, home health services that are not covered in part A, and other services such as durable medical equipment and ambulance services. In addition, Part B covers certain self-administered oral cancer and anti-nausea drugs, erythropoietin, immunosuppressives used after organ transplantation, and clotting factors for hemophilia. In general, beneficiaries have a 20% copayment for drugs they receive under their part B benefit with CMS paying for the remaining 80% of the drug cost.[4]

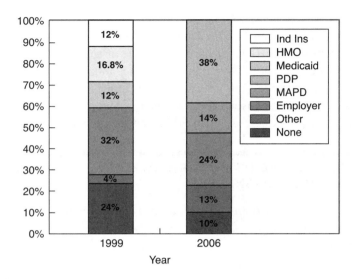

FIGURE 19-3 Percent of Medicare Beneficiaries with Drug Coverage, by Primary Source of Coverage, 1999 versus 2006.
Source: Rxperts Inc, 2008. Based on Program Information for Medicare Section III.A. Page 54, CMS, June 2002 and Medicare Data Update, Prescription Drug Coverage among Medicare Beneficiaries, Kaiser Family Foundation, June 2006. Available at http://www.kff.org/medicare/upload/7453.pdf. Accessed 3 November 2008.

Throughout the 1990s, the Inspector General of DHHS and the General Accounting Office (GAO) studied actual drug prices paid by providers and others, and generally concluded that the Medicare program paid more than other purchasers in both the public and private sectors. These studies also found that prescribing decisions related to the use of Part B covered drugs made by physicians in specialty areas were often influenced by the margin retained between the actual acquisition price paid and the amount reimbursed by Medicare on the basis of average wholesale price (AWP). As a result, Congress decided that Medicare should reimburse an amount closer to the marketplace reality. Thus, in 2005 CMS phased out the previous AWP payment schedules for part B drug reimbursement and moved to an average sales price (ASP) plus 6% methodology, and in 2006 added a competitive acquisition program (CAP) as an alternate system for physicians to acquire part B covered products.

ASP PLUS 6% METHODOLOGY

Beginning in 2005, providers billing Medicare for a covered part B drug only are reimbursed at a rate of ASP plus 6% for the drug product. Additional fee schedules are in place to reimburse the physician for the administration of the agent via infusion or injection. The ASP plus 6% rate for each drug is based on data provided by the manufacturers to CMS on a quarterly basis. The ASP is calculated for each region of the country. ASP incorporates all aspects of product sales, including any rebates, volume discounts, and any other discounts that a manufacturer extends to customers. However, pricing discounts offered to other government programs such as Veterans Affairs, Department of Defense, and 340B pricing are excluded from the ASP calculation.

The calculation of ASP is difficult because multiple discounts and rebates may apply to a single pharmaceutical product, and these discounts and rebates are constantly changing based upon payment, timing, market share, volume and a host of other factors. Although the ASP price is calculated regularly, it is still an average price. As such, smaller purchasers may not have the purchasing power to obtain product at or below the CMS reimbursable amount, creating a dynamic where some providers may believe they can no longer provide certain part B covered therapies without losing money.

COMPETITIVE ACQUISITION PROGRAM

Beginning July 2006, physicians who administer drugs in their offices to Medicare beneficiaries under Medicare's Supplementary Medical Insurance Program (Part B) had the option of obtaining many of these drugs under a new voluntary CAP. The CAP for Part B drugs and biologicals is only for injectable and infused drugs currently billed under Part B that are administered in a physician's office. CAP is a voluntary program that offered physicians an option to acquire drugs from one or more CMS vendors who were selected through a competitive bidding process.[7] For 2006 through 2008, Bioscript, Inc. is the only approved CAP vendor. Beginning in 2009, the CAP program is to be suspended until a new CAP vendor can be identified.

CAP, if re-instituted, would offer an option especially attractive to physicians who cannot purchase products at or below the ASP plus 6% rate, allowing them to provide patient treatment without having to purchase and bill for the product itself. Based on the 2008 rules, once a physician has elected to participate in CAP, they must obtain all drugs on the CAP drug list from their chosen drug vendor until the following year when they can either re-enroll or remove themselves from the program. Vendors are responsible for supplying the product to the physician ready for patient administration and then billing CMS for the product cost based on their negotiated contract. In addition, the CAP vendor(s) is also responsible for collecting any applicable patient deductibles and coinsurance from the beneficiaries. For those drugs that cannot be provided by the physician's CAP vendor, physicians must continue to purchase and bill Medicare under the ASP plus 6% system.[7]

NEW MEDICARE PRESCRIPTION DRUG BENEFITS (PART D)

DISCOUNT CARD PROGRAM

In June 2004, most Medicare recipients, with the exception of those also eligible for Medicaid, became eligible to purchase a discount card that reduced their drug costs by a reported 8% to 61%, depending on the specific drug, card program, and location of the pharmacy.[8] This card program was an effort to provide assistance to seniors between enactment of the MMA legislation and the date the full prescription drug benefit took effect in 2006. As beneficiaries began to enroll in the new Part D benefit, the card program was phased out with a final date of operation of May 2006.

MEDICARE PART D PRESCRIPTION BENEFIT

The new Medicare prescription drug benefit implemented in January 2006 allows all Medicare beneficiaries, including the dual eligible enrollees, to obtain prescription drug coverage by selecting a stand alone prescription drug program (PDP) or a Medicare Advantage Prescription Drug program (MAPD) with prescription benefits. PDPs offer drug-only coverage for beneficiaries in traditional FFS Medicare, while MAPD plans cover all Medicare benefits, including prescription drugs. This new benefit is intended to provide coverage for prescription therapies not currently covered under the Medicare Part A or B benefit, although several categories of agents are specifically excluded from coverage, including:

- Agents when used for anorexia, weight loss, or weight gain
- Agents when used to promote fertility
- Agents when used for cosmetic purposes or hair growth
- Agents when used for the symptomatic relief of cough or colds
- Prescription vitamin and mineral products (except prenatals and fluoride)
- Non-prescription medications
- Barbiturates
- Benzodiazepines
- Covered agents where the manufacturer requires the direct purchase of a test or monitoring device
- Erectile dysfunction agents

While Medicare excludes these agents from payment, plans can choose to include some or all of these agents as supplemental or enhanced benefits, and also may cover over-the-counter agents at no cost to the enrollee.

The specific language of the Part D benefit also excludes any drug that is available under Part A or Part B, although there are multiple examples of agents that could be covered under Part B or D depending on the specific condition being treated and/or how the agent is administered. For example; immunosuppressants would be covered under Part B if the beneficiary received a transplant through their Medicare coverage but would be covered under part D for any other reason; epogen is covered under Part B for ESRD patients but under Part D for all other diagnoses; inhaled solutions for use with nebulizers are Part B, but hand-held multi-dose inhalers of the same active ingredient are Part D.

MEDICARE DRUG BENEFIT DESIGNS

There are 34 PDP and 26 separate MAPD regions.[3] The original legislation states that each beneficiary will have a choice of at least two Medicare drug benefit programs within their region; with at least one program being a PDP. Organizations offering the Part D benefit either as a PDP or MAPD bid to provide services regionally and must bear financial risk for the benefit. If two offerings are not available in a given region, CMS has the option to use "fallback" plans, where CMS will bear insurance risk. In 2008, along with more than 1,800 MAPD plan offerings a total of 1,824 PDPs are available across the 34 PDP regions nationwide.[9,10] In general, beneficiaries in most states have a choice of at least 50 stand-alone PDPs and multiple MAPD plans.

The initial standard prescription drug benefit in 2006 offered an average premium of $25.93 per month and an annual deductible of $250.00. After the deductible is met, the enrollee would pay a 25% coinsurance based on the cost of the prescription for drugs between $251.00 and $2,250 dollars. The beneficiary would then be responsible for payment of any prescription drug above $2,250.00 until the total out-of-pocket expenditures—including the deductible, copay, and full cost drugs—have reached $3,600.00. After this threshold is met, the beneficiary would pay only 5% of the cost of any additional prescription medication needs with the insurer paying the balance. The 2006 program also allowed for subsidies for low-income beneficiaries to offset the costs of monthly premiums, deductibles levels, coinsurance, and out-of-pocket limits, such that enrollees below 135% of poverty level pay no more than $5.35 per brand-name prescription with no premium or deductible, full gap coverage, and no copayment once they have reached the annual catastrophic coverage level.[9] **Table 9-1** shows the initial estimated standard drug benefit under Medicare Part D for calendar years 2006–2013.

For 2008, the base average monthly beneficiary premium is $30.14.[10] The standard benefits were adjusted to a $275 deductible lower than initially estimated, and 25% coinsurance up to an initial coverage limit of $2,510 in total drug costs, followed by a coverage gap where enrollees pay 100% of their drug costs until they have spent $4,050 out-of-pocket.[11]

Organizations can offer the basic benefit or one that is considered "actuarially equivalent" and also may offer enhanced benefits that reduce the deductible, copay levels, and/or monthly premium.

Out of the 266 firms that participated in the 2006 Medicare Part D market, ten companies accounted for 72% of Part D enrollment.[12] Two organizations—UHC PacifiCare (United) and Humana—dominate the Part D marketplace. Seven of the top ten Part D sponsor organizations have a presence in both the PDP and MAPD markets. In 2006, stand-alone PDPs attracted a greater share of Part D enrollment than MA-PD plans. This trend continues in 2008 with 17.4 million enrollees in PDP plans and 8 Million in MAPD programs.[9] The higher PDP enrollment could be due to several factors: Nearly 90% of beneficiaries were in Medicare's traditional FFS program prior to 2006, and stand-alone PDPs are designed to supplement traditional Medicare. Beneficiaries had wider access to PDPs offered by national or near-national Part D sponsors; and more than seven million low-income beneficiaries are auto-enrolled into PDPs,

TABLE 19-1   Estimated Standard Drug Benefit under Medicare Part D for Calendar Years 2006–2013

Calendar Year	Annual Deductible ($)	Average Coinsurance Between Deductible and Initial Coverage Limit (%)	Initial Coverage Limit ($) Program Spending at Limit ($)	Initial Coverage Limit ($) Beneficiary Spending at Limit ($)	Total Spending at Limit ($)	Coinsurance Between Initial Coverage Limit and Catastrophic Threshold (%)	Catastrophic Threshold ($) Out of Pocket Spending at Threshold ($)	Catastrophic Threshold ($) Total Spending at Threshold ($)	Catastrophic Coinsurance Above Threshold (%)
2006	250	25	1,500	750	2,250	100	3,600	5,100	5
2007	275	25	1,646	824	2,470	100	3,950	5,596	5
2008	300	25	1,808	903	2,710	100	4,350	6,158	5
2009	325	25	1,946	974	2,920	100	4,650	6,596	5
2010	350	25	2,115	1,055	3,170	100	5,050	7,165	5
2011	380	25	2,265	1,135	3,400	100	5,450	7,715	5
2012	410	25	2,460	1,230	3,690	100	5,900	8,360	5
2013	445	25	2,666	1,334	4,000	100	6,400	9,066	5

Source: Rxperts Inc., 2007. Based on data from CBO: A Detailed Description of CBO's Cost Estimate for the Medicare Prescription Drug Benefit, 7/2004. Available at http://www.cbo.gov/ftpdoc.cfm?index=5668&type=0&sequence=2. Accessed 15 July 2008.

accounting for more than 40% of all PDP enrollees. **Table 19-2** shows the top ten Medicare Part D organizations in 2007.[13]

Because of the way the new benefit is designed, some Medicare eligibles will fare much better and others could fare much worse under the Part D program. Members with low prescription needs (< $2,000 per year) who currently pay full cost for their medications will likely see a significant reduction in their prescription expenses. Enrollees with significant prescription needs (> $5,000 per year) and limited or no current prescription coverage will also see a reduction in their overall drug expenses. However, enrollees with moderate expenses ($2000–$4000) may find themselves trapped within the 100% payment gap and pay as much or more than they did prior to the benefit. Additionally, enrollees with generous drug benefits today through a retiree program or other insurance will likely see an increase in the amount they pay towards their prescriptions if their current programs are phased out in favor of the Part D benefit. To minimize the reduction of enhanced benefits offered by employer retiree programs, tax-free subsidies are available to employers who maintain drug coverage for retirees.

In future years, the deductible, annual limit, and out-of-pocket expense limits will continue to be adjusted based on the annual percentage increase in the average per-capita expenditure for prescription drugs for all Medicare beneficiaries. Medicare beneficiaries are able to access Web-based tools through the CMS Web site to assist them in determining their potential savings under the new Part D program, compare their benefits and costs based on plan options available to them, and assist with completing the enrollment process.

TABLE 19-2   2007 Medicare Part D Enrollment by Top 10 Parent Organizations

Plan Name	PDP Lives in Millions	MA-DP Lives in Millions	Total Lives in Millions
UHC-Pacificare	4.65	1.24	5.89
Humana Inc.	3.45	1.09	4.53
Wellpoint Inc.	1.21	0.24	1.45
Member Health Inc.	1.15	0.00	1.15
WellCare Health Plans Inc	0.97	0.10	1.07
Kaiser Permanente	0.00	0.83	0.83
Coventry Health Care Inc.	0.70	0.09	0.79
Universal American Financial Corp.	0.49	0.06	0.55
Health Net Inc.	0.34	0.20	0.54
Medco Health Solution Inc.	0.30	0.00	0.45

Source: Rxperts Inc. 2008, based on data from Overview of Medicare Part D Organizations Plans and Benefits by Enrollment in 2006 and 2007. Available at http://www.kff.org/medicare/upload/7710.pdf. Accessed 25 September 2008.

MANAGEMENT OF THE MEDICARE PRESCRIPTION DRUG BENEFIT

Medicare beneficiaries are highly dependent on prescription drugs to manage their acute and chronic medical conditions. More than 40% of seniors are taking five or more prescription agents and 54% visit more than one physician to manage their various illnesses.[3] Management of the prescription drug process is important to plan sponsors not only because providing prescription drug coverage to seniors is a major expense but, more importantly, because adequate use of medications can reduce the costs of other medical care such as hospitalizations.

Under an unmanaged prescription drug delivery system, seniors do not receive the monitoring, education, and consultation about their prescriptions that they need. This lack of education can harm seniors' health and cost billions of dollars. In the mid-1990s, the GAO cited pharmacists for not providing better utilization review of beneficiaries' medications. A GAO study found that close to 20% of Medicare patients were using at least one prescription drug that was potentially unsuitable.[13]

To manage the financial risk under the new benefit, plans will need to rely on two areas: reduced drug prices and strong utilization management. Plans are encouraged to secure rebates, discounts, or other price concessions from drug manufacturers through negotiations. Beneficiaries are to be offered access to the negotiated prices in the form of subsidies, lower premiums, or lower copayments at the point of sale. Plans will be required to disclose their aggregate price concessions, not rebates, on an individual drug-by-drug basis. Under the Part D benefit, any discounts offered to plans on products covered under their benefit program will not be subject to Medicaid best price. As a result, CMS expects that prices offered by pharmaceutical manufacturers to program sponsors will be lower than what is currently offered to State Medicaid programs. This assumption may or may not be realized as the program progresses.

To manage utilization, plans may use formularies, tiered copay structures, mail-order service, prior authorization, step therapy, mandatory generics, and other techniques to manage the financial risk of the benefit. However, the actual benefit design offered must pass a CMS-enforced "actuarial equivalence" test to assure the benefit is not actuarially different from the standard Part D drug benefit.

DRUG FORMULARIES

The new Medicare drug benefit expressly permits the use of drug formularies by plans that offer the drug benefit. The plan must develop a Pharmacy and Therapeutics (P & T) Committee with at least one practicing physician and one practicing pharmacist with expertise in the care of the elderly or disabled and free of conflict with respect to the sponsor and the plan, and with the majority of members being physicians or pharmacists. Plans are expected to review treatment protocols, products, and procedures related to their formularies at least once a year.

The formulary must in general include at least two drugs within each pharmacologic category and one drug within each key drug type as defined and updated by the U.S.

Pharmacopoeia (USP) annually. In 2006, there were a total of 41 therapeutics categories and 118 key drug types. For 2008, both therapeutic categories and key drug types increased to 50 and 192, respectively.[15] Additionally, CMS is requiring that all or substantially all of the drugs in the antidepressant, antipsychotic, anticonvulsant, anticancer, immunosuppressant, and HIV/AIDS categories be included in the plan's formulary. While not all drugs within the other pharmacologic classes need to be covered by the plan, the P & T Committee will be required to base formulary decisions on the safety and efficacy of the product, the strength of the scientific evidence, and standards of practice including assessing peer-reviewed medical literature, randomized clinical trials, pharmacokinetic studies, outcomes research data, and other information as appropriate. In addition, program sponsors may wish to consider "Potentially Inappropriate Medications for the Elderly According to the Revised Beers Criteria" when developing their formulary (**Table 19-3**).[16] USP Formulary Guidelines for Medicare Part D can be accessed through the USP Web site (http://www.usp.org/aboutUSP/).

Plans can add or remove drugs from the formulary during the benefit year but must provide appropriate notice to the membership affected and must provide an exception

TABLE 19-3 Agents Eligible for Part D Coverage That May Be Inappropriate for Use in the Elderly by Generic Name

A	disopyramide	K	P
amiodarone	doxazosin	ketorolac	pentazocine
amitriptyline	doxepin		perphenazine-
amphetamines		M	amitriptyline
	E	meperidine	piroxicam
C	ergot mesyloids	mesoridazine	promethazine
carisoprodol	estrogens	metaxalone	propantheline
cascara sagrada	ethacrynic acid	methocarbamol	propoxyphene and
chlorpheniramine		methyldopa	combination
chlorpropamide	F	methyldopa-	products
chlorzoxazone	fluoxetine	hydrochlorothiazide	
clonidine		methyltestosterone	
cyclandelate	G		R
cyproheptadine	guanadrel	N	reserpine
	guanethidine	nifedipine	
D		nitrofurantoin	
dessicated thyroid	H		T
dexchlorpheniramine	hydroxyzine	O	thioridazine
dicyclomine	hyoscyamine	orphenadrine	ticlopidine
digoxin		oxaprozin	trimethobenzamide
dipyridamole	I	oxybutynin	tripelennamine
	indomethacin		
	isoxsuprine		

Sources: Rxperts, Inc., 2007. Based on Beers Criteria for potentially inappropriate medication use in older adults; Frick D.M., Cooper J.W., Wade W.E., et al. Updating the Beers criteria for potentially inappropriate medication use in older adults. *Arch Intern Med.* 2003; 163(122): 2716-2724.

process to members to request coverage of non-formulary agents as well as deviations from step protocols or standard copayment levels due to medical necessity.

PHARMACY NETWORK

Under the Part D benefit, program sponsors are to secure the participation of pharmacies within their network that distribute drugs directly to patients in a sufficient number to make access to covered benefits convenient for the beneficiary as defined by the Secretary of the DHHS. Plans must include any pharmacy willing to participate under the network terms with at least 90% of beneficiaries living on average within two miles of a pharmacy in urban service areas, five miles in suburban areas, and 15 miles in rural areas. Plans must permit enrollees to receive the same benefits through any network pharmacy (mail or retail) with any higher charges through the retail pharmacy to be paid by the beneficiary. Organizations offering Part D benefits also must include a sufficient number of pharmacies that can provide medications in packaging specific for long-term care facilities and intravenous products for home care administration.

DRUG UTILIZATION REVIEW AND MEDICATION THERAPY MANAGEMENT

Under the new Part D benefit, benefit sponsors need to provide a drug utilization management program, quality assurance measures, medication therapy management programs, and programs to control fraud, waste, and abuse. Mandated drug utilization review (DUR) and the medication therapy management (MTM) program will help ensure that drugs are used to "optimize therapeutic outcomes through improved medication use, and to reduce the risk of adverse events, including adverse drug reactions,"[17] in certain high-risk patients. The intent of these programs is to provide additional counseling and drug use oversight to Medicare beneficiaries with multiple chronic diseases, on multiple medications, and who are likely to incur annual drug costs of over $4,000 per year.[17]

While details of the specific drug therapy management program(s) are left to the individual Part D provider, task groups comprised of personnel from leading managed care organizations, including the Academy of Managed Care Pharmacy (AMCP), have suggested that components of any MTM program would likely include:[18]

- Performing or obtaining necessary assessments of the patient's health status
- Formulating a medication treatment plan
- Selecting, initiating, modifying, or administering medication therapy
- Monitoring and evaluating the patient's response to therapy, including safety and effectiveness
- Performing a comprehensive medication review to identify, resolve, and prevent medication-related problems, including adverse drug events

- Documenting the care delivered and communicating essential information to the patient's other primary care providers
- Providing verbal education and training designed to enhance patient understanding and appropriate use of his/her medications
- Providing information, support services, and resources designed to enhance patient adherence with his/her therapeutic regimens
- Coordinating and integrating medication therapy management services within the broader healthcare management services being provided to the patient

While many of these interventions can be executed in a cost-effective manner through telephonic and mail-based initiatives, there are likely certain interventions that should most effectively be made through a face-to-face encounter with a qualified pharmacist.

ELECTRONIC PRESCRIBING

In an effort to prevent medication errors, lower costs, and improve the quality and efficiency of the Part D benefit, electronic prescribing provisions have also been written into the Medicare Modernization legislation passed in 2003. Part D sponsors are required to comply with e-prescribing standards, must have an e-prescribing program, and must support electronic prescribing once standards are in place.

Initial standards were adopted by CMS prior to the end of 2005 and were subjected to pilot testing in 2006. Final standards for e-prescribing were released in April 2008 with the expectation that all PDP and MAPD plan sponsors will be compliant with the standards by April 2009.[19]

CONCLUSION

As the U.S. population ages, the membership in Medicare plans will increase. There will be challenges in managing the prescription "biotechnology" pharmaceuticals, electronic prescribing technologies, increasing healthcare utilization, and shrinking budgets. Pharmacists involved in managing Medicare prescription drug programs will face the challenges of managing appropriate utilization and must be able to measure how using cost-effective medications can improve quality of care and decrease overall medical costs. The addition of a prescription drug benefit to Medicare by the federal government will create enormous pressures on pharmacy benefit programs to achieve the cost control objectives, but also will create enormous opportunities to the organizations participating in the new Part D program. Additionally, pharmacotherapy in the elderly may present great opportunities for disease management and pharmaceutical care due to this population's greater use of drugs, higher potential for adverse effects and interactions, and age-related alterations in physiology.

REFERENCES

1. United States Census Bureau, *2005 American Community Survey*. Available at http://factfinder.census.gov/servlet/STTable?_bm=y&-geo_id=01000US&-qr_name=ACS_2006_EST_G00_S0101&-ds_name=ACS_2006_EST_G00_ Accessed 15 Sept 2008.

2. United States Department of Health and Human Services, Health, *United States 2007 with Chartbook on Trends in the Health of Americans;* Available at http://www.cdc.gov/nchs/data/hus/hus07.pdf#fig01. Accessed 16 September 2008

3. Kaiser Family Foundation and Medicare Chartbook. Available at http://www.kff.org/medicare/upload/Medicare-Chart-Book-3rd-Edition-Summer-2005-Report.pdf. Accessed 23 September 2008

4. Centers for Medicare & Medicaid Services, *Medicare & You 2008*. Available at http://www.medicare.gov/Publications/Pubs/pdf/10050.pdf. Accessed 23 September 2008.

5. Senior Journal 2008, *Medicare Says Projected Cost of Part D Drug Program Continues to Drop*. Available at http://www.seniorjournal.com/NEWS/MedicareDrugCards/2008/8-01-31-MedicareSays.htm. Accessed 23 September 2008.

6. The Henry J. Kaiser Family Foundation. Medicare Advantage Fact Sheet. March 2004. Available at http://www.kff.org/medicare/upload/Medicare-Advantage-Fact-Sheet.pdf. Accessed 25 September 2008.

7. Department of Health and Human Services, Center for Medicare and Medicaid Services. *Press Releases: Competitive Acquisition Program Interim Final Rule (CMS-1325-IFC)*. Available at http://www.cms.hhs.gov/apps/media/press/release.asp?Counter=1492. Accessed 15 July 2008.

8. Health Policy Alternatives, Inc. Medicare Drug Discount Cards: A *Work In Progress, Executive Summary*. July 2004. Available at http://www.kff.org/medicare/upload/Medicare-Drug-Discount-Cards-A-Work-in-Progress-Executive-Summary.pdf. Accessed 23 September 2008.

9. Hoadley J, Hargrave E, Cubanski J, et al. *Medicare Prescription Drug Plans in 2008 and Key Changes Since 2006: Summary of Findings*. Available at http://www.kff.org/medicare/upload/7762.pdf. Accessed 23 September 2008.

10. Hoadley J, Thompson J, Hargrave E, et al. *Medicare Part D 2008 Spotlight: The Coverage Gap*. Available at http://www.kff.org/medicare/upload/7707.pdf. Accessed 23 September 2008.

11. Center for Medicare & Medicaid Services. *2008 Part D Notification*. Available at http://www.cms.hhs.gov/MedicareAdvtgSpecRateStats/downloads/PartDAnnouncement2008.pdf. Accessed 23 September 2008.

12. Cubanski J., Neuman P., Status report on Medicare Part D enrollment in 2006: analysis of plan-specific market share and coverage. *Health Aff.* 2007; 26(1): W1-W12.

13. Overview of Medicare Part D Organizations, Plans and Benefits by Enrollment in 2006 and 2007. Available at http://www.kff.org/medicare/upload/7710.pdf. Accessed 25 September 2008.

14. United States General Accounting Office. Prescription Drugs in the Elderly: Many Still Receive Potentially Harmful Drugs Despite Recent Improvements. GAO Letter Report, March 1996. Available at http://www.gao.gov/archive/1995/he95152.pdf. Accessed 25 September 2008.

15. United States Pharmacopeia. *Medicare Prescription Drug Benefit Model Guidelines Revisions*. Available at http://www.usp.org/hqi/mmg/revisions.html. Accessed 24 September 2008.

16. Frick D.M., Cooper J.W., Wade W.E., et al., Updating the Beers criteria for potentially inappropriate medication use in older adults. *Arch Intern Med.* 2003; 163(22): 2716-2724. Erratum 2004; 164(3): 298; Comment 2004; 164(15): 1701.

17. Medicare Part D Medication Therapy Management (MTM) Programs 2008 Fact Sheet. Available at http://www.cms.hhs.gov/PrescriptionDrugCovContra/Downloads/MTMFactSheet.pdf. Accessed 25 September 2008.

18. Academy of Managed Care Pharmacy. *Medication Therapy Management Services*. Available at http://amcp.org/amcp.ark?pl=AB430072. Accessed 23 September 2008.

19. Department of Health and Human Services, Centers for Medicare and Medicaid Services. *e-Prescribing Overview*. April 2008. Available at http://edocket.access.gpo.gov/2008/pdf/08-1094.pdf. Accessed 25 September 2008.

SUGGESTED READING

United States Department of Health and Human Services, Health, *United States 2007 with Chartbook on Trends in the Health of Americans.* Available at http://www.cdc.gov/nchs/data/hus/hus07.pdf#fig01. Accessed 16 September 2008.

Congressional Budget Office. *A Detailed Description of CBO's Cost Estimate for the Medicare Prescription Drug Benefit.* July 2004. Available at http://www.cbo.gov/ftpdoc.cfm?index=5668&type=0& sequence=2. Accessed 15 July 2008.

Mays J. and Brenner M., Actuarial Research Corporation, Neuman T., Cubanski J., Claxton G., The Henry J. Kaiser Foundation, *Estimates of Medicare Beneficiaries' Out-of-Pocket Drug Spending in 2006, Modeling the Impact of the MMA.* November 2004. Available at http://www.kff.org/medicare/loader.cfm?url=/commonspot/security/getfile.cfm&PageID=48943&tr=y&auid=758027. Accessed 25 September 2008.

THE VALUE OF PHARMACEUTICALS

ALBERT I. WERTHEIMER
THOMAS M. SANTELLA

INTRODUCTION

Over the last century, the advancements that have taken place regarding new and better pharmaceutical products are nothing less than astounding. As a result of almost unimaginable effort, today we have pharmaceuticals for almost every condition, drugs that work quickly or that can be released slowly to extend treatment. As a result of much innovation, we now have drugs that more accurately target the problem site and act with fewer side effects. The real total value of pharmaceuticals, however, comes not just in the form of better acting drugs, but also in other typically unrealized forms. Pharmaceuticals are valuable mostly because they improve peoples' health, but they also aid the entire nation by increasing worker productivity, reducing the number of workdays lost to illness, and most importantly, improving overall quality of life. A review of the various benefits of pharmaceuticals bodes well for the industry proving their history of constant improvement.

INDIVIDUAL ADVANCES IN MAJOR CONDITIONS

Over the past several decades, the progress that has been made in regards to new and increasingly effective pharmaceutical treatments are nothing less than astonishing. Some of these include: an enormous expansion of antiviral medications to treat HIV/AIDS; the creation of new antibiotics such as oxazolidones; a significant improvement in the way asthma is treated; advances in the tailoring of beta blockers, calcium channel blockers, and angiotensin converting enzyme (ACE) inhibitors individualizing and revolutionizing the treatment of hypertension; new antidepressants with fewer side effects; and vast improvements in diabetes treatment. The list continues with countless examples creating a seemingly limitless progression of innovation and more effective pharmaceutical products.

ASTHMA

There are approximately 17 million asthmatics in the United States, and asthma prevalence, morbidity, and mortality are increasing, not only in our country but around the world. Data show that treatment for upper airway diseases is associated with a reduced frequency of asthma-related emergency department visits. There are two major forms of medication for asthma: those that either relieve symptoms or prevent asthma attacks. Both forms of medication aim to avoid permanent damage to the lungs. The introduction of inhaled steroids via metered dose inhalers (MDI) has brought relief for numerous patients and minimizing their complications of long-term steroid use. Furthermore, patients now have the option of taking a pill to prevent asthma attacks. Future research includes treatments that stimulate the production of Th1, an anti-IgE monoclonal antibody (MoAb), which lessens severe asthma symptoms, exacerbations, and the need for rescue medications. Other future innovations are in progress including a promising asthma vaccine against the respiratory syncytial virus (RSV), which could be available in just three years.

FUNGAL INFECTIONS

With the rise in incidence of AIDS and the increasing number of patients undergoing cancer therapy, the number of fungal infections has dramatically increased, fueling the rapid development of powerful anti-fungals. Amphotericin B deoxycholate, the gold standard for the treatment of serious fungal conditions, has been available since 1960. Since then, there have been many improvements; the lipid formulation was approved in 1995, which didn't have the kidney toxic profile of its old predecessor, a factor that had limited its use in the past. Flucytosine, available since 1973, is the only antimetabolite drug having antifungal activity. It still remains in clinical use as a part of combination therapy. Newer classes of antimetabolites have emerged since then, such as the azoles (fluconazole and itraconazole) and the squalene epoxidase inhibitors (terbinafine), with major advantages including reduced toxicity, enhanced efficacy, and shorter duration of therapy. The newest class of agents is the echinocandins, which block fungal cell wall synthesis and are indicated for patients unresponsive to the older agents. Future developments include Pradimicins-benanomicins, which are generally fungicidal, Nikkomycin, a quinone that interrupts the exoskeletal structure synthesis, and Mycopres, a synthetic peptide that acts earlier in the fungal lifecycle than amphotericin B. As our understanding of fungal infections expands and new treatment options become available, the recommendation for therapy is likely to change, offering treatments with less toxicity and greater, more potent fungal activity.

ALLERGIC RHINITIS

Compared to the classic antihistamines, the newer second-generation antihistamines offer a much brighter hope of effective treatment. Their efficacy, lack of side effects, and longer duration of action are significant improvements. These second generation antihistamines have greater, more rapid absorption in the gastrointestinal tract and thus work more quickly and have a longer duration of action. The recent, more improved, third generation antihistamines are as effective as the previous generation but have no cardiac side effects. Azelastine nasal spray was approved in 2000, providing patients with an alternative option of increased convenience.

RHEUMATOID ARTHRITIS

Arthritis and other rheumatic conditions are among the most prevalent chronic conditions in the United States, affecting approximately 38 million people. Arthritis treatments have come a long way since the 1960s. Treatments were first geared towards pain relief but not in preventing the inflammation itself. It wasn't until the 1980s that disease-modifying drugs were made available. The DMARDs work to reduce the body's own defense mechanisms and prevent it from attacking its own cells. Recently, Biological Response Modifiers were developed targeting tumor necrosis factor (TNF), one of the hormones that activates cells responsible for inflammation. One future direction of treatment approaches involves a T-cell regulatory protein called BMS188667 that acts as a potent inhibitor of cells that launch the immune response. Pralnacasan, an interleukin-1β converting enzyme (ICE) inhibitor, has been proven to significantly reduce inflammation processes. Humira (adalimumab) was the first human monoclonal antibody approved by the U.S. Food and Drug Administration (FDA) for reducing the signs and symptoms of arthritis and inhibiting the progression of structural damage in adults with moderately to severely active rheumatoid arthritis.

DEPRESSION

Besides electric shock treatment, antidepressant therapy once included opium and various other addictive drugs. Monoamine oxidase (MAO) inhibitors were the first class of drugs specifically designed for depression. Since then, antidepressants have advanced tremendously and have safer and far fewer side effects. Still, further research is in development for antidepressants with novel modes of action. Under current investigation is the first and only norepinephrine reuptake inhibitor (NRI) in the United States called Reboxetine, which has fewer side effects than selective serotonin reuptake inhibitors (SSRIs) and is safer for the elderly. Also under investigation is a compound that blocks the "substance P" protein, which is believed to be involved in mood regulation.

DIABETES

Insulin was the first, and has remained the primary means of treatment for Type 1 diabetes ever since it was first successfully used in 1922. Diabetes treatment was improved upon with the advent of synthetic human insulin and several different classes of antidiabetic medications. The future brings promise of inhaled insulin and insulin administered in the form of a pill or patch. All of these advances will dramatically improve patients' compliance and well-being. The second-generation sulfonylureas are at least 100 times more potent on a weight basis and appear to produce fewer side effects than the first-generation agents.

IMMUNOLOGICAL DISORDERS

Immunosuppressive therapy is responsible for great strides in the prevention of organ rejection. Corticosteroids have been the backbone of maintenance immune suppression since the early 1960s. The development of azathioprine in 1957 led directly to the use of immunosuppressant drugs in patients with kidney grafts, resulting in the one-year survival of related donor transplants reaching 80% in 1963. The next major advance was the discovery in the late 1970s of cyclosporine, which is now the front-line immunosuppressant drug. The most significant progress made in the past three decades has been with macrolide immunosuppressants, which selectively inhibit T cells. Each of these treatments with various mechanisms of action is effective in treating different types of transplants. Potential therapies target donor antigen presentation as peptide or protein moieties or immunomodulation by highly selective monoclonal antibodies or cell infusions.

SCHIZOPHRENIA

Antipsychotic medications have been available since the mid-1950s and have appeared to help a vast number of patients improve. Though available on the market as treatment for other conditions, a number of atypical antipsychotic drugs were approved for schizophrenia over the last two decades. Clozapine was the first of this kind and has been shown to be more effective than other antipsychotics; however, periodic blood work is needed due to the risk of agranulocytosis. The atypical antipsychotics developed after clozapine have shown a decreased incidence of side effects.

HIV/AIDS

Years into the modern era of HIV/AIDS treatment, which began in 1995 with highly effective AIDS drugs, the outlook for people with HIV infections continues to improve. Expansion of the number of classes of antiviral medications made possible a shift from monotherapy to combination therapy with two or more classes. The revolutionary practice of combination therapy is called highly active anti-retroviral therapy (HAART) and dramatically increases survival and decreases mortality. HAART has, for many, turned HIV into a chronic controllable illness.

INFECTIOUS DISEASES

Treatment with antibiotics essentially began in the 1950s. Over time, antibiotics have revolutionized health care, saving millions of lives and lengthening life expectancies. The newest antibiotics are the oxazolidonones, which have a unique mechanism of antibacterial action and activity bacteria, with multiple resistances to other antibiotics. Linezolid was the first antibiotic agent introduced for the treatment of methicillin-resistant *Staphylococcus aureus* (MRSA) infections, for which there were otherwise very limited treatment options. Currently, daptomycin is being developed and is the first product of a new class of antibiotics called lipopeptides. New antibiotics are being reconstructed from older versions so that they will continue to be active against resistant bacteria. Phage therapy may prove an effective future treatment, a therapy that uses viruses to attack specific bacteria and also has proven to be effective against MRSA. Even with new antibiotics, however, resistant bacteria remain a formidable adversary. Hopefully, with greater patient awareness, increased discretion in dispensing, and use in combination with the development of new treatments, further resistance should be minimal.

LIPID METABOLISM DISORDERS

Numerous medications are now available to help lower levels of cholesterol and triglycerides while increasing the levels of good cholesterol, high density lipoprotein (HDL). Statins, or HMG-CoA (hydroxymethylglutaryl coenzyme A) reductase inhibitors, were a major advancement and have become the most widely prescribed class. They are safe, effective, and convenient. Recently, Zetia® was approved, which has a different method of action than any of the previously available drugs. Future innovations involve the reverse lipid transport (RLT) pathway, which is responsible for removing excess cholesterol and other lipids from arterial walls and other tissues and eliminating them from the body. Two of the agents in this class, ETC-216 and ETC-642, have proven safe and well tolerated at all dose levels tested. Another innovation involves the regulation of elimination and absorption of dietary cholesterol. Three proteins, retinoid, farensoid and liver X receptors, have been identified and act as a biological switch to rid the body of cholesterol and inhibit lipid absorption.

HYPERTENSION

An estimated 50 million or more Americans have high blood pressure. Diuretics, discovered in the 1960s, are to this day an effective treatment option. Other options include beta blockers, calcium channel blockers, and ACE inhibitors. Today, there are many treatment options available utilizing single agents or various combinations of agents, which individualize treatment to each patient's unique medical condition. There has been research in which the genomic region, containing WNK kinases, has been linked to hypertension. Overactivity of these enzymes can expand blood volume and raise blood pressure. This research is paving the way for antihypertensive treatments that utilize a different blood-pressure–regulating pathway.

THE OVERALL PICTURE

Clinicians, patients, and administrators are all greatly affected by pharmaceutical treatment innovations and improvements in the latest therapies and drugs. We learn about these products through continuing educational offerings and corporate promotions as well as reference works and professional publications such as peer-reviewed journal articles. The opinion of clinicians, administrators, and patients concerning these treatment innovations and improvements can be nothing less than gratitude and wonderment.

When we reflect on the progress in most therapeutic areas, we find a record of unrelenting research, improvement, and innovation within the pharmaceutical industry. It has generated a continuing flow of new products that surpass their predecessors in both safety and efficacy. The only logical conclusion to make is that the improvement of pharmaceutical drugs and treatments will continue to progress as an escalating continuum of progress.

INCREASED WORKER PRODUCTIVITY

While there is little doubt that pharmaceuticals for many conditions are drastically better today than even two decades ago, research has shown that better drugs yield significant results in terms of worker productivity. One of the greatest costs associated with illness comes from the cost of lost worker productivity. Days spent off the job and even days spent on the job but in poor health have a tremendous effect on the productive capacity of the nation. A relatively new area of research has found that many classes of drugs reduce the overall indirect costs of illness. As one article stated, "The evidence is very good for about a dozen classes that pharmaceuticals reduce productivity losses caused by respiratory illnesses (i.e., asthma, allergic disorders bronchitis, upper respiratory infections, and influenza), diabetes, depression, dysmenorrheal, and migraine."[1]

The literature centering on the connection between pharmaceuticals and worker productivity is duplicitous. New non-sedating antihistamines have been shown to actually increase worker productivity by 5% when compared to sedating antihistamines. Another study found that improved anti-asthma agents, specifically beta agonists, can reduce the number of school/work days missed by 57%. New and improved antidepressants also have helped people to stay on the job. The use of triptans (serotonin receptor agonists), a relatively new class of drugs used to treat migraines, have proved equally beneficial in terms of increasing worker productivity. The result of better influenza vaccines on worker illness and work lost has been studied extensively; all significant studies have demonstrated the positive effects of influenza vaccine in lowering lost work days.

Clearly, one of the major benefits of pharmaceuticals is their ability to curb illness so that people can work, or control unwanted symptoms so that people can work better. Even more impressive than the numerous articles detailing pharmaceuticals' positive effect on work, other studies indicate that the costs of the new drugs are actually dwarfed by the dollar gains attributable to more time worked. According to one study, for example, "under very conservative assumptions, the estimates indicate that the value of the increase in ability to work attributable to new drugs is 2.5 times as great as expenditure on new drugs."[2]

BENEFITS OF NEW DRUGS/DRUG FORMULATIONS

The advantages of incremental improvements on already existing drugs are paramount to overall increases in the quality of health care. As the pharmaceutical industry has developed, classes of drugs have expanded to provide physicians with the tools they need to treat diverse patient groups. While critics claim that there are too many drugs, drugs based on incremental improvements often represent advances in safety and efficacy, along with providing new formulations and dosing options that significantly increase patient compliance. From an economic standpoint, expanding drug classes represent the possibility of lower drug prices as competition between manufacturers is increased. Additionally, pharmaceutical companies depend on incremental innovations to provide the revenue that will support the development of more risky "block-buster" drugs. Policies aimed at curbing incremental innovation ultimately will lead to a reduction in the overall quality of existing drug classes and may ultimately curb the creation of novel drugs.

CARDIOVASCULAR DRUG IMPROVEMENTS

Whether an ACE inhibitor, beta blocker, or calcium channel blocker to reduce blood pressure, an antiplatelet agent to prevent clotting, or a statin to lower cholesterol, pharmaceuticals constitute a critical part of cardiovascular disease (CVD) prevention. Among the literature are countless examples of the cost-effectiveness of the various drugs used to prevent CVD.

Pharmacological interventions are principally employed to reduce the known risk factors. These agents include those to reduce blood pressure, the cholesterol and triglyceride agents, and those to prevent platelet aggregation. There is more recent literature, although based on less evidence, to use anti-inflammatory agents and folic acid.

STATINS

The use of statins to lower lipid levels represents a major breakthrough in the prevention of CVD. The effectiveness of the class as a whole has been studied and proven. For example, early clinical trials indicated that statin therapy resulted in a 13% reduction in CHD mortality and a 10% decrease in total mortality. Additionally, it has been found that statins are effective in reducing overall low density lipoprotein-C (LDL-C) levels by 20% to 46% while increasing HDL-C levels by 5% to 10%.

There is little doubt then, that the use of statin therapy in at-risk patients can reduce the prevalence of CVD and extend life expectancy, but at what cost? While there is no consensus on the value of human life, the cost effectiveness of pharmaceuticals is often measured in the cost for one year-of-life-saved (YOLS). Very generally, experts have indicated that medications that cost less than $40,000 are affordable while those of $75,000 are not. Many studies have found statins to be cost-effective. For example, a 1989 study found that treatment with low-dosage lovastatin cost $20,000 per YOLS.[3] The cost of statin therapy, however, is quite diverse as well as dependent on individual risk factors. In one examination of many cost-effectiveness studies involving statins, it was found that the YOLS ranged from $1,800 to $40,000 in patients with pre-existing coronary artery disease (CAD) and from $15,000 to $1 million for patients without pre-existing CAD.[4] Nevertheless, the great majority of studies indicate that statins are cost-effective and reduce the overall risk of CVD by 23% to 36%.[5,6]

ANTIHYPERTENSIVES

The cost effectiveness of the various drugs, including ACE inhibitors, beta blockers, and calcium channel blockers, is undisputed. As one article states, "[beta]-Blockers have been well investigated and have demonstrated positive outcomes related to the prevention of cerebrovascular events and in those patients with compelling indications such as prior MI or heart failure . . . The profile of calcium channel antagonists also includes evidence of risk reduction in controlled trials of ISH . . . As a class, ACE inhibitors provide an antihypertensive option that is well tolerated, is applicable to indications such as diabetic nephropathy, heart failure and post-MI [myocardial infarction] conditions, and requires an uncomplicated administration regimen."[7] Indeed, many studies have demonstrated the cost effectiveness of antihypertensive therapies. In particular, MacMahon et al. reviewed 17 different studies and found that blood pressure reduction of 5.8 mm Hg led to a 38% reduction in fatal and nonfatal stroke, an 8% reduction in coronary heart disease, and an 11% reduction in total mortality.[8] Similarly, the Framingham Heart Study found that long-term treatment of hypertension significantly reduced the CVD mortality rate in men from 43% to 31% and in women from 34% to 21%.[9] These results appear with great consistency within the literature, where controlling blood pressure generally results in a 20% reduction in the incidence of CHD and a 37/38% reduction in stroke.[10] The cost savings of antihypertensive treatments has been demonstrated as well. In one trial, for example, that examined the cost-effectiveness of beta blocker therapy with either metoprolol or carvedilol in addition to conventional therapy for patients with heart failure, the incremental cost-effectiveness ratio was found to be $8,394 per life-year gained (LYG).[11] In a study using data from the Randomized Aldactone Evaluation Study (RALES), it was found that "spironolactone therapy during the first 35 months of follow-up in RALES increased quality-adjusted survival time without increasing costs."[12] Another study found that aldosterone blockade with eplerenone decreased mortality in patients with left ventricular systolic dysfunction and heart failure after acute myocardial infarction, with cost-effectiveness ratios among three data sets including the Framingham Heart Study, the Saskatchewan Health database, and the Worcester Heart Attack Registry, at $13,718, $21,876, and $10,402 per LYG, respectively.[13] In yet another study, treatment with ACE inhibitors reduced the number and length of hospital stays, thus reducing costs. That study also indicated that many prime candidates for treatment with ACE inhibitors go without them. Furthermore, the study suggested that if treatment with ACE inhibitors increased from 55% to 80% of all chronic heart failure (CHF) patients, a cost savings of $615 per patient would result.[14]

Studies examining ACE inhibitors such as ramipril and perindopril have demonstrated the multiple ways in which such drugs are cost effective. Pharmacoeconomic analyses conducted through the Heart Outcomes Prevention Evaluation (HOPE) study as well as the EUROPA study indicated that cost savings through ACE intervention can accrue due to savings based on cost per life-year gained, savings from reduced hospitalizations costs, and savings from an overall reduction in CVD risk.

In an economic evaluation of the HOPE study in Germany, conducted from the Statutory Health Insurance (SHI) perspective, the goal was set to determine the cost effectiveness of ramipril versus placebo, when added to the medication regimen of high risk patients. The study was conducted for both a general population sample and a subgroup of patients with diabetes. The study found, after 4.5 years, that the incremental-cost effectiveness ratio of ramipril versus placebo was $3,585 and $2,187 per LYG for the respective population samples. These results led to the conclusion that "ramipril is likely to be cost effective in secondary prevention of cardiovascular events from the perspective of the SHI (third party payer)."[15] In another economic evaluation of data from the HOPE study, the analysts looked at the connection between ramipril and hospital costs. Compared to placebo, the study found that hospital costs were reduced for patients in the ramipril group.[16] Still a third study, also based on the HOPE study, was conducted to estimate the direct cost savings attributable to the decreased risk of stroke associated with ramipril. Among the studies findings was that ramipril reduced the risk of stroke by 32% for high risk cardiovascular patients. Further, the study found that after four years, the use of ramipril resulted in 21 fewer strokes among the sample group at a cost savings of $52,861.[17] In a similar evaluation, the EUROPA study conducted by the European Society of Cardiology found that treatment with perindopril among high risk patients reduced the risk of cardiovascular events by 20%. Accordingly, economic considerations were taken into consideration to determine the costs per LYG for patients in the Netherlands, France, Italy, and Poland. The study concluded that, with a range of 2,536 to 8,904 (euros)/LYG, the use of perindopril was cost effective for all countries examined.[18]

ANTIPLATELETS

As with other CVD therapy options, the use of antiplatelets to avoid MI and stroke has proven to be very cost effective. A host of studies have been aimed at comparing the respective cost-effectiveness of various antiplatelet options as well as combination therapy. For example, a series of randomized controlled trials was conducted, aimed at determining the cost effectives of using clopidogrel in addition to aspirin to prevent cardiovascular events. The prospective studies, Clopidogrel in Unstable Angina to Prevent Recurrent Events (CURE), Percutaneous Coronary Intervention sub study of CURE (PCI-CURE), and Clopidogrel for the Reduction of Events During Observation (CREDO) each demonstrated the utility of prevention using antiplatelet therapy. The studies concluded that the cost per YOLS were $6,173, $$5,910, and $3,685, respectively.[19] Studies aimed solely at the use of aspirin have shown it to be an effective strategy as well. One study, for example, found that the use of aspirin to prevent MI in patients with a history of unstable angina saved from $5,703 to $5,761 per avoided event.[20] Whether a single or combination therapy, it is generally recognized that the use of antiplatelets ultimately reduces the risk of thrombotic events, particularly stroke and MI, by about 25%.[21]

ADVANCES IN DRUG FORMULATIONS

Since the dawn of modern medicine, there has been a continual search for new, improved ways to administer medicinal products. An early example is the invention of the syringe during the Civil War in the United States, which enabled intravenous morphine injections for the quick relief of pain. Over the last 50 years, drug delivery technology has been considerably enhanced. The 1950s brought the first microencapsulated drug particles, and in the 1960s polymers began to be utilized to deliver drug products into the body. By the 1980s, transdermal delivery became a reality; transepithelial delivery systems were developed in the 1990s. The current decade has seen the advent of liposomal systems for the delivery of peptides and other large molecule drugs and biologics.

These novel drug delivery methods offer substantial clinical advantages, including "reducing dosing frequency and improved patient compliance; minimized . . . fluctuation of drug concentrations and maintenance of drug concentrations within a desired range; localized drug delivery; and the potential for reduced side effects.[22]

Although tablets, capsules, ointments, aerosols, injectables, and liquids remain the primary modes of drug delivery, they are increasingly enhanced by and embedded with technology that allows them to work at a desired rate of delivery, sustain drug concentration within an optimal therapeutic range, maximize the efficacy-dose relationship, minimize frequent dosing, and improve patient adherence.[23]

The principal drawback of traditional forms of dosage is the lack of control of delivery, which can lead to a number of undesired results. For many drugs, rapid release equates to fast absorption and while this is often necessary or intended, it also may increase adverse effects or require frequent dosing. By controlling the rate at which the drug is released, advanced dosage systems can reduce the number of necessary doses, making a drug more convenient, which tends to enhance adherence and effectiveness.

Transdermal delivery is one approach to achieving controlled release of medication. In avoiding hepatic first-pass metabolism, transdermal patches allow drug delivery over longer periods of time. Transdermal patches also enable more efficient delivery of drugs with limited oral bioavailability. Patch formulations now are available for a wide variety of medications, including birth control and smoking cessation medications, fentanyl, clonidine, nitroglycerin, lidocaine, oxybutynin, and testosterone. In many of these cases, transdermal delivery is preferable to oral administration because it lessens the side effects these drugs sometimes cause.

PHILANTHROPIC EFFORTS

In recent years, the pharmaceutical industry has been severely criticized with respect to its philanthropic efforts. On the contrary, pharmaceutical companies not only engage in philanthropy on a large scale but when compared to other major industries in the United States, lead the way both in monetary and product donations. A numerical analysis of the state of philanthropy in the United States shows that the pharmaceutical industry contributes a major portion of its resources to societal improvement annually both here and abroad. The common belief is that large industries simply donate money or large quantities of goods to impoverished or ailing people. While this is certainly true in most cases, the pharmaceutical industry goes beyond this type of charity. Pharmaceutical companies do provide money and medicine to those in need but, perhaps more importantly, they provide training to recipients so that their donations will be used with maximum effectiveness. The pharmaceutical industry spends about $30 billion a year on research and development. The industry has established guidelines and is currently and constantly engaged in a debate to improve the quality and effectiveness of drug donation programs. Many pharmaceutical companies have divisions of their companies devoted to philanthropy. This analysis of pharmaceutical philanthropy will show that the pharmaceutical industry is highly active and generous in its charitable contributions.

According to a year 2000 Annual Conference Board Study,[24] pharmaceutical companies donated approximately $882.7 million U.S. dollars; $242.4 million dollars of that amount was donated as hard cash while $640.2 million was donated in the form of medicine, some as drugs and some as medical training. Total pharmaceutical profits for this same year totaled $6.8 billion. This means that the pharmaceutical industry gave away approximately 12% of its annual income to philanthropic activities.[25] Obviously, some companies contribute more than others. **Table 20-1** shows the donations of five of the largest pharmaceutical manufacturers in 1999.

The pharmaceutical industry is one of America's top industries not only in terms of profitability and new product development but also in terms of philanthropic activity. Indeed, the pharmaceutical industry leads U.S. industry in charitable giving despite that it is a relatively small industry compared to many others. The industry donates significantly

TABLE 20-1   Top Five Pharmaceutical Company Donors

Pharmaceutical Company	Donations (millions)
1. Merck	$190.3
2. Johnson and Johnson	$146.3
3. Pfizer	$106.3
4. Eli Lilly	$102.8
5. Proctor & Gamble	$ 60.6

Source: The Taft Group, published in the 1999 edition of *Giving USA—An Annual Report on Philanthropy.*

to developing nations where their assistance is most desperately needed. It also has established organizations and guidelines to make the donation process more efficient and effective. Finally, the pharmaceutical industry's philanthropic history is progressive. It is expected that American pharmaceutical companies will continue to develop their philanthropy programs and increasingly donate larger amounts of resources in both cash and product worldwide, which will make our world a healthier place to live.

IMPROVING QUALITY OF LIFE

There is little doubt that improving drug interventions stands in direct relationship to the effectiveness of care and ultimately to the most important patient health indicator: quality of life. New drugs that better stabilize hypertensive patients, control cholesterol or sugar levels for diabetes patients; drugs that help eliminate migraines or stop allergies without unwanted side effects; antipsychotics that control depression; and vastly improved HIV treatments all significantly and positively affect overall quality of life. In some cases, quality of life may be measured simply, perhaps only better masking a patient's condition allowing them to work or function normally. In other cases, new and better drug interventions may extend a patient's life while allowing them to live more comfortably and healthily.

But the problem remains of how we measure changes in quality of life due to drug interventions. In recent years, many researchers have worked to quantify the impact of drugs on quality of life with bountiful results. Cost-utility studies have yielded many positive results; for example, Warfarin therapy to prevent stroke, immunosuppressive drugs for kidney transplant patients, and mood-altering drugs for patients with depression. As one review of the literature states, these interventions "provide good value in the sense that they produce health benefits for relatively little cost or may actually save money for the healthcare system."[26] But what dollar value constitutes cost-effectiveness? How do you measure the value of extending someone's life or allowing them to live healthier lives? Typically, $50,000 to $100,000 per quality adjusted life year (QALY) is considered a good value. Of course, these numbers are highly dependent on individual circumstances; one might argue that it is worth $500,000 or $1 million to save the life of a child, but unreasonable to pay such an amount for someone over 90 years old. As evident from this exaggerated scenario, measuring drugs in terms of their quality of life benefits often rests on philosophical pretensions. Regardless, it is difficult to argue that the extension of a person's life is only worth so much. Debate over whether particular drug interventions are cost-effective and whether they yield worthwhile results will likely continue, as will the development of still better and more effective pharmaceuticals.

CONCLUSION

The benefits of pharmaceuticals and of the pharmaceuticals industry are in many cases as clear as day, yet in other instances, may be subtle, shown in improvements such as a better formulation, an extended release capsule, or cheaper alternatives. The benefits also go beyond base matters of drug effectiveness as pharmaceuticals directly impact worker productivity and quality of life. The success of the industry can be seen as a benefit as its health translates to greater philanthropic results. Overall, better medicines mean better lives for patients and a healthier nation. Fortunately, these benefits are growing exponentially.

REFERENCES

1. Burton W., Morrison A., Wertheimer A., Pharmaceuticals and worker productivity loss: a critical review of the literature. *J Occup Environ Med.* 2003; 45(6), 610-621.
2. Lichtenberg F., Availability of new drugs and Americans' ability to work. *J Occup Environ Med.* 2005; 47(4): 373-380.
3. Goldman L., Weinstein M.C., Goldman P.A., Williams L.W., Cost effectiveness of HMG-CoA reductase inhibitor for primary and secondary prevention of coronary heart disease. *JAMA* 1991; 265: 1145-1151.
4. Peterson A.M., McGhan W.F., Pharmacoeconomic impact of non-compliance with statins. *Pharmacoeconomics.* 2005; 23(1): 13-25.
5. Beghi E., Frigeni B., Beghi M., et al., A review of the costs of managing childhood epilepsy. *Pharmacoeconomics.* 2005; 23(1): 27-46.
6. Grover S.A., Ho V., Lavoie F., et al., The importance of indirect costs in primary cardiovascular disease prevention: can we save lives and money with statins? *Arch Intern Med.* 2003; 163(3): 333-339.
7. Dunn E.C., Small R.E., Economics of antihypertensive therapy in the elderly. *Drugs Aging.* 2001; 18(7): 515-525.
8. MacMahon S.W., Cutler J.A., Furberg C.D., et al., The effects of drug treatment for hypertension on morbidity and mortality from cardiovascular disease: a review of randomized controlled trials. *Prog Cardiovasc Dis* 1986; 29(Suppl. 1): S99-S118.
9. Sytkowski P.A., D'Agostino R.B., Belanger A.J., et al., Secular trends in long-term sustained hypertension, long-term treatment, and cardiovascular mortality. The Framingham Heart Study 1950 to 1990. *Circulation* 1996; 93(4): 697-703.
10. Pardell H., Tresserras R., Armario P., Hernandez del Rey R., Pharmacoeconomic considerations in the management of hypertension. *Drugs* 2000; 59(Suppl. 2): 13-20.
11. Levy A.R., Briggs A.H., Demers C., O'Brien B.J., Cost-effectiveness of beta-blocker therapy with metoprolol or with carvedilol for treatment of heart failure in Canada. *Am Heart J.* 2001; 142(3): 537-543.
12. Glick H.A., Orzol S.M., Tooley J.F., et al., Economic evaluation of the randomized aldactone evaluation study (RALES): treatment of patients with severe heart failure. *Cardiovascular Drugs Ther.* 2002; 16(1): 53-59.
13. Weintraub W.S., Zhang Z., Mahoney E.M., et al. Cost-effectiveness of eplerenone compared with placebo in patients with myocardial infarction complicated by left ventricular dysfunction and heart failure. *Circulation.* 2005; 111(9): 1106-1113.
14. Glick H., Cook J., Kinosian B., et al., Costs and effects of enalapril therapy in patients with symptomatic heart failure: an economic analysis of the studies of the left ventricular dysfunction (SOLVD) treatment trial. *J Cardiac Fail.* 1995; 1: 371-380.
15. Schadlich P.K., Brecht J.G., Rangoonwala B., Huppertz E., Cost effectiveness of ramipril in patients at high risk for cardiovascular events: economic evaluation of the HOPE (Heat Outcomes Prevention Evaluation) study for Germany from the Statutory Health Insurance Perspective. *Pharmacoeconomics.* 2004; 22(15): 955-973.
16. Ostergren J.B., Bjorholt I., Andersson F., Kahan T., Pharmacoeconomic impact of HOPE. *Int J Clin Pract Suppl.* 2001; Jan(117): 19-21.
17. Carroll C.A., Coen M.M., Rymer M.M., Assessment of the effect of ramipril therapy on direct health care costs for first and recurrent strokes in high-risk cardiovascular patients using data from the Heart Outcomes Prevention Evaluation (HOPE) study. *Clin Ther.* 2003; 25(4): 1248-1261.
18. Niessen L.W., Redekop W.K., Deckers JW, et al., Cost-effectiveness of perindopril compared to placebo to prevent cardio-vascular events in stable coronary heart disease. *European Society of Cardiology Annual Meeting*, Stockholm, Sweden; 2005; September 5.

19. Weintraub W., Jonsson B., Bertrand M., The value of clopidogrel in addition to standard therapy in reducing atherothrombotic events. *Pharmacoeconomics*. 2004; 22(Suppl. 4): S29-S41.

20. Marissal J.P., Selke B., Lebrun T., Economic assessment of the secondary prevention of ischaemic events with lysine acetylsalicylate. *Pharmacoeconomics*. 2000; 18(2): 185-200.

21. Sarasin F.P., Gaspoz J.M., Bounameaux H., Cost-effectiveness of new antiplatelet regimens used as a secondary prevention of stroke or transient ischemic attack. *Arch Intern Med*. 2000; 160(18): 2773-2778.

22. Rosen H., Abribat T., The rise and rise of drug delivery. *Nat Rev Drug Disc*. 2005; 4(5): 381-385.

23. Chien W., Lin S., Optimisation of treatment by applying programmable rate-controlled drug delivery technology. *Clin Pharmacokinet*. 2002: 41(15): 1267-1299.

24. Kao A., *Corporate Contributions in 2000*. New York: Conference Board; 2001.

25. Neumann P., Sandberg E., Bell C., et al., Are pharmaceuticals cost-effective? A review of the evidence. *Health Aff*. 2000; 19(2): 92-109.

26. Burton, W., Morrison, A., Wertheimer, A., Pharmaceuticals and worker productivity loss: a critical review of the literature. *J Occup and Environ Med*. 2003; 45(6): 610-621.

Chapter 21

MEDICATION THERAPY MANAGEMENT

DENISE KEHOE

INTRODUCTION

Medication therapy management (MTM) is an emerging service that is approached from various perspectives and fulfills multiple needs in the marketplace. MTM programs focusing on medication therapy problems show improved clinical and financial outcomes.[1–3] Organizations interested in the future of medication management created a consensus document outlining important features of a sound MTM program as well as operational aspects that an optimal MTM program encompasses.[4] Aligned incentives focus on the patient, thus allowing service interventions to be directed to the best clinical, humanistic, and economic outcomes.

Disease management (DM) and MTM contribute various pieces to the healthcare puzzle. These services provide synergies that otherwise would not be realized with the same impact if applied separately. When DM, case management, and MTM are adopted separately, they create misalignment for payers and confusion for patients. MTM Core Elements for pharmacists and other healthcare professionals have been established by the American Pharmacists Association (APhA) and National Association of Chain Drug Stores Foundation (NACDS).[5] Vendors providing MTM services continue to evolve along with the adoption of services by health plans and various payors in the marketplace. Technology plays an integral role in the success of MTM. The future of health care will be brighter as MTM becomes commonplace. The healthcare synergies created by adoption of collaborative care continue to drive positive clinical, economic, and humanistic outcomes for all involved.

DEFINITION OF MTM AND ELIGIBILITY CRITERIA

The Academy of Managed Care Pharmacy convened a group of stakeholders including PBMs, health plans, stand-alone MTM companies, and integrated health systems to address future features of MTM as well as operational aspects of MTM programs. The document defines *medication therapy management programs* as healthcare programs developed by health plans and other entities that focus on improving therapeutic outcomes for patients. *MTM services* are those components of a MTM program delivered by healthcare professionals.[6]

Eleven national pharmacy organizations created a definition for MTM services, and defined MTM as follows:[7]

Medication Therapy Management is a distinct service or group of services that optimize therapeutic outcomes for individual patients. Medication Therapy Management Services are independent of, but can occur in conjunction with, the provision of a medication product. Medication Therapy Management encompasses a broad range of professional activities and responsibilities within the licensed pharmacist's, or other qualified health care provider's, scope of practice. These services include but are not limited to the following, according to the individual needs of the patient:

a. Performing or obtaining necessary assessments of the patient's health status;
b. Formulating a medication treatment plan;
c. Selecting, initiating, modifying, or administering medication therapy;
d. Monitoring and evaluating the patient's response to therapy, including safety and effectiveness;
e. Performing a comprehensive medication review to identify, resolve, and prevent medication-related problems, including adverse drug events;
f. Documenting the care delivered and communicating essential information to the patient's other primary care providers;
g. Providing verbal education and training designed to enhance patient understanding and appropriate use of his/her medications;
h. Providing information, support services, and resources designed to enhance patient adherence with his/her therapeutic regimens;
i. Coordinating and integrating medication therapy management services within the broader healthcare-management services being provided to the patient.

A program that provides coverage for Medication Therapy Management Services shall include:

- Patient-specific and individualized services or sets of services provided directly by a pharmacist to the patient.[a] These services are distinct from formulary development and use, generalized patient education and information activities, and other population-focused quality assurance measures for medication use.
- Face-to-face interaction between the patient[a] and the pharmacist as the preferred method of delivery. When patient-specific barriers to face-to-face communication exist, patients shall have equal access to appropriate alternative delivery methods. Medication Therapy Management programs shall include structures supporting the establishment and maintenance of the patient-pharmacist relationship.
- Opportunities for pharmacists and other qualified healthcare providers to identify patients who should receive medication therapy management services.
- Payment for Medication Therapy Management Services consistent with contemporary provider payment rates that are based on the time, clinical intensity, and resources required to provide services (e.g., Medicare Part A and/or Part B for Current Procedural Terminology & Resource-Based Relative Value Scale).
- Processes to improve continuity of care, outcomes, and outcome measures.

The 2003 Medicare Modernization Act (MMA) mandates all Medicare Part D plan sponsors to offer MTM services to beneficiaries who meet threshold requirements. Eligible patients in this program must:

- Have multiple chronic diseases (number of diseases quantified by the plan sponsor).
- Have multiple covered Part D medications (number of medications quantified by plan sponsor).
- Incur annual costs for Part D medications exceeding a specified level decided by the Secretary of Health and Human Services.

---

[a] In some situations, MTM services may be provided to the caregiver or other persons involved in the care of the patient. Approved July 27, 2004 by the Academy of Managed Care Pharmacy, the American Association of Colleges of Pharmacy, the American College of Apothecaries, the American College of Clinical Pharmacy, the American Society of Consultant Pharmacists, the American Pharmacists Association, the American Society of Health-System Pharmacists, the National Association of Boards of Pharmacy, the National Association of Chain Drug Stores, the National Community Pharmacists Association and the National Council of State Pharmacy Association Executives. Organization policy does not allow NABP to take a position on payment issues.

Plan sponsors have discretion on how their MTM offering is provided.

There is confusion about the definition and what it implies from the patient's perspective. Patients who qualify with one Medicare sponsor may leave that Part D sponsor and may need to meet different criteria, including medication regimens following various formulary variations, based on the thresholds created by the new Part D sponsor. Confusion to users and providers of the services continues when an unfamiliarity with medication therapies impacting patient care enter the equation.

The path that includes pharmacists in their role of medication experts as part of the healthcare team looks optimistic. The Centers for Medicare and Medicaid Services (CMS) currently allow plans the liberty to decide what MTM looks like within their organization. Plans can define how and by what means their patient members receive services. Most plans currently comply with the MTM requirements by sending out mailers and/or offering telephonic case management services. Plans currently are only required to report eligibility information and limited patient data to CMS. Clinical interventions and improved patient care has yet to be addressed by CMS. Many health plans around the country are concerned that a large percentage of MTM opportunities remain undelivered due to the mismatch of technology systems and the current needs around MTM. Data are not updated regularly; systems are archaic and/or have perverse incentives for case management. Employees cannot fully perform their duties due to decreased access and lack of technology as well as an inability to work with pharmacists, the medication expert. Many case management companies do not require pharmacist intervention when complex medication therapies arise because the current technology does not allow medication evaluation as a parameter of care. The case manager is allowed to use discretion when faced with MTM interventions, including complex drug regimens. Many case management organizations currently underutilize pharmacists to their full capacity. The current manner in which systems are set up does not allow for pharmacist involvement.

PHARMACY FOCUS

Pharmacists continually face changes in the way their pharmacy services are acknowledged in the marketplace. The dynamics facing the practicing pharmacist are complex. There are many areas impacting the pharmacist working directly with patients. Pharmacists spend much of their time dispensing the appropriate product or medication to patients.

In the business model through which managed care organizations (MCOs) and PBMs maintain focus on the medication costs, the dispensing fee has been the only additional fees paid to pharmacies. For years, the profit margins for medications were high enough that consulting patients and clinical and pharmaceutical care were offered as part of the prescription process. The Omnibus Budget Reconciliation Act of 1990 (OBRA '90) non-funded mandate required pharmacies to offer counseling to patients receiving Medicaid prescriptions. Payment for services for these Medicaid patients has been attached to the product dispensed, as the dispensing fee. As MCOs and their PBMs create distribution networks, and competitive margins persist for pharmacies, pharmacy owners are beginning to see the value of pharmacist services as part of assisting with improved profits in the overall business model. The service model is in the early adopter stage. Most retailers remain attached to dispensing the product as the aging baby boomer generation grows in number and the resulting demand on the corner drug store for pharmaceutical products continues to rise.

The senior population is booming in the United States. Patient numbers in this age group are exploding, with most requiring more medications with complex medication regimens. Thus, the need for pharmacist services is growing. Because the CMS adopted senior medication services as MTM, guidance for health plans and payors continues to evolve with pharmacist expertise as an invaluable piece to this puzzle.[8]

CMS is working toward addressing services currently provided by payors to their enrollees. Organizations affiliated with quality, such as the Pharmacy Quality Alliance (PQA), are contributing to the quality solution.[9] Payors are now looking at projected 2009 and 2010 data to define and evaluate the efforts and successes since the inception of the CMS program in January 2006. While preliminary reports are coming in for health plans, self-insured employers are seeing and implementing valuable programs similar to that of the Asheville project[10] and other pharmacist-led MTM programs and services. The future depends on how pharmacists and the pharmacy industry address the immediate opportunity. Health plans and PBMs recognize that their focus continues to be on point-of-sale (POS) edits, step therapy, and prior authorizations (PAs) to pursue quality patient care at the lowest cost. The paradigm shift occurs when pharmacists show the continuous value of their clinical service interventions. The impact is multifaceted and includes humanistic, economic, and clinical outcomes.

MANAGED CARE ORGANIZATIONS

As MCOs reach their goals by optimizing costs while addressing patient needs, pharmacy is underutilized as part of the entire healthcare arena. Many barriers affect the practicing pharmacist's ability to work within health plans. Pharmacists are not considered mid-level providers of services. One example is an endocrinologist who valued the work of a clinical pharmacist and preferred sending 80% of patients in his practice to a clinical pharmacist to monitor their medication therapies. This endocrinologist then had the time to focus on the 20% of patients who needed the immediate skills of the specialist physician.[11]

The number of primary providers continues to decrease throughout the United States. Pharmacists throughout our country are working at a grassroots level to engage payors to embrace them as qualified medication experts and allow pharmacists with clinical expertise to provide services.

LEGISLATIVE

Patients living with diabetes came to the patient care center in which the author practiced and described the work we did together to lower their HbA1c levels. Many patients described that after working with the clinical pharmacist, they now understood their medication therapies. The patients gained an understanding of the value of insulin and how they could overcome the denial they faced by living with diabetes. Many healthcare policymakers may be unaware of the educational level of pharmacists and their expertise as a pharmacotherapy expert. Pharmacy as a profession must continue reaching out to educate our legislators about the enormous value of the profession. Pharmacists are underutilized and have capabilities above and beyond making sure the right drug gets into the right bottle with the right directions at the right time and of course at the right price. In their role as medication experts, pharmacists show cost savings to the healthcare system when included as part of the healthcare solution.

Currently, legislation has been introduced in Congress in the form of House Bill 5780, which would acknowledge pharmacists as providers of healthcare services under Medicare Part B. Practicing pharmacists and others are engaged in medication reimbursement that continues to be scrutinized by payors, including Medicare, Medicaid, and health plans.

ALIGNED INCENTIVES

Pharmacy benefit managers continue to align incentives based on the product: medications (see Chapter 4). While many health plans realize the product is separate from the service in pharmacy, most organizations have not implemented clinical services from pharmacists outside of their health plan. Of those health plans that have implemented these changes, they actualize savings that is over and above what DM and case management have shown to date.

DISEASE MANAGEMENT HISTORY AND CASE STUDIES

Disease management success is a holistic approach based on reaching out to patients and reporting event-driven parameters that include coordinating care, supporting the appropriateness of care, and patients' adherence to the therapeutic plan, to name a few examples. Adherence may be either the traditional view of medication adherence or the persistence a patient demonstrates while adhering to a prescribed treatment therapy that is non-drug related.

Disease management programs, primarily developed by MCOs, usually provide a multidisciplinary approach to patient care. Physicians work with a group of mid-level providers, such as pharmacists, nurses, and behavioral health therapists (psychologists), as well as respiratory therapists and dieticians. These professionals bring an aspect of care to patients qualifying for services. Most services identify patients in an opt-in, opt-out, or a combination of the two programs. MTM services customarily focus on chronic diseases due to the immediate cost avoidance savings shown with healthcare provider interventions. DM customarily does not require multiple disease state qualifications in order to provide the services, as CMS Part D requirements mandate. The theme of DM is to empower patients by educating them to take control of their own health care. Common DM interventions include telephone scheduling of office visits and date/time follow-up reminders.

Medication review and monitoring are areas where DM can assist with the overall care of patients. DM is a collaborative effort with other providers that can measure results of interventions, show outcomes in patient care, and target patients who benefit from the program services. DM ends after the case manager reviews the list of medications the patient takes. A few DM companies transfer patients to pharmacists who then review complex medication therapies. Generally, DM organizations check whether patients are taking their medications and, if so, confirm they are taking medications as prescribed.

Disease management companies may become more effective by including MTM services and medication reviews that focus on increased therapeutic outcomes by raising the level of appropriate medication use that supports the current treatment plan. When including MTM in the healthcare loop, patients and the entire healthcare team benefit by helping patients to reach their goals and truly understand their medication regimens as well as the importance of persistence and monitoring parameters. The scope of expertise a medication expert brings to the table makes a DM program a full-service product offering because the MTM program focuses and probes into the individual's medication therapy. Leveraging technology and objective measurements, including medical and pharmacy data along with laboratory and self-reported data, assists the pharmacist in making efficient medication therapy recommendations and implementing changes collaboratively with prescribers and patients.

The verdict is still out on the success of DM programs. Data interpretation varies based on how the information is evaluated. Health plans and employers are adopting more consumer-based initiatives that incent individuals to take control of their own health care. As health plans embrace the value of medication therapy, the win–win will be seen by all involved, especially the patient.

AETNA CASE STUDY

Many DM companies have prudent and patient-accepted access to healthcare information. When this includes the aforementioned medical and pharmacy data along with laboratory and self-reported data, these companies are able to risk-stratify patients for outreach and target those with a need. Here, the leveraging technology can create the algorithm that standardizes need and the most appropriate outreach strategy.

Example: Drug, Condition Plus Insight   Through using an algorithm that documents appropriate angiotensin converting enzyme (ACE) inhibitor utilization, an integrated system shows the lack of prescription claims for the ACE inhibitor adjudicated for a patient who has a valid diagnosis for congestive heart failure. This algorithm shows the current treating physician who is either the cardiologist, family practitioner, or internist. This sentinel event allows a pharmacist to outreach to the treating physician and validate the need for such an agent. Plus, this interaction adds insight to the lack of medication prescription therapy if the medication was discontinued on the patient's own volition *or* addresses the need for such a product when considering accepted guidelines. This need is amplified when the patient also has diabetes. In that example, metrics of success are the validation of a need for pharmacotherapy, consideration of the specific drug for the individual patient to treat his/her condition, and the resumption of the drug in the patient's drug regimen. Short- and long-term medication adherence would be another to measure to insure that the patient benefits from appropriate utilization.

Example: Drug, Condition Plus Insight Humanistic   In the previous example, an algorithm from an integrated health company pinpointed the need for outreach using an algorithm dependent upon medical, pharmacy, and laboratory claims and data. However, less sophisticated algorithms may only need to center on medication adherence. One such managed care experience identified the lack of drug claims for a member who by drug proxy had a cardiovascular condition. Upon outreach to the patient, the pharmacist was made aware that the spouse, who was the patient's caregiver, recently died. The patient saw no need to refill his complex drug medication. With this information, the pharmacist was able to outreach to the internist and cardiologist to make them aware of the situation, coordinate a continuity of visits and somatic care, plus refer the patient to a behavioral health DM program that dealt with grief for the patient's benefit. All of these outreaches were made possible and merely supportive of the healthcare team's concurrent review because of the proactive participation of the pharmacotherapy specialist.

CLINICAL PROGRAMS

Currently, health plan MTM programs include centralized call centers with combined mailers to patients as a form of service. Many health plans agree that the missing link is the pharmacy component. The one thing patients continue to need and take is their medications. The issue is whether patients are empowered to understand their disease and follow recommendations made by providers. Case management companies provide case managers with the ability to override and decide whether a medication issue is addressed and if the medication therapy should be resolved by a medication expert, when a medication management opportunity appears. Currently, pharmacists are not considered a regular part of the resolution of care. Organizations that include pharmacists have a limited number of pharmacists and still allow case management to make a decision as to whether a patient needs to speak with a pharmacist. However, this is one area where pharmacists have the ability to assist by not only addressing and resolving MTM issues, but also showing a cost savings associated with the interventions. When organizations realize the incredible value of including a medication expert in the healthcare arena above and beyond a dispensing function, everyone will win.

MEDICATION THERAPY MANAGEMENT SERVICES

The American Pharmacists Association and the National Association of Chain Drug Stores Foundation developed a MTM Core Elements Service Model, which includes a workflow diagram depicting how the patient care process integrates with MTM service delivery. The overall goal is to include the pharmacist throughout the process of medication management and engage patients in self-managing their medications. In the model, the medication therapy review is followed by an intervention and/or referral to an appropriate team member. The patient is empowered by being provided with "collateral" that includes a personal medication record and a medication-related action plan, which the pharmacist then uses to document and communicate any future activity, including communication with others involved with that patient's care.

There are variations in delivering the service model but the core elements remain the same (**Figure 21-1**). The dynamic components are twofold: active involvement of the patient and the ability to collaborate with other healthcare providers who interact with the patient. As you can see in the center of Figure 21-1, referrals, interventions,

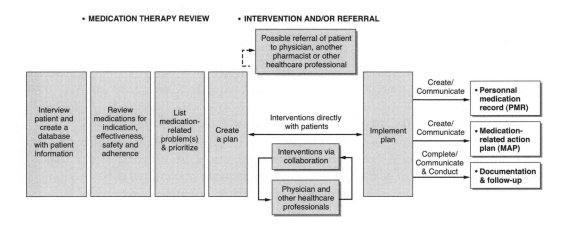

FIGURE 21-1 Core Elements of the MTM Service Model, Version 2.0, March 2008.

MTM core elements (◊) interfaces with the patient care process to create an MTM service model.

and collaboration with providers take place within the model. Overall, the goal is to effectively integrate MTM services into patients' overall health care by facilitating transitions of care to ensure a seamless process.

MTM services are made available to patients from both private and public sector payors, including self-insured employers, state Medicaid programs, and Medicare. Because MTM services are required for targeted beneficiaries in the Medicare Part D benefit, the evolution of MTM under Part D is being followed closely. To date, MTM program providers have used various delivery methods, including face-to-face visits, telephonic interventions, and educational mailings, or a combination of those methods. Most prescription drug programs (PDPs) and Medicare Advantage Prescription Drugs (MAPDs) are providing MTM services to eligible beneficiaries using in-house providers to deliver services telephonically or by sending educational mailings to beneficiaries. A small number of plans contract directly or use MTM vendors to contract with community pharmacists to provide MTM services. Community pharmacists deliver the services face-to-face or telephonically.[12] Developing the evidence to support various delivery methods and outcomes of MTM services will be important in establishing the value pharmacists bring to MTM for payors and other key stakeholders.

APhA compiled two national surveys to evaluate strategies for MTM service implementation and the value of these services to pharmacist providers and payors.[5,6] The pharmacy profession's consensus definition of MTM was used for both surveys, and the delivery models included face-to-face and telephonic interactions, but not mailings.

In the pharmacist provider survey, respondents were asked to indicate the importance of factors influencing their decision to implement or not implement MTM services (**Figure 21-2**). Those pharmacists who chose to implement MTM services did so because of patient needs, their responsibility as a healthcare provider, and the need to improve healthcare quality. Barriers for those pharmacists who have not yet implemented MTM services include inadequate time, insufficient staffing levels, heavy dispensing loads, and difficulty in documentation and billing for MTM services.

Another consideration in the delivery of MTM services is the training/credentialing requirement for MTM providers. Currently, there is wide variation in the training/ credentials required of MTM providers that ranges from no requirements to training on documentation software to completion of certificate training programs or Board of Pharmaceutical Specialties (BPS) certification. Some pharmacists are independently completing certificate training programs and obtaining additional certifications for the delivery of their MTM services. This professional engagement is in line with other healthcare professionals who enhance their abilities by obtaining credentials designed to assess competence. As the healthcare system continues to acknowledge pharmacists' value, pay-for-performance and other incentives likely will be used to assess the quality and consistency of care delivered and provide the support needed to expand these services within the profession.

Reasons to Implement	Reasons Not to Implement

Highest Importance

Reasons to Implement:
- Patient needs
- Responsibility as healthcare provider
- Recognized need to improve healthcare quality
- Contribution to healthcare team
- Professional satisfaction
- Reducing healthcare system costs
- Primary business mission
- Reducing health insurer costs
- Provider needs
- Need for other revenue sources
- Competitive pressure
- Decreased prescription volume

Reasons Not to Implement:
- Inadequate time
- Insufficient staffing levels
- Heavy dispensing activities
- Difficult billing
- Inadequate training/experience
- Cumbersome documentation
- Inadequate space
- Unsupported by management
- Technology barriers
- Too few patients to justify cost
- Difficult to determine patient eligibility
- Unable to collect needed information
- Patients not interested in participation
- Physicians resistant
- Not needed for eligible patients

Lowest Importance

FIGURE 21-2 Factors Influencing Pharmacists to Participate in MTM Services.
Source: Schommer, J.,Planas, L., Johnson, K, Doucette, W. APhA Medication Therapy Management Digest: Perspectives on MTM Implementation. © 2008 by the American Pharmacists Association and National Association of Chain Drug Stores Foundation. All rights reserved. Reprinted with permission. No part of this publication may be reproduced, stored in a retrieval system, or transmitted in any form, or by any means, electronic, mechanical, photocopying, recording, or otherwise, without prior permission of the National Association of Chain Drug Stores Foundation and the American Pharmacists Association.

UNDERSTANDING PAYOR NEEDS

Payors are using a variety of methods to address the need to provide MTM services throughout the country. In telephone interviews of payors known to provide MTM services as a covered benefit, the top three barriers experienced in providing MTM services in the marketplace include: 1) patient's lack of perception of need of the services; 2) lack of physician's and other healthcare provider's acceptance of MTM services; and 3) insufficient providers of MTM services to meet needs. Some payors also expressed skepticism that services would produce tangible outcomes for payors and patients, and concern that costs to implement such services would exceed expected benefits (**Figure 21-3**).

Payors want to implement the best offering for their contracted clients. The most common enrollment strategy for payors in this survey was an opt-out program (44% of payors)

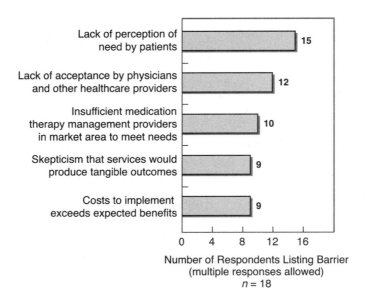

FIGURE 21-3 Potential Payor Barriers to Offering MTM Services.
Source: Schommer, J.,Planas, L., Johnson, K, Doucette, W. APhA Medication Therapy Management Digest: Perspectives on MTM Implementation. © 2008 by the American Pharmacists Association and National Association of Chain Drug Stores Foundation. All rights reserved. Reprinted with permission. No part of this publication may be reproduced, stored in a retrieval system, or transmitted in any form, or by any means, electronic, mechanical, photocopying, recording, or otherwise, without prior permission of the National Association of Chain Drug Stores Foundation and the American Pharmacists Association.

that automatically enrolls eligible beneficiaries into an MTM service benefit. Enrolled patients can then decide, at their discretion, whether they want to participate in the service.

Implementing successful enrollment strategies impact the viability of an MTM program. As payors continue to realize the value of MTM service interventions, people living with costly health conditions will receive medication management as a standard service, just as they currently would receive physical therapy or other mid-level services.

As patients gain an understanding of the importance of receiving valuable medication management services, they become empowered by realizing that their medications are an integral part of their overall state of health.

With limited budgets for all healthcare services, a dual collaborative effort focused on patient empowerment and education in conjunction with medication therapy is becoming an appropriate targeted service among the wide range of services provided within the healthcare system. MTM will continue to show overall savings to the healthcare system when included as part of overall medical care. Payors continue to pursue a variety of models of care for MTM, including: opt-out, where all patients have access; opt-in, where pre-identified patients are eligible; and combinations of the two programs. The verdict as to the best model is yet to be seen (**Figure 21-4**).

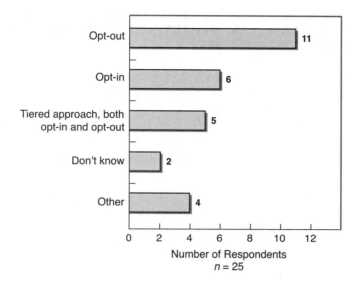

FIGURE 21-4 Payor Attitudes to MTM Enrollment Strategies.

Source: Schommer, J.,Planas, L., Johnson, K, Doucette, W. APhA Medication Therapy Management Digest: Perspectives on MTM Implementation. © 2008 by the American Pharmacists Association and National Association of Chain Drug Stores Foundation. All rights reserved. Reprinted with permission. No part of this publication may be reproduced, stored in a retrieval system, or transmitted in any form, or by any means, electronic, mechanical, photocopying, recording, or otherwise, without prior permission of the National Association of Chain Drug Stores Foundation and the American Pharmacists Association.

QUALITY

Health plans throughout the country strive to obtain an excellent rating from the National Committee for Quality Assurance (NCQA). A higher rating for a health plan affords plans to gain market share from employers who are looking for the best care for their employees. The PQA and other quality-related organizations are beginning to look at quality measures for pharmacy, including MTM services. PQA in collaboration with NCQA released an initial starter set of 15 quality measures and developed template report cards to report quality information to pharmacists and the public.[15] Several demonstration projects are underway to examine implementation of the measures in real-world settings by gathering feedback from pharmacists on the utility of performance report cards.

The quality parameters focus on economic, humanistic, and clinical outcomes. As the quality alliance evolves, the Agency for Healthcare Research and Quality (AHRQ), the NCQA, and the National Quality Forum (NQF) are engaged in evaluating, validating, and endorsing the pharmacy measures to bring greater quality to patient health care.

DISEASE MANAGEMENT/CASE MANAGEMENT/MEDICATION THERAPY MANAGEMENT IN QUALITY INITIATIVES

Disease management and MTM can go hand-in-hand. What better way to assist the system as well as the patient than to allow medication experts to address medication treatment and other DM factors, and then use case management (CM) work with patients to follow up on office visits, obtain labs, and other modes of treatment and care? This is a holistic strategy. Combining Health Plan Employee Data and Information Set (HEDIS) measures with other pharmacist-specific quality measures will allow for effective assessment of the quality of care delivered. As consumerism grows and the demand of care shifts to the patient to be responsible for their own care, pharmacists fill a unique niche as the only medication experts in the patient care loop (**Figure 21-5**).

The health plans in the APhA survey reported variability in the quality indicators used to evaluate MTM services. Some payors relied on HEDIS measures as well as patient

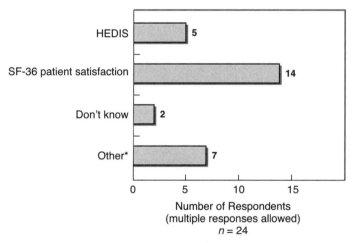

Number of Respondents
(multiple responses allowed)
n = 24

HEDIS = Healthcare Effectiveness Data Information Set.
SF-36 = Short Form-36 Health Survey.

*Other indicators included: the Short Form-8 Health Survey, the number of patients achieving the intended goals of therapy, and measures that were developed internally.

FIGURE 21-5 Impact of MTM Services on Healthcare Quality Measures.

satisfaction surveys in order to assess the success of health plan quality. As the healthcare system continues to incorporate MTM services, these quality parameters and others yet to be developed will become a prominent need when assessing the value of health plans throughout the country.

TECHNOLOGY

Payors are tapping into data. In order to improve performance measures, data are needed. Data are a foundational need for successful programs, including MTM. The days of siloed claims (those claims only used within one division) data are coming to a halt. The three primary needs for an MTM are: 1) integrated data systems to track MTM services; 2) data collection to monitor MTM services; and 3) analysis to compare key areas of care that decrease medical complications. MTM integrated data systems focus on clinical pharmacy parameters and allow pharmacists to make the most impact to the entire healthcare system in their role as medication experts. MTM integrated products assist pharmacists in providing physicians and other healthcare providers the best care to patients. Integrated pharmacy data systems, such as PharmMD, allow pharmacists leverage and electronic information availability regarding patients who need MTM assistance. Important metrics—such as medical claims including diagnosis; pharmacy claims; laboratory data; survey results including health risk assessments; and self-reported data including over-the-counter medications, herbals, and vitamins—allow for informed recommendations to assist patients, prescribers, and other healthcare providers. In turn, this improves overall healthcare quality, increases patient satisfaction for the MTM, and provides cost effectiveness that supersedes current system savings of providers without that information.

Self-insured employers are readily embracing integrated MTM data systems. Change is happening on a grassroots level as employers are finding ways to save money by leveraging technology and pushing the envelope in health care. Health plans already collect claims data. Many health plans throughout the country still have paper medical claims and or several different systems housing their claims data. As the need to streamline patient care increases, health plans are realizing the value of merging the data and warehousing it for future analysis. The unique feature of MTM technology providers is its clinical rule sets that streamline pharmacy MTM and provide collaborative and efficient methods of care.

MTM SERVICES PROVIDERS: CASE STUDY OF PHARMMD

Health plans are beginning to appreciate the value of technology and pharmacy infrastructure. The author is employed by PharmMD, one of the most robust pharmacy infrastructure vendors providing MTM. PharmMD combines state-of-the-art technology that focuses on quality. PharmMD realizes that clinical and consultant pharmacists provide a level of service that is in line with payor needs. The company offers services for Medicare, Medicaid, and other government entities as well as employers and commercial business. Most self-insured employers are getting on board with this concept because of escalating premiums and the realization that pharmacists are valuable and integral providers of services.

PharmMD addresses medication needs based on three basic categories: misuse, underuse, and overuse of medications. Within each of these categories are subcategories outlining specific interventions and drug therapy problems pharmacists intervene and impact from clinical, humanistic, and economic parameters.

Misuse of medications includes potentially harmful high-risk medications taken by the elderly. This intervention type is associated with a dispensing event. A list of high-risk inappropriate medications is triggered and a network pharmacist facilitates communications with the prescriber and patient to convey the clinical rationale for the intervention. In addition, metrics including medical claims, laboratory tests, adverse drug reactions, therapy doses, and patient self-reported data are evaluated.

Underuse of medication includes adherence and persistency. This intervention enhances patients' medication regimen, as intended by the prescriber. PharmMD Solutions focuses on patient therapy (based on a dispensing event) and those patients who are late for chronic medications. The PharmMD facilitates patient consultations regarding persistence/adherence and address persistence related issues either face-to-face or via telephone contact.

Overuse of medication includes polypharmacy. This process identifies client qualified candidates, who are those taking multiple medications for chronic diseases as well as pain management and specialty medications.

PharmMD leverages technology and focuses on providing a quality network of pharmacists as well as a clinical resolution center to provide robust services that empower patients, decrease overall expenditures including hospitalizations, and analyze all metrics available to gain a clear picture of the patient in order to provide the best service levels. PharmMD services sit between PBMs and payors to provide services above and beyond First Data Bank edit messaging, which allows PBMs to send messages to pharmacies upon adjudication explaining information about a particular claim. The services tap into and filter the metric data through proprietary clinical rules, national guideline standards, evidence-based medicine, and client-specific needs.

Figure 21-6 illustrates the cost savings realized for one client cohort over a one-year period. The medication interventions are defined as medication misuse, underuse, or overuse. Patients who fall into these categories are connected with a pharmacist who evaluates the drug therapy problem, and then addresses and resolves the issue on behalf of the patient. The types of interventions vary. Some patients visit multiple physicians who do not regularly communicate about that patient's overall care and prescribed prescription therapies. Many patients have only one consistent, accessible healthcare provider: their local pharmacist within the community. Often patients are not on appropriate medications and even may be taking too many medications. Pharmacists are able to review medication therapies, intervene as medication experts, and empower patients to understand their disease and treatment regimen. Patients take ownership of their individual medica-

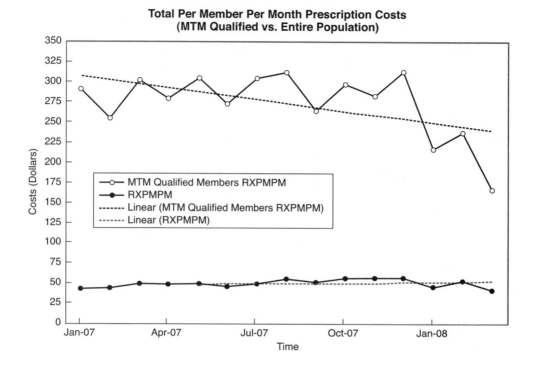

FIGURE 21-6   Impact of MTM Services on Annual Pharmacy Costs.
Source: ©PharmMD, 2008.

tion therapy. Payors traditionally have never realized the value that medication interventions bring to the system and the scope of savings is minimally documented. PharmMD works collaboratively with other healthcare team members to deliver medication-related interventions as part of the collaborative function of health care. **Figure 21-7** shows the impact of MTM services on medical costs for one cohort.

Although PharmMD knows that not all medical spending is directly correlated to the efforts of the medication interventions, when a pharmacist has all metrics available, including medical claims, laboratory data, pharmacy claims, and patient self-reported data, a more robust intervention can be actualized and provided to optimize patients' health. The medical spend is impacted by the positive efforts of pharmacy. An example are those patients who are diagnosed with depression and continually use the medical system; repeat unnecessary visits to the physician occur due to not uncovering the side effect profile of the prescribed medications. Pharmacist interventions, in this example, allow the appropriate medication to be optimized so that it works best for the patient. The pharmacist then empowers the patient to realize the value of taking the medication regularly throughout the

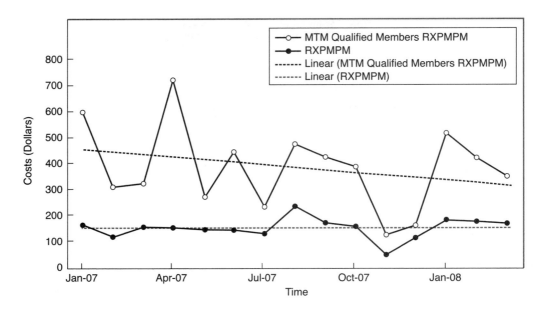

FIGURE 21-7 Impact of MTM Services on Medical Costs for One Client (MTM Qualified vs. Entire Population).
Source: ©PharmMD, 2008.

84-day period, which is a standard of care, in order to actualize the true value and effectiveness of the medication.

In-patient admissions are another area that pharmacy and medication therapy impacts (**Figure 21-8**). An example is patients who are living with asthma who continually end up in the emergency room because they are not on the appropriate medication. There is a direct relationship of pharmacy medication use, and spend, to the medical use, and spend, within a healthcare system. PharmMD works within the scope and guidelines of the client needs and focuses interventions to optimize care of every patient.

Table 21-1 demonstrates potential projected MTM savings for specific medical conditions. Overall, the savings seen for hospitalizations can be prevented by truly tapping into the most underutilized healthcare profession: pharmacy. MAPD can integrate metric data that examine the overall impact of patient care and the role and impact of medication management on hospitalizations. The impact pharmacists have on healthcare is astounding. Health plans that look past the product and incorporate the services pharmacists are capable of providing, in order to optimize care, give patients what they are looking for in health care. As health plans continue to adopt a true clinical model of care, quality, and efficiency, overall healthcare savings will continue to be actualized.

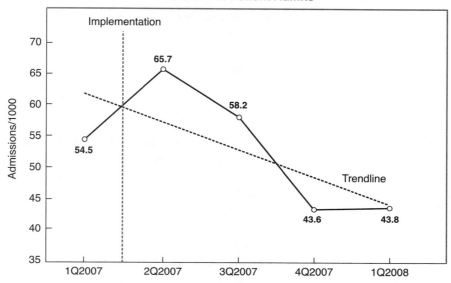

FIGURE 21-8   Impact of MTM Services on In-Patient Admissions.
MTM services results provided to a large self-insured employer group.
Source: ©PharmMD, 2008.

TABLE 21-1   Projected MTM Savings for Specific Medical Conditions

Diagnosis Category	Population 50,000	Population 100,000
CHF	$ 2,758,673.50	$ 5,517,347.00
COPD/Asthma	$ 2,200,920.50	$ 4,401,841.00
Diabetes long term complications	$ 467,008.50	$ 934,017.00
Hypertension	$ 91,415.00	$ 182,830.00
Total Savings Proposed	$ 5,518,017.50	$ 11,036,035.00

The following are assumptions regarding savings using PharmMD's pharmacist–led national MTMS program:

- Prevalence rate is higher than hospitalization rate
- Change percent (impact) may vary based on several factors
- Numbers are based on average discharge rate per diagnosis
- DRG information from actual plan data targets specific recommendations and impacts that fit your needs

Source: ©PharmMD, 2008. Hospital savings based on projected MTM services through internal analysis and information.

CLINICAL PHARMACIST OPPORTUNITIES

There are many examples of clinical pharmacy activities within various MCOs. Many health plan pharmacists oversee prior authorizations, drug utilization review, and network needs and issues. Clinical pharmacists working in managed care organizations realize that pharmacists practicing within the community, including consultants, are able to provide a quality service and document and report the results to save overall costs in the system.

HEALTHSPRING

Medication therapy management is moving to more robust levels throughout the country. Pharmacists' ability to impact care positively by addressing formulary management, drug utilization review, and following guidelines and best practices in the industry are becoming more evident within overall health plan strategies. Development underway will include clinical pharmacists as part of the healthcare team and working collaboratively with specialists and primary providers.

One popular health plan is HealthSpring, a public company directed towards the Medicare Advantage benefits market. In their organization, the pharmacist is acknowledged as the medication expert and works side-by-side with the physicians. The company's goal is to move into a realm where the physician diagnoses the patient and the pharmacist—as the medication expert—reviews all metrics, provides the appropriate medication, and encourages the patient with education to take appropriate medication properly and persistently. This seems to be a true partnership. As this program shows success, their plan is to scale this model throughout the health plan industry.

NEW MEXICO

Two states, New Mexico and North Carolina, recognize clinical pharmacists as providers, and the professional designation in these states allows for pharmacists to provide advanced services and payment. The New Mexico insurance authority acknowledged pharmacist clinicians as providers and pharmacists with this designation are allowed payment by health plans under this state provision. Health plans in this state employ as well as contract with pharmacist clinicians.[17] There are significant savings shown by utilizing pharmacists with advanced clinical expertise. Ernest Dole, one of several progressive pharmacist clinicians making a difference in patient care in New Mexico, continues to bring value to the healthcare system he serves. At his pain clinic he brings:

- Efficient care, positive clinical outcomes including patient satisfaction, and cost savings to the healthcare system.
- A cost savings for a pharmacist-operated pain clinic showed an annual savings of more than $450,000. This is actual savings to the health plan.
- A reduction in reported pain scores was observed and maintained across visits over time. In all cases, the change was in the desired direction, averaging about a one point reduction in patient pain scores; data were statistically significant in all cases.

PRESBYTERIAN HEALTH PLAN

Prior to the implementation of Medicare Part D, Presbyterian Health Plan (PHP) already had a robust Medicare D Medication Therapy Management (MTM) program in place. Presbyterian Health Plan was one of the few surviving Medicare Risk contractors remaining in the managed care industry on the "eve" of Medicare Part D. The MTM program, which was implemented in 1992, was credited with survival of the Medicare Risk program by "keeping seniors on their medications and out of the higher cost centers of care." PHP, having recognized the benefits of MTM, began a strategic imperative to "expand beyond Medicare" in 2007. The basic principles of MTM are applicable to disease management, employee wellness programs, and case management of high risk patients irrespective of age or disease state. PHP MTM initiatives beyond Medicare D include:

- MTM expanded to support Diabetes Disease Management Initiatives for all high risk diabetics not in good control irrespective of line of business (i.e. Commercial, Medicaid and Medicare) in 2007.
- Expanded to support all Disease Management Initiatives for CHF, hypertension, and asthma in 2008.
- Expanded to support all members in case management and care coordination in 2006.
- MTM expanded to support Employer Wellness Initiatives for high profile employer groups (2007-2008).
- Ongoing MTM expansion for PHP Disease Management Initiatives for CHF, hypertension, and asthma (2008-2009).
- Developed case tracker IS tool to manage data and interventions and report outcomes in 3rd Quarter of 2008.
- Other potential areas currently being evaluated include oncology and chronic pain management.

Success for MTM programs at PHP includes a clinical pharmacist-led CHF program. Louanne Cunico, a PHP clinical pharmacist, initiated a CHF program within a large medical group. Louanne evaluated and provided the following savings actualized in 2003, in which collaborative efforts with physicians and pharmacists in an ambulatory setting provided:

- Savings due to decreased admits of approximately $383,278.77 over a six month period
- Savings due to decreased Emergency Room visits of approximately $13,770.00 over a six month period
- Overall annual savings of $25.55 per member per month (pmpm) savings for 2003

There are more interventions and savings pharmacists are bringing to health plans in New Mexico. Health plans in this state acknowledge the value of the added credential and clinical expertise of pharmacists. These health plans are implementing advanced programs that have pharmacists working with physicians as a collaborative partner in health care. Clinical pharmacists providing quality standards to health plans are ready to be acknowledged as providers of service under Medicare Part B, just as other mid-level providers such as physician assistants and nurse practitioners.

MEDICATION THERAPY MANAGEMENT AND DISEASE MANAGEMENT

Medication therapy management provides a solid backdrop to DM. Many disease management managers have relationships with patients. An MTM provider (e.g., PharmMD) reaches out to providers and works to implement appropriate therapies. Many updates and empowerment occurs with DM managers and these can be worked in tandem. These services provide and optimize the best therapies to patients.

MEDICAL DIRECTOR ROLE

More medical directors are realizing the value pharmacists bring to the table. MCOs that have champions (i.e., early adopters) are beginning to work toward data warehousing and merging all of the historical metrics. Laboratory values, self-reported data, medical claims, pharmacy claims, and other metrics allow for providers to make better informed decisions and assist patients who are unfamiliar with the healthcare industry. Many medical directors understand that analyzing overall budgets—pharmacy and medical combined—and connecting the effects of one to another, truly impact the overall healthcare dollar.

As standards of care for pharmacy evolve, medical directors will continue to look for ways to implement valuable tools that allow their care to impact patients more effectively.

FUTURE OF PHARMACY

The future of pharmacy is lush with opportunities. Of course, the commodity—the drug product—always will remain important. As health plans realize the most underutilized healthcare provider, the medication expert (the pharmacist), is prepared to assist with the overall health care of patients, everyone wins from a quality as well as financial perspective. MTM services, especially those focused on the pharmacist-specific interventions, will continue to grow and become commonplace as a valuable asset to optimizing patient care, and show the value of consistent care, including the medication.

Pharmacists provide more than products. The clinical pharmacist keeps up with the latest developments in medication therapies, develops skills and niche service offerings such as specialty pharmacy medication in order to provide patients with the best service and quality. Savings from clinical pharmacists who provide services continue to rise. The entire healthcare system benefits by including pharmacy MTM as part of the portfolio of services and care patients should expect when using healthcare systems.

As pharmacists continue to develop professionally, the need for inter-rater reliability will become more important in the marketplace. The pharmacy profession must develop and implement strategies to address this need. As quality organizations such as AHRQ and NCQA refine benchmarks for service, the profession must become more efficient in order to provide for such a wide array of patients needing their services. As MTM grows, health plans will realize the value of opt-out programs and the need to allow all patients the access and ability to participate in this emerging service.

Acknowledgment

The author wishes to acknowledge the contributions of Michael J. Arizpe, Anne Burns, Larry Georgopoulos, Tim Sawyers, and Marissa Schlaifer.

REFERENCES

1. Schumock G.T., Butler M.G., Meek P.D., et al., Evidence of the economic benefit of clinical pharmacy services. *Pharmacotherapy.* 2003; 23(1): 113-132.

2. Ditusa L., Luzier A.B., Brady P.G., et al., A pharmacy-based approach to cholesterol management. *Am J Manag Care.* 2001; 7(10): 973-979.

3. Blakely S.A. and Hixson-Wallace J.A., Clinical and economic effects of pharmacy services in a geriatric ambulatory clinic. *Pharmacotherapy.* 2000; 20(10): 1198-1203.

4. Sound Medication Therapy Management Programs (version 2.0 with validation study). *J Man Care Pharm.* 2008 Jan; 14(1 Suppl B): S2-44.

5. Medication therapy management in pharmacy practice: core elements of an MTM service (version 2.0). *J Am Pharm Assoc.* 2008;48:341-53).

6. Sound Medication Therapy Management Programs (version 2.0 with validation study). *J Academy of Managed Care Pharmacy.* 2008;14(1): 1-46.

7. Bluml B.M., Definition of medication therapy management: development of profession-wide consensus. *J Am Pharm Assoc (Wash).* 2005; 45(5): 566-572.

8. Schommer J., Planas L.G., Johnson K.A., Doucette W.R., Pharmacist provided medication therapy management provider perspectives (part 1): provider perspectives in 2007. *J Am Pharm Assoc (Wash).* 2008; 48: e36-e45.

9. Pharmacy Quality Alliance (PQA), *PQA Recommended Measures—2007.* Available at http://www. pqaalliance.org/files/PQA_MeasureDescriptions ForDemonstrations.pdf. Accessed 24 July 2008.

10. Fera T,, Bluml BM, Ellis W.M, et al. The Diabetes Ten City Challenge: Interim clinical and humanistic outcomes of a multisite community pharmacy diabetes care program. *J Am Pharm Assoc.* 2008;48:181–190.

11. Schommer J., Planas L.G., Johnson K.A., Doucette W.R., Pharmacist-provided medication therapy management: provider perspectives (part 1) 2007. *J Am Pharm Assoc (Wash).* 2008; 48:e36-e45.

12. Touchette D.R., Burns A.L., Bough M.A., Blackburn J.C., Survey of medication therapy management programs under Medicare Part D. *J Am Pharm Assoc (Wash).* 2006; 46: 683.

13. Medication therapy management in pharmacy practice: core elements of an MTM service (version 2.0). *J Am Pharm Assoc.* 2008;48:341-353.

14. Sound Medication Therapy Management Programs (version 2.0 with validation study). *J Academy of Managed Care Pharmacy* 2008;14(1):1-46.

15. Pharmacy Quality Alliance (PQA), *PQA Recommended Measures—2007.* Available at http://www. pqaalliance.org/files/PQA_MeasureDescriptions ForDemonstrations.pdf. Accessed 24 July 2008.

16. Sound Medication Therapy Management Programs (version 2.0 with validation study). *J Academy of Managed Care Pharmacy* 2008;14(1): 1-46.

17. Dole E.J., Murawski M.M., Adolphe A.B., et al., Provision of pain management by a pharmacist with prescribing authority. *Am J Health-Syst Pharm.* 2007; 64(1):85-89.

Chapter 22

PHARMACIST CAREER OPPORTUNITIES IN MANAGED CARE

CLAIBORNE E. REEDER
DARLENE M. MEDNICK

INTRODUCTION

The U.S. healthcare system continues to evolve at a rapid pace. The size of the U.S. population is growing, demand for health care is increasing, technological advances in medicine are occurring exponentially, and healthcare costs are rising each year. Since the early 1980s, insurers, employers, and healthcare payors have been searching for ways to deliver high quality care at affordable costs. Managed care emerged as a strategy to cope with this dilemma. Today's pharmacist faces a new healthcare environment that is heavily influenced by managed care. This new environment presents many new career options and opportunities for pharmacists.

PHARMACIST ROLES IN MANAGED CARE

Pharmacists who work in managed care organizations (MCOs), such as health plans and pharmacy benefit management companies (PBMs), are responsible for delivery of the prescription drug benefit to over 250 million people. The prescription drug benefit typically includes a broad range of clinical and drug management services in addition to the responsibility for delivery of the drug product.

Managed care pharmacy is a critical component of managed health care. While initially focusing on controlling the cost of pharmaceuticals, the role of the managed care pharmacist has expanded greatly to encompass providing comprehensive pharmaceutical care to a population of individuals. The goal of providing pharmaceutical care requires a team of creative, visionary pharmacists and a dedicated support staff. While the role of the managed care pharmacist still includes the efficient distribution of medicines, the expanded role includes many exciting career opportunities.

The new roles for pharmacists that have emerged in the managed care sector require creativity and a redefinition of the professional work domain.[1] In this new practice culture, pharmacists are expected to:

1. Shift their primary interest and attitudes from product to patient (individual and populations of patients).
2. Focus on prevention and wellness as well as providing for a continuum of care across time and place.
3. Provide high-quality, cost-effective care that is responsive to patient needs and preferences.
4. Adapt to the changing healthcare environment by developing new skills and competencies.

With its emphasis on reducing costs and improving outcomes, managed care is influencing and will continue to influence pharmacy work. Once largely ignored by managed care, drug therapy—the most frequently used form of medical intervention—is now the focus of intensive cost reduction and quality improvement measures. This is due not only to the escalating cost of pharmaceuticals but also to the high costs associated with drug morbidity and mortality. The recently enacted Medicare Part D prescription drug benefit requires medication therapy management (MTM) programs. MTM programs have been described as a "distinct service or group of services that optimize outcomes for individual patients" that "are independent of, but can occur in conjunction with, the provision of a medication product."[2]

While most other professions have changed in response to the growth in managed care, in many important ways pharmacy has found itself ahead of the managed care curve. Due in large part to early adoption of technological innovations such as pharmacy computer systems, personal digital assistants (PDAs), and electronic claims submission, pharmacy began its own evolution in parallel to the emergence of managed care. In large part, the impact of managed care on pharmacy practice has been to escalate a process that was already in motion.

Clearly, the United States is moving toward a system where all care will be "managed." The growth in private and public health insurance programs, like Medicare and Medicaid, has concentrated the payment for services in the hands of third parties and not individual patients. These large payors are demanding *value* for the money they expend and evidence that the care is not only efficient, but also of high quality. In such a system, pharmacists perform a variety of functions directly related to comprehensive drug therapy management or indirectly supporting the cost-effective design, application, and assessment of drug therapy management within the system. Clearly, pharmacists working in managed care will continue to serve in many of the roles and responsibilities of non-managed care pharmacists such as responsibility for the delivery of safe and appropriate medicines. To be successful in managed care, however, pharmacists will need different knowledge, attitudes, skills, and behaviors.

SKILLS FOR MANAGED CARE PRACTICE

Managed care has produced some unique variations in traditional pharmacy practice. Pharmacists continue to be patient pharmacotherapy champions, working to achieve optimum pharmaceutical outcomes. However, managed care offers a unique mix of business and clinical opportunities. Managed care systems attempt to integrate the cost and quality of care aspects of all delivery components to evaluate their interaction and contribution to overall patient outcomes. Beyond the basic pharmacy skills needed to optimize patient therapeutic outcomes, there are a number of other skills that will make pharmacists highly desirable in managed care. Among this enhanced skill set are:

- General business and financial management skills
- Oral and written communication and presentation skills
- Sales and marketing skills
- Computer skills including database management and analysis
- Understanding of information system applications
- Understanding of pharmacoeconomic principles and applications
- Basic clinical and outcomes research design and application skills

These skills will enhance a pharmacist's ability to pursue novel career paths in managed care. As illustrated in the example job descriptions in the next section, elements of these skills are in most position requirements in managed care pharmacy.

MANAGED CARE PHARMACIST JOB FUNCTIONS

Depending on the size and scope of the organization, the managed care pharmacist may be involved in several activities or focused primarily on one or two functions. Functions typically performed by managed care pharmacists fall into seven general categories.[3]

1. Drug distribution and dispensing
2. Patient safety
3. Clinical program development
4. Communication with patients and providers (prescribers and pharmacists)
5. Drug benefit design
6. Business management
7. Cost management

DRUG DISTRIBUTION AND DISPENSING

Managed care organizations may own and operate their own pharmacies (in-house pharmacies) or contract with a network of community pharmacies to deliver the drug benefit. In the case of in-house pharmacies, the pharmacist is actually providing the drug in addition to an array of comprehensive pharmacy services. Pharmacists in this environment typically have access to integrated patient information systems, so they are able to provide an enhanced set of clinical services beyond direct dispensing and counseling. Kaiser Permanente is a good example of an MCO that owns and operates its own pharmacies as part of a fully integrated healthcare system.[4]

In the case of contracted or "network" pharmacies, managed care pharmacists may be involved in designing and implementing the drug benefit. This could entail claims adjudication, eligibility determinations, prior authorization, and clinical appropriateness of medicines. The managed care pharmacist also may be involved with the dispensing pharmacist and the prescriber in facilitating use of formulary medications or resolving potential adverse consequences of medication use.

Last, an MCO may use a centralized mail order facility to deliver part of its drug benefit, especially for maintenance medications. Pharmacists in mail order distribution centers may be involved in managing the operations of the facility, assuring service quality, monitoring adherence to legal and practice standards, and assessing the appropriate use of therapy.

PATIENT SAFETY

Patient safety is a primary concern for the pharmacist anytime a medicine is prescribed and dispensed to a patient. Adverse consequences of medication use can result from contraindications or sensitivities to the drug itself or from inappropriate combinations of medicines (*polypharmacy*). The cost of adverse drug events to society are enormous and in large part preventable. Ernst and Grizzle have estimated that in 2000, the cost of drug-related morbidity exceeded $177 billion.[5] By analyzing prescription data during the claims adjudication process, managed care pharmacists are able to prevent many drug-related problems. When a potential problem is identified, the managed care pharmacists can interact with other pharmacists, prescribers, or the patient to resolve the problem. This important job function is known as Drug Utilization Review (DUR). As part of their jobs, managed care pharmacists may also be involved in prior authorization (PA) and quality assurance (QA) activities as well as clinical monitoring programs.

CLINICAL PROGRAM DEVELOPMENT

Quality improvement is at the core of the philosophy of managed care. In an effort to continually improve the quality of patient care, managed care pharmacists are involved in clinical program development (see Chapter 21). In this role, pharmacists use their clinical and analytical skills to scientifically evaluate and select the most effective and efficient treatments for the population of patients they serve. Managed care pharmacists serve on Pharmacy and Therapeutics (P & T) Committees where they apply the principles of evidence-based medicine to the formulary development process. These same skills also are used to develop disease management programs to help improve the treatment outcomes of patients with chronic conditions, such as diabetes, asthma, and heart failure.

COMMUNICATION WITH PATIENTS AND PROVIDERS

Information management is a critical component of patient care. A lack of continuity in patient care and information sharing may result in sub-optimal patient outcomes. Managed care pharmacists are actively involved in communications with prescribers, pharmacists, and patients that are intended to improve the quality and appropriateness of care. These communications require excellent verbal and written communication skills on the part of the pharmacist. Managed care pharmacists provide patients with educational materials, information on their medication history, and answer eligibility and benefit questions. Communications with prescribers and pharmacists may involve questions of potential drug interactions, duplicate therapies, eligibility, and formulary coverage.

PLAN BENEFIT DESIGN

Design of the prescription drug benefit involves determining the level of coverage and types of services that should be included. Managed care pharmacists are involved in deciding the type of formulary (open vs. closed) the health plan will use, the amounts of any cost-sharing provisions (copayments and deductibles), how the drug benefit will be delivered (in-house pharmacy, network pharmacy, mail order, or some combination), and the types of clinical programs that might be included. To accomplish its goal of high quality, cost-effective pharmacy services, drug benefit design requires sound clinical judgment coupled with good business skills.

BUSINESS MANAGEMENT

Managed care pharmacists who work primarily on the "business side" of their organization interact with employers, pharmacies, and pharmaceutical manufacturers to develop networks, assist with prescription benefit design issues, and establish contracts. One of the tools that managed care uses to control benefit cost is to negotiate with pharmaceutical firms for discounts on their products and with pharmacy networks for a favorable dispensing and service fee. Pharmacists in this role must have excellent communication skills and business acumen as well as a strong clinical practice background.

COST MANAGEMENT

Closely related to the business management role in managed care is the cost management role for pharmacists. Prescription benefit costs are managed within the context of providing high quality care. The objective is to provide access to the most cost-effective therapies in terms of their impact of treatment on total utilization and cost in the plan. Pharmacists who have responsibility for managing costs must understand the inter-relationship of appropriate medication use and the use of other healthcare resources. To be effective, these pharmacists must understand the principles of pharmacoeconomics, health outcomes research, and evidence-based medicine, and think of the prescription benefit from a "system" perspective. Managing pharmacy costs is more than obtaining the lowest drug price; it also includes developing and implementing programs that help assure appropriate medication use, such as treatment guidelines, protocols, and disease management initiatives.

CAREERS IN MANAGED CARE

A review of current job descriptions for pharmacists practicing in managed care reveals an interesting array of job titles and position descriptions (**Table 22-1**).

The following examples of job descriptions illustrate the duties and skills needed for a position in managed care pharmacy.

EXAMPLE 1. CLINICAL PHARMACIST AT REGIONAL HEALTH PLAN, INC.

Job Responsibilities: Primary responsibilities of the clinical pharmacist include, but are not limited to, the following:

- Develops and evaluates all clinical programs such as prior authorization guidelines, clinical interventions, and disease management programs.
- Provides drug information and clinical support to all medical areas of Regional Health Plan.
- Develops and prepares the agenda, monographs, and other materials for P & T Committee meetings.
- Develops formulary prescribing guidelines for oral and injectable medications.
- Participates in the quality improvement initiatives of the organization.
- Develops utilization and cost forecasts for drugs in the development pipeline.
- Supports the development of the new Part D Medicare formularies, required utilization management tools, Medication Therapy Management Services program, and the UM/QA programs.
- Develops coverage management programs focused on patient and physician educational activities, automated reporting functions, and online pharmacy editing processes.

Skill or Experience Requirements: The candidate must have a Doctor of Pharmacy degree and be eligible for licensure in the state. Post-graduate degree or residency is preferred. Applicants must work well in team environments, possess strong verbal and written communication skills, and be self-directed.

EXAMPLE 2. CLINICAL PHARMACOTHERAPY SPECIALIST AT LOCAL HEALTH PLAN

Job Responsibilities: Primary responsibilities of the Clinical Pharmacotherapy Specialist include, but are not limited to, the following:

- Possesses strong clinical skills in evaluating medication therapy and recommending appropriate drug treatments for the Medicare population.

- Implements the MTMS component for the Part D benefit.
- Creates care guidelines for the nursing staff and is able to provide guidance to nursing case managers.
- Serves as the subject matter expert on drug therapies, particularly in the elderly.
- Ensures that any medication management programs are appropriately implemented on an individual basis.
- Directs communications with physicians, pharmacists, nurses, and patients to resolve drug related problems or benefit issues.

Skill or Experience Requirements: The candidate must have a Registered Pharmacist (R.Ph.) or Doctor of Pharmacy (Pharm.D.) degree with two to five years of direct clinical experience in drug therapy management. Applicants must work well in team environments and possess strong verbal and written communication skills. Candidates are expected to be capable of providing strategic direction, evaluating reports related to monitoring program activity and be self-directing. Certification in Geriatric Pharmacy as well as knowledge of geriatric pharmacy and Medicare guidelines are a plus. The individual must be capable of providing educational training to nursing or other staff as needed.

TABLE 22-1   Examples of Managed Care Pharmacy Job Titles

Benefit Management
Call Center Clinical Operations
Clinical Account Management
Clinical Program Development
Clinical Program Pharmacist
Contracting (Manufacturer)
Drug Information Specialist
Formulary Manager
Formulary Services Manager
Mail Service Dispensing
Network Contracting and Relations
Pharmacoeconomics and Outcomes Research
Pharmacotherapy Specialist
Prior Authorization Manager
Quality Assurance
Retail Pharmacy Network Management
Sales and Marketing
Specialty Pharmaceuticals Management

EXAMPLE 3. PHARMACOECONOMIC RESEARCH SPECIALIST AT NATIONAL PHARMACY BENEFIT MANAGER

Job Responsibilities: Primary responsibilities of the Pharmacoeconomic Research Specialist include, but are not limited to, the following:

- Provides leadership within the company for research design and statistical methodology used in modeling and outcomes studies.
- Develops and executes health data strategic plans, policies, and procedures for analysis.
- Develops and executes statistical/analytical procedures, processes, and data reports that support internal business activities.
- Applies appropriate research design and statistical procedures utilized in internal studies.
- Develops and participates in presentations and consultations to internal business constituents and pharmaceutical company departments.

Skill or Experience Requirements: Successful applicant must hold the Doctor of Pharmacy degree and Master's degree in statistics, economics, health services research, or related field. Candidate must possess pharmacoeconomic and applied outcomes research skills using both retrospective and prospective study designs. A strong analytical/quantitative background in health services research, health economics, econometrics, continuous quality improvement (CQI) and quality assurance (QA) methods, medical informatics, statistics, and multivariate analyses is required. Experience with data mining tools and decision tree software applications are needed. Healthcare experience is required; pharmaceutical industry experience is beneficial. The candidate must be proficient in using Excel, Word, and SAS software programs.

EXAMPLE 4. MEDICATION USE MANAGEMENT CLINICAL PHARMACIST

Primary Job Responsibilities: Primary responsibilities of the Medication Use Management Clinical Pharmacist include, but are not limited to, the following:

- Identifies, develops and maintains clinical criteria for standard and client-specific prior authorization programs.
- Develops and maintains prior authorization policies and procedures manual.
- Trains sales and account management staff on prior authorization programs.
- Develops medication monographs and therapy-class reviews as necessary.
- Assists in retrospective drug utilization review and in the development of related clinical intervention criteria.
- Assists in the development and support of the organization's Pharmacy and Therapeutics Committee.
- Serves as a preceptor and mentor for pharmacy students, interns, and residents.
- Assists in miscellaneous clinical projects as required.

Job Requirements: Successful candidate must possess strong clinical, verbal, and written communication skills, be flexible, creative, adaptive to a changing environment, and self-directing. Excellent organizational skills and orientation to detail are necessary. The candidate must be able to perform and manage multiple projects simultaneously. Strong analytical and problem-solving skills and ability to work with Microsoft Office, especially Word and Excel, software programs are needed. Candidate must demonstrate good interpersonal skills and ability to work as part of a team.

CONCLUSION

Managed care has become a major component of healthcare delivery in the United States. With the growth of Medicare and Medicaid, coupled with a rapidly aging population, the expansion of managed care is likely to continue. While managed care presents pharmacists with enormous challenges, it also offers many opportunities for pharmacists to participate in novel professional experiences and practice their profession in unique ways. As part of the managed care team, pharmacists are able to provide comprehensive pharmaceutical care while having the opportunity to assume numerous positions with increasing responsibilities.[6]

As with pharmacists who practice in other settings, managed care pharmacists are responsible for the safe, appropriate, and cost-effective use of medications. Managed care pharmacists must not only be excellent clinicians; they also must be problem solvers, analysts, and effective communicators. The job responsibilities and requirements presented in this chapter illustrate the breadth and scope of those who practice managed care pharmacy. A career in managed care pharmacy offers pharmacists the opportunity to work with healthcare providers and payors to determine the most effective and efficient pharmaceutical treatments for their patients. It is truly an exciting and upwardly mobile career.

Acknowledgments

The authors wish to acknowledge the contributions of the Academy of Managed Care Pharmacy (AMCP) to this chapter. Their publication entitled, "The Roles of Pharmacists in Managed Health Care Organizations," served as the framework for this section and was an invaluable resource in our writing. This publication is available online at http://www.amcp.org.

Thanks to all our friends and colleagues who shared information about their jobs and others available in managed care pharmacy. The materials included in the "Careers in Managed Care" section were gleaned from conversations and correspondence with these people and is an amalgam of job titles and descriptions.

REFERENCES

1. Trinca C.E., Pharmacist Career Path Opportunities in Managed Care. In Navarro R.P., ed. *Managed Care Pharmacy Practice*. Gaithersburg, MD: Aspen Publishers, Inc.; 1999: 497-505.
2. Bluml B.M., Definition of medication therapy management: development of professionwide consensus. *J Am Pharm Assoc (Wash)*. 2005; 45(5): 566-572.
3. Academy of Managed Care Pharmacy (AMCP). *The Roles of Pharmacists in Managed Health Care Organizations*. Available at http://www.amcp.org/content/pr/roles.cfm. Accessed 25 July 2008.
4. Kaiser Permanente, homepage. Available at https://www.kaiserpermanente.org/. Accessed 25 July 2008.
5. Ernst F.R. and Grizzle A.J., Drug-related morbidity and mortality: updating the cost-of-illness model. *J Am Pharm Assoc (Wash)*. 2001; 45: 192-199.
6. American Association of Colleges of Pharmacy. Managed Care Pharmacy. Available at http://www.aacp.org/site/tertiary.asp?TRACKID=&VID=2&CID=1397&DID=3679. Accessed 08 August 2008.

Chapter 23

ETHICAL ASPECTS OF PHARMACY PRACTICE IN MANAGED CARE

MILA ANN AROSKAR

Managed care systems challenge the professional practice and values of pharmacists and other health professionals. Evolving arrangements for the financing and delivery of health care that focus primarily on cost containment or stockholder interests bring new urgency to ethical issues and create ethical challenges related to policy development, protection of patient confidentiality, conflict of interests, and the allocation of finite financial and other resources such as time and professional expertise.

This chapter provides pharmacists with resources that help them to manage ethical problems and concerns. Pharmacists are encouraged to practice *preventive ethics*, defined as the early identification and management of ethical concerns that may, and sometimes do, escalate into ethical or legal crises. Use of a proactive approach to ethically troubling patient care and policy decisions helps to prevent ethical crises. It also assists pharmacists to prevent harm to patients and to preserve their well-being, protect the integrity of healthcare professionals, and enhance the overall mission of healthcare organizations.

This chapter has four major sections. The first section provides examples of ethical issues and concerns that pharmacists may face. The second is a brief discussion of ethical and professional values. The third examines ethical principles and concepts drawn from the *Code of Ethics for Pharmacists* that are fundamental to professional practice. The fourth section is a brief review of selected resources that may guide pharmacists, individually and collectively, as they respond to the ethical issues and questions identified earlier in this chapter. Working as a healthcare professional in managed care organizations (MCOs) requires both reflection and the use of resources such as professional codes to determine one's ethical obligations and to maintain one's personal and professional integrity.

EXAMPLES OF ETHICAL ISSUES AND CONCERNS

Pharmacists who practice in managed care settings are involved in many situations that raise ethical questions. Concern for the ethical aspects of practice includes discernment of the right action(s) when available choices conflict or one's professional obligations are unclear. Professional standards of practice provide essential but not sufficient guidance; often no ready-made answers exist in a particular situation and use of a thoughtful decision making process is required.

Ethically troubling situations that require decision making by individual practitioners as professionals and employees in managed care plans may be characterized in the following ways:

1. There are conflicts of goals, values, obligations, loyalties, interests, or needs in responding to a patient or developing an organizational drug policy.
2. There are ethical principles or values at stake, such as trust and trustworthiness, respect for persons as individuals and as interdependent members of communities, avoidance of harm or minimization of harm, responsibility and accountability, personal and professional integrity, and justice as fairness.
3. The situation involves the feelings and values of all of the stakeholders.
4. Ethically supportable decisions and actions may require broad-based, interdisciplinary discussion.

Some general issues in managed care that require ethical reflection include the for-profit status of health plans and services, stewardship of financial and professional resources (e.g., time for patient counseling, determination of member pharmacy benefits, balancing of patient/population/community benefits, and financial incentives for providers), due process for patients and providers, allocation of scarce or very expensive lifesaving drugs, and informed consent and decision making. Everyday examples of ethical concerns for pharmacists include:

- Allocation of time for patient counseling to address worries of health plan members on fixed incomes who are forced to pay increased out-of-pocket costs for medications that control serious chronic health problems
- Protecting the privacy of prescription data for individuals who are viewed by the organization as members of a population group
- Filling prescriptions for less expensive generic drugs for patients who have responded favorably to more expensive drugs when the pharmacist knows that the less expensive drug is not as effective or potentially has additional adverse side effects
- Dealing with health plan policies that limit information given to patients regarding the drug coverage in their health insurance policy or healthcare plan, so-called *gag rules*

When gag rules are in place, pharmacists may worry about adequately informed consent and decision making for treatment and the potential for deceiving patients when there are plan limitations on the information they receive. Moral struggles occur as a pharmacist decides how to manage these issues and maintain personal and professional integrity, realizing that the health plan may retaliate if one challenges existing policy and practice.

The most urgent ethical concerns often focus on MCOs that are for-profit and investor owned, such as health plans owned by insurance companies. There has been a noteworthy shift in managed care generally over the past two decades from not-for-profit independent health maintenance organizations (HMOs) to for-profit organizations in various configurations. In 1985, not-for-profit HMOs outnumbered for-profit HMOs by two to one. By 1994, this ratio was already reversed and now the majority of patients receive their health care in some form of managed care.

Policy analyst Reinhard Priester examined these trends in relation to their jeopardizing healthcare goals of promoting efficiency, expanding access, improving quality, preserving freedom of choice, and protecting patient advocacy.[1] Priester's preliminary assessment demonstrated that relatively little is known about the impact of managed care arrangements on these essential goals. He acknowledged that managed care has the potential to both improve the healthcare system and interfere with the achievement of important health goals. He concluded that growth in the rapidly expanding for-profit sector is especially troubling from three perspectives. First, the values of the marketplace often conflict fundamentally with the values and goals of healthcare professionals and traditional healthcare institutions. Second, the push to enroll more Medicare and Medicaid recipients in managed care plans has resulted in an influx of high-risk persons into these plans. Third, some of these plans are inadequately prepared to respond to the health needs of Medicaid enrollees and individuals on Medicare, such as Medicaid enrollees with chronic mental illnesses or Medicare enrollees who have several comorbidities.[1 p60-61]

A major ethical concern about for-profit health plans involves the use of profits, which is a crucial issue when considering the ethical principle of justice as fairness. Making a profit is not automatically unethical; in fact, profits are essential for maintenance and improvement of services. What is ethically problematic is the use of so-called *profits*. Whether health plan profits are used to improve services, to enrich stockholders, or to help achieve some mix of these goals is ethically significant.

John Worthley, a professor of public administration, wrote that conflicts of duties and obligations in everyday professional practice are the rule rather than the exception. This perspective has not received much attention in bioethics because the focus has been on the more dramatic, headline-grabbing issues and dilemmas such as abortion or assisted suicide. Ethical aspects are considered by Worthley to be part of any interaction in which one person is in a position of power in relation to another person and makes decisions that affect the well-being of that other person. Health professionals often hold such positions of power in their relationships with patients.[2] For example, if a patient who is an identified HIV-infected addict seeks information about the composition of a drug, a pharmacist might wonder what this individual plans to do with the information. The pharmacist is troubled, wondering what she can and should do to meet her ethical obligations as an advocate for patients and her social responsibilities to the community.

While managed care is often depicted as a "bad guy," particularly in geographical areas where it is the primary mode of healthcare financing and delivery, ethical issues also existed under fee-for-service medical care. Issues such as overtreatment and overtesting often involved ethical debates about harms and benefits for patients. Additionally, ethical issues were focused more on direct patient care and less on the economics of health care. Until the early 1980s, Medicare and Medicaid reimbursement for patient care was unquestioned, and many individuals carried health insurance through their place of employment. Now, most employers either seek ways to cut their costs of health insurance or are self-insured. This reality means an increased financial burden for many employees and their families.

Ethical issues in pharmacy practice also may be considered in the context of the increasing attention that is being paid to organizational ethics in bioethics and medical ethics. The rationale for paying attention to the broader organizational context of ethical issues and the economics of health care is drawn from four sources. The first source is empirical data that show that the organizational structures and cultures within which health care is delivered influence recognition of ethical issues and how they are managed.[3] The second is the radical change, in many geographic markets, from fee-for-service to a variety of managed care arrangements with reimbursement based on capitation. A third is the increasing emphasis on teamwork in delivery of health care. Several types of health professionals with their own codes and ideologies work together and must juggle often conflicting values and goals for patient care. A fourth source is the development of accreditation requirements that mandate attention by healthcare organizations to ethics problems and issues. For example, the Joint Commission on Accreditation of Healthcare Organizations (JCAH) has mandated requirements for organizations to develop standards with implementation processes and mechanisms such as ethics committees to manage the organization's "relationships with patients and the public in an ethical manner."[4(p35)]

In summary, pharmacy practice is confronted with both old and new ethical challenges as the structures for financing and delivery of healthcare services evolve and technologies provide new, costly, and challenging delivery modes for health services, including pharmaceutical products and services such as patient counseling and education in a cost-containment environment.

ETHICAL VALUES: THEIR PLACE IN PHARMACY PRACTICE

Ethical values are fundamental to professional practice. Yet not all values are ethical values. Personal and organizational values can be economic, business oriented, social, ethnic, or religious. Conflicting societal values in our country and a continuing focus on individual rights force people to ask fundamental questions about the values that should guide decisions and actions by individual healthcare professionals and healthcare organizations.

Values are ideals, attitudes, beliefs, and commitments that are basic to how people conduct their lives. Even though individuals do not often talk explicitly about values and generally take them for granted, values inform daily decisions and actions. They help individuals appraise their own decisions and actions and those of others. Different types of values—such as respect for persons, educational achievement, earning a good living, maintaining one's health, and practicing prevention—influence our perceptions of the world. Because many values guide thinking and behavior, they are not always congruent, and people are often not able to realize all their values simultaneously. Personal values related to the importance of material goods in a person's life may well conflict with values related to a belief that healthcare benefits should be distributed fairly. The economic value of controlling spiraling healthcare costs often conflicts with the social and ethical value of providing access to adequate health care for all in need.

Given the focus on the economic values of cost containment and efficiency in managed care systems, pharmacists and the pharmacy profession must ask themselves whether there are ethical and professional values that must be preserved in any type of institutional arrangements that deliver health care and health-related activities. This is not to argue that economic and business values are unimportant. Healthcare systems cannot survive without an economic base. But humane and respectful health care also requires clarity about the ethical and value-based foundations that support healthcare services in a pluralistic society. Values such as advocacy for individual patients reflect assumptions, ideas, and beliefs about what members of the pharmacy profession consider to be important and worth fighting for in emerging managed care systems that emphasize health care as a for-profit business. The professional code of ethics serves as a guide for ethical values in pharmacy practice.

In the early 1990s, an interdisciplinary group of health professionals, academics, and community representatives conducted a study of values that do and should underlie healthcare delivery and financing in the United States. Recommendations based on this study include a "new" values framework that could be used as a benchmark for healthcare reform proposals and evolving managed care arrangements. This "new" values framework balances more social or community-oriented values with values that focus on individual rights that still take precedence over the more socially oriented values of the common good and health of the public. The framework also points to the underlying values, including economic and ethical values that are at stake or that conflict in realizing both public health and personal health (medical) care goals in our society.[5]

The "old" values identified in this study, that is, those that have influenced U.S. health care since World War II, are professional autonomy, including clinical autonomy of practitioners and regulatory autonomy of the professions; patient autonomy, that is, respect for patients' rights to make informed healthcare decisions, including the right to refuse care; consumer sovereignty that includes freedom to choose an insurance plan and one's own physician; patient advocacy, which combines a mix of values, including care, service, and patient interests as the first priority; high-quality care; and access to care for more people. Although these values were never fully realized in health care, they have served as ideals. Physician autonomy is recognized in this report as the value realized to the greatest degree in the past. Even this value has been eroded in managed care arrangements that constrain clinical decision making and emphasize cost containment.[5 p80-88]

Jeremy Kassirer, former editor of the *New England Journal of Medicine*, warned about the possible consequences if medicine develops a population- or group-based ethic to replace the traditional medical ethic of commitment to individual patients. He rejects an ethic based on groups and driven by market forces because it may turn physicians into economic agents rather than healthcare professionals. For instance, patients would not be able to trust physicians who are viewed as agents of insurance plans rather than as advocates for individual patients. Patients might view pharmacists the same way.[6]

The proposed "new" values framework for U.S. health care retains the old values, redefines and reorders them, and adds more community-oriented values and goals. Two sets of values are identified in the framework: essential values and instrumental values. They may be used as benchmarks for evaluation of managed care health plans that include cost, quality, and access as part of a mission statement but, in reality, focus primarily on cost containment. One value set is presented as *essential* values. These are the foundational values that should underlie health care. The second set is *instrumental* values that contribute to achieving the essential values.

According to the Priester report, there are five *essential* values without which any healthcare system would be deficient: fair access, quality, efficiency, respect for patients, and patient advocacy. *Fair access* for individuals ensures access to an adequate level of health care. This does not automatically mean that each individual will receive the same level of services. It does mean that a floor level of "adequate care" is defined through public policy that permits but does not define higher levels of care.[5 p92-94] In 1983, the President's Commission for the Study of Ethical Problems in Medicine and Biomedical and Behavioral Research concluded that the ultimate responsibility for ensuring access to health care rests with the federal government.[7] Still, universal access has not been attained; over 40 million U.S. citizens are uninsured or lack adequate access to health care at any given point in time.

Quality of care incorporates maximizing the likelihood of desired health outcomes for individuals and populations, care that is consistent with current and emerging professional knowledge, and care that is provided in a humane and respectful way. The value of *efficiency* focuses on achieving desired healthcare outcomes—that is, the greatest benefit for the lowest cost—a more utilitarian ethical approach. Efficiency joins economic and ethical values by recognizing that societal resources for health care are finite and should be allocated in a fair way for all.

Respect for patients incorporates elements of respectful and dignified treatment, protecting confidentiality of patient information, and patient access to information for informed decision-making about medical care and treatment. *Patient advocacy* asserts that healthcare providers should promote the best interests of their patients within established and recognized constraints based on finite healthcare resources. This is a significant modification of the traditional medical ethic of doing everything possible for individual patients, a modification that worried Kassirer.[6] Advocacy also encompasses promotion of the fair use of resources to meet the needs of individuals and groups that have historically been left out of the healthcare system.

Priester discussed *instrumental* values as those values that are important to realizing the essential values.[5] p98-103 These include traditional values of provider autonomy and consumer sovereignty and "new" values of personal responsibility, social solidarity, social advocacy, and personal security. *Personal responsibility* includes both individual and institutional aspects. For instance, individuals should share in the cost of their care to the extent possible to encourage prudent use of healthcare services. Personal freedom and responsibility are included in the framework to indicate that individuals should be encouraged to take greater control over behaviors that influence their health. The institutional aspect of personal responsibility requires that providers and the healthcare system enable individuals to take greater control over their health. Inherent in the concept of personal responsibility is the recognition that barriers such as lack of education or limited financial resources often make it difficult for individuals to take more responsibility for their health. Pharmacists and other health professionals are in key positions to recognize those barriers and to work toward achieving the conditions in which better health can be realized, including promotion of healthy environments.

Social solidarity involves enhancement of a commitment to community that includes all members of society in the healthcare system. Socioeconomic, racial, and class differences should not be reflected in health care. The healthcare system should help to ensure that individuals as community members are not abandoned when they need health care. This value emphasizes attention to the common good, a traditional value in public health activities. Efforts to achieve fairness and equity in access to and availability of healthcare services attempt to realize this value through public policy. *Social advocacy* supports enhancement of the public's health, particularly advocacy for the most vulnerable and the underserved.

The instrumental value of *personal security* refers to the healthcare system's protection of an individual's peace of mind. This is accomplished through meeting healthcare needs and attention to financial security, which is meeting healthcare needs without personal impoverishment. Medicare and Medicaid, under continuing threat, are national examples of legislation to address concerns of the elderly and other populations for meeting their healthcare needs without going bankrupt. Generally, personal security has not been valued in U.S. healthcare policy as it has in other places such as the Scandinavian countries.

While the *Code of Ethics for Pharmacists* focuses on advocacy for individual patients, the code also speaks to responsibilities to communities and society and to an obligation to "seek justice in the distribution of health resources."[8] p2 This provision of the code is important to consider as healthcare plans focus their priorities and policies on risk factors and health needs of populations or enriching their stockholders. Pharmacists may fulfill this obligation in several ways, such as participation in health policy development, health education of the public, or in organizations that serve the most vulnerable populations. These activities, traditionally those of public health, are also part of enabling individuals to take more responsibility for their own health. Support for values of social advocacy and solidarity reaffirm our interrelatedness as human beings who are both autonomous moral agents and interdependent members of society.

In summary, the values framework discussed in the Priester report[1] may be used to guide public debate and policy development for delivery of personal medical and pharmacy services and for realization of the public health goal of ensuring the conditions within which people can be healthy. The latter goal incorporates a comprehensive view of health services to individuals and populations at risk and determination of the impact of the environment on the health status of individuals and communities. Health policies and systems that do not reflect these realities are impoverished and fail to respect all members of the human community.[9]

Pharmacists are positioned in healthcare organizations and in communities to realize that all people are vulnerable to the vagaries of illness and to the impact of unhealthy environments and workplaces. Pharmacists have professional knowledge and experience that can be used to influence the distribution of health resources in an equitable way. While the pharmacists' professional code states that the primary obligation is to individual patients, their obligations also extend to communities and the broader society. These ethical obligations support the involvement of pharmacists in efforts to achieve fairness for all in meeting healthcare needs and reducing human suffering through participation in organizational and public policy development.

ETHICAL PRINCIPLES AND CONCEPTS IN PHARMACY PRACTICE

The values discussed in the previous section are reflected in this discussion of ethical principles and concepts drawn from the *Code of Ethics for Pharmacists*.[8] A key ethical concept in the code is trust. It is especially important to pay attention to this concept in evolving managed care arrangements because it has faded in contemporary healthcare institutions, as evidenced by malpractice suits and increasingly adversarial relations between healthcare professionals and the public. Trust is characterized by philosophers Beauchamp and Childress as confidence in and reliance on the ability and moral character (trustworthiness) of another person to "act with the right motives in accord with moral norms."[10 p469] Trustworthiness is a critical ingredient in the relationships between pharmacists and patients so that a patient can depend upon a pharmacist's behavior to be in the patient's best interests rather than solely a health plan's financial interests.

Three traditional ethical principles are reflected in the *Code*. They are: respect for autonomy; beneficence, which incorporates the principle of nonmaleficence; and justice. *Respect for autonomy* can be expanded to the broader principle of respect for persons. This broader principle requires attention to two dimensions. One is respect for autonomy as self-determination or self-governance, which is a major focus in discussions of bioethics.

The second dimension is respect for persons as interconnected and interdependent members of the human community. With the focus in managed care on populations, this dimension enriches the discussion of respect for autonomy and requires attention to the reality that many decisions made by individuals influence the well-being of others. This dimension has not received the attention that it needs in past bioethics writings and discussions. One consequence is that healthcare practitioners often focus solely on respect for self-determination with limited attention to the potential consequences of decisions that patients and others make in healthcare settings or to including significant others such as families in decision making if the patient wishes. Cultural differences in ways of making decisions about medical care and treatment have drawn attention to this important and realistic aspect of respect for persons. With their focus on population-based care, managed care arrangements are required to pay some attention to this aspect, even if it is not made explicit.

The principle of *beneficence* can be discussed as incorporating two aspects. One aspect is providing benefits; the second is avoiding or preventing harm (principle of *nonmaleficence*). Sometimes the principles are discussed as two separate principles. In this chapter, they are discussed together, as part of a spectrum extending from not inflicting harm to providing specific benefits; in fact, avoiding or preventing harm is a form of a benefit, even though patients may not always recognize this as a benefit. By withholding key information, for instance, a pharmacist affects the decision-making capacity and well-being of a patient or colleague; provision of that information prevents potential harm and promotes more informed decisions. Considerations of both beneficence and nonmaleficence express important ethical values in the face of managed care arrangements that withhold benefits or mandate other actions that cause potential harm to vulnerable patients or jeopardize professional integrity. The negative duty to avoid harm generally takes priority over provision of benefits, other things being equal, in situations where the two seem to conflict.

Further aspects of beneficence include the balancing of harms or costs and the benefits that promote and maintain health or reduce suffering. Costs are not solely financial. Costs may be anything that detracts from human health and well-being, such as physical pain and suffering, psychological pain, or opportunity costs such as giving up one's career to become the caregiver for a family member suffering with Alzheimer's disease. Because costs are often difficult to quantify, they are sometimes referred to as risks, that is, possible future harms.

Consideration of the principle of *justice* as fairness is fundamental to evolving managed care arrangements, whether it is discussed explicitly or not. While there is no consensus on what constitutes justice in our society or in healthcare organizations, the failure to consider justice and fairness issues hampers organizational and public discussions of ethically responsible policy for financing and delivery of health care. While most people probably agree that lack of access to basic health care for millions is unjust, there is no agreement on what constitutes a just healthcare system or how one could be developed.

Several ways of looking at justice from the perspectives of moral and political philosophy can inform the kinds of choices that are involved in development of health care and related policy such as individual justice, social justice, distributive justice, and intergenerational justice. Distributive justice in health care involves the fair distribution of costs and benefits when resources are finite and the goal is fair distribution. Benefits take several forms such as access to adequate information for decision making about a recommended drug treatment. As noted earlier, burdens or costs also may take several forms, including the time involved in education to assist patients in making better informed decisions.

Treating people in similar circumstances similarly is an important goal in seeking justice as fairness. Yet individuals are often treated differently solely because of their race or socioeconomic status. Such reasons for treating people differently are not ethical or just. To morally justify treating individuals or groups differently, relevant differences between them must be considered. Differences may include age, individual need, individual effort, ability to pay, societal contribution, or contract. Age is a very controversial criterion for distributing health care as it may lead to unfair discrimination—an example is withholding costly high-technology care at the end of life. Ability to pay is problematic as a basis for treating people differently because people do not choose the socioeconomic circumstances into which they are born or their genetic profiles. Both influence health status. Different bases for distribution are used in different contexts, such as welfare payments, which are based on need, while jobs and promotions are usually distributed on the basis of individual achievement or merit.[10 p331]

Individual need, generally described as *medical necessity* in managed care settings, is a commonly invoked basis for distribution of benefits. One issue in using the concept of need to justify differential treatment is how to distinguish needs from demands or desires. *Fundamental needs* may be defined as needs for something without which one will be harmed. For example, impoverished elderly individuals may have to choose between two fundamental needs: spending money for food or spending money for drugs critical to treatment of a serious chronic illness such as diabetes. Personal security, an important value in the framework presented earlier, is at stake in this and similar situations.

Philosopher John Rawls provides another starting point for considering the goal of treating similar people similarly in the fair distribution of health care, including access to needed pharmaceutical products and services. According to Rawls, principles of justice are concerned with "primary social goods" such as income, wealth, liberty, opportunity, and bases for self-respect.[11] While Rawls makes no claim that his ideas can be directly applied to societal issues such as access to health care, one of his proposed principles is particularly relevant for those individuals and populations who are vulnerable by virtue of their health or socioeconomic status. The principle states that inequalities may be allowed only to improve the condition of the least fortunate or the most vulnerable in a society. These individuals or groups should be in a normative position in any society that claims to treat people fairly. Basic rights and obligations then proceed from the notion of fairness for the least advantaged.[11] While the most socially advantaged may still benefit under this principle, consequences for the least advantaged must always be considered explicitly in public policy development. Using this principle, for-profit and not-for-profit managed care arrangements must pay attention to their social responsibilities to the least-advantaged. Using income inequalities and ability to pay as screening devices for access to healthcare services is ethically unjustifiable under this view of justice as fairness. Skimming healthier individuals for a patient base also becomes ethically problematic for healthcare organizations when adequate provisions are not made by society for care of the chronically and seriously ill, who run the risk of being abandoned.

Bioethicist Ezekiel Emanuel proposes four principles for the just allocation of healthcare resources in order to improve justice within American health care when society has no overall consensus on what constitutes justice.[12]

He claims that these principles, dealing with access and allocation as two dimensions of justice, will be helpful because they are already widely accepted in managed care and are related to justice because they bear on *how* allocation decisions are made. The four broad principles are: improving health should be the primary goal; patients and members should be informed; patients and members should have the opportunity to consent; and conflicts of interest should be minimized. While these principles do not provide ready-made answers in a particular situation, they do provide general criteria for assessing decisions and actions where issues of justice and fairness are at stake in managed care arrangements.

This brief discussion of trust, respect for persons, beneficence, and justice as fairness can be used as a resource by individual pharmacists and the profession collectively to further discern and reflect on their ethical obligations in managed care organizations and systems. Philosophers Beauchamp and Childress remind us that "disunity, conflict, and moral ambiguity" are pervasive aspects of our moral lives in community that also include ". . . untidiness, complexity, and conflict."[10 p107] These realities affirm the interdependence and interconnectedness of human beings, which is a significant part of the principle of respect for persons as pharmacists, along with other health professionals, and patients' struggle to resolve moral conflicts in making individual and policy decisions.

RESOURCES FOR MANAGING ETHICAL CONCERNS IN PHARMACY PRACTICE

As evolving managed care environments raise new and difficult professional challenges for pharmacists, ethically justifiable responses must be developed to support the integrity of the individual healthcare provider and the integrity of healthcare services and systems. There are several types of organizational and professional support available for pharmacists who seek to improve the ways in which they manage their ethical concerns. These mechanisms are not always readily available, but new technologies such as the Internet make ethics education more accessible than ever before.

PROFESSIONAL CODE OF ETHICS

A readily available general guide on ethics for pharmacists is the *Code of Ethics for Pharmacists* (mentioned earlier) adopted by the American Pharmaceutical Association.[8] While most professional codes express fundamental values and obligations of the profession, individuals often find that codes are not very helpful in responding to specific situations and value conflicts. Healthcare professionals who find this frustrating must remember that codes are not designed for that particular purpose. But professional codes do serve as starting points for reflection on ethical concerns and make public the ethical commitments of a profession. Sometimes just being aware of the tenets of a professional code and using them as a benchmark in an ethically troubling situation will provide enough guidance to cause an individual to reconsider an action that might be taken without ethical reflection. Acting with honesty and integrity in professional relationships is one provision of the pharmacists' code that might give an individual pause if he or she thinks that deceiving a colleague justifies a desired end. Just thinking about the potential consequences and human costs that might arise from deceiving a colleague may prevent such behavior. One consequence is the potential loss of trust and confidence if one's colleague suspects or discovers the deceit. Trust between colleagues is essential for good working relationships and is not to be tossed aside lightly. Sometimes professionals can decide whether one proposed action is better ethically than another by thinking about whether they would want to tell their families or a television news reporter about all possible actions that one is considering.

DECISION-MAKING GUIDES

Many decision-making guides have been developed to assist pharmacists and others with ethical dilemmas. General elements of these guidelines include: review of the overall situation; identification of the "facts" of the situation and the information needed, such as the patient's values and goals for treatment, response to specific drugs, and any relevant legal information; identification of other affected parties or stakeholders who will receive the benefits and bear the burdens or costs of the pharmacist's decision; specific ethical issues or conflicts in the situation; possible options for action and each action's ethical justification; and identification of foreseeable consequences and practical constraints (legal, economic, political, etc.) of each option. Once these steps have been taken, individuals may take action or follow up on recommendations, assess the situation, and clarify how what has been learned may help in similar situations in the future, and identify any implications for policy assessment and development. Using such a decision-making framework will not guarantee a single right answer, but it will help a person develop an ethically justifiable response based on thoughtful reflection and analysis and may help him or her to reject some possible choices for action. These guidelines for moral reasoning can be used in combination with the *Code of Ethics for Pharmacists* to develop responses for examples of ethical issues provided earlier in the chapter, such as protection of patient privacy and assuring informed decision making.

ORGANIZATIONAL MECHANISMS, REQUIREMENTS, AND GUIDELINES

Pharmacists in many hospitals and healthcare systems, including HMOs, have access to ethics committees and ethics education programs for assistance in dealing with actual or potential ethical concerns. Ethics committees generally have three overall functions: education, consultation, and policy development and review. They may be composed of physicians, nurses, social workers, clergy, bioethicists, and administrators. Some institutional ethics committees include laypeople and legal counsel. Pharmacists also serve on ethics committees in some MCOs or use existing committees for consultation.

Regulatory statements such as those promulgated by the JCAH require that their accredited organizations must have a code of ethical behavior that addresses business practices such as marketing, transfer and discharge, and billing. In addition, they are required to develop mechanisms such as ethics committees to respond to ethical issues in patient care and in the work of health professionals. Some hospitals employ only an ethics consultant because they do not want an interdisciplinary committee to serve in this capacity. Other institutions such as nursing homes, long-term care facilities, and home care agencies sometimes have an ethics committee or access to a committee or a consultant if they are part of a larger healthcare system. Community-wide ethics committees or networks also exist in some geographic areas.

Three organizations have developed guidelines for managed care that incorporate ethical values. They are the Midwest Bioethics Center, the Coalition for Accountable Managed Care, and the National Academies of Practice Interdisciplinary Association of Professionals. The Midwest Bioethics Center developed a document entitled, *Ethical Issues in Managed Care: Guidelines for Clinicians and Recommendations to Accrediting Organizations.*[13] This document emphasizes the need to create an ethical corporate culture; addresses the rights and responsibilities of members, providers, and plans in managed care; and links concerns for ethics with quality. This document is used for guidance across the country by the JCAH and other groups, including managed care plans. Members of the task force that developed these guidelines used the ethical principle of respect for persons to ground their reflection and development of recommendations. The recommendations in this document respect societal pluralism, provide ethical guidance for resource allocation, and point to the need for managed care organizations to pay attention to social responsibilities such as pro bono care.

The Coalition for Accountable Managed Care, composed of physician, medical, health, and hospital organizations, developed *The Principles for Accountable Managed Care.*[14] These principles are meant to apply to all types of managed care plans and provide a missing dimension to discussions of managed care by public and private policy makers. The principles include: promotion of access to services without discrimination in enrollment; provision of quality care through clinical excellence; identification of and response to needs of communities through community accountability and commitment to community service, including provision of care to persons unable to pay, the community's underserved, and high-risk patients; health system improvement and participation in community public health initiatives; provision of consumer information, education, and choice; governance of plans that is representative of the interests and needs of populations and the community as well as the enrolled population; and financial responsibility, which includes the budgeting of adequate resources to carry out previously described principles.

The National Academies of Practice, including Pharmacy, developed *Ethical Guidelines for Professional Care and Services in a Managed Care Environment*, which are broad guidelines, founded on patient advocacy and protection of patient welfare. They recognize that "virtually all managed care plans tend to shift financial risk from payers to health professionals"[15 p1] with the potential to create ethical conflicts because of a tension between economic considerations and patient-focused care. Professionals are then caught in clashes between prudent use of resources, professional standards of care, and their commitment to patients. The National Academies of Practice takes the strong position that it is unethical to compromise patient care to satisfy financial objectives. Examples of benefits that all providers should offer include: patient access to appropriate professional services; patient satisfaction with those services; flexible use of clinical guidelines so that practitioners' decisions are not hampered; and provision of professional expertise beyond primary care as determined by the complexity of the patient situation. There are also strong positions taken on disclosure of information. Practitioners, including pharmacists, should be able to offer patients the information and options for care and services that are needed for informed decision making based on the patient's right to informed consent and decision making. Health professionals should not be hampered by economic restrictions or contractual prohibitions such as gag rules that restrict provision of information to plan coverage only.

In summary, individual pharmacists and the profession have several resources available to assist them in managing ethical conflicts and concerns in managed care settings.

CONCLUSION

Pharmacists are confronted with new and troubling ethical issues in evolving managed care systems. Discussions of values, principles, and concepts can help pharmacists confront situations that require ethical reflection for their resolution. Resources such as the professional code of ethics and guidelines developed by professional organizations and accrediting bodies such as the JCAH can be useful for individual pharmacists and for education programs provided by professional associations and organizations. Pharmacists do not have to search alone for solutions to their ethical problems. Resources in this chapter provide a starting place for managing ethical issues that confront pharmacists, other health professionals, and patients in managed care settings in more proactive and preventive ways.

REFERENCES

1. Priester R., Value based formulas for purchasing. Does managed care offer value to society? *Manag Care Q.* 1997; 5(1): 57-63.

2. Worthley J.A., *The Ethics of the Ordinary in Healthcare.* Chicago: Health Administration Press; 1997: 4-10.

3. Chambliss D., *Beyond Caring: Hospitals, Nurses, and the Social Organization of Ethics.* Chicago: University of Chicago Press; 1996: 182-183.

4. *Comprehensive Accreditation Manual for Hospitals.* Oakbrook Terrace, IL: Joint Commission on Accreditation of Healthcare Organizations; 1996: 35.

5. Priester R., A values framework for health system reform. *Health Aff.* 1992; 11(1): 84-107.

6. Kassirer J., Managing care—should we adopt a new ethic? [Editorial] *N Engl J Med.* 1998; 339(6): 397-398.

7. President's Commission for the Study of Ethical Problems in Medicine and Biomedical and Behavioral Research. *Securing Access to Health Care.* Washington, DC: U.S. Government Printing Office; 1983: 5. Available at http://bioethics.gov/reports/past_commissions/securing_access.pdf. Accessed 27 July 2008.

8. *Code of Ethics for Pharmacists (revised).* Washington, DC: American Pharmaceutical Association; 1994: 2.

9. Aroskar M.A., Exploring ethical terrain in public health. *J Public Health Manag Pract.* 1995; 1(3): 16-22.

10. Beauchamp T.L., Childress J.F., *Principles of Biomedical Ethics,* 4th ed. New York: Oxford University Press; 1994.

11. Rawls J., *A Theory of Justice.* Cambridge, MA: Harvard University Press; 1971: 62-80.

12. Emanuel E.J. Justice and Managed Care: Four Principles for the Just Allocation of Health Care Resources. *Hast Cent Rep.* 2000; 30(3): 8-16.

13. Biblo J., Christopher MJ, Johnson L, et al. *Ethical Issues in Managed Care: Guidelines for Clinicians and Recommendations to Accrediting Organizations.* Kansas City, MO: Midwest Bioethics Center; 1995: 11-20.

14. Coalition for Accountable Managed Care. *Principles for Accountable Managed Care.* Washington, DC; 1997: 5-12.

15. National Academies of Practice, *Ethical Guidelines for Professional Care and Services in a Managed Care Environment.* Edgewood, MD; 1999: 1-3.

SUGGESTED READING

Emanuel E.J., Justice and managed care: four principles for the just allocation of health care resources. *Hast Cent Rep.* 2000; 30(3): 8-16.

Lisi D.M., Ethical issues for pharmacists in managed care. *Am J Health-Syst Phar.* 1997; 54(9): 1041-1042, 1045.

Randel L., Pearson S.D., Sabin J.E., et al. How managed care can be ethical. *Health Aff.* 2001; 20(4): 43-56.

Resnik D.B., Ranelli P.L., Resnik S.P., The conflict between ethics and business in community pharmacy: what about patient counseling? *J Bus Ethics.* 2000; 28(2, part 2): 179-186.

<table>
<tr><td>

Chapter

24

</td><td>

POLITICS, PUBLIC POLICY, AND NATIONAL HEALTHCARE REFORM: MEDICARE AND THE MEDICARE MODERNIZATION ACT OF 2003

</td></tr>
</table>

ALAN LYLES

Politics is the art of the possible.
Otto von Bismarck, 1867

———

The dream of reason did not take power into account.
Paul Starr, 1982

INTRODUCTION

The Medicare Modernization Act of 2003 was a victory of politics and expediency and, ironically, a success claimed by the political party least associated with expanding Medicare benefits. Health programs and public benefits expansion have been traditionally issues championed by the Democratic Party, while the Republican Party conventionally has advocated fiscal discipline and the responsibility of states for health and welfare programs. With U.S. spending on health care at $2 trillion in 2005 and 16% of Gross Domestic Product (GDP),[1] the politics of health care are intense, often quite narrow, and include ideology, pragmatism, and self-interest.

In 1973, Republican President Richard Nixon signed the Health Maintenance Organization (HMO) Act to control the rate of growth in healthcare costs. In 1983, Republican President Ronald Reagan advanced the Prospective Payment System (Diagnosis Related Groups) for hospitals using the purchasing power of the Medicare program to restrain hospital cost increases.[2] President Reagan also signed the Consolidated Omnibus Budget Reconciliation Act of 1985 that established a resource-based relative value scale (RBRVS) for physician payments and created the Physician Payment Review Commission (PPRC), both of which were distinctly not pro-market approaches. The Omnibus Budget Reconciliation Act of 1989, also signed by a Republican President (George H.W. Bush), included a Medicare fee schedule to restrain expenditures for physicians' services.[3]

How was it that in 2003, a Republican President signed into law the Medicare Modernization Act (MMA) containing a prescription drug benefit[4] that the Congressional Budget Office estimated to cost $395 billion over its first ten years? Answering this question requires a brief review of American constitutional democracy and its core values. MMA's specific features and how they were implemented are a result of the federal legislative process, political party platforms and coalitions, and interest group pressures.

Today's politics and health policy continue the divisions and reflect the structures that emerged from the colonial period. The former American colonies were primarily localities and states and only secondarily units of a new nation. From the beginning, distrust of a strong central government influenced the division of powers between the states and the developing federal government.

BACKGROUND: POLITICAL VALUES, FEDERALISM, AND THE LEGISLATIVE PROCESS

STATE VERSUS FEDERAL AUTHORITIES: DUAL SOVEREIGNTY

The Articles of Confederation, the first experiment with a national government model, was a provisional structure during the American Revolution that gave so little power to the new central government that it failed in the post-war period. A new Constitution emerged from the Constitutional Convention of 1787, but even then passage by the states was uncertain; many were concerned that in joining this new union they would be giving up too much of their autonomy. The stronger federalism contained in the new Constitution could only be achieved through the voluntary consent of the recently independent states to cede some authorities to this federal government. There was marginal enthusiasm for this new Constitution; many believed that it took power that legitimately resided and that should remain in the states. For example, Article I, Section I boldly states: "All legislative Powers herein granted shall be vested in a Congress of the United States, which shall consist of a Senate and House of Representatives."[3] To secure states' support for the ratification of the Constitution, ten amendments to the Constitution (the "Bill of Rights") explicitly protecting individual freedoms and setting additional limits to federal versus state authorities were promised.

The eventual Constitution and its amendments provided a federal government with only those powers essential to the functioning of an independent nation and which the states were willing to delegate to it; some examples are national defense, and foreign and diplomatic relations. Federalism in the American experience recognizes federal and state powers over the same individuals and the same regions but the specific authorities differ. Much of the federal government's role in health care has developed under legislation that uses funding incentives to encourage states to participate in programs when the federal government lacks authority to compel them to do so.

The Ninth Amendment clarified the range of individual freedoms protected under the Constitution: "The enumeration in the Constitution, of certain rights, shall not be construed to deny or disparage others retained by the people."[3] Concerns regarding the protection of states' rights prompted the Tenth Amendment, which explicitly recognizes that limited federal powers come from the states: "The powers not delegated to the United States by the Constitution, nor prohibited by it to the States, are reserved to the States respectively, or to the people."[5] It is this Amendment that retained state authority over police powers; that is, health, education, welfare, and law enforcement, among other functions.[6] Consequently, a national health policy could not be imposed on the states by the federal government but only implemented indirectly, such as through financing medical services.

LEGISLATION AND POLITICS AT THE NATIONAL LEVEL

Having experienced the consequences of unchecked centralized power as colonists, the designers of the new government were careful to establish a foundation that would prevent that in the new Union. Their solution was separation of powers and a system of checks and balances between the branches of government and even within the Congress. This structure was intended to minimize the risk of the ascendancy of any one branch of government, or faction. However, it makes change difficult and major change very difficult. Thus, partitioning power promotes stability and the status quo, as radical legislative change would require the concurrence of many groups, at least some of whom would likely have divergent interests and serve as a restraint on the others.

Consequently, most legislative initiatives do not become law because interests differ more often than they align and robust coalitions are difficult to create. Successful bills must pass through the stages of introduction by a sponsor in the Congress, with assignment to committee(s) and possibly subcommittee(s). Bills may span the jurisdictions of more than one committee, so the choice of the primary committee to which the bill is assigned can influence the legislative outcome. Committees are the working units of the legislature. They may hold hearings, add amendments, produce a report(s), and vote on a measure or "table it," meaning that it is effectively no longer active. Appointment as a committee chairman confers both status and authority, giving a strong opportunity to advance legislation consistent with a Chair's and her/his party's goals and to retard the legislative agenda of the opposing party. In the Senate, a bill voted out of Committee may then be scheduled for consideration and a possible vote. In the event of a tie, the Vice-President casts the tie-breaking vote, giving a slight edge to the Administration's political party.

In the House of Representatives, however, a positive Committee vote leads to consideration by the Rules Committee, which is responsible for scheduling debate on the bill, the length of that debate and whether amendments from the floor would be permitted. Only then can the bill be brought before the House. In effect, the Rules Committee acts as a gatekeeper, and can prevent action on bills that may have majority support but are not supported by the leadership. This Committee can further control legislation by when it schedules votes and by prohibiting amendments from the House floor; in the 108th United States Congress (January 3, 2003–January 3, 2005), 72% of bills brought to the floor prohibited the addition of amendments.[7] Commenting on the one day in which they had to read the 415 page MMA bill, Representative Nita Lowey (D-NY) said, "There was no way that every member of Congress could hold up their right hand and say, 'I read every page of that bill before the vote.'"[7]

Even if a bill were to be introduced in both chambers in the same form, it is unlikely that changes to the bill would be the same in each. A Conference Committee is used to reconcile these differences and produce a bill in the final form that is returned to each chamber for a vote. Traditionally, the Conference Committee has accepted the portions of the bill on which there was agreement and worked to resolve the areas where there was disagreement, but did not introduce new features not previously debated.[7] Based on the Conference Committee report and the revised bill, the House and the Senate vote on the final version. If the legislation is successful at this stage, then the President may sign it or veto it and the bill does not become law (other details omitted; for a full discussion, see The Library of Congress[8]). If the President does veto the bill, a 2/3 majority in each chamber can successfully override the President's veto and the bill will still become law. There could be a constitutional challenge to the law and if the Supreme Court hears the case it may uphold the law or it may declare the law to be unconstitutional and void it.

POLITICAL PARTIES

In practice, elected officials' political party affiliation strongly determines the fate of legislation, and, if successful, its contents. A divided government exists when the majority political party differs between the House and the Senate or between the Congress and the President. A unified government exists when the majorities of both houses are from the same party as the President. While there is dispute on which form results in more legislative accomplishments, Coleman argues persuasively that political party cohesion in a united government overcomes many of the Constitution's structural impediments to legislative action.[9] One way this occurs is that Committee Chair assignments are based on majority party membership. In addition, Conference Committee assignments and the composition of the conference committees are determined by political party, with the majority party having greater representation. A unified government provides unusual opportunities to implement a party's legislative agenda. For example, working with a unified Republican Party government, President Bush did not veto any legislation until his fifth year in office.[10] Conversely, a divided government poses numerous obstacles to legislative actions.

INTEREST GROUPS, LOBBYING, AND INFLUENCE

Interest group activities and lobbying to influence public policy are often viewed as political perversions that corrupt open discourse and unbiased consideration of the balance among individual, group, and public preferences. Yet these activities are at the heart of representative democracy; they express the people's will without trampling minority or dissenting group rights. Interest group politics embody the acceptance of, if not respect for, political pluralism, which is a fundamental characteristic of government and health policy development in the United States. Pluralism recognizes legitimately differing views both on issues appropriate for policy intervention and, if so, the appropriate mechanisms for those interventions. This contest of views is often reflected in the political process to achieve their resolution, one that relies on the formation of groups with shared interests, the articulation of those interests, and compromise when competing groups are sufficiently powerful or influential to block an interest group's preferred action.

In writing to persuade ratification of the Constitution, Madison anticipated modern concerns about interest groups, lobbyists, and undue influence on government actions. In the *Federalist No. 10*, he addressed the ". . . mischiefs of factions . . . By a faction, I [Madison] understand a number of citizens, whether amounting to a majority or a minority of the whole, who are united and actuated by some common impulse of passion, or of interest, adversed to the rights of other citizens, or to the permanent and aggregate interests of the community . . ."[11] Madison saw factions (interest groups) as a threat to individual liberty, but argued that they could not be removed without the loss of that liberty. Thus, he continued, a republic must rely on representative government and many factions, so many that there would be a likelihood that no one would dominate.

Some of the ways in which modern interest groups attempt to influence legislators are through the use of issue advertisements, campaign contributions, and lobbyists. President Clinton's Health Security Act of 1993 encountered interest group opposition by the *Coalition for Health Insurance Choices*, a group financed substantially by the Health Insurance Association of America (HIAA). A memorable series of advertisements paid for by the *Coalition for Health Insurance Choices* featured 'Harry and Louise' with Louise grimly saying, "There's got to be a better way," and an announcer following with, "Things are going to change, and not all for the better . . . The Government may force us to pick from a few health care plans designed by Government bureaucrats."[12] The campaign was noted for its originality and for its effectiveness in swaying public opinion in the direction of HIAA's opposition to the Health Security Act.[13]

CAMPAIGN CONTRIBUTIONS

The United States Federal Election Commission has an online, searchable database of campaign finance disclosures by political candidates.[14] In addition, watchdog groups and investigational reports provide a view on the flow of funds around particular issues, politicians, and political parties. The scale of these contributions suggests a relative ability to assure that a perspective or set of interests receive thorough consideration. For the period 1989 to 2006, the American Federation of State, County & Municipal Employees was the leading donor to federal campaigns at $38.1 million; the American Medical Association was 11th with $24.2 million; the American Hospital Association was 40th with $13.6 million; Blue Cross Blue Shield was 44th at $12.8 million; Pfizer was 58th with $11.2 million; GlaxoSmithkline was 78th with $8.5 million; and Eli Lilly was 87th at $7.8 million, just slightly behind the American Academy of Ophthalmology, which was 84th at $8 million.[15]

The Center for Responsive Politics also divides the campaign contributions by the recipient political party, suggesting where the donors see the best potential for legislators with a perspective more consistent with their interests. In the past, contributions and relationships existed between interest groups and both major political parties, even if the relationship tilted to one of them. However, two substantial changes occurred in recent years that have altered that practice: 1) House Majority Leader Tom Delay's (a.k.a. *The Hammer*) *Pay-to-Play* criterion, and 2) the now infamous *K Street Project*, which associated the Republican Party with lobbying firms on K Street in Washington as a strategy of aggressive fundraising. According to Fred Wertheimer, Democracy 21 president, the way these worked is that, "If you want to do business with Republicans, you have to give your money to Republicans—and not give any money to the Democrats—and you have to hire Republicans from the Hill to be your lobbyists."[16] Melanie Sloan, of Citizens for Responsibility and Ethics in Washington (CREW), explained the 2005 dynamic in the pendulum of financial corruption that passes between the Democratic and Republican parties: "It would be difficult to bribe a Democrat, particularly a Democrat in the House, because they can't deliver anything . . . You need to have power to abuse it."[16] The net result has been a far more partisan approach to interest group representation and effective lobbying, even when it does not cross legal boundaries.

When issues are not contested or if the contest is not close, lobbying is less intense (and lucrative). However, when there are strong, divided positions on the desirability or the content of legislation, the intensity increases. When the potential sums of money involved are very large, it escalates even more. These were the conditions in the Congress just prior to the MMA's passing. According to Robert M. Hayes, a consumer activist, "It became a feeding frenzy."[17]

From 1990 through the 2006 federal election cycles, pharmaceutical manufacturing monies peaked in 2000 and 2002, with 72% of it going to Republican Party candidates.[18] Viewing data from the Center for Responsive Politics during this period provides a consistent pattern of Congressional donations going to incumbents rather than to the wider field of candidates. The Bipartisan Campaign Reform Act of 2002, also known as the McCain-Feingold Act after its lead sponsors, was intended to reduce the corrosive effects of special interest influence secured through donations. It focused mainly on regulation of soft money contributions, which in principle were to support parties and not specific candidates, but money is fungible so in practice it had become a source of unregulated monies.[19]

LOBBYISTS

In addition to direct contributions to political campaigns, interest groups retain the services of lobbyists to advance their legislative agenda. According to an investigative report by the *Boston Globe*, "The dearth of debate and open dealing in the House [of Representatives] has given a crucial advantage to a select group of industry lobbyists who are personally close to decision-makers in Congress."[20] From the *Boston Globe's* report, expenditures for the top ten lobbyists for the Medicare bill are seen in **Table 24-1**.

TABLE 24-1 **Expenditures of the Top Ten Lobbyists in 2004**

Donor	Amount ($ in millions)
American Association of Retired Persons (AARP)	$20.9
American Medical Association (AMA)	$17.3
Pharmaceutical Research and Manufacturers of America (PhRMA)	$16.0
American Heart Association	$12.5
Merck & Co., Inc.	$7.5
National Committee to Preserve Social Security and Medicare	$6.8
America's Health Insurance Plans	$5.8 [pre-merger]
Bristol-Myers Squibb Company	$5.3
The Seniors Coalition	$5.3
GlaxoSmithKline	$5.0

Source: Milligan S., "Closed, for Business." *Boston Globe* Special Series. October 3, 2004. And Rowland C., "Medicare bill: a study in D.C. spoils system." *Boston Globe* Special Series. October 5, 2004. Chart available at http://www.boston.com/news/specials/closed_for_business/chart_medicare_top/. Accessed 30 July 2008.

One way a lobbyist can advance a group's interests is by influencing a legislator's use of *earmarks*. The Office of Management and Budget defines an earmark as, ". . . *funds provided by the Congress for projects or programs where the congressional direction (in bill or report language) circumvents the merit-based or competitive allocation process, or specifies the location or recipient, or otherwise curtails the ability of the Administration to control critical aspects of the funds allocation process.*"[21] The 2004 Consolidated Omnibus Spending Bill, the last prior to the 2004 elections, included 7,931 earmarks that added an estimated $10.7 billion to the budget.[22]

A BRIEF HISTORY OF MEDICARE

The context of the times creates opportunities for health policy initiatives or barriers forcing retrenchment and delay. The Great Depression in the United States brought Franklin Delano Roosevelt to the Presidency in 1933, with his New Deal and promise of an active federal role in the economy and social programs. President Roosevelt, a Democrat, convened a Committee on Economic Security in 1934 to examine and make recommendations regarding the elderly, the unemployed, medical, and health insurance. However, health insurance was not included in the ensuing Social Security Act of 1935. In the interim, the American Medical Association's "House of Delegates once again denounced compulsory health insurance and any lay control of medical benefits in relief agencies . . . but . . . accepted voluntary insurance plans for medical service, so long as the plans were under the control of county medical societies and followed American Medical Association (AMA) guidelines."[23] A tightening economy during the mid-to late 1930s led to infighting among federal agencies for priority funding, creating an additional barrier to passage of health insurance and its position relative to the priorities of existing agencies and their portfolios.

As unemployment surged from 14.3% in 1937 to 19.0% in 1938,[24] there were growing concerns that the New Deal programs were failing to address the economic depression of the 1930s. Voters expressed their views in the 1938 Congressional elections, returning a Congress that had bipartisan resistance to extensions of the New Deal or social welfare programs. The growing prospect of war shifted attention and funding from domestic to international concerns. Despite the introduction of the Wagner-Murray-Dingell bill for universal, comprehensive national health insurance in 1943 [p.280], President Roosevelt's assessment was that, "We can't go up against state medical societies; we just can't do it."[25] The bill died in committee but was reintroduced by President Truman, also a Democrat, in 1945. "Immediately after the President's [Truman's] message, the National Physician's Committee, a professional lobby set up in 1938 to receive contributions mainly from the drug industry, sent out an emergency bulletin calling upon doctors to resist the program."[23 p281-282]

The 1946 mid-year elections returned a Republican majority, who "charged that national health insurance was part of a larger socialist scheme."[23 p284] A Democratic majority in Congress—although conservative—was restored and the Democratic Party candidate for president won a surprising re-election in 1948.[26]

The late 1940s saw a convergence of factors internal and external to health care that illustrate the difficulty of major change in national healthcare policy:

1. A growing concern about international communism;
2. The Labor movement's shift from strong support of government health insurance to negotiating to expand employment-based private insurance;
3. Rising unemployment;
4. Concerted opposition by the AMA, which established a $4.5 million fund from a special per member fee against "the enslavement of the medical profession" by the Wagner-Murray-Dingell bill in Congress.[21]

The AMA spent $1.5 million in 1949 on a campaign to mobilize opinion against government health insurance, which was "at that time the most expensive lobbying effort in American history."[22] This campaign against President Truman's proposal successfully capitalized on the fears of the time by characterizing government health insurance as socialized medicine, an association that has proven durable and beneficial to the profession.[23 p285] Compounding these difficulties in developing a government health insurance policy agenda, President Truman's support of civil rights alienated southern Democrats. General Dwight Eisenhower, a declared opponent of government health insurance, was elected in 1952 and the move for expanded health insurance coverage ceased being a priority. Senator Joseph McCarthy's anti-Communism agenda in the 1950s further marginalized government health insurance.

Using his considerable skills from the Senate and House of Representatives, President Lyndon Johnson secured passage of the Social Security Amendments Title XVIII (Medicare) and, with a powerful assist from the House Ways and Means Chairman Wilbur Mills, Title XIX (Medicaid). It was intentional, not accidental, that prescription drugs were excluded as a Medicare benefit initially because of their "unpredictable and potentially high costs."[27]

Over the years, both political parties have proposed changes that received strong opposition from interest groups. Mr. Caspar Weinberger, Secretary of Health, Education and Welfare under Republican President Nixon, proposed in 1973 paying for prescription drugs at "the lowest cost at which the drug is generally available unless there is a demonstrated difference in therapeutic effect."[28] The Omnibus Budget Reconciliation Act of 1990 (OBRA90) created the Medicaid Drug Rebate Program.[29] Under this program, manufacturers gave a rebate to the federal government based on the difference between the price charged Medicaid programs and the best price charged to other purchasers of their drugs. In Federal Fiscal Year 2001 alone, this program returned approximately $4.9 billion from pharmaceutical manufacturers.[30] Two decades after Secretary Weinberger's proposal, President Clinton's Consumer Choice Health Security Act of 1993 would have required rebates from manufacturers, but not from generic manufacturers or for those enrolled in managed care plans, and would have given the Secretary of the Department of Health and Human Services the authority to negotiate drug prices.[31] For numerous reasons, this act was not passed. These experiences crystallized Pharmaceutical Research and Manufacturers' (PhRMA) position favoring private plans versus Medicare as the vehicle for a drug benefit and, based on the Medicaid rebate experience, that the federal government not be a direct purchaser or payor for pharmaceuticals.

Nonetheless, there was, for a brief time, prescription drug coverage under the Medicare Catastrophic Coverage Act (MCCA), passed in 1988 and repealed in 1989.[32] The political lessons from this experience influenced lawmakers who would later consider a Medicare drug benefit. MCCA was designed to meet the needs of the most desperate Medicare beneficiaries, those with catastrophic illness, and to be "budget neutral," that is, it could not add net costs to the federal budget. Thus it had two features that would prove to be fatal politically: 1) in any given year only one-fifth of beneficiaries would qualify for the catastrophic benefit, and 2) its funding relied on means testing (intra-generational transfers) of Medicare beneficiaries. Because most Medicare beneficiaries did not directly benefit from the program, and those with higher incomes generally had prescription drug coverage and thus would not need this more costly benefit, the program was ripe for organized opposition and was rescinded when it came. A tipping point was reached when the evening news showed Representative Daniel Rostenkowski (D-Ill), Chair of the House Ways and Means Committee and 31-year representative of the 8th Congressional District in Illinois, being chased from the Copernicus Senior Citizens Center by dissatisfied Medicare beneficiaries and cowering in his car.[23 p284]

The 1965 Medicare bill provided hospital and physician benefits with payment arrangements (fee-for-service) that retained the autonomy and support of providers and yet encouraged utilization and fueled cost increases. From the beginning, program cost forecasts consistently underestimated actual expenditures. The costs from the addition of benefits for end-stage renal disease (ESRD), for example, greatly exceeded even the highest initial estimates. These experiences created a wariness among fiscal and political conservatives against expanding the program any further—particularly with growing federal deficits—and, if possible, to scale back or eliminate it.

PROCESS AND HISTORY CONVERGE IN THE MMA OF 2003

Serious consideration of a Medicare program expansion to include prescription drugs was only possible because of a federal budget surplus. The transient federal surplus in the late 1990s allowed the possibility both of improving the long-term solvency of the Medicare program and of expanding it to include some form of a prescription drug benefit.

The federal budget deficit of $290 billion in 1992 had been resolved and the surplus of $125 billion in 1999 grew to $236 billion in the election year 2000.[33] However, by 2002 the budget had a deficit of $157.8 billion; in 2003, the deficit was $377.6 billion and in 2004 it increased further to $412.7 billion.[30] If a drug benefit were not passed using the provisional budget for it in the 2004 budget resolution, the growing deficit assured that there would not be a second chance. President Clinton announced his plan for such a benefit in June 1999, supporting marketplace competition but rejecting means-testing for payments or raising the Medicare qualification age.[34] Clearly, the politics of domestic social programs had a limited opportunity to achieve results.

Passage of the Medicare Prescription Drug, Improvement, and Modernization Act of 2003 (subsequently shortened to the Medicare Modernization Act [MMA]) was described by John Iglehart as, "a pure power play."[35] With a unified government, the Republican Party controlled the committee chairs, conference committee majority, and the Administration. Even this was almost not enough. Resistance came from across the political spectrum and for differing reasons. Mollifying the opposition required creative incentives, timing, and political force.

The Critical Committees and their Chairs for the 108th Congress were 1) the Senate Finance Committee, chaired by Senator Chuck Grassley (R-Ia) with ranking Democrat Max Baucus (D-Mt); and 2) two critical committees in the House of Representatives: the House Energy and Commerce Committee, chaired by Rep. William R. (Billy) Tauzin (R-La); and the powerful House Ways and Means Committee, Chaired by Rep. Bill Thomas (R-Calif). These Chairman appointments assured 1) a preference for prescription drug coverage through private plans, and 2) that rural patient and provider interests would receive intense consideration.

In March 2003, President Bush proposed a *Framework to Modernize and Improve Medicare*, identifying $400 billion over ten years, but requiring beneficiaries to join a private health plan to obtain a prescription drug coverage. The Senate Finance Committee rejected major provisions of the President's *Framework*, offering instead prescription drug benefits in the traditional Medicare fee-for-service program and in private preferred provider organization (PPO) plans. The Committee reported a bill, S. 1, the Prescription Drug and Medicare Improvement Act, and it was passed by the Senate on June 27, 2003. Reflecting Senators

Grassley and Baucus' rural home state allegiances, the Senate bill provided the Medicare program as a guarantee and fall back if there were not at least two private plans in a region. The drug benefit would begin in 2006 but the Committee provided for a drug discount card in the interim. Although not insurance, the discount drug card program included a $600 allowance for low-income beneficiaries. The House Committees with relevant jurisdiction passed a Medicare drug plan, also on June 27, that retained means-testing for catastrophic expense coverage; it succeeded by one vote.[36] Representative Jo Ann Emerson (R-Mo), who wanted to include the authority for importation of prescription drugs, cast the decisive vote in favor of the House measure when she received assurances that her proposal would be considered later, in a separate bill.[29]

The Conference Committee to reconcile the two bills began work in August 2003.

Representative Bill Thomas (R-Calif) chaired a Committee of ten Republicans and seven Democrats, although Senators Grassley and Baucus, who supported the measure, were the only Democrats allowed to participate in the Conference Committee discussions; the other Democrats were excluded from all but the first and last meetings. Representative Edward J. Markey (D-Mass), an excluded Democrat conferee, was reported to have said that he found out what was in the bill from lobbyists.[17]

The House and Senate versions of the Medicare bill differed substantially and, with positioning for the 2004 election already begun in 2003, it forced the White House to decide which bill to support. Senator Grassley said that the Administration's decision would indicate whether it believed California or Iowa was more important to re-election of President Bush; similarly he contrasted his bill with House Rep. Bill Thomas' approach as, "I'm legislating for 2010; he's legislating for 2004."[37]

On November 17, 2003, the American Association for Retired Persons (AARP), the powerful association for Americans over 50 years old and retirees, announced its support for the Medicare drug benefit. Although traditionally an ally of the Democratic Party's agenda, AARP saw a gain for its membership in the expansion of the Medicare program.[33] AARP's support was linked to including incentives for employers to continue offering prescription drug benefits for retirees. Later, however, it complained about the growth in Part B premiums caused by the MMA and urged removing the premium penalty for late enrollment.[38]

When the Conference Committee reached an impasse after months of work, House Speaker Dennis Hastert and Senate Majority Leader Bill Frist intervened to broker a compromise and liberate the bill from the Committee. The bill came before the House again, in its final form, on November 22, 2003. In a process that generally takes 15 minutes, the roll call vote for this legislation took two hours and fifty-one minutes—a record. The delay provided time for President Bush, by telephone, and Speaker Hastert in person to convince swing voters to support the legislation. Ultimately, the promises and compromises resulted in the bill's being passed by a vote of 220 for it and 215 against it.[35]

The Senate vote on the final form of the bill was also in doubt, and had to overcome a procedural objection to voting on it at all because its projected costs were larger than the total provided for it in the 2004 budget resolution.[39] Senator Frist marshaled one more than the 60 votes needed to overcome this objection and called for a vote on the bill. Despite the drama during the Senate vote regarding the forecasted costs of the drug benefit, the Department of Health and Human Services (DHHS) Actuary's ten-year cost estimate made on June 11, 2003, was subsequently revealed to have been even higher: $551.5 billion.[40,41] Had this information been made available prior to voting, it is likely that the legislation would not have passed. According to David Walker, Comptroller General of the United States, "the new prescription drug benefit . . . is one of the largest unfunded liabilities ever undertaken by the federal government."[42] In a reported e-mail to his colleagues, Richard S. Foster, chief Medicare actuary, wrote in March 2004, "I'm perhaps no longer in grave danger of being fired, but there remains a strong likelihood that I will have to resign in protest of the withholding of important technical information from key policy makers for political reasons."[43]

Iglehart's review identified major financial incentives to secure support from key constituencies: employers (~$89 billion in tax credits for continuing to offer retirees prescription drug benefits if they were already doing so), physicians (repeal of the 4.5% fee decreases scheduled for 2004 and 2005, replacing them with a 1.5% increase), rural providers (~$20 billion), state governments (~$16 billion in 2002 dollars by shifting dual-eligible enrollees to the federal program), health plans (a 10.6% increase in payments in 2004, and a ~$12.5 billion 'stabilization fund' to be used at the discretion of the Secretary DHHS to maintain private plan participation in all regions).[35] When viewed in its entirety, the range and depth of funds to make the legislation a reality are breathtaking.

In addition to the financial incentives, certain features of the MMA were designed to appeal to legislative preferences of key members of Congress and interest groups: to enlist votes for passage, not to create coherent policy or to facilitate implementation. As Kravitz observed, ". . . *political compromise often begets convoluted policy, but the Medicare drug benefit is particularly complex.*"[44] Consequently, there are elements of the MMA that address concerns of those who were against expansion of the program based on political philosophy and that the estimated increase in Medicare costs would not be fiscally responsible. Some required that their specific interests be addressed in order to give their support (e.g., physician fee increases versus scheduled cuts, Health Savings Accounts clearly provide a stimulus to new brokerage accounts and insurance products). Others believed that it did not go far enough in addressing the gaps in the program and needs of society; for them, the premiums and deductibles for these plans would be sliding scale and modified if any of the co-payments were for low income beneficiaries.

Approximately two months after President Bush signed the MMA into law and one year before the end of his congressional term, Representative William Tauzin resigned the House Energy and Commerce Committee chairmanship.[45] Former Representative Tauzin became President and Chief Executive Officer of the PhRMA, a public policy advocacy group for pharmaceutical and biotechnological research companies, effective January 3, 2005.[46] As a former Member of the House of Representatives, Mr. Tauzin would have privileges to be on the House Floor and to use the House gym, although explicit lobbying in these locations by former Members is prohibited. According to Democratic Representative Nancy Pelosi, "If you want to know the price of selling seniors down the river, it is approximately about $2 million a year, if you want to hire the manager of the bill on the floor of the House of Representatives."[45]

To achieve the maximum political benefit from passing this legislation, the MMA included an interim Medicare-approved drug discount card program; Medicaid enrollees were excluded. The discount drug card program spanned June 1, 2004 to December 31, 2005, and was immediately followed by the actual drug benefit on January 1, 2006. For qualified low-income beneficiaries this program provided a waiver of the enrollment fee and a $600 credit each year to be applied to the purchase of prescription drugs. Potential savings with these cards were estimated to be 11% to 18%, though even for those who would clearly benefit from the Transitional Assistance ($600 credit) enrollment lagged.[47]

OUTCOMES: IDEOLOGICAL AND PRAGMATIC

Safety

a. The Institute of Medicine: MMA charged the Institute of Medicine with performing "a comprehensive study . . . of drug safety and quality issues in order to provide a blue print for system-wide change," which was achieved, and a final report issued on July 20, 2006.[46] In addition, the Institute of Medicine study of health insurance performance measures, payment incentives, and performance improvement programs under Medicare's Quality Improvement Organization (QIO) Program was completed in March 2006.[49]

b. Drug Importation: The Department of Health and Human Services Task Force chaired by Surgeon General Carmona concluded, "In sum, this report finds that American consumers currently purchasing drugs from overseas are generally doing so at significant risk," that most savings would go to intermediaries and consumer savings would be modest, perhaps 1% to 2%.[50] The American Pharmacists Association (APhA), "applauds the extensive analysis of a complex issue by the Department of Health and Human Services' (HHS) Task Force on Importation,"[51] and the Academy of Managed Care Pharmacists (AMCP) similarly rejects importation until adequate safety data can be provided.[52] Ironically, the promise of legislation permitting drug importation was what had convinced Rep. Jo Ann Emerson (R-Mo) to give the deciding one-vote margin for passage of the MMA bill in the House of Representatives prior to going to the Conference Committee.

c. Medicare Health Support (initially known as the Chronic Care Improvement Program): MMA provides a three-year pilot project in the fee-for-service program to improve quality and achieve cost savings for the care of beneficiaries with congestive heart failure and/or complex diabetes. Participation by beneficiaries is voluntary. If targets are reached after 2½ years, the Secretary HHS can expand the program.

d. Medication Therapy Management Services: The MMA required drug therapy management for high risk and high cost Medicare beneficiaries, identifying these services as, "furnished by a pharmacist and that is designed to assure, with respect to targeted beneficiaries described in clause (ii), that covered part D drugs under the prescription drug plan are appropriately used to optimize therapeutic outcomes through improved medication use, and to reduce the risk of adverse events, including adverse drug interactions."[4] While this recognition was an advance for pharmacists, it left two main open issues: what are MTMSs exactly and how will their payment be determined? The pharmacy profession took the initiative and the Pharmacy Services Technical Advisory Coalition (consisting of the American Pharmacists Association, the National Association of Chain Drug Stores, and nine other organizations) defined an operational model for MTMS. It consists of Medication Therapy Review, a patient's personal medication record, a medication action plan, intervention and referral, and documentation and follow-up.[53] Regarding payment, CMS' position is that the fees for MTMS are included in a plan's administrative costs, that CMS will not establish a fee schedule for MTMS, and pharmacists must negotiate payment with the PDPs.[54] The inadequacy of this arrangement led John A. Gans, the American Pharmacists Association Executive Director, to propose to the Senate Finance Committee on February 6, 2007 that MTMS services be removed as a benefit from Medicare Part D and placed as a separate professional service under Part B.[55]

Modernization and Savings

a. Premiums, Deductibles, and Coinsurance: The basic design for the MMA drug benefit is a consequence of the restriction that the plan cost no more the $400 billion over its first decade. This led to a model against which proposed providers must be actuarially equivalent. Under this plan, in 2006 estimated premiums would be $35 per month with a $250 deductible. Once that annual deductible was met, there was 25% coinsurance for the next $2,850. At this point there was a $2,800 gap without coverage, the so-called *doughnut hole*. If a Medicare beneficiary still has qualified drug expenses at this point a catastrophic coverage provision provides program payment of 95% of expenses. To get to the catastrophic coverage level, however, Medicare beneficiaries must pay out-of-pocket $3,600 before that coverage. The premiums and deductibles are annual amounts indexed to the cost of increase in Medicare drug expenses. For Medicare beneficiaries on fixed incomes, this essentially assures that these costs will increase faster than their incomes.

September 22, 2005 was designated as "Doughnut Hole Day" to dramatize the gap in drug coverage; this was the day when the average Medicare beneficiaries would reach the point of no coverage until they pay an additional $2,800.[56]

b. e-Prescribing[57]:   e-Prescribing builds on existing foundation standards and is optional for physicians and pharmacists, but participating drug plans were required to have the capability to support it. As part of the e-Prescribing initiative, Medco Health Solutions performed an evaluation of the Southeastern Michigan Electronic Prescribing Initiative, one of the largest e-Prescribing programs, and a pilot project with four organizations: RAND Corporation and the New Jersey e-Prescribing Action Coalition; Brigham and Women's Hospital; SureScripts, Brown University and vendors; and, for long-term care facilities assessment, Achieve Healthcare Information Technology.[58] On April 17, 2007,

HHS Secretary Michael Levitt reported that, "electronic prescribing improves efficiencies while helping to eliminate potentially harmful drug interactions and other medication problems . . . It also solves the problem of hard-to-read handwritten prescriptions. Additionally, such health information technologies promote affordability by allowing physicians to know which medications are covered by their patients' Part D plans."[59] The pilots also identified standards that were not yet ready for broad use, such as detailed instructions for patients and prior authorization information. Additional information is in the article by Bell and Friedman.[60]

c. Formularies: Instead of having the Medicare program directly negotiate with pharmaceutical manufacturers, the MMA relies on formularies developed by private prescription drug plans (PDPs) and Medicare Advantage Prescription Drug (MAPD) plans. The oversight of this is consistent with public sector reliance on private sector standard setting or accreditation organizations. Using a model for formularies developed by the United States Pharmacopeia,[61] CMS reviews plan formularies. In addition, CMS must determine "that the design of the plan and its benefits (including any formulary and tiered formulary structure) are [not] likely to substantially discourage enrollment by certain part D eligible individuals under the plan."[62]

d. Pay for Performance (P4P):   To accommodate concerns that Medicare was not achieving optimal results for its medical care payments, a range of pay-for-performance initiatives were required. In collaboration with numerous partners, CMS is examining P4P initiatives for hospital care, physicians, the use of information technology, patient safety, chronic illness case management, high cost beneficiaries, ESRD, and disease management programs.[63] Early reports on these initiatives suggest modest improvements in the quality indicators, however, returns on investment are yet to be determined as to whether there are more effective mechanisms of achieving these results.[64-66]

e. Fraud and Abuse: To control costs and provide the oversight desired by the legislature, MMA required eight Medicare Drug Integrity Contractors (MEDICs) who would perform data mining and analysis to identify possible fraud and abuse, and refer such cases to law enforcement.[67]

Demonstration Projects   Influential conservative legislators who opposed expansion of the Medicare program held out for direct competition between private plans and traditional fee-for-service Medicare. The compromise to obtain their votes for the MMA was a pilot demonstration for six years, starting in 2010, in no more than six Metropolitan Statistical Areas chosen by the Secretary of HHS. The program, called the *Comparative Cost Adjustment Demonstration*, would create competition, but the feasibility of identifying the pilot regions and actually implementing this program is doubtful.

Private Health Plan Participation   The preference of key legislators, interest groups, and the Administration for a private or pro-competition component to the MMA had to address the

Medicare+Choice experience. Under that earlier program to encourage enrollment in private plans, there was initially an increasing number of private plans participating in Medicare only to see a 50% drop in participating plans[68] from 1998 to 2003. This occurred despite increases in the payments to these plans through the Balanced Budget Refinement Act of 1999 (BBRA) and the Benefits Improvement and Protection Act of 2000 (BIPA).[68] Consequently, the MMA contained a 10.6% payment increase effective March 2004 and an additional $12.5 billion 'stabilization fund' for further incentives to private plan participation to be used at the discretion of the Secretary DHHS.[35] The success of this approach in attracting private plans has meant that the fall-back provision of Medicare was not required but has led to some complaints from beneficiaries about confusion resulting from the proliferation of plans and choices. Among the 80% of Medicare beneficiaries who reported that they would not enroll in a drug plan or were not sure if they would as of November 2005, 37% said that it was too complicated.[69] A critical open question is what private plans will do once the excess payments and subsidies disappear: will they once again withdraw from participation, and of so, what are the implications for this benefit?

Concern about potential conflicts of interest led to the restriction on what pharmacists can and cannot do in advising Medicare beneficiaries on which Medicare plan to select. Pharmacists can advise on which plans contain the best formulary for the medications a patient may be taking; however, pharmacists may not advise on which specific plan a patient should select. The rationale was that pharmacists might have a financial interest in a specific plan and guide Medicare beneficiaries to that plan. For 2007, America's Health Insurance Plans (AHIP), the National Association of Chain Drug Stores (NACDS), and the National Community Pharmacists Association (NPA) worked together to develop the *Medicare Prescription Drug Plan Guide: How to Choose Your 2007 Plan* to assist beneficiaries in selecting a prescription drug plan under their Medicare benefits. It is an attempt to address the frustration beneficiaries have when trying to compare and select plans based on so many different variables.[70]

Reducing the Risk of Adverse Selection   A politically charged feature of the MMA is the penalty for Medicare beneficiaries who delay in participating in this voluntary prescription drug benefit program. The insurance industry was concerned that elective timing on when a beneficiary joins a drug plan could result in moral hazard and adverse selection, making utilization assumptions and premium calculations based on them unreliable. Therefore, legislators permitted a grace period from the start of the program on January 1 until May 15, 2006, but imposed a 1% per month penalty on those enrolling after that date. For people who deferred until the second year of the program, this could add up to 17% to their premiums, and would remain with them for as long as they were in the program. This is one of the immediate points of political friction with the Democratic party vowing to rescind this provision.

To discourage employers from directing their retirees to the Medicare program for prescription drug benefits, MMA provided tax credits for them to continue to offer their drug benefit. In addition, to encourage retirees enrolled in those plans to remain in them, the penalty for late enrollment applied to others would be waived for those who had been in actuarially equivalent retiree prescription drug plans. A survey of employers who accepted the drug subsidy in 2006 reported that 44% would **not** allow retirees who enroll in a Medicare drug plan to re-enroll in an employer plan. The percentage of them who were likely to continue offering retiree drug benefits and accepting the employer subsidy in 2007 was 82% but only 50% as they looked toward 2010.[71]

Prescription Drug Coverage for Dually Eligible Beneficiaries   Responsibility for covered out-patient prescription drugs for persons dually eligible for Medicaid and Medicare passed from states to the federal government under the MMA. Recognizing the difficulty of noti-fying all of the dually eligible persons and obtaining their required voluntary enrollment; they were auto-enrolled in qualified plans. The attraction of this shift for states was tem-pered by two features.

First, dislocations that occurred when this vulnerable population was transferred from state Medicaid plans, which provided a wide selection of medication options to physicians, to private plans that used restrictive formularies: some patients were dropped from rosters and could not obtain their chronic medications; others found that their prescribed medica-tion(s) was not on the formulary of the plan in which they were enrolled. As Dr. Joshua Sharfstein, Commissioner of Health for Baltimore City noted, "If one person switches, it's an insurance issue. When 28,000 people switch on one day, it's a public health issue."[72]

Second, the anticipated windfall to state budgets from savings on the costs of drugs for these persons did not materialize. Under a provision known as the *phased-down state contri-bution*, states would pay the federal government based on a formula for the portion of the drug expenses that they would have paid had the enrollees remained a state responsibility. For 2006 the state was ~$6.6 billion, a non-trivial sum.[73] States saw this as a *clawback*, and that it overestimated state costs and their payment to the federal government. An immediate unanticipated adverse consequence is for states to have to begin to restrict the criteria to qualify as an optional dual-eligible; this was already seen in Florida and Mississippi.[74]

SPECULATION

Public policies shift over time, sometimes taking a more regulatory approach, sometimes a more market-based approach. For the foreseeable future, it appears that the United States will be relying more on market-based solutions, through collaborations between the pub-lic and private sectors.

Implementation concerns did not guide or dictate the features in the MMA; conse-quently, there are ill-defined provisions and time-limited features that cause friction to one group or another. Given the difficulty of policy change, it is unlikely that an open debate on changes to the MMA to remove or resolve these features will occur unless a fiscal crisis demands it. Even if the current shift to a Democratic majority in Congress continues into the next election, the essential features of the MMA may not change materially. Once a debate began, reform proposals would be difficult to contain. Even those who disagree with some or most of the program see some benefits from it, benefits that might be at risk in an open debate on its reform.

If the past is a guide, the most critical single factor that could influence healthcare policy in the future would be fundamental campaign finance reform and non-partisan enforcement. The fiscal requirements of effective political campaigns create incentives contrary to unbiased representation. Until the conflicts-of-interest these donations establish are removed, there can be no coherent health policy based first on the nation's needs as a whole.

DISCLOSURE

The author is a registered voter unaffiliated with a political party.

REFERENCES

1. Department of Health and Human Services (DHHS), Centers for Medicare and Medicaid Services, *National Health Expenditure Data*. Available at http://www.cms.hhs.gov/National HealthExpendData/02_NationalHealthAccounts Historical.asp#TopOfPage. Accessed 30 July 2008.

2. Mayes R., The origins, development, and passage of Medicare's revolutionary prospective payment system. *J Hist Med Allied Sci.* 2007; 62(1): 21-55.

3. Culbertson R.A. and Lee P.R., Medicare and physician autonomy. *Health Care Financ Rev.* 1996; 18(2): 115-130. Available at http://www.ssa.gov/history/pdf/MedicarePhysicalAutonomy.pdf. Accessed 30 July 2008.

4. Medicare Prescription Drug, Improvement, and Modernization Act of 2003 (MMA), Public Law 108-173. Available at http://www.ustreas.gov/offices/public-affairs/hsa/pdf/pl108-173.pdf. Accessed 30 July 2008.

5. The National Archives, The Charters of Freedom, Bill of Rights. Available at http://www.archives.gov/national-archives-experience/charters/bill_of_rights_transcript.html. Accessed 30 July 2008.

6. Wing, K.R., Chapter 2: "The Power of State Governments in Matters Affecting Health," in *The Law and the Public's Health*. Chicago, IL: Health Administration Press; 1999.

7. Milligan S., "Back-Room Dealing a Capitol Trend: GOP Flexing its Majority Power." *Boston Globe*, October 3, 2004.

8. The Library of Congress. *How Our Laws Are Made*. Available at http://thomas.loc.gov/home/lawsmade.toc.html. Accessed 30 July 2008.

9. Coleman J.J., Unified government, divided government, and party responsiveness. *Am Politic Sci Rev.* 1999; 93(4): 821-835.

10. Babington C., "Stem Cell Bill Gets Bush's First Veto." *Washington Post*, July 20, 2006; page A04.

11. Madison J., *Federalist Essay No. 10: The Union as a Safeguard Against Domestic Faction and Insurrection*. November 23, 1787. The Avalon Project at Yale University. Available at http://www.yale.edu/lawweb/avalon/federal/fed10.htm. Accessed 30 July 2008.

12. Kolbert E., "New Arena for Campaign Ads: Health Care." *New York Times*, October 21, 1993. Available at http://query.nytimes.com/gst/fullpage.html?res=9F0CE6D7163DF932A15753C1A965 958260&sec=health&spon=&pagewanted=2. Accessed 30 July 2008.

13. Goldsteen R.L., Goldsteen K., Swan J.H., Clemena W., Harry and Louise and health care reform: romancing public opinion. *J Health Politic Policy Law* 2001; 269(6): 1325-1352.

14. United States Federal Election Commission. *Campaign Finance Reports and Data*. Available at http://www.fec.gov/disclosure.shtml. Accessed 30 July 2008.

15. The Center for Responsive Politics. *Heavy Hitters. Top All Time Donors, 1989-2008*. Available at http://www.opensecrets.org/orgs/list.asp?order=A. Accessed 30 July 2008.

16. Ciole Z., "Corruption and the politics of pay-to-play: Mantle of scandal worn by GOP was Dems' a decade ago." *San Francisco Chronicle*, December 4, 2005.

17. Rowland C., "Medicare Bill a Study in D.C. Spoils System." *Boston Globe*, October 5, 2004. Available at http://www.boston.com/news/nation/articles/2004/10/05/medicare_bill_a_study_in_dc_spoils_system/. Accessed 30 July 2008.

18. The Center for Responsive Politics. *Pharmaceutical Manufacturing: Long-Term Contribution Trends*. Available at http://www.opensecrets.org/industries/indus.asp?cycle=2006&ind=H4300. Accessed 30 July 2008.

19. Federal Election Commission. *Campaign Finance Law Quick Reference for Reporters. Major Provisions of the Bipartisan Campaign Reform Act of 2002*. Available at http://www.fec.gov/press/bkgnd/bcra_overview.shtml. Accessed 30 July 2008.

20. "The Globe's Major Findings." *Boston Globe*, October 3, 2004. Available at http://www.boston.com/news/nation/articles/2004/10/03/the_globes_major_findings/. Accessed 30 July 2008.

21. Office of Management and Budget. *OMB Guidance to Agencies on Definition of Earmarks*. Available at http://earmarks.omb.gov/earmarks_definition.html. Accessed 30 July 2008.

22. Taxpayers for Common Sense. *TCS Statement on the Omnibus Spending Bill*. Available at http://www.taxpayer.net/search_by_tag.php?action=view&proj_id=447&tag=Earmarks&type=Project. Accessed 14 August 2008.

23. Starr P., The Social Transformation of American Medicine. New York: Basic Books; 1982. ISBN 0-465-07934-2.

24. U.S. Census Bureau, *Statistical Abstract of the United States: 2003*. Table No. HS-29. Employment Status of the Civilian Population: 1929 to 2002. Available at http://www.census.gov/statab/hist/HS-29.pdf. Accessed 30 July 2008.

25. Blum J., *The Morgenthau Diaries: Years of War 1941-1945*. Boston, MA: Houghton-Mifflin; 1967: 72. Quoted in Starr P., *The Social Transformation of American Medicine*. New York: Basic Books; 1982. ISBN 0-465-07934-2.

26. Social Security Online. Social Security History. Chapter 3: The Third Round 1943-1950. Available at http://www.ssa.gov/history/corningchap3.html. Accessed 30 July 2008.

27. Marmor T.R., *The Politics of Medicare*, 2nd ed. New York: Aldine de Gruyter. 2000. Cited in Oliver T.R., A political history of Medicare and prescription drug coverage. *Milbank Q*, 2004; 82(2): 283-354.

28. Silverman M. and Lee P.R., *Pills, Profits and Politics*. Berkeley, CA: University of California Press; 1976: 168. Cited in Oliver T.R., Lee P.R., Lipton H.L., A political history of Medicare and prescription drug coverage. *Milbank Q*. 2004; 82(2): 283-354.

29. *Omnibus Budget Reconciliation Act of 1990*, P.L. 101-508 (5 November 1990).

30. Tepper C.D. and Lied T.R., Trends in Medicaid prescribed drug expenditures and utilization. *Health Care Financ Rev*. 2004; 25(3): 69-78. Available at http://www.cms.hhs.gov/HealthCareFinancingReview/Downloads/04springpg69.pdf. Accessed 30 July 2008.

31. The Medicare Payment Advisory Commission (MedPAC). Report to the Congress: Selected Medicare Issues. Medicare beneficiaries and prescription drug coverage. June 2000. Available at http://www.medpac.gov/publications/congressional_reports/Jun00%20Ch1.pdf. Accessed 30 July 2008.

32. Moon M., *Medicare NOW and in the Future*, 2nd Ed. Washington, DC: The Urban Institute Press; 1996. ISBN-10: 0877666539.

33. Budget of the United States Government. Historical Tables. Fiscal Year 2007. Table 1.1—Summary of Receipts, Outlays, and Surpluses or Deficits (–): 1789–2011. Available at http://www.whitehouse.gov/omb/budget/fy2007/pdf/hist.pdf. Accessed 30 July 2008.

34. Goldstein A., "Clinton to Seek Modest Medicare Drug Benefit." *Washington Post* Medicare Special Report, June 29, 1999, p. A1. Available at http://www.washingtonpost.com/wp-srv/politics/special/medicare/stories/medicare062999.htm. Accessed 30 July 2008.

35. Iglehart J., The new Medicare prescription-drug benefit—a pure power play. *N Engl J Med.* 2004; 350(8): 826-833.

36. Oliver T.R., A political history of Medicare and prescription drug coverage. *Milbank Q.* 2004; 82(2): 283-354.

37. Samuel T., "The Capitol (Hill) Gang: Big issues, looming deadlines—and everyone's fighting everyone." *U. S. News and World Report*, November 9, 2003. Available at http://www.usnews.com/usnews/news/articles/031117/17repub.htm. Accessed 30 July 2008.

38. The Commonwealth Fund. Washington Health Policy Week in Review: September 20, 2004. *Medicare Cost Wars—Day 284.* Available at http://www.commonwealthfund.org/healthpolicyweek/healthpolicyweek_show.htm?doc_id=239737. Accessed 30 July 2008.

39. O'Sullivan J., Chaikind H., Tilson S., et al., Overview of the Medicare Prescription Drug, Improvement, and Modernization Act of 2003. Congressional Research Service. Updated December 9, 2003. Available at http://leahy.senate.gov/issues/seniors/CRSoverviewofprescriptiondrug.pdf. Accessed 30 July 2008.

40. Stolberg S.G. and Pear R., "Mysterious Fax Adds to Intrigue Over Drug Bill." *New York Times*, March 18, 2004.

41. Office of Management and Budget. Table S–13. Outlay Impact of Prescription Drug and Medicare Improvement Act of 2003 (P.L. 108–173). Available at http://www.whitehouse.gov/omb/budget/fy2005/tables.html. Accessed 30 July 2008.

42. Snow J.D. 2004 Financial Report of the United States Government. Available at http://fms.treas.gov/fr/04frusg/04frusg.pdf. Accessed 30 July 2008.

43. Pear R., "Senate Backs Medicare Pick After Promise On Imports." *New York Times*, March 13, 2004.

44. Kravitz R.L. and Chang S., Promise and perils for patients and physicians. *N Engl J Med.* 2005; 353: 2735-2739.

45. Stolberg S.G. "Lawmaker's Plans to Lobby Raise Issue of Crossing Line." *New York Times*, February 7, 2004, p. A12.

46. Pharmaceutical Research Manufacturers of America. Press Release: PhRMA Names Tauzin President, CEO. December 15, 2004. Available at http://www.phrma.org/news_room/press_releases/phrma_names_tauzin_president,_ceo/. Accessed 30 July 2008.

47. Kaiser Family Foundation. *Medicare Drug Discount Cards: A Work in Progress.* Available at http://www.kff.org/medicare/loader.cfm?url=/commonspot/security/getfile.cfm&PageID=44514. Accessed 30 July 2008.

48. Institute of Medicine of the National Academies. *Identifying and Preventing Medication Errors.* Available at http://www.iom.edu/?id=22526&redirect=0. Accessed 30 July 2008.

49. Leavitt M.O., *Report to Congress: Improving the Medicare Quality Improvement Organization Program—Response to the Institute of Medicine Study.* 2006. Available at http://www.cms.hhs.gov/QualityImprovementOrgs/downloads/QIO_Improvement_RTC_fnl.pdf. Accessed 30 July 2008.

50. Department of Health and Human Services. *HHS Task Force of Drug Importation. Report on Prescription Drug Importation.* December 2004. Available at http://www.hhs.gov/importtaskforce/Report1220.pdf. Accessed 30 July 2008.

51. American Pharmacists Association. News Release. December 22, 2004. Available at www.pharmacist. com. Accessed 15 August 2008.

52. Academy of Managed Care Pharmacy. Prescription Drug Reimportation. Position approved by the Board of Directors August 2000 and Revised February 2003. Available at http://www.amcp.org/amcp.ark?p=AA45A93A. Accessed 30 July 2008.

53. American Pharmacists Association and National Association of Chain Drug Stores Foundation. Medication Therapy Management in Community Pharmacy Practice: Core Elements of an MTM Service (Version 1.0). *J Am Pharm Assoc.* 2005; 45: 573-579.

54. American Society of Consultant Pharmacists (ASCP). Medicare Drug Benefit Questions and Answers. Available at http://www.ascp.com/advocacy/briefing/upload/MedicareQnA.pdf. Accessed 30 July 2008.

55. Gans J.A., Communication to Senators Max Baucus and Charles Grassley. February 7, 2007. Available at http://www.pharmacist.com/AM/Template.cfm?Section=Issues&Template=/TaggedPage/TaggedPageDisplay.cfm&TPLID=107&ContentID=16720. Accessed 21 August 2008.

56. Wolf R., "More Patients Fall Into a Hole in Drug Benefit." *USA Today*, July 26, 2006. Available at http://www.usatoday.com/news/health/2006-07-26-drug-hole_x.htm. Accessed 30 July 2008.

57. Department of Health and Human Services, Centers for Medicare and Medicaid Services. *Electronic Prescribing Standards Announced to Make Medicare's New Prescription Drug Benefit Easier and Safer.* November 1, 2005. Available at http://www.hhs.gov/news/press/2005pres/20051101.html. Accessed 30 July 2008.

58. Department of Health and Human Services, Centers for Medicare and Medicaid Services. *Pilot Project Launched to Expand Electronic Prescribing.* January 17, 2006. Available at http://www.hhs.gov/news/press/2006pres/20060117a.html. Accessed 30 July 2008.

59. Department of Health and Human Services, Centers for Medicare and Medicaid Services. *HHS Issues Report To Congress On e-Prescribing: Electronic Prescribing to Cut Errors and Costs.* April 17, 2007. Available at http://www.hhs.gov/news/press/2007pres/04/pr20070417b.html. Accessed 30 July 2008.

60. Bell D.S. and Friedman M.A., E-Prescribing and the Medicare Modernization Act of 2003. *Health Aff.* 2005; 24(5): 1159-1169.

61. United States Pharmacopeia. *Medicare Model Guidelines.* Available at http://www.usp.org/hqi/mmg/. Accessed 30 July 2008.

62. Department of Health and Human Services, Centers for Medicare and Medicaid Services. Medicare Modernization Act Final Guidelines— Formularies. Guidelines for Reviewing Prescription Drug Plan Formularies and Procedures. Available at http://www.cms.hhs.gov/PrescriptionDrugCovContra/Downloads/FormularyGuidance.pdf. Accessed 30 July 2008.

63. Department of Health and Human Services, Centers for Medicare and Medicaid Services. *Medicare "Pay For Performance (P4P)" Initiatives.* Available at http://www.cms.hhs.gov/apps/media/press/release.asp?Counter=1343. Accessed 30 July 2008.

64. O'Kane M.E., Performance-based measures: the early results are in. *J Manag Care Pharm.* 2007; 13(2 Suppl B): S3-S6.

65. Mehrotra A, Pearson SD, Coltin KL, et al., The response of physician groups to P4P incentives. *Am J Manag Care.* 2007; 13(5): 249-255.

66. Lindenauer P.K., Remus D., Roman S., et al., Pay for performance in hospital quality improvement. *N Engl J Med.* 2007; 356(5): 486-496.

67. Department of Health and Human Services, Centers for Medicare and Medicaid Services, *CMS Fact Sheet. The New Prescription Drug Program: Attacking Fraud and Abuse.* October 7, 2005. Available at http://www.cms.hhs.gov/apps/media/press/factsheet.asp?Counter=1693&intNumPerPage=10&checkDate=&checkKey=&srchType=1&numDays=3500&srchOpt=0&srchData=&keywordType=All&chkNewsType=6&intPage=&showAll=&pYear=&year=&desc=false&cboOrder=date. Accessed 30 July 2008.

68. Kaiser Family Foundation. Medicare Fact Sheet: Medicare+Choice. April 2003. Available at http://kff.org/medicare/upload/Medicare-Choice-Fact-Sheet-Fact-Sheet.pdf. Accessed 30 July 2008.

69. The Kaiser Family Foundation and Harvard School of Public Health, *Kaiser Family Foundation Survey November 2005: The Medicare Drug Benefit: Beneficiary Perspectives Just Before Implementation.* Chart 6. Available at http://www.kff.org/kaiserpolls/upload/The-Medicare-Drug-Benefit-Beneficiary-Perspectives-Just-Before-Implementation-Chartpack.pdf. Accessed 30 July 2008.

70. America's Health Insurance Plans, National Association of Chain Drug Stores and the National Community Pharmacists Association. *Medicare Prescription Drug Plan Guide: How to Choose Your 2007 Plan.* Available at http://www.healthdecisions.org/guide/about_us.html. Accessed 30 July 2008.

71. Kaiser Family Foundation. Kaiser/Hewitt 2005 Survey on Retiree Health Benefits—Chartpack. *Prospects for Retiree Health Benefits.* December 2005. Available at http://www.kff.org/medicare/7440.cfm. Accessed 30 July 2008.

72. Salganik M.W., "City to aid Medicare launch; Health agency to monitor seniors' needs as drug plans shift." *Baltimore Sun,* December 21, 2005, p. 1D.

73. Kaiser Commission on Medicaid and the Uninsured. *An Update on the Clawback: Revised Health Spending Data Change State Financial Obligations for the New Medicare Drug Benefit.* March 2006.

Available at http://www.kff.org/medicaid/upload/7481.pdf. Accessed 30 July 2008.

74. Kaiser Family Foundation. Smith V., Gifford K., Ellis E., Wiles A., *Medicaid Budgets, Spending and Policy Initiatives in State Fiscal Years 2005 and 2006: Results from a 50-State Survey*. October 2005. Available at http://www.kff.org/medicaid/upload/Medicaid-Budgets-Spending-and-Policy-Initiatives-in-State-Fiscal-Years-2005-and-2006-report-executive-summary.pdf. Accessed 30 July 2008.

Chapter 25

INTERNATIONAL OPPORTUNITIES FOR PHARMACISTS IN MANAGED CARE

NORRIE THOMAS
ALBERT I. WERTHEIMER

The concept of managed care was developed in the United States and has spread to several other countries. American health insurance companies are doing business in Australia, Canada, and in parts of Asia and Western Europe. In addition, the tools of managed care are being used by health insurers from both the private sector as well as the public sector. These managed care tools include the use of formularies, multiple copayment levels, prospective drug utilization review (DUR), audits and retrospective DUR, physician report cards, and a whole host of incentives and disincentives to encourage cost-effective prescribing. When possible, formulary decisions are based upon pharmacoeconomic considerations as well as clinical characteristics of the drug products.

This chapter features some of the more interesting characteristics that are to be found in the drug sectors in Canada and Australia, with mention of several other countries where interesting and innovative practices have developed. The chapter does not intend to describe the pharmaceutical benefit schemes found throughout the world, but rather highlights a few very interesting and innovative systems where there are lessons to be learned for those in the United States.

UNITED KINGDOM

NATIONAL INSTITUTE FOR HEALTH AND CLINICAL EFFECTIVENESS

The National Health Service (NHS) in the United Kingdom formed the National Institute for Health and Clinical Effectiveness (NICE) in 1999 as an independent organization responsible for providing guidance on the use of medications. The role of NICE is to provide patients, health professionals, and the public with authoritative, robust, and reliable guidance on "best practice." Guidance covers both 1) individual health technologies; including medications, medical devices, diagnostic techniques, and procedures specifically as they relate to pharmacy management techniques, and 2) NICE procedures clinical guidelines.

Guidance provided by NICE is sometimes referred to as the *fourth hurdle*, which is an additional barrier that the pharmaceutical industry must face in order to gain market entry and reimbursement for their products. The pharmaceutical industry must demonstrate not only safety, efficacy, and quality (the first three hurdles) but also clinical effectiveness (the fourth hurdle). A new product must demonstrate that it is better than currently available alternatives—including no treatment as well as clinical effectiveness—to address the question: "Does the new product offer value for the price?" NICE is the most organized and effective group of its kind to influence medication decisions. The United States managed care market does not have a similar national mechanism to establish clinical effectiveness, although individual health plans and pharmacy organizations all provide a similar role through their formulary decision-making procedures. However, the NHS has always been a managed care organization (MCO) using the three elements of disease management: knowledge based on the economic burden of disease, a coordinated delivery system, and a quality assessment audit process.[1]

In 1993, Australia became the first healthcare system to develop formal regulations governing the advising to the health minister about reimbursement. (The Canadian Providence of Ontario began economic evaluation of drugs in 1994.) The introduction of NICE in 1999 is the most important fourth hurdle development in United Kingdom and is fast becoming the model for all of Europe. Taylor et al.[2] stated that the promise of cost effectiveness comparisons was to improve reimbursement decisions, but these authors recommended greater transparency in the process and open collaboration with manufacturers to eliminate costly submissions and to identify the effectiveness questions most likely to impact reimbursement. In general, they concluded that the effect of the fourth hurdle has not improved the quality of evidence, has not provided a fixed threshold to support decision making, and the effect on drug prices has been minimal. Although differences in decision making will continue, it may be time for a convergence in economic guidelines. They recommend improving the process by initiating standardization of cost-effectiveness in pharmaceutical decisions in Europe, and they cite questions regarding the process of value based drug comparisons.[2]

Fourth hurdle value-based drug comparisons are used not to price a medication but as a method to determine the status of a drug, for example, defining them by preferred, restricted use, or excluded. The problem is that *value* is a relative term. The United Kingdom's NICE addresses this challenge by providing guidance on treatments for NHS patients. Cost-effectiveness is one factor, and NICE has determined guidance based on quality-adjusted-life-year (QALY). Regardless of the NICE recommendation, patients cannot be denied treatments if need can be provided.[3]

In the United Sates, the Academy of Managed Care Pharmacy (AMCP) introduced a format for formulary decision making that incorporates cost effectiveness as a major criterion. The AMCP format mirrors national formulary systems (like NICE) except in a decentralized manner that is more suited for the U.S. healthcare system, and it has become a critical tool important in bringing cost-effectiveness methods to reimbursement decisions. There is the risk that this type of decision making is just a screen for cost containment; however, cost-effectiveness methods also highlight under-use and lack of technology adoption when clearly indicated.[4]

Use of cost effectiveness information has evolved in the United Kingdom. There are obvious strengths and weaknesses of the NICE process. Strengths include the use of an explicit and economic approach to clinical effectiveness as well as transparency. In addition, the committee structure employed by NICE includes representation by the public and patient advocacy groups, pharmacy, medical, and economic expertise. The economic analysis completed by NICE examines the relationship of new treatment in comparison to "no treatment" and "usual care." "Usual care" includes the use of generics and over-the counter medications, which is a definite strength of the NICE review process.

One major weakness of NICE is its difficulty to implement decisions. To assist with NICE recommendations, there seems to be an increasing role for community pharmacists to work as advisors to physicians.[5] In comparison, while the U.S. managed care cost-effectiveness review process completed on an organizational level may not be as robust in terms of overall economic analysis, or as transparent, the ability to implement reimbursement policy based on economic analysis by design is far easier to implement.

A number of authors have published papers that portend future changes within NICE and how the fourth hurdle will change to address the ever increasing challenges of pharmacy innovation, cost, and value.[6-10] As NICE continues to influence drug decision-making in the United Kingdom and Europe, there also will be an impact on the use of cost effectiveness assessment in the United States.

COST EFFECTIVENESS SHOULD BE CONDUCTED THROUGHOUT THE DRUG CYCLE

Langley[6] posited that cost effectiveness should become a natural process during the entire drug cycle, not just at product launch. He recommended that cost effectiveness measurement become an integral part of drug development. The value for money argument, the fourth hurdle, can become an antidote for clinical optimism (which has a direct impact on sales and marketing), and provide the basis for the performance of new products and formulary position acceptable to the manufacturer and the entity making reimbursement decisions. Affordability is the key hurdle in achieving reimbursement, and NICE process and guidelines influence affordability decisions.

Manufacturers must be ready to demonstrate that their products provide value for money over alternatives, including "not treatment."[7]

BUDGET ANALYSIS: AN ADDED CRITERION

As additional innovation and higher costs impact pharmacy budgets, funding decisions will compete between the same resource dollars. Cohen et. al.[8] argue that budget analysis become an additional NICE criterion. They define budget impact in terms of the drug costs/value across the entire healthcare budget, not just the pharmacy budget. A NICE request estimates on budget impact.

INTEGRATE REIMBURSEMENT DECISIONS AND RESEARCH

Another major weakness of NICE, as discussed by Claxton and Sculpher,[9] is the lack of integration between reimbursement decisions and research. NICE does not have the authority to request research, but each year NICE can identify three research priorities. As NICE and the research committees begin to work together, the intention is that reimbursement decisions and clinical practice will become more integrated. The authors strongly recommend that reimbursement authorities have the authority to direct research questions and priorities, or base coverage decisions on the need for additional research.[9]

INTERNATIONAL DIFFUSION: FOURTH HURDLE SCRUTINY

The presence of early warning activity for new technology and national coverage decision-making (e.g., NICE) have a mixed association with the adoption of innovation in clinical practice.[10] A single state agency controlling expenditure through a fourth hurdle process has a greater impact on diffusion (both positive and negative) than multiple schemes. Study results reported by Packer et al.[10] clearly show a huge difference between several European countries in their adoption of new technology; the patterns vary significantly, and this gulf between the evidence-based ideal and reality will lead to continual fourth hurdle scrutiny.

Healthcare delivery differences between the United States and the United Kingdom may cloud the belief that the two systems are too varied to be compared; however, both countries face the same challenges—value, quality and innovation—and there is much for the United States to learn from NICE.[10] As NICE changes and evolves, its strengths and weaknesses will provide the U.S. managed care pharmacy industry with essential lessons as well as unique ideas for improvement.

CANADA

Perhaps one of the most interesting and original features in Canadian health care is the Patented Medicine Prices Review Board (PMPRB). The Board was created in 1987 under the Canadian patent act as an independent quasi-judicial tribunal. It limits the prices set by manufacturers for all patented medicines, new and existing, that are sold in Canada either under prescription-only status or as over-the-counter. The purpose of the Board is to ensure that Canadian prices are not excessive. Patents are granted for a period of 20 years in Canada. Nearly all branded products are patented, at least in the beginning of their life, and some brand-name products and generic drugs are no longer under patent protection. The Board reviews the ex-factory prices at which medicines are sold to wholesalers, hospitals, and pharmacies but it does not have any jurisdiction over prices charged by wholesalers or retailers, nor over the professional fees charged by pharmacists.

Under the regulations, patentees are required to report information on the introductory prices and sales of new patented medicines within 60 days of the date of the first sale, and to continue to file detailed information on prices and sales of each patented drug for the first and last six months, and each year for as long as the drug remains patented.

Prices are set so that the cost of therapy is in the range of the cost of therapy for existing drugs sold in Canada used to treat the same disease. In addition, breakthrough drug prices are limited to the median of the prices for the same drugs charged in other specified industrial countries that are set out in the patented medicines regulations. At the moment these are: France, Germany, Italy, Sweden, Switzerland, the United Kingdom, and the United States. Existing patented drug prices cannot increase by more than the Consumer Price Index (CPI) and the price of a product in Canada can never be the highest in the world.

When Board members find that the price of the patented drug appears to exceed these guidelines and where the criteria for commencing an investigation are met, Board staff will conduct an investigation to determine the facts. An investigation can result in a voluntary compliance undertaking (VCU) by the patentee to reduce the price and to pay excessive revenues, or in a public hearing and remedial action. After an investigation has been completed, one of three outcomes are completed:

1. The file may be closed when it is concluded that the price was within the guidelines.
2. A voluntary compliance will be undertaken by the manufacturer to reduce the price and to take other measures to comply with the guidelines.
3. A public hearing is held to determine whether the price is excessive and, if so, there is an issuance of a remedial order by the Board.

It is interesting to note that the PMPRB does not have the authority to prevent the sale of a patented medicine based on its price nor to remove it from the market. However, if a price is found to be excessive, the manufacturer is provided an opportunity to lower the price and/or to make a payment to the Canadian government. The PMPRB has no authority to regulate research and development. Its mandate is to report on all research and development. In addition, it made a public commitment that the brand name pharmaceutical industry would increase its research and development expenditures by 10% as a percentage of sales by 1996. In 2002, the research and development to sales ratio was 9.9%.

The PMPRB reports annually to Parliament on its activities, including price trends of patented and all medicines and on research and development expenditures as reported by the pharmaceutical patent-holding companies. It should be noted that this definition of patented medications includes vaccines, topical preparations, anesthetics, diagnostic products, and products used *in vivo* regardless of the delivery mechanism. Section 82 of the Patent Act requires a patentee to notify the PMPRB of its intention to offer a drug product for sale and the date on which the sale is expected to begin. A new drug is assigned a drug information number (DIN). Then prices are compared to other products within that same DIN category.

The PMPRB in association with patients and other interested parties have developed various tests to determine whether the price of the drug product is within their guidelines.

The *reasonable relationship test* considers the association between the strengths and the price of the same medicine in the same or comparable dosage forms. The *therapeutic class comparison test* compares the price of the DIN under review with the prices of DINs that are clinically equivalent and sold in the same market at prices that the Board considers reasonable. The *international price comparison test* compares the average transaction price of the DIN under review with the publicly available ex-factory prices of the same medicine sold in countries listed in the regulations.

The Board differentiates between a breakthrough drug product that is the first to be sold in Canada that effectively treats a particular illness or addresses a particular indication of a disease. A drug product constituting a substantial improvement is one that, relative to other drug products sold in Canada, provides substantial improvement in therapeutic effects and will provide significant savings to the Canadian healthcare system.

An investigation will commence if one or more of the following three criteria are met:

1. The introductory price is 5% or more above the maximum non-excessive price.
2. Excess revenues in the introductory period of $25,000 or more are discovered.
3. Complaints with significant evidence are presented to the Board.

CANADIAN HEALTH CARE IN SUMMARY

The Canadian system effectively uses a panel that enables all relevant stakeholders to be involved in the decision-making process and sets criteria for price characteristics of patented drugs sold in the Canadian market. The rules and policies are all known in advance and there is an open (transparent) scheme for monitoring the conduct of the industry. Appeals, processes, and other mechanisms are available. While there are a number of complaints periodically from pharmaceutical companies, the overall impression from viewing this topic from a variety of sources is that it is fair as well as objective, and accomplishes its goal of maintaining pharmaceutical prices within Canada at a level considered a to be non-excessive.

AUSTRALIA

Australia was the first nation to require pharmacoeconomic information in order for a drug to be listed on the national drug benefit publication, so that it could be prescribed at a reduced price to the patient. This has been the case in Australia since 1953. The Pharmaceutical Benefits Scheme (PBS) has been the model from which a number of other national health programs and managed care as well as health insurance organizations have used features. Approximately 80% of all prescriptions dispensed in Australia are subsidized under the PBS. The typical patient might pay $30.70 for most PBS medicines or $4.90 if he or she has a concession card. In comparison, the Australian government pays the remaining portion of the price of the product. In a typical year, around 170 million prescriptions are covered under the Australian PBS system. This equates to about eight prescriptions per person per year in Australia. The cost of operating the PBS is approximately $6 billion per year.

Australian citizens have subsidized access to more than 600 medicines, available in 1800 forms marketed as 2600 differently-branded items. In recent years, the expense of the program has increased at a rate of 2.7% per year, which is considerably less than the increasing costs in most other prescription drug benefit plans around the world. In order to maintain a price level among the lowest in developed countries, the Australian government is about to reduce the prices of pharmaceutical products even more in the coming year. This change will affect products that are in a competitive market, where patent protection has ended and multiple generic products are available. In addition to mandated price decreases that began in August 2008, there will be a price drop of 2% per year for three years from medicines where competition between brands is low and a one-time price drop of 25% where there is a high level of competition between brands.

Reference pricing will continue for medicines that belong to groups of products that are interchangeable between patients. Of interest to pharmacists will be the plan to pay pharmacies an additional $.40AUD per prescription when that prescription is processed using PBS online. It is expected that this incentive will encourage more pharmacists to join the Web-based program and thereby create efficiencies in the administration of the PBS system. Dispensing fees increased on August 1, 2008 in addition to an incentive payment of $1.50 each time a medicine is dispensed that costs the patient no more than the standard copayment amount. The government is committed to making available the full range of products listed in the PBS scheme in all pharmacies in Australia. This is done through the creation of a community services obligation funding pool, where $23 million a year will be added to assure availability of products throughout the country.

In the system today, approximately 450 medicines require a pre-approval telephone call to Medicine Australia by the physician. It is planned that 200 of these products in the very near future will no longer require such a telephone call in order to be prescribed. Also, a community education campaign is to be designed to promote the benefits of generic medicines; the campaign will build on previous initiatives to ensure that consumers and health professionals are aware of the safety, health, and economic benefits of generic medicines.

Australia is one of the few countries that lists approved uses for many of its products. In addition, the benefits scheme publication lists restrictions regarding certain products that are not to be used at all for certain conditions or are only to be used when other products have been used unsuccessfully. As a result of these activities within the PBS, Australia maintains one of the lowest average price levels for pharmaceuticals of any developed country.

It is well-known that the multinational pharmaceutical manufacturers have periodically threatened not to market certain products in Australia, claiming that they cannot be sold profitably at the price that would be granted by the PBS. Yet we see most all of the products sold in the other developed countries available for sale in Australia. This may not be the case in the future as further price regulations come into effect that are intended to lower pharmaceutical product prices further.

It was considered beyond the scope of this chapter, but anyone interested in this fascinating social experiment is encouraged to read more about the PBS. It is composed of a number of committees, councils, and task forces that study prices in other countries and compare the clinical outcomes to the proposed price in Australia. There is an opportunity for manufacturers to appeal decisions and, while most interested parties claim that they are not completely happy with the system, it appears that it does function reasonably well from nearly all perspectives. The manufacturer is required to complete a two-page form when a drug is about to be marketed in Australia providing cost and financial information to the authorities.

AUSTRALIAN HEALTH CARE SUMMARY

A nearly 60-year-old plan that regulates the use and price of pharmaceutical products and that is paid for by a government health system continues to function in Australia. It is being updated and streamlined so that it can continue to play an important role in maintaining access to superior products at the lowest possible cost to the Australian population. It is fair to say that the Australian drug benefits scheme is probably the most invasive in impact on physician prescribing and drug use anywhere in the world. It appears that Australian physicians and pharmacists have become accustomed to this level of government involvement, and patients appear to be satisfied with the balance of price and services.

CONCLUSION

As seen in this chapter, the principles and tools of managed care are being applied to improve the quality and efficiency of the drug benefit throughout the world. While this chapter described three very diverse examples of how countries chose to deal with their drug programs, the results are similar in that each has an efficient, useful, and high-quality drug benefit program.

Every month, additional countries and insurance organizations are adopting related techniques to keep inferior products out of their formularies and to obtain the best prices for those products selected to be included. While only three countries have been highlighted in this chapter, pieces of these healthcare strategies are seen with growing frequency in Mexico, Israel, France, Sweden, Japan, New Zealand, Spain, and in about 40 other countries today.

REFERENCES

1. Lawrence M. and Williams T., Managed care and disease management in the NHS. (Editorial) *BMJ*. 1996: 313(7050): 125-126.
2. Taylor R.S., Drummond M.F., Salkeld G., Sullivan S.D., Inclusion of cost effectiveness in licensing requirements of new drugs: the fourth hurdle. *BMJ*. 2004; 329: 972-975.
3. Jacobson G., Pharmaceuticals pricing: US and European strategies. *European Affairs*. Summer/Fall 2007; 8(2-3).
4. Neumann P., Evidence-based and value-based formulary guidelines. *Health Aff*. 2004; 23(1): 124-134.
5. Silcock J., Raynor T., Petty D., The organization and development of primary care pharmacy in the United Kingdom. *Health Policy*. 2004; 67(2): 207-214.
6. Langley P., Focusing pharmacoeconomic activities: reimbursement or the drug life cycle? *Curr Med Res Opin*. 2004; 20(2): 181-186.
7. Paul J., and Trueman P., Fourth hurdle reviews, NICE, and database applications. *Pharmacoepidemiol Drug Saf*. 2001; 10: 429-438.
8. Cohen J., Stolk E., Niezen M., The increasingly complex fourth hurdle for pharmaceuticals. *Pharmacoeconomics*. 2007; 25(9): 727-734.
9. Claxton K., Sculpher M.J., Using value of information analysis to prioritize health research: some lessons learned from recent UK experience. *Pharmacoeconomics*. 2006; 24(11): 1055-1068.
10. Packer C., Simpson S., Stevens A., International diffusion of new health technologies: a ten-country analysis of six technologies. *Int J Technol Assess Health Care*. 2006; 22(4): 419-428.
11. Pearson S., and Rawlins M., Quality, innovation, and value for money: NICE and the British National Health Service. *JAMA*. 2005; 294(20): 2618-2622.

SUGGESTED READING

Australian Government, Department of Health and Ageing, *About the PBS*. Available at http://www.pbs.gov.au/html/consumer/pbs/about. Accessed 31 July 2008.

Health Canada, Patented Medicine Prices Review Board, *About the PMPRB*. Available at http://www.pmprb-cepmb.gc.ca/english/View.asp?x=175&mp=87. Accessed 31 July 2008.

Henry D., Hill S., Harris A., Drug prices and value for money: the Australian Pharmaceutical Benefits Scheme. *JAMA*. 2005; 294(20): 23-30.

National Institute for Health and Clinical Excellence, homepage. Available at https://www.nice.org.uk. Accessed 31 July 2008.

Wagner J. and McCarthy E., International differences in drug prices. *Annu Rev Public Health*. 2004; 25: 475-495.

Wertheimer A. and Smith M., *International Drug Regulatory Mechanisms*. Binghamton, NY: Haworth Press; 2003.

FUTURE OF MANAGED CARE PHARMACY PRACTICE

KIM A. CALDWELL

All progress requires change. But not all change is progress.
John Wooden, UCLA Basketball Coach 1948–1975

INTRODUCTION

Basketball great, Coach John Wooden delivered two strong thoughts in the quote above; for those of us in pharmacy, these messages could serve as constant reminders of our future. Perhaps as much as any other segment of the healthcare delivery team, pharmacists/pharmacy must change, we must progress. Purchasers of pharmacy products and services—including the federal government, employers, state governments, third-party organizations, and individuals—want more than they are getting today for their pharmacy dollars. Regulatory boards are beginning to anticipate and demand more and better care from the pharmacy providers. Most importantly, pharmacists are recognizing that today's service is not all that it can be . . . should be . . . will be.

NOW IS THE TIME FOR CHANGE

Time for change has arrived. Opportunities abound and challenges call out, but what is unclear is whether we, as pharmacists, are paying attention. Managed care pharmacy practice in the future will be the center position—the hub of the wheel—as we view the delivery of pharmacy products and services. These are my humble opinions. Hopefully, this chapter will offer some thought-provoking material for you, the reader, to consider. Different opinions are welcome and sought. Bigger dreams and better-defined templates are wished for. Action is mandatory.

Before we begin, you are asked to indulge me in a little experiment. The following works better when the audience (that's you) can listen with eyes closed and imagination wide-open. Because closed eyes makes reading difficult, we will just put more emphasis on the imagination portion.

In your mind's eye, imagine three separate video screens, each ready to display a visual of the streaming story being told. As each scene is described, use your imagination to the fullest. Be clear in your thoughts.

Screen 1: Picture a very busy clinic setting in which several physicians make it their business to deliver progressive, evidence-based, leading-edge medicine to their patient population. The majority of patients have passed the age of 66 years and most have been diagnosed with three or more chronic disease states. At the time of this story, best practices have dictated that the physicians should focus on (a) diagnosing, (b) educating, and (c) treatment. Prescribing has been proven to be best performed by other professionals trained to interpret the physicians' diagnosis notes in concert with a thorough review of the patient's history. She writes the prescriptions.

Screen 2: Here you should visualize a modern waiting room furnished with moderate, yet comfortable chairs, tables, lamps, plants, and reasonably current magazines. Only a couple of people are waiting as the office staff is efficiently scheduling patient visits. In this office, a third-party payor identifies the patient's need for intervention. This professional will determine the activity as specific by his patient's circumstance. The outcomes from this type of healthcare intervention have been validated to improve patient health conditions, improve patient quality of life, reduce overall healthcare costs associated with the patient, and have been added to the standard of practice for many insured.

Screen 3: (Your imagination will have to stretch a little in this setting.) The site is a large, open office with multiple workstations complete with highly sophisticated computer hardware and drawers full of healthcare data. In the center of the room is a large conference table . . . warm, inviting oak wood is well hidden by the stacks of paper and reference books. In the chairs, the professional men and women sit listening to their colleague describe her study. The evidence has once again pointed to the fact that a slight increase in patient compliance with the selected antihypertensive medication has caused a dramatic reduction in emergency room (ER) visits.

Do you still see the three screens? Can you make out the professionals, each in his or her own practice setting? Can you? Now, imagine that there are no pharmacists involved.

IT'S OUR FUTURE: WE SHOULD HAVE SOME SAY IN WRITING THE PLAN

Okay—none of us want to see that happen, but it could. Other professional groups are waiting in the wings today to take our place. They are ready, willing, and capable of delivering on many of the issues we are only talking about. Healthcare quality improvement is a major focus—but cost containment and patient-centric healthcare availability is perhaps even bigger—especially when one considers the political wars of recent years. How can we avoid these results? What might trigger positive thoughts? Let's see:

The story viewed on Screen 1 speaks to the issue of pharmacists prescribing. More likely than not, you have engaged in discussion with others about the subject; perhaps you are one of the believers that this is a wave of progress for tomorrows' pharmacists. I see some merit to the argument that because pharmacists have substantial knowledge in values and risks linked to therapeutic categories, classes, and individual, unique medications, it follows that pharmacists would be less likely to erroneously prescribe a product. But I don't think that we really want to go there. If pharmacists prescribe the medication, what group will serve as the final check, that is, the point of validation? Instead of moving pharmacists as a unit into the prescribing role, let's consider broadening our role as drug information expert, educator, and advisor. In the future, pharmacists will have the opportunity to directly assist physicians in the thorough evaluation of the very unique, very potent pharmaceuticals of the day. A few may actually generate prescriptions, but I'm hopeful that the prescribers will be handling that chore via an electronic system carried neatly in his/her pocket.

Screen 2 displayed a future office for medication therapy management (MTM) interventions. It won't be time for many of these offices until managed care pharmacy leaders and retail pharmacy practitioners get over their disputes of the late 1990s and early 2000s. It is time to put those differences on a shelf so that there is room on the table for open collaboration among professionals. MTM properly delivered can be the hole in the wall that allows the profession of pharmacy to move beyond the mechanics of dispensing into new, magnificent, valued roles in the healthcare models. Pharmacists are clearly best at gaining trust and confidence from the patients (beneficiaries) and their caregivers. Additionally, pharmacists have the trust and appreciation from other practitioners such as physicians, nurses, and support staff.

This is a big deal. Pharmacists should be actively engaged in person-to-person interventions with the selected MTM candidates. Managed care plans and pharmacy benefit managers (PBMs) are frequently the decision-makers as to whom, how, and what will be provided in MTM programs. The two must meet! Someday in the future, pharmacists will be billing the government and other third-party payors for services rendered; perhaps the payment will be based upon outcomes obtained or on a percent of savings generated. What matters is that the door is open for pharmacists and pharmacy to enter the new world of responsible MTM.

Let's say that we've agreed to accept the responsibility and that ambulatory pharmacists have come to terms with PBMs and MCOs relating them to specific roles and reimbursement. Is that all that's needed? Hardly. Responsibility attracts risk and liability. This particular responsibility requires re-tooling of old practice sites such as retail pharmacies. Boards of Pharmacies will have to reevaluate the ability, training, function, and use of support staff such as registered pharmacy technicians. Structures will have to be rebuilt to accommodate more talking with patients in private and less interference from outside sources. And none of this will happen unless the pharmacists involved can prove to the payors that indeed quality improvement and healthcare cost containment were achieved. How does that happen? See Screen 3.

In the Screen 3 display, we found well-trained professionals engaged in the analysis of drug data and perhaps associated data from other healthcare activities like hospital stays, ER visits, and physician office visits. This isn't necessarily a new science, but we are on the edge of a new, huge gold mine of data. Today, several organizations make it their business to collect samples of pharmacy data, run various analysis reports on those data, and market the results from the analysis. Frequently, pharmacists are not major players in this process. That means that although data studies are ongoing, the eyes and minds that view the raw data, participate in the handling of the data runs, and interpret the various stages of analysis results are not the eyes and minds of the drug experts. One could imagine that pharmacists might view the situations differently than an actuary or an accountant or even a physician. Terms such as benefit design, tier structure, utilization management tools, adherence, persistence, compliance, and daily average consumption are words of second nature for pharmacists.

When the Medicare Part D data are finally available to CMS, they will be able to do many things well: pay claims, validate the Part D Plans' adherence to specified formulary and benefit design, and verify elements of the originally submitted Part D Plan Bid, among other things. The staff at CMS will be able to analyze many factors related to initial oversight of the very large and cumbersome Part D program. But they may not be able to share the results. In fact, unless authorized, it's unclear whether CMS will be able to blend the data from Part A, B, and D to form a broad data set to study and analyze appreciable results. I am convinced that it will happen sooner rather than later.

Outside of CMS, non-government groups have been formed to study quality, value, cost, and other topics related to data mines such as this one. They too believe that there is a future story in healthcare outcomes waiting to be told. They also believe that authorization to combine data will come and those studies will follow. What is unclear is how many pharmacists have been brought into or will be part of those groups. Who will study the data?

I have believed for years (as have many of the readers) that a dollar spent on appropriate pharmaceuticals and pharmacy services is the *best* dollar spent in health care. The problem is that millions of dollars and multiple years later, no one has been able to prove or disprove that theory. Why? Well for the most part, it comes down to the fact that the consumers of healthcare services and products (including pharmacy and pharmaceuticals) jump from program to program, payor to payor, formulary to formulary, benefit design to . . . well you get the idea. Part D's birth delivered the opportunity for something different. This is a benefit that may be altered a little here and there in the future, but a benefit that will not change significantly. This is a pharmacy program for a very large, predictable population. No previous study has involved a very large population, focused on a similar benefit model, with similar formulary requirements, with similar disease states such as the Medicare Part D study will provide.

Given the fact that the compilation of Parts A, B, and D should paint a fairly complete picture, this is the chance to prove the value of today's pharmaceutical products and services or it will disprove the same. Who better to sit at center court in the game of pharmacy data than highly trained, data-savvy pharmacists? In this case, managed care pharmacists hold a significant edge, but they must stand up to be recognized as viable players in developing and analyzing these new studies. Evidence-based medicine decisions will be one of the many benefits resulting from properly utilized drug analysis studies. Rebirth of benefit designs and tier structures may be other outcomes. Innovative drug design and development might be a product of the evidence gathered, studied, and shared.

IMPACT OF A GROWING PHARMACIST SHORTAGE

There were 3 billion prescriptions written in 2006 during a pharmacist shortage. Consider the implications when we reach 4 billion prescriptions annually by 2010. Thinking smarter, planning more wisely, and acting faster will be mandates. It doesn't hurt that the United States is seeing a growth in the number of pharmacy schools and the number of graduates per year, but these alone will not solve the workflow issues.

So, where do we go from here? Earlier, the need for increased use of registered, certified technicians was mentioned. This is an increasingly important factor to consider, but don't go meekly down that path. These support staff members must be well-trained, mandatory registration (or similar) with the state's governing body must be required, and pharmacists should never relinquish the final check/final responsibility for prescriptions dispensed. Even with a well-structured plan, incorporating technicians into the process won't be enough to handle the increased volume of patients.

Automation, technology, structured procedures, and sub-contractor assistance are all possible tools for pharmacies of the future. Consider the slowly growing advent of *central-fill* pharmacies in different regions of the country. Evidence suggests improvement in volume of processed prescriptions with the partnerships involved in the central-fill system. For those unclear on the concept, an example would be a chain of pharmacies owned by a single entity utilizing a daily truck delivery system from a single-source warehouse. The company potentially could open a closed-door pharmacy in or near the warehouse for the sole purpose of filling refill prescriptions for the other store pharmacies. These pharmacies (if allowed by local regulation) could transfer prescriptions into the central pharmacy, have the refills processed, and then receive the completed prescription back in the originating store as a final product also by transfer. State laws about this business operation may vary. It works if the patient/customer has previously indicated that the refill won't be picked up until at least one day following the order. It also might be possible for the central pharmacy to deliver prescriptions by mail if so requested.

Upside? There are several possible "wins" with this process. The originating pharmacy lessens their daily load; the central-fill pharmacy has fewer outside distractions and less likelihood of system problems that might allow an error; the volume generated by the central-fill potentially allows better inventory turns, less expired product, and improved purchasing power. Managed care programs should consider the value of network pharmacy providers partnering with central-fill locations (their own or sub-contracted). Additionally, the MCO might want to consider the need to audit the filling process and billing mechanics involved with using the central-fill partner. This could be a plus for both sides.

MAIL SERVICE PHARMACY: IS NOW THE TIME TO RESTRUCTURE THAT BUSINESS?

Often one hears retail pharmacists complaining about things that seem to be caused by MCOs and PBMs. Let's take the time to review some of the issues and think about possible cause/effect/repair. First, mail order pharmacy competition is hurting the retail pharmacy business. Mandatory or mail order preferred pharmacy benefits are unfair business practice. Let's dissect this issue. Those pharmacists complaining about the mail order competitors are the same pharmacists complaining that they can hardly keep up with the large volume of prescriptions flowing through their operations, the number of technical issues (e.g., formulary compliance, prior authorizations, patient counseling), and other obstacles such as compounding and long-term care. These are the same pharmacists who want to take on the challenge (and time commitment) of MTM. Fact: there is a pharmacist shortage. Fact: mail order fills don't typically exceed 15% of the total annual prescription volume. Fact: there is likely to be an increase of one billion pharmacy prescriptions per year by the year 2010. Therefore, if the mail order business was to disappear, the ability for the current retail pharmacy force to successfully handle the load is questionable at best.

So how do we fix the issue? Perhaps the leaders in pharmacy, especially those trained in managed markets and PBM processes, should rethink which prescriptions are appropriate for mail order processing. What if mail centers limited their business to those products identified as chronic care validated by a physician's diagnosis and only following original fills elsewhere. Additionally, mail centers appear best suited for specialty products and high cost therapies; both require focused attention on inventory control and timely delivery of product and support. While this might alter the volume equation in one direction or another, it probably will control the cost of goods for the third-party purchaser while allowing the ambulatory pharmacists more time for the delivery of patient services.

Second, retail pharmacists complain that they receive too little reimbursement for the services provided. In fact, the reimbursement is for the purchase of the product as the third-party payor is anticipating that the pharmacy will automatically provide the minimum service necessary to deliver the product correctly as ordered by the prescriber. This process has been all over the table, and it will never be resolved as is currently delivered. So, what if a new model was considered for the future? Continue to purchase the product at the current low profit structure, but add meaningful reimbursement for services provided. No, I don't mean add dollars for nothing new, but offer logical reimbursement for the services previously discussed above. MTM doesn't have to be a Medicare Part D limitation. There is significant thought and study to support direct patient interventions for high use and high-risk patient populations. If structured thoughtfully, it is possible that the patient will receive better care, be more adherent, more compliant, and better controlled on their original, lower-dose therapy. It would seem likely that an appropriate partnership with the pharmacists could lead to appropriate generic use and potential formulary support. This seems to fit with the "solution" to the mail order issue.

Third, pharmacists in retail settings have a valid complaint that they spend too many hours attempting to settle insurance issues such as non-formulary, prior authorization, step-edits, and therapeutic switches. This is an opportunity for MCO and PBM pharmacy teams. The sooner structured programs can entice the prescribing population to significantly join the electronic world, the sooner the hassles will diminish. It's clear that HHS/CMS is driving toward the successful implementation of electronic prescribing in the future; demo projects were created to identify the next load of standards and requirements. As of 2008, standards are in place for the electronic prescribing, transmission, clarifying, etc. There is a problem, however; these standards technically only apply to patients eligible to be Medicare and non-controlled products covered by Medicare Part D. That said, MCO and PBM organizations have much to gain by encouraging physician buy-in and pharmacy compliance. Formulary compliance, appropriate tracking of prescriptions written verses prescriptions filled, adherence and compliance monitoring, online prior authorization systems, and multiple provider tracking are just a few of the positive rewards for the third-party payor. Besides, the retail pharmacy won't complain as much.

IMPACT OF EXTERNAL FORCES

TECHNOLOGY

Beyond what we do within the profession of pharmacy, developments external to the profession will take place as they always have in the past. Just as the computer enables prospective DUR, inventory management, and automated record keeping, new future developments will move practice further down the road of innovation. Here are a few examples.

Genotyping and Phenotyping   Individualized drug therapy will come about after a database can hold genotyping and phenotyping characteristics of patients. So, when a patient needs an antihypertensive agent, his or her physician will know which of the products on the market is compatible with their enzyme system characteristics.

Biotechnology Coming of Age   Today we have only a handful of biotech products that include interferon, human growth hormone, recombinant insulin, erythropoietin, and a few others. But soon, that number will explode as results of the last two or three decades of biochemical research begin to pay dividends. These agents are proteins or peptides and therefore are not likely effective in the oral route. Who will operate "shooting galleries" where patients stop in for a two minute injection by appointment. Will pharmacy grab this opportunity or lose it to other healing professions?

Also, the biotech revolution can spell the demise of the synthetic (small molecule) chemistry in the pharmaceutical industry. Think about it. Most of our current drugs are maintenance therapies to control—not cure—chronic diseases. But if we could insert materials to enable the pancreas to again produce effective insulin, no one would require external insulin or the oral antidiabetic agents. This concept could be applied to the situation for gout, hypertension, clotting disorders, depression, and arthritis, among other diseases.

Perhaps in the 1970s, only a few hundred persons knew how to prepare monoclonal human insulin, but that is not so today where literally tens of thousands of biochemists around the world are capable of producing equivalent quality biotechnology agents. This will influence prices, competition, education, and other services to the professions.

Drug ATMs like vending machines will dispense refills in the beginning and new prescriptions later. Such automation, the use of technicians, and successful biotech products may cause severe repercussions for the pharmacy humanpower situation. It also could make redundant some of the 30 new pharmacy faculties that have been established during the past half-decade.

Developments in artificial intelligence and Internet capability may completely revise the nature and functioning of the healthcare delivery system. In the near future, the MCO patient phoning a clinic for a physician's appointment will be directed to a Web site where a series of questions will be posed to the patient. ("Does it always hurt, or just hurt when you are standing?") This algorithm will provide the differential diagnosis and the Web site will direct the patient to the appropriate next source of care, which may be a pharmacy for some over-the-counter medications, or the clinic's imaging department, or home for a rest.

LEGISLATION AND HEALTH POLICY

Just about everyone knows that the current continuing education system is not functional. What older practitioners fear will probably come to pass: an every five or ten year re-licensure examination. To demonstrate continuing competence, the practitioner must pass the examination.

And lastly, the few state laws that require PBMs to divulge their costs and financial transactions can be expected to continue and grow, with at least 40 states joining in that movement thus far. In simple terms, this means that PBMs will be forced to develop new business models.

AUTHOR'S CAVEAT

We futurists could be 100% wrong in our projections, but it is always fun to think about possible options for the future of our business and to speculate what might be happening on a global scale.

GET INVOLVED IN THE SYSTEM: VOICE OPINIONS, VOTE, AND STAND YOUR GROUND

Managed Care Pharmacy and *Pharmacy Benefit Managers*: these are not ugly terms. Sometimes we need to hear that message. In the 1950s, virtually all of pharmacy was governed by the independent pharmacy mindset. In the 1970s and 1980s, the chain pharmacy began to be the competitive dark horse as they wedged their way onto the pharmacy scene. By the 1990s, MCOs and PBMs were sharing the right to be the dark side of pharmacy. Soon, those in the pharmaceutical industry received the naming "award." The truth is, none of them represents the dark side of pharmacy. All present an opportunity for the brotherhood/sisterhood of pharmaceutical care as we share our talents, time, heart, and lives with those outside of our profession. Each member of the pharmacy world would benefit by saving the energy spent squabbling among themselves and present a united front for the real battles in our legislative houses, courtrooms, newspapers, theatres, and across foreign borders. Remember the theory: the appropriate dollar spent on pharmaceutical products and services is the best dollar spent in health care.

AMCP GLOSSARY OF MANAGED CARE TERMS

A

AAPCC—*See Adjusted Average Per Capita Cost.*

AAPPO—*See American Association of Preferred Provider Organizations.*

Access—A patient's ability to obtain medical care determined by the availability of medical services, their acceptability to the patient, the location of health care facilities, transportation, hours of operation, and cost of care.

Accounts Receivable—The balance of money owed to a client by others.

Accreditation—Accreditation programs give an official authorization or approval to an organization by comparing it with a set of industry-derived standards.

ACF—*See Ambulatory Care Facility.*

Actuaries—The insurance professionals who perform the mathematical analysis necessary for setting insurance premium rates.

Adherence—Formerly referred to as compliance. The ability of a patient to take their medication or follow a treatment protocol according to the directions for which it was prescribed; a patient taking the prescribed dose of medication at the prescribed frequency for the prescribed length of time.

Adjudication—The process of completing all validity, process, and file edits necessary to prepare a claim for final payment or denial.

Adjusted Average Per Capita Cost (AAPCC)—used by the Centers for Medicare & Medicaid Services (CMS) as the calculation for the funds required to care for Medicare recipients; risk contract reimbursement is based on 95% of the AAPCC fee-for-service (FFS) expenditures on a 5-year rolling average for a county or parish; the 122 AAPCC actuarial stratification includes factors for age, sex, Medicaid eligibility, institutional status, the presence of end-stage renal disease, and whether a person has both Part A and Part B of Medicare; CMS uses these rates to make monthly payments to contractors that agree to accept risk and treat Medicare patients; *see also Medicare Risk.*

Adjusted Community Rating—*See Rating, Adjusted Community Rating.*

Adjustment—A credit or debit amount appearing at the carrier/group level on claims and administrative fee invoices sent to plan sponsors or at a claim level on adjustment advice sent to pharmacies. An adjustment can result from claims processing and/or billing errors (e.g., incorrect dispensing fee paid, incorrect pharmacy paid, incorrect administration fee billed, wrong carrier/group billed). An adjustment can also be processed against a general ledger account (e.g., bad debt or error).

Administrative Costs—The costs assumed by a managed care plan for administrative services such as claims processing, billing, and overhead costs.

Administrative Services Only (ASO) Contract—A contract under which a third party administrator (TPA) or an insurer agrees to provide administrative services to an employer in exchange for a fixed fee per employee.

Adverse Event—Any harm a patient suffers that is caused by factors other than the patient's underlying condition.

Adverse Selection—A particular health plan, whether indemnity or managed care, is selected against by the enrollee, and thus an inequitable proportion of enrollees requiring more medical services are found in that plan.

Agency for Healthcare Research and Quality (AHRQ)—Formerly the Agency for Health Care Policy and Research (AHCPR); created by Congress in 1989 to conduct federal research into technology assessment and outcomes management and to develop practice guidelines for public dissemination. AHRQ is perhaps best known for funding the patient outcomes-based research trials that form the basis for its practice guideline efforts.

AHCPR—*See Agency for Healthcare Research and Quality.*

AHRQ—*See Agency for Healthcare Research and Quality.*

Alignment of Incentives—A phrase used to describe the relatively new economic arrangements of sharing between physicians and hospitals that creates an incentive for physicians to accept capitation.

Allowable Cost—From the context of a federally qualified Health Maintenance Organization (HMO)—the direct and indirect costs, including normal standby costs incurred, that are proper and necessary for efficient delivery of needed healthcare services, including provider costs, and costs for marketing, enrollment, membership, and operation of the HMO, that are peculiar to healthcare prepayment organizations.

ALOS—*See Average Length of Stay.*

Alternative Delivery Systems—An expression used to describe all forms of healthcare delivery systems other than traditional fee-for-service (FFS) indemnity health care. Just about all managed care organizations are called alternative delivery systems.

Ambulatory Care—Health services delivered on an outpatient basis. If the patient makes the trip to the doctor's office or surgical center without an overnight stay, it is considered ambulatory care, but if he or she is treated at home, it is not.

Ambulatory Care Facility (ACF)—A medical care center that provides a wide range of healthcare services, including preventive care, acute care, surgery, and outpatient care, in a centralized facility. Also known as a medical clinic or medical center.

American Association of Preferred Provider Organizations (AAPPO)—The national trade association for Preferred Provider Organizations (PPOs), founded in 1983. There are currently over 1,200 members. The mission statement of the AAPPO is "to provide direction and assistance to and for PPOs and their partners in managed care through education, information, research, and advocacy."

Ancillary Services—Auxiliary or supplemental services, such as diagnostic services, home health services, physical therapy, and occupational therapy, used to support diagnosis and treatment of a patient's condition.

Antikickback Statute—Forbids referral kickback remuneration of any kind for Medicare and Medicaid, imposing criminal sanctions; kickbacks cannot be solicited, taken, or offered for business involving the purchase or lease of healthcare goods or services.

Any Willing Provider Laws (AWPLs)—Requires managed care organizations to grant network enrollment to any provider who is willing to join, as long as they meet provisions outlined in the plan; the central issue is the fairness of physician de-selection by a plan, and conversely the plan's ability to reduce medical costs by eliminating overuse of physicians; multiple state laws challenge and establish policy.

Appeal—A formal request by a covered person or provider for reconsideration of a decision, such as a utilization review recommendation, a benefit payment or administrative action.

Arbitration—In the event of dispute or difference in opinion arising out of agreements between certain plans and reinsurers, or between other entities, the parties typically agree that such disputes will be submitted to and settled by arbitration in accordance with an authority such as the Bermuda Arbitration Act of 1986, which is considered to be the sole means by which disputes will be resolved.

ASO—*See Administrative Services Only Contract.*

Assignment of Benefits—The payment of medical benefits directly to a provider of care rather than to a member; generally requires either a contract between the health plan and the provider, or a written release from the subscriber to the provider allowing the provider to bill the health plan; the transfer of one's interest or policy benefits to another party.

Assumption of Financial Risk—The risk a Health Maintenance Organization (HMO) bears on behalf of its members; according to CFR-42, each HMO must assume full financial risk on a prospective basis for the provision of basic health services, except that it may obtain insurance or make other arrangements to cover the following: for the cost of providing an aggregate value of more than $5,000 to an enrollee in any year; the cost of legitimate out-of-area care; for not more than 90% of the amount by which its costs for any fiscal year exceed 115% of its income; and to cover risk for its participating providers.

Attrition Rate—Disenrollment expressed as a percentage of total membership; a plan with 40,000 members with a 2% attrition rate per month would need to gain 800 new members each month to retain the initial 40,000 covered lives.

Authorization—As it applies to managed care, authorization is the approval of care, such as hospitalization. Preauthorization may be required before admission takes place or care is given by non-HMO providers.

Average Cost (or Benefit)—The average cost (or benefit) for a unit of output (e.g., one day in a hospital for one patient) is the total cost (or benefit) of one unit of output divided by the total units of output.

Average Cost per Claim—A financial amount, representing the sum of the medical charge and administrative charge for services provided within the categories of admissions, physician services, and outpatient claims.

Average Length of Stay (ALOS)—calculated as the average number of patient days of hospitalization for each admission, expressed as an average of the population within the plan for a given period of time.

Average Wholesale Price (AWP)—The published average "cost" of a drug product paid by the pharmacy to the wholesaler. This price is specific to drug strength or concentrating dosage form, package size, and manufacturer or labeler. The average wholesale price of each drug is maintained on the National Drug Code (NDC) master file. This price is used to calculate the upper limit of payment available under a plan.

Average Wholesale Price (AWP) Discount—A cost-containment program implemented to reduce drug program costs for plan sponsors without influencing cardholders. As AWP no longer always equals the actual cost of a drug to the pharmacy, by applying a discount to AWP, a new upper limit of payment is established and savings are realized by the plan sponsors. An example is a plan sponsor with a plan that allows average wholesale price less 10% (AWP-10%).

AWP—*See Average Wholesale Price.*

AWPLs—*See Any Willing Provider Laws.*

B

Balance Billing—The practice of a provider billing a patient for all charges not paid for by the insurance plan, because those charges are above the plan's UCR (usual, customary, and reasonable) practice or may be considered medically unnecessary; plans are increasingly prohibiting providers from balance billing except for allowed copays, coinsurance, and deductibles.

Benchmarking—A method of identifying the level of performance that can be related to specific outcomes of a particular procedure, intervention, or process. The goal is to identify "best practices." Benchmarking is frequently used as a quality improvement (QI) initiative.

Beneficiary (Insured)—The primary person receiving the benefit coverage. This information is maintained on the eligibility file of the plan sponsor. If the client can provide the information, dependent names are also maintained.

Benefit Design—A process of determining what level of coverage or type of service should be included within a health plan or specific product, at specified rates of reimbursement, based on a multiple of relatively unstandardized and often unique factors, such as market pressure, cost, clinical effectiveness and medical evidence, legislated mandate, medical necessity, and preventive value; *see also Covered Services.*

Benefit Package—Services an insurer, government agency, health plan, or an employer offers under the terms of a contract.

Best Practices—Actual practices, in use by qualified providers following the latest treatment modalities, which produce the best measurable results on a given dimension.

Blended Rating—*See Rating, Blended Rating.*

Brand-Brand Interchange—Dispensing one brand name product for another brand name product marketed by another manufacturer.

Brand Drug—The drug manufacturer whose name is listed on the application to the FDA for approval of a new drug.

Brand Name—The trademarked name of the drug that appears on the package label.

Broker—A salesperson who has obtained a state license to sell and service contracts of multiple health plans or insurers, and who is ordinarily considered to be an agent of the buyer, not the health plan or insurer.

C

Capitation—A per-member monthly payment to a provider that covers contracted services and is paid in advance of its delivery. In essence, a provider agrees to provide specified services to Health Maintenance Organization (HMO) members for this fixed, predetermined payment for a specified length of time (usually a year), regardless of how many times the member uses the service. The rate can be fixed for all members or it can be adjusted for the age and sex of the member, based on actuarial projections of medical utilization.

Cardholder (Insured or Beneficiary)—The primary person receiving the benefit coverage in whose name the card is issued. This information is maintained in the eligibility file. If the client can provide the information, dependent names are also maintained.

Carrier/Group—The combination used to signify both the plan sponsor (carrier) and the specific group under it. An example of a carrier/group would be:

0007/0023

0007-Carrier-ABZ Insurance Co.

0023-Group-The Marley Company

Carrier Name—This term is used to identify any plan sponsor—the underwriter of an insured account or the company name of a self-administered account. This name is often used on management reports sent to the plan sponsor.

Carrier Number—An assigned 4-digit number that identifies the plan sponsor (insurance company, self-administered account, third-party administrator, multiple employer trust, health maintenance organization). A plan sponsor may have more than one carrier number.

Carve-Out Pharmacy Benefit—The prescription coverage benefit that is removed from the primary health care coverage plan and handled by another company (e.g., a Pharmacy Benefits Manager [PBM]). Within a capitation environment, a type of service not included as an agreed service to be provided within the contract, therefore carved out within the per member per month (PMPM) or pricing structure for certain categories of health care services (typically high-volume, high-cost, or areas where specialty expertise can reduce costs for that segment, such as behavioral, lab, podiatry, X-ray, or transplants), not subject to discretionary utilization, and not included within the capitation rate; may also be created when a provider cannot or will not provide some segment of care, or is unavailable during periods of time when care may still be needed; normally a carve out is warranted because there is special expertise and improved cost-effectiveness in a segment of care, versus lumping the segment in with an overall pricing.

Case Management—The process whereby a healthcare professional supervises the administration of medical or ancillary services to a patient, typically one who has a catastrophic disorder or who is receiving mental health services. Case managers are thought to reduce the costs associated with the care of such patients, while providing high-quality medical services.

CDHP—*See Consumer Directed Health Plan.*

Centers for Medicare & Medicaid Services (CMS)—Formerly known as the Health Care Financing Administration (HCFA); the federal agency responsible for administering Medicare and overseeing states' administration of Medicaid and the Office of Prepaid Healthcare Operations and Oversight (OPHCOO), which in turn oversees Health Maintenance Organizations (HMOs).

Certificate of Coverage (COC)—The basic document listing all healthcare benefits within the plan, as required by state law to reflect the contract as negotiated between employer and plan and shared with the employee.

Certificate of Insurance—Document delivered to an individual that summarizes the benefits and principal provisions of a group insurance contract.

Certification—Certification is the official authorization for use of services.

Claim—Information submitted by a provider or covered person to establish that medical services were provided to a covered person, from which processing for payment to the provider or covered person is made.

Claims Adjudication—*See Adjudication.*

Claims Review—The method by which an enrollee's healthcare service claims are reviewed before reimbursement is made. The purpose of this monitoring system is to validate the medical appropriateness of the provided services and to be sure the cost of the service is not excessive.

Clinical Care Pathway—A clinical protocol that lists steps and timing for the management of a specific disease, condition, or procedure; the goal being standardization in treatment, elimination of duplication of services, and improved patient outcomes.

Clinical Practice Guidelines—A utilization and quality management mechanism designed to aid providers in making decisions about the most appropriate course of treatment for a specific clinical case.

Closed Formulary—A type of formulary that limits the number of prescription drugs reimbursed by the plan.

COB—*See Coordination of Benefits.*

COBRA —*See Consolidated Omnibus Budget Reconciliation Act of 1985.*

COC—*See Certificate of Coverage.*

Coinsurance—The percentage of the costs of medical services paid by the patient. This is a characteristic of indemnity insurance and PPO plans. The coinsurance usually is about 20% of the cost of medical services after the deductible is paid.

Community Rating—*See Rating, Community Rating.*

Complaint—Any circumstance where a member expresses dissatisfaction about any aspect of a care or service within the managed care organization, with a provider, or other members that does not rise to the level of a formal grievance. Complaints are usually generated by a telephone call or inquiry that is generally the result of a misunderstanding or misinformation and may be resolved informally. An unresolved complaint or a succession of related complaints may become a grievance. *See also Grievance.*

Compliance—More accurately referred to as adherence; the ability of a patient to take their medication or follow a treatment protocol according to the directions for which it was prescribed; a patient taking the prescribed dose of medication at the prescribed frequency for the prescribed length of time.

Concurrent Review—A screening method by which a healthcare provider reviews a procedure performed or hospital admission performed by a colleague to assess its necessity.

Consolidated Omnibus Budget Reconciliation Act of 1985 (COBRA)—Federal legislation that made amendments to the Medicare and Medicaid programs. This act is best known for its establishment of a Physician Payment Review Commission, which makes recommendations to Congress on Medicare Part B reimbursements for services. It included a component that required employers to offer former employees the opportunity to purchase continuation of healthcare coverage under the employer's medical plan.

Consumer Directed Health Plan (CDHP)—A health plan that allows beneficiaries more direct control over medical decisions and costs. Typically, this type of plan consists of several tiers—a health spending account funded by the employer that can be rolled over from year to year. Generally, a "defined contribution," such as a specific dollar amount is placed in this account by the employer for the employee. The deductible is funded by the employee and used after the health spending account is exhausted; and health insurance is triggered after the deductible is met. Employees also may fund medical reimbursement accounts to pay for their share of expenses. *See also Defined Contribution and/or High Deductible Health Plan.*

Continuous Quality Improvement (CQI)—A comprehensive philosophy of continuously improving the quality of a product or service by constantly monitoring operations, correcting problems, and implementing systems to better assist customers. It is a comprehensive approach for improving overall organizational performance and it challenges the traditional way of doing business. It contends that most quality problems involve procedures and strategies (i.e., the process) and are not the fault of individuals.

Continuum of Care—Clinical services provided during a single inpatient hospitalization or for multiple conditions over a lifetime. It provides a basis for evaluating quality, cost, and utilization over the long term. A spectrum of healthcare options, ranging from limited care needs though tertiary care, which has become the focus for an integrated delivery system to provide the appropriate expertise for the patient without providing a more expensive setting than necessary.

Coordination of Benefits (COB)—A system whereby responsibility for claims is determined for a person who is covered by multiple insurers. Under this system, each person with multiple coverages has primary and secondary insurance based on a set of industry rules. COB rules are designed to prevent duplicate payments for the same service.

Copayment—A nominal fee charged to an insured member to offset costs of paperwork and administration for each office visit or pharmacy prescription filled; a cost-sharing arrangement in which a covered person pays a specified charge for a specific service, such as a fixed dollar amount for each prescription received; (e.g., $5.00 per generic prescription, $10.00 per preferred brand name prescription, and a higher charge such as $25.00 for a non-formulary product.)

Copay Amount—The amount insured members must pay each time they receive a prescription or medical care using their benefit.

Cosmetic—A drug used to improve complexion, or to enhance beauty.

Cost Benefit—Cost-benefit analysis expresses the outcomes of therapies (e.g., the benefits) in monetary rather than physical units.

Cost Containment—A program to decrease the overall costs of a drug, medical benefit, or health care.

Cost-Effectiveness—Usually considered as a ratio, the cost-effectiveness of a drug or procedure, for example, relates the cost of that drug or procedure to the health benefits resulting from it. In health terms, it is often expressed as the cost per year per life-year saved or as the cost per quality-adjusted life-year saved.

Cost Sharing—A method of reimbursement for healthcare services that holds the patient responsible for a portion or percentage of the charge, with an attending strategy to serve as a means of reducing utilization; normally includes an annual deductible amount; *see also Coinsurance.*

Cost Shifting—The redistribution of payment sources. Typically, cost shifting occurs when a discount on provider services is obtained by one payer and the providers increase costs to another payer to make up the difference.

Covered Lives—Refers to the number of persons who are enrolled within a particular health plan, or for coverage by a provider network; includes enrollees and their covered dependents.

Covered Services—A written healthcare benefit document that outlines the benefit package to be provided to either individual beneficiaries or a purchasing group or employer, with a corresponding sum for each service; services specified for beneficiaries by an insurer, the Centers for Medicare & Medicaid (CMS), or equivalent state program for Medicaid entitlements, in a benefit plan or managed care contract; specific services and supplies for which the federal or commercial payer will provide reimbursement. These may consist of a combination of mandatory and optional services within each state.

CPT—*See Physician's Current Procedural Terminology.*

CQI—*See Continuous Quality Improvement.*

Credentialing—Examination of a physician or other healthcare provider's qualifications to determine if he or she is entitled to clinical privileges at a hospital or to see insured individuals at a managed care organization.

Criteria—Systematically developed statements that can be used to assess the appropriateness of care, services, and/or outcomes.

D

DAW —*See Dispense as Written.*

Decision Tree—The decision tree, the fundamental analytic tool for decision analysis, is a way of displaying the temporal and logical sequence of a clinical decision problem. Its form highlights three structural components: the alternative actions that are available to the decision maker; the probabilistic events that follow from and affect these actions, such as clinical information obtained or the clinical consequences revealed; and the outcomes for the patient that are associated with each possible scenario of actions and consequences.

Deductible—A fixed amount of healthcare dollars of which a person must pay 100% before his or her health benefits begin. Most indemnity plans feature a $200 to $500 deductible and then pay up to 100% of money spent for covered services above this level.

Defined Contribution—An employer allocates a fixed amount of money to each employee. The employee uses those funds to purchase healthcare coverage. This shifts the responsibility for payment and selection of healthcare plans from the employer to the employee. *See also Consumer Directed Health Plan.*

Dependent—An enrolled health plan member who has coverage tied to that of the sponsor; may be a spouse or an unmarried child, or a stepchild or legally adopted child of either the employee or the employee's spouse, whose primary domicile is with the employee, except for other arrangements as approved by the plan; often dependent children status is also delineated by those under the age of 18, or children attending college full-time under a specified age.

Dependent Coverage Code—Allows the plan sponsor to control the type of coverage each cardholder receives.

DESI—*See Drug Efficacy Study Implementation.*

Diagnostic and Treatment Codes—Special codes that consist of a brief, specific description of each diagnosis or treatment and a number used to identify each diagnosis and treatment, for example, Physician's Current Procedural Terminology (CPT) codes.

Diagnosis-Related Groups (DRGs)—A Yale University-derived system of classification for 383 inpatient hospital services based on principal diagnosis, secondary diagnosis, surgical procedures, age, sex, and presence of complications; this system is used as a financing mechanism to reimburse hospital and selected other providers for services rendered; used to describe patient mix in hospitals and to determine hospital reimbursement policy. A standard flat rate per procedure is derived from this scale, which is paid by Medicare for its beneficiaries, regardless of the cost to the hospital to provide that service.

Direct Costs—Direct costs are those that are wholly attributable to the service in question—for example, the services of professional and paraprofessional personnel, equipment, and materials.

Disease Management—A philosophy toward the treatment of the patient with an illness (usually chronic) that seeks to prevent recurrence of symptoms, maintain high quality of life, and prevent future need for medical resources by using an integrated approach to health care. Pharmaceutical care, continuous quality improvement, practice guidelines, and case management all play key roles in this effort, which should result in decreased healthcare costs as well.

Disease Management Measures—Indicators of a health plan's success in treating the entirety of a disease across the continuum of care—related to the family of outcome measures that treat the disease as opposed to managing health; may include measures for major diagnostic categories (hypertension, diabetes, heart disease), primary care (patient satisfaction with service, utilization of preventive services, illness episodes per 1,000), specialty care (diagnosis—specific health status scores), acute care episodes (Average Length of Stay [ALOS] per major Diagnostic-Related Group [DRG] categories, surgeries per 1,000 readmission rates) or rehab and recovery (patient compliance, DRG-specific health status scored).

Dispense as Written (DAW)—A notation used by a physician that will determine whether or not generic substitution is to occur when a prescription is filled. The dispensing pharmacist translates the notation of the physician when submitting a claim for payment using one of the ten DAW codes listed below (numeric values are assigned to each code for computer entry using online claims adjudication systems):

0 = No Product Selection Indicated
This is the field default value used for prescriptions when product selection is not an issue. Examples include prescriptions written for single source brand products and prescriptions written using the generic name and a generic product is dispensed.

1 = Substitution Not Allowed by Prescriber
This value is used when the prescriber indicates, in a manner specified by prevailing law, that the product is to be dispensed as written.

2 = Substitution Allowed-Patient-Requested Product Dispensed
This value is used when the prescriber has indicated, in a manner specified by prevailing law, that generic substitution is permitted but the patient requests the brand product. This situation can occur when the prescriber writes the prescription using either the brand or generic name and the product is available from multiple sources.

3 = Substitution Allowed-Pharmacist-Selected Product Dispensed
This value is used when the prescriber has indicated, in a manner specified by prevailing law, that generic substitution is permitted and the brand product is dispensed because the dispensing pharmacist using his/her professional judgment has determined that the brand product is the drug of choice.

4 = Substitution Allowed-Generic Drug Not in Stock

This value is used when the prescriber has indicated, in a manner specified by prevailing law, that generic substitution is permitted and the brand product is dispensed since a currently marketed generic is not stocked in the pharmacy. This situation exists due to the buying habits of the pharmacist, not because of the unavailability of the generic product in the marketplace.

5 = Substitution Allowed-Brand Drug Dispensed as a Generic

This value is used when the prescriber has indicated, in a manner specified by prevailing law, that generic substitution is permitted and the pharmacist is utilizing the brand product as the generic entity.

6 = Override

This value is used by various claims processors in very specific instances as defined by that claims processor and/or its client(s).

7 = Substitution Not Allowed-Brand Drug Mandated by Law

This value is used when the prescriber has indicated, in a manner specified by prevailing law, that generic substitution is permitted but prevailing law or regulation prohibits the substitution of a generic product even though generic versions of the product may be available in the marketplace.

8 = Substitution Allowed-Generic Drug Not Available in Marketplace

This value is used when the prescriber has indicated, in a manner specified by prevailing law, that generic substitution is permitted and the brand product is dispensed since the generic is not currently manufactured or distributed or is temporarily unavailable.

9 = Other

This value is reserved and currently not in use. The National Council for Prescription Drug Programs (NCPDP) does not recommend use of this value at the present time. Please contact NCPDP if you intend to use this value and document how it will be utilized by your organization.

Dispensing Fee—Contracted rate of compensation paid to a pharmacy for the processing/filling of a prescription claim. The dispensing fee is added to the negotiated formula for reimbursing ingredient cost.

Doctor Number—An identification number used primarily by Health Maintenance Organizations (HMOs) to uniquely identify each physician in their network in order to facilitate rejection of claims received for services rendered by a nonparticipating physician. (The HMO may elect to use the physician's Drug Enforcement Administration (DEA) number in lieu of their own HMO doctor number.) This doctor number is also reported back to the HMO, or any client receiving prescription utilization reports, on their end-of-month reports.

Documentation—Detailed descriptions of relevant participants, evidence, assumptions, rationale, and analytic methods used in determining quality of care.

DRG—*See Diagnosis-Related Groups.*

Drug Efficacy Study Implementation—A study of drugs by the Federal Food and Drug Administration (FDA) that rates certain drugs as not safe and effective and experimental or investigational in nature. To comply in part with the 1962 amendments to the Food, Drug and Cosmetic Act, the FDA contracted in 1966 with the National Academy of Sciences/ National Research Council to study drugs approved between 1938 and 1962 from the standpoint of efficacy. The DESI program evaluated over 3000 separate products and over 16,000 therapeutic claims. By 1984, the FDA had completed final regulatory action on 3,443 products; of these, 2,225 were found to be effective, 1,051 were found not effective, and 167 were pending. The ineffective drugs were designated as DESI drugs and the Omnibus Budget Reconciliation Act of 1981 prohibited payment for these drugs by Medicaid programs and under Medicare Part B.

Drug Formulary—*See Formulary.*

Drug Mix—An evaluation of the type of drugs prescribed by an individual or defined population. The drug mix may reveal the rate of new drug adoption by reviewed physicians.

Drug Use Evaluation (DUE)—An evaluation of prescribing patterns of physicians to specifically determine the appropriateness of drug therapy.

Drug Utilization Review (DUR)—A system of drug use review that can detect potential adverse drug interactions, drug-pregnancy conflicts, therapeutic duplication, drug-age conflicts, etc. There are three forms of DUR: prospective (before dispensing), concurrent (at the time of prescription dispensing), and retrospective (after the therapy has been completed). Appropriate use of an integrated DUR program can curb drug misuse and abuse and monitor quality of care. DUR can reduce hospitalization and other costs related to inappropriate drug use.

DUE—*See Drug Use Evaluation.*

DUR—*See Drug Utilization Review.*

E

EDI—*See Electronic Data Interchange.*

Edits—Criteria that, if unmet, will cause an automated claims processing system to "reject" a claim for further/manual review.

Effectiveness—When used in the research setting, clinical effectiveness reflects how a particular treatment performs in an actual practice environment. It differs from clinical efficacy because, for example, patients receiving a product in a typical medical practice may have comorbidities that might alter the ability of a medication to achieve its intended effect; the actual effects of treatment resulting from the drug under "real life" conditions. (e.g., patients not always remembering to take their doses, physicians often not prescribing the lowest

Food and Drug Administration (FDA) recommended doses, side effects not all controlled, etc). "Head to head" effectiveness studies with similar medications are preferable.

Efficacy—The ability of a treatment to achieve the desired results under ideal study conditions. Most clinical drug trials are performed under these conditions, in which, for instance, ideal patients are selected to test a product's ability to treat infection; the *potential* effects of treatment resulting from the drug under *optimal* circumstances (e.g., patients all taking their doses at the right times, physicians prescribing correct doses, side effects appropriately monitored, etc). Efficacy studies are typically the foundation of new drug submissions to the Food and Drug Administration (FDA). Studies that compare the efficacy of similar drugs, rather than just efficacy compared to placebo, are preferable.

Electronic Claim—Insurance claim submitted to the carrier by a central processing unit, tape diskette, direct data entry, direct wire, dial-in telephone, digital fax, or personal computer download or upload. *See also Electronic Data Interchange.*

Electronic Data Interchange (EDI)—The electronic transfer of claims data or other information between two or more healthcare organizations; payers and providers are making an increased use of EDI.

Electronic Medical Record (EMR)—An automated, online medical record that is available to any number of providers, ancillary service departments, pharmacies, and others involved in patient treatment or care as a result of computer technology that stores, processes, and retrieves patient clinical and demographic information upon request of the user.

Eligibility List—A list that shows the eligible enrolled members for healthcare services and supplies, including their effective date.

Eligible Employee—Health plan contracts outline requirements for an employee to meet eligibility requirement in the health plan, which are based on factors such as full-time or part-time employment as stipulated in the contract.

Employee Retirement Income Security Act of 1974 (ERISA)—A federal law that regulates employer-sponsored benefit plans and restricts state government from regulating these plans. This law mandates reporting and disclosure requirements for group life and health plans with relevant guidance on the sponsorship, administration, minimum record retention period, servicing of plans, some claims processing, appeals regulations, and minimum mandatory clinical benefits.

EMR—*See Electronic Medical Record.*

Encounter—A healthcare visit of any type by an enrollee to a provider of care or services.

Encounter Record—Another word for a claim; also refers to a patient visit information record in a capitation system.

Enrollee—Any person eligible, as either a subscriber or dependent, in an employee benefit plan. *See also Beneficiary and/or Member.*

EOB—*See Explanation of Benefits.*

EPO—*See Exclusive Provider Organization.*

ERISA—*See Employee Retirement Income Security Act of 1974.*

Exception Report—A list of items (i.e., procedures, drugs, physicians, etc.) that do not conform to defined limits of acceptability. For example, a drug utilization exception report may list all patients that use a higher number of prescriptions than allowed by plan guidelines.

Exclusions—Drugs not covered under the pharmacy benefit of the health plan. Examples of drug exclusions include cosmetic and fertility drugs, investigational drugs, and over-the-counter (OTC) products. Specific examples include amphetamine and non-amphetamine appetite suppressant drugs.

Exclusive Provider Organization (EPO)—The EPO is a form of a preferred provider organization in which patients must visit a caregiver who is on its panel of providers. If a visit to an outside provider is made, the EPO will offer limited or no coverage for the office or hospital visit.

Experience Rating—*See Rating, Experience Rating.*

Experimental Drugs—Experimental drugs are those currently under investigation and not yet approved for use by the Food and Drug Administration (FDA) for any indication. There is not enough accumulated scientific data to establish medically appropriate use of the drug for treatment of a disease. However, FDA has established programs to allow patients with an immediately life-threatening disease "early access" to new treatments. Since patients who have exhausted standard therapeutic options may be willing to accept additional risks and potentially dangerous side effects from drug products still under study, these programs allow patients access to investigational drugs.

Explanation of Benefits (EOB)—A statement the health plan submits to the member and the provider that indicates: who provided the care, the kind of covered service or supply received, the allowable charge and amount billed, the amount the health plan paid, how much of the deductible has been paid, and the cost-share. It also gives the reason for denying a claim.

F

FDA—*See Food and Drug Administration.*

FDA 1P Drugs—The Food and Drug Administration (FDA) classifies investigational new drug applications (INDs) and new drug applications (NDAs) to assign review priority on the basis of the drug's chemical type and potential benefit. Drugs assigned a "1P" classification contain an active ingredient that has never been marketed in the United States and appears to represent an advance over available therapy. The FDA gives these drugs an expedited review and a more rapid decision is made regarding approval for the indication of use as suggested by the manufacturer.

Fee-for-Service (FFS)—Traditional provider reimbursement, in which the physician is paid according to the service performed. This is the reimbursement system used by conventional indemnity insurers. The full rate of charge for a patient without any type of insurance arrangement, discounted arrangement, or prepaid health plan.

Fee Schedule—A comprehensive listing of fees used by either a healthcare plan or the government to reimburse physicians and other providers on a fee-for-service (FFS) basis.

FFS—*See Fee-for-Service.*

First-Dollar Coverage—A feature of an insurance plan in which there is no deductible, and therefore the plan's sponsor pays a proportion or all of the covered services provided to a patient as soon as he or she enrolls.

Food and Drug Administration (FDA)—The federal agency that reviews drug products for safety and efficacy. A drug may not be marketed in the United States unless it has received approval from the FDA.

Formulary—A specific list of drugs that are included with a given plan for a client. A continually updated list of medications, related products and information, representing the clinical judgment of physicians, pharmacists, and other experts in the diagnosis and/or treatment of disease and promotion of health. Types include closed formulary, negative formulary, and open formulary.

Formulary Management—An integrated patient care process that enables physicians, pharmacists, and other healthcare professionals to work together to promote clinically sound, cost effective pharmaceutical care. The formulary management process provides the managed healthcare system with the ability to objectively discriminate between superior and marginally effective drug products.

Formulary System—An ongoing process whereby a healthcare organization, through its physicians, pharmacists and other healthcare professionals, establishes policies on the use of drugs, related products, and therapies, and identifies drugs, related products, and therapies that are the most medically appropriate and cost effective to best serve the health interests of a given patient population.

G

Gatekeeper—Most Health Maintenance Organizations (HMOs) rely on the primary-care physician (PCP), or "gatekeeper," to screen patients seeking medical care, and effectively eliminate costly and sometimes needless referral to specialists for diagnosis and management. The gatekeeper is responsible for the administration of the patient's treatment, and this person must coordinate and obtain authorization for all medical service's laboratory studies, specialty referrals, and hospitalizations. In most HMOs, if an enrollee visits a specialist without prior authorization from his or her designated primary-care physician, the enrollee must pay for medical services.

Generic Substitution—In cases in which the patent on a specific pharmaceutical product expires and drug manufacturers produce generic versions of the original branded product, the generic version of the drug (which is theorized to be identical to the product manufactured by a different firm) is dispensed even though the original product is prescribed. Some managed care organizations and Medicaid programs mandate generic substitution because of the generally lower cost of generic products. There are state and federal regulations regarding generic substitutions.

Grievance—Complaint from a member, which is initially addressed as appealed, or formal written complaint, generally of a more complex or sophisticated nature than a Complaint. Grievances may be administrative or medical in nature. Administrative grievances are generally those related to benefit determination, eligibility, satisfaction with the delivery of services, or coverage issues. Medical grievances relate to providers, quality management, medical care services, or policy and procedures dealing with medical care delivery. *See also Complaint.*

Group-Model HMO—*See Health Maintenance Organization, Group Model.*

H

HCFA—*See Centers for Medicare & Medicaid Services.*

HDHP—*See High Deductible Health Plan.*

Health Alliances—Also known as regional health alliance, these entities are purchasing pools that are responsible for negotiating health insurance for employers and employees. Alliances use their leverage as a large healthcare purchaser to negotiate contracts.

Health Care Financing Administration (HCFA)—*See Centers for Medicare & Medicaid Services.*

Health Insurance Portability and Accountability Act of 1996 (HIPAA)—A federal law that outlines the requirements that employer-sponsored group insurance plans, insurance companies, and managed care organizations must satisfy in order to provide health insurance coverage in the individual and group healthcare markets. It establishes national standards for electronic healthcare transactions and national identifiers for providers, health plans, and employers. It also addresses the security and privacy of health data.

Health Maintenance Organization (HMO)—A form of health insurance in which its members prepay a premium for the HMO's health services, which generally include inpatient and ambulatory care. For the patient, it means reduced out-of-pocket costs (i.e., no deductible), no paperwork (i.e., insurance forms), and only a small copayment for each office visit to cover the paperwork handled by the HMO. There are several different types of HMOs.

   Group Model—In the group-model HMO, the HMO contracts with a physician group, which is paid a fixed amount per patient to provide specific services.

The administration of the group practice then decides how the HMO payments are distributed to each participating physician. This type of HMO is usually located in a hospital or clinic setting and may include a pharmacy. These physicians usually do not have any fee-for-service (FFS) patients.

Hybrid Model—A combination of at least two managed care organizational models that are melded into a single health plan. Since its features do not uniformly fit one model, it is called a hybrid.

Independent Practice Association (IPA) Model—The individual practice association contracts with independent physicians who work in their own private practices and see fee-for-service (FFS) patients as well as HMO enrollees. Physicians belonging to the IPA guarantee that the care needed by each patient for whom they are responsible will fall under a certain amount of money. They guarantee this by allowing the HMO to withhold an amount of their payments (usually about 20% per year). If, by the end of the year, the physician's cost for treatment falls under this set amount, then the physician receives his entire "withhold fund." If the opposite is true, the HMO can then withhold any part of this amount, at its discretion, from the fund. Essentially, the physician is put "at risk" for keeping down the treatment cost. This is the key to the HMO's financial viability.

Network Model—A network of group practices under the administration of one HMO.

Point-of-Service (POS) Model—Sometimes referred to as an "open-ended" HMO. The point-of-service model is one in which the patient can receive care either by physicians contracted with the HMO or by those not contracted. Physicians not contracted with the HMO who see an HMO patient are paid according to the services performed. The patient is incentivized to use contracted providers through the fuller coverage offered for contracted care.

Staff Model—The staff-model HMO is the purest form of managed care. All of the physicians in a staff-model HMO are in a centralized site, in which all clinical and perhaps inpatient services and pharmacy services are offered. The HMO holds the tightest management reigns in this setting, because none of the physicians traditionally practice on an independent fee-for-service (FFS) basis. Physicians are more likely to be employees of the HMO in this setting, because they are not in a private or group practice.

Health Plan Employer Data and Information Set (HEDIS)—The result of a coordinated development effort by the National Committee for Quality Assurance (NCQA) to provide a group of performance measures that gives employers some objective information with which to evaluate health plans and hold them accountable; HEDIS helps ensure that plans and purchasers of care are speaking the same language when they are comparing value and accountability (HEDIS™ is a registered trademark of NCQA.)

Health Promotion Programs—Preventive care programs designed to educate and motivate members to prevent illness and injury and to promote good health through lifestyle choices, such as smoking cessation and dietary changes. Also known as wellness programs.

Health Savings Account (HSA)—A tax-sheltered savings account that may be used by beneficiaries covered by high deductible health plans to pay for routine healthcare expenses. Money remaining in the account at the end of the year may be used in the succeeding year.

HEDIS—*See Health Plan Employer Data and Information Set.*

High Deductible Health Plan (HDHP)—A medical plan that has specified minimum limits for the annual deductible and maximum limits for out-of-pocket expenses. An HDHP must have a minimum deductible of $1,000 for individual coverage or $2,000 for family coverage. Annual out-of-pocket expenses must not exceed $5,000 for individual coverage or $10,000 for family coverage. The amounts for deductible and out-of-pocket maximum will be indexed annually for inflation in $50 increments.

HIPAA—*See Health Insurance Portability and Accountability Act of 1996.*

HMO—*See Health Maintenance Organization.*

HMO Act—a 1973 federal act (42 U.S.C., 300 et seq.) outlining requirements for federal qualification of Health Maintenance Organizations (HMOs), consisting of legal and organizational structures, financial strength requirements, marketing provisions, and healthcare delivery; the voluntary status of "federally qualified" is sought in order to gain credibility with employers, and the chance to gain covered lives from dual choice mandates that require employee access to such plans.

Home Care—In contrast with inpatient and ambulatory care, home care is medical care that would ordinarily be administered in a hospital or on an outpatient basis; however, the patient is not sufficiently ambulatory to make frequent office or hospital visits. In these patients, intravenous therapy, for example, is administered at the patient's residence, usually by a healthcare professional. Home care reduces the need for hospitalization and its associated costs.

Horizontal Integration—Also called specialty integration; health entities that contain multiple groupings of similar care components along the continuum of care, with financial incentives for alignment into the larger group (such as multiple hospitals, or sub-acute care facilities, long-term care, home health, or behavioral health components), are combined in a system with the purpose of increased contracting leverage or increased chances of survival due to economies of scale and elimination of redundant overhead staff or function; *see also Vertical Integration.*

Hospice—A healthcare facility that provides supportive care for the terminally ill.

Hospital Alliance—A group of hospitals that have joined together to improve competitive positions and reduce costs by sharing common services and developing group purchasing programs.

HSA—*See Health Savings Account.*

I

IBNR—*See Incurred But Not Reported Expenses.*

ICD-9-CM—*See International Classification of Diseases, 9th Revision, Clinical Modification.*

Incurred But Not Reported (IBNR) Expenses—This term refers to financial accounting of all services that have been performed but have not yet been invoiced or recorded.

Indemnity Insurance—Traditional fee-for-service (FFS) medicine in which providers are paid according to the service performed.

Indirect Costs—Indirect costs are usually termed overhead costs; they are the costs shared by many services concurrently. For example, maintenance, administration, equipment, electricity, and water.

Institute of Medicine (IOM)—The mission of the Institute of Medicine is to advance and disseminate scientific knowledge to improve human health. Established in 1970 by the National Academy of Sciences, the Institute, upon its own initiative, identifies issues of medical care, research, and education. It provides objective, timely, authoritative information and advice concerning health and science policy to government, the corporate sector, the professions, and the public.

Insurance Company (Plan Sponsor)—A client, also referred to as a carrier, who underwrites the insurance for individual groups. The insurance company signs the contract and is financially responsible for all bills incurred by groups insured by them. Each insurance company is assigned a unique insurance code and can generally tailor the program for their individual groups.

Insured—*See Beneficiary.*

Integrated Healthcare Systems—Healthcare financing and delivery organizations created to provide a "continuum of care," ensuring that patients get the right care at the right time from the right provider. This continuum of care from primary care provider to specialist and ancillary provider under one corporate roof guarantees that patients get cared for appropriately, thus saving money and increasing the quality of care.

International Classification of Diseases, 9th Revision, Clinical Modification (ICD-9-CM)—A statistical classification system consisting of a listing of diagnoses and identifying codes for reporting diagnosis of health plan enrollees identified by physicians; coding and terminology to accurately describe primary and secondary diagnosis and provide for consistent documentation for claims; the codes are revised periodically by the World Health Organization; since the Medicare Catastrophic Coverage Act of 1988, ICD-9 is mandatory for Medicare claims.

Intervention—Educational, directive (e.g., formulary or prior authorization), or consultative communications between providers, especially pharmacists to physicians.

IOM—*See Institute of Medicine.*

IPA (Independent Practice Association)—*See Health Maintenance Organization, IPA Model.*

J

JCAHO—*See Joint Commission on Accreditation of Healthcare Organizations.*

Joint Commission on Accreditation of Healthcare Organizations (JCAHO)—Formerly JCAH (Joint Commission on Accreditation of Hospitals); an accreditation body for clinics, hospitals, home care, other medical facilities, and health networks; the seal of approval by this nonprofit agency is the goal of most for-profit, public, and even federal or military facilities, and its approval may be contractually mandated by Health Maintenance Organizations (HMOs) for network hospitals.

K

Kassebaum-Kennedy Health Coverage Bill—The name of legislation passed in August 1996, which began on July 1, 1997; the bill primarily benefits those who already have insurance but suddenly lose or change jobs, and also benefits the self-employed or employees of small businesses, and those who leave jobs with insurance and want to buy an individual policy; portability and fixed premiums are guaranteed for those who change jobs, as long as they have been insured for 12 months (regardless of whether they quit, are fired, or are laid off).

L

Length of Stay—The number of consecutive days a patient is hospitalized.

Life Style Drugs—Drugs designed to improve the quality of life or extend the normal life span, and generally do not treat a life-threatening disease. These may include drugs that would successfully restore or improve sexual potency, restore hair growth, allow acute treatment to prevent conception (so-called morning-after pill), or reverse the effects of aging.

Lives—Refers to the number of lives, or people, or members of a health plan or Pharmacy Benefit Manager (PBM) that are eligible for coverage or benefits. Includes both subscribers and dependents. *See also Plan Member.*

Long-Term Care—Services ordinarily provided in a skilled nursing, intermediate-care, personal-care, supervisory-care, or eldercare facility.

M

MAC—*See Maximum Allowable Cost.*

Mail-Service Drug Program—A growing number of Health Maintenance Organizations (HMOs) and Pharmacy Benefit Management (PBM) companies affiliated with corporations or federal contracts use mail-service drug programs to ensure their members have timely access to discount rate drugs.

Managed Behavioral Health Organization (MBHO)—An organization that provides behavioral health services by implementing managed care techniques.

Managed Care Organization (MCO)—A generic term applied to a managed care plan; also called Health Maintenance Organization (HMO), Preferred Provider Organization (PPO), Exclusive Provider Organization (EPO), although the MCO may not conform exactly to any of these formats.

Managed Competition—One type of health care reform that may correct the inequalities of the healthcare delivery system through increased competition. Health plans compete on the basis of cost and other factors; healthcare purchasers have information at their disposal that allows them to compare competing health plans across several dimensions of performance. Purchasers then choose a plan using the comparative data.

Managed Health Care—The sector of health insurance in which healthcare providers are not independent businesses run by, for example, the private practitioner, but by administrative firms that manage the allocation of healthcare benefits. In contrast with conventional indemnity insurers, which did not govern the provision of medical services and simply pay for them, managed care firms have a significant say in how the services are administered so that they may better control healthcare costs. Health Maintenance Organizations (HMOs) and Preferred Provider Organizations (PPOs) are examples of managed care organizations.

Management Service Organization (MSO)—A form of integrated health delivery system. An MSO purchases certain hard assets of a physician's practice and then provides services to that physician at fair market rates. Usually formed as a means to contract more effectively with a managed care organization. The MSO does not need to be a hospital. Also called physician practice management or physician management corporation.

Mandatory Generic Substitution—A pharmacy benefit management tool that mandates the use of a generic equivalent drug product whenever one is available. Prescribers must justify the use of a brand-name product over the use of its generic equivalent.

Manual Rating—*See Rating, Manual Rating.*

Maximum Allowable Cost (MAC)—A cost management program that sets upper limits on the payment for equivalent drugs available from multiple manufacturers. It is the highest unit price that will be paid for a drug and is designed to increase generic dispensing, to ensure the pharmacy dispenses economically, and to control future cost increases.

Maximum Out-of-Pocket Costs—The limit on total member copayments, deductibles, and coinsurance under a benefit contract; sometimes health plans will specify that copays be excluded from consideration.

MBHO—*See Managed Behavioral Health Organization.*

MCO—*See Managed Care Organization.*

Medicaid—An entitlement program of medical aid provided by the federal government and administered at the state level to provide preventive, acute, and long-term benefits with little or no patient cost share, with benefits according to established criteria for the poor, aged, blind and disabled, and aid to dependent children. The federal government matches the states' contribution on a certain minimal level of available coverage. The states may institute additional services, but at their own expense.

Medicaid Prudent Pharmaceutical Purchasing Act (MPPPA)—Enacted as part of the Omnibus Budget Reconciliation Act of 1990 (OBRA '90), MPPPA provides that Medicaid must receive the best discounted price of any institutional purchaser of pharmaceuticals. Thus, drug companies provide rebates to Medicaid that are the difference between the discounted price and the price at which the drug was sold.

Medical Center/Medical Clinic—*See Ambulatory Care Facility.*

Medical Loss Ration (MLR)—The amount of revenues from health insurance premiums that is spent to pay for the medical services covered by the plan. Usually referred to by a ration, such as 0.96—which means that 96% of premiums were spent on purchasing medical services.

Medical Protocols—Medical protocols are the guidelines physicians are asked to follow to achieve an acceptable clinical outcome. The protocol provides the caregiver with specific treatment options or steps to follow when faced with a particular set of clinical symptoms or signs or laboratory data.

Medically Necessary Services—Services or supplies as provided by a physician or other healthcare provider to identify and treat a member's illness or injury, which, as determined by the payor, are consistent with the symptoms, diagnosis, and treatment of the member's condition; in accordance with the standards of good medical practice; not solely for the convenience of the member, member's family, physician, or other healthcare provider; and furnished in the least intensive type of medical care setting required by the member's condition.

Medicare—A national program of health insurance that has been operated by the Centers for Medicare & Medicaid Services (CMS) on behalf of the federal government since its creation by Title XVIII-Health Insurance for the Aged in 1965 as an amendment to the Social Security Act, which provides health insurance benefits primarily to persons over the age of 65 and others who are eligible for Social Security benefits, and covers the cost of hospitalization, medical care, and some related services.

> **Part A**—An insurance program (also called Hospital Insurance program) that provides basic protection against the costs of hospital and related post-hospital services for: individuals age 65 or over and eligible for retirement benefits under the Social Security or Railroad Retirement System. Part A pays for inpatient hospital, skilled nursing facility (SNF), and home health care; the Hospital Insurance program is

financed from a separate trust fund, primarily funded with a payroll tax levied on employers, employees, and the self-employed; *see also Medicare*

Part B—The Medicare component that provides benefits to cover the costs of physicians' professional services, whether the services are provided in a hospital, a physician's office, an extended-care facility, a nursing home, or an insured's home.

Part D—The Medicare component that provides benefits to cover the costs of outpatient prescription drugs. Benefits will commence on January 1, 2006, and will be administered through private health plans.

Medicare Advantage—Previously called Medicare+Choice. Legislation in which Medicare expanded the number of eligible private and public entity risk contractors, as part of the Balanced Budget Act of 1997 in which current Health Maintenance Organizations (HMOs) and competitive medical plans (CMPs) are automatically transitioned but must comply with new rules, while Provider-Sponsored Organizations (PSOs) also are allowed to accept Medicare risk. Applications to become a Medicare+Choice demonstration site first began in 1995 as a way to encourage metropolitan areas with high numbers of Medicare eligibles, yet low percentages of Medicare HMO penetration, to develop new HMO constructs (and to test the receptivity of beneficiaries to enroll in a broad range of options) to help reduce healthcare costs. Medicare+Choice plans must be state licensed as risk-bearing entities except those PSOs that obtain three-year federal waivers from state licensure.

Medicare+Choice—*See Medicare Advantage.*

Medicare Plus—the name given to one draft alternative to traditional Medicare, which was outlined in the Medicare Preservation Act of November 1995 and also in the congressional budget reconciliation bill (H.R. 2491), featuring the beneficiary's choice of any plan available where they live, to include fee-for-service (FFS), coordinated care through Health Maintenance Organizations (HMOs), Preferred Provider Organizations (PPOs), Point of Service (POS) plans, and Provider Services Networks (PSNs), a $6,000 deductible plan with a medical savings account, union or association plans; the congressional budget office predicted savings of $27 billion if 24% of eligible persons enrolled by 2002.

Medicare Risk—Generic name give to either the product or classification of managed care delivery in support of any of the Centers for Medicare & Medicaid Services (CMS)-sponsored programs that involve an element of risk, providing care for members age 65 and older; a Medicare managed care contracting basis used in contrast to the previous fee-for-service (FFS) cost contracting.

Medicare SELECT—A Medicare supplement that uses a preferred provider organization to supplement Medicare Part B coverage.

Medigap—Insurance provided by carriers to supplement the money reimbursed by Medicare for medical services. Since Medicare pays physicians for services according to their own fee schedule, regardless of what the physician charges, the individual may be required to pay the physician the difference between Medicare's reimbursable charge and the physician's fee. Medigap is meant to fill this gap in reimbursement, so that the Medicare beneficiary is not at risk for the difference. Also referred to as a Medicare Supplement Policy.

Member—A participant in a health plan who makes up the plan's enrollment.

Member Services—The broad range of activities that a managed care organization and its employees undertake to support the delivery of the promised benefits to members and to keep them satisfied with the company.

Mental Health Parity Act (MHPA)—A law that prohibits group health plans from applying more restrictive annual and lifetime limits on coverage for mental illness than for physical illness.

MHPA—*See Mental Health Parity Act.*

MLR—*See Medical Loss Ratio.*

Modified Community Rating—*See Rating, Adjusted Community Rating.*

MPPPA—*See Medicaid Prudent Pharmaceutical Purchasing Act.*

MSO—*See Management Services Organization.*

Multidisciplinary—Representative of all affected healthcare professionals.

N

National Committee for Quality Assurance (NCQA)—Independent, private-sector group that was jointly formed by AMCRA and GHAA in 1979 to promote QA, standards, performance measures, review procedures of Health Maintenance Organizations (HMOs) and similar types of plans, and render an accreditation; NCQA is becoming a hallmark of quality for HMOs and similar types of plans.

National Council for Prescription Drug Programs (NCPDP)—An organization that promotes standardization and efficiency within the third-party prescription drug program industry and provides accurate and reliable information as to third-party prescription drug programs.

National Drug Code (NDC)—A unique 11-digit code given to drugs that identifies the labeler, product, and package size. It is used to identify the medication in prescription drug claims.

NCPDP —*See National Council for Prescription Drug Programs.*

NCQA—*See National Committee for Quality Assurance.*

NDC —*See National Drug Code.*

Network—The group of physicians, hospitals, and other medical care professionals that a managed care organization has contracted with to deliver medical services to its members.

Network-Model HMO—*See Health Maintenance Organization, Network Model.*

Non-Formulary Drugs—Drugs not included in the formulary. Health plans that use formularies have policies in place to give physicians and patients access to non-formulary drugs where medically appropriate.

Non-Participating Provider—A term used to describe a provider that has not contracted with the managed care organization to be a participating provider of health care.

O

Off Label Use—The use of a drug for clinical indications other than those stated in the product labeling approved by the Food and Drug Administration (FDA). For example, a drug that has received FDA approval for the treatment of certain types of cancer (ovarian, bladder, breast) may be used to treat another type of cancer (pancreatic).

OOP—*See Out-of-Pocket Costs.*

Open Enrollment—A period during which a managed care organization allows persons not already enrolled to apply for plan membership.

OTC—*See Over-the-Counter Drug.*

Out-of-Pocket (OOP) Costs—The share of health services payments paid by the enrollee.

Outcome—Also called health outcome, or the result of a process of prevention, detection, or treatment; an indicator of the effectiveness of healthcare measures upon patients; *see also Outcomes Measurement.*

Outcomes Management—A clinical outcome is the result of medical or surgical intervention or nonintervention. Managed care is now attempting to better manage the clinical outcomes of their enrollees to increase patient and payer satisfaction while holding down costs. It is thought that a database of outcomes experience will help caregivers see which treatment modalities result in consistently improved outcomes for patients. Outcomes management will, as a natural consequence, lead to medical protocols.

Outcomes Measurement—Method of systematically monitoring a patient's medical or surgical intervention or nonintervention together with the associated responses, including measure of morbidity and functional status; findings from outcomes studies enable managed care entities to outline protocols according to their findings; *see also Outcome.*

Outcomes Research—Studies that evaluate the effect of a given product, procedure, or medical technology on health or costs. Outcomes research information is vital to the development of practice guidelines.

Outlier—One who does not fall within the norm; typically used in utilization. A provider who uses either too many services or too few services (for example, anyone whose utilization differs 2 standard deviations from the mean on a bell curve) is termed an outlier.

Outpatient Care—Treatment that is provided to a patient who is able to return home after care without an overnight stay in a hospital or other inpatient facility.

Over-the-Counter (OTC) Drug—A pharmaceutical that may be sold without federal or state prescription requirements, and may be purchased without a doctor's order; coverage for selected OTC drugs is a benefit option in some plans.

P

P & T Committee—*See Pharmacy and Therapeutics Committee.*

Participating Provider—A healthcare provider who participates through a contractual arrangement with a healthcare service contractor, HMO, PPO, IPA or other managed care organization.

Payer—*See Plan Sponsor.*

PBM—*See Pharmacy Benefit Management Companies.*

PCP—*See Primary Care Physician/Provider.*

Peer Review—A system in which the appropriateness of healthcare services delivered by a provider to health plan members is evaluated by a panel of medical professionals. *See also Professional Review Organization.*

Per Diem Reimbursement—Reimbursement of a institution, usually a hospital, based on a set rate per day rather than on charges. Per diem reimbursement can be varied by service (e.g., medical/surgical, obstetrics, mental health, and intensive care) or can be uniform regardless of intensity of services.

Per Member Per Month—Often used in the context of pharmacy or medical costs; the cost of providing a particular medical service stated as the average cost to provide that service to one member for one month.

Per Member Per Year—The cost of providing a particular medical service stated as the average cost to provide that service to one member for one year.

Performance Measures—Methods or instruments used to estimate or monitor how a healthcare provider's actions conform to criteria and standards of quality.

Pharmaceutical Care—A concept in providing health care defined by Hepler and Strand in 1990; it is a strategy that attempts to utilize drug therapy more efficiently to achieve definite outcomes that improve a patient's quality of life. A pharmaceutical care system requires a reorientation of physicians, pharmacists, and nurses toward effective drug therapy outcomes. It is a set of relationships and decisions through which pharmacists, physicians, nurses, and patients work together to design, implement, and monitor a therapeutic plan that will produce specific therapeutic outcomes.

Pharmacy and Therapeutics (P & T) Committee—An advisory committee that is responsible for developing, managing, updating, and administering the drug formulary system. P & T Committees are comprised of primary care and specialty physicians, pharmacists, and other healthcare professionals. Committees may also include nurses, legal experts, and administrators.

Pharmacy Benefit Design—Contractually specifies the level of coverage and types of pharmaceutical services available to health plan members. A sound pharmacy benefit design balances patient care outcomes, costs, quality, risk management, and provision of the services that beneficiaries expect. The pharmacy benefit design establishes coverage parameters and sets liability limits.

Pharmacy Benefit Management (PBM) Companies—Organizations that manage pharmaceutical benefits for managed care organizations, other medical providers or employers. PBMs contract with clients interested in optimizing the clinical and economic performance of their pharmacy benefit. PBM activities may include some or all of the following: benefit plan design, creation/administration of retail and mail service networks, claims processing and managed prescription drug care services such as drug utilization review, formulary management, generic dispensing, prior authorization and disease and health management.

Pharmacy Carve Out—Within a capitation environment, pharmacy supplies and services are often provided through a carve out from the per member per month (PMPM) or pricing structure for a specified range of coverage; the most competitive regional pharmacy subcontractors, or national pharmacy benefit managers (PBMs), are capable of delivering these requirements at a savings for a commercial population; *see also Pharmacy Benefit Management Companies.*

Pharmacy Services Administrative Organization (PSAO)—An organization that is dedicated to providing prescription benefits to enrollees of managed care plans by using existing community pharmacies. The PSAO contracts as a provider group with the managed care organization so that the individual pharmacies receive negotiating representation in numbers and the prepaid health plan does not have to provide the capital necessary to start, own, and operate its own pharmacy department.

PHO—*See Physician-Hospital Organization.*

Physician Practice Management (PPM) Organization—A variant of a Management Services Organization (MSO), but are physician only—not hospital. For-profit PPMs often purchase physician practices and sign multi-year contracts with physicians. PPM provides management for all support functions.

Physician's Current Procedural Terminology (CPT)—Unique sets of five-digit codes that identify the medical service or procedure performed by physicians and other providers; the system of coding for physicians' services, established by the CPT Editorial Panel of the American Medical Association (AMA), has become the industry coding standard for reporting.

Physician-Hospital Organization (PHO)—A type of integrated healthcare system that in its simplest form is an organization that collectively commits both physicians and the hospital to payer contracts. They sometimes use existing Independent Practice Association (IPA) structures or individual physician contracting. In its most effective form, the PHO must commit the entire physician and hospital panel, without an opt-out, to the PHO organization.

Plan Member—Refers to number of lives, or people, or members of a health plan or Pharmacy Benefit Manager (PBM) that are eligible for coverage or benefits. Includes both subscribers and dependents; *see also Lives*.

Plan Sponsor—The company that assumes financial responsibility for an insured group. A plan sponsor can be an insurance company, third-party administration, or the company itself, if the company is self-insured.

PMPM—*See Per Member Per Month.*

PMPY—*See Per Member Per Year.*

Point of Service HMO—*See Health Maintenance Organization, POS Model.*

Pool—*See Risk Pool.*

POS—Point of sale or point of service. *See Health Maintenance Organization, Point-of-Service Model.*

PPM—*See Physician Practice Management Organization.*

PPO—*See Preferred Provider Organization.*

Practice Guidelines—Also called practice parameters or medical protocols. Physicians may be required to follow these in order to obtain the best clinical outcome. The guideline provides the caregiver with specific treatment options or steps to follow when faced with a particular set of clinical signs or symptoms or laboratory data. The protocols can be very flexible in nature or very rigid. They are designed through an accumulated database of clinical outcomes.

Preadmission Certification—The practice of reviewing claims for hospital admission before the patient actually enters the hospital. This cost-control mechanism is intended to eliminate unnecessary hospital expenses by denying medically unnecessary admissions.

Preferred Provider Organization (PPO)—A managed care organization in which physicians are paid on a fee-for-service (FFS) schedule that is discounted, usually about 10% to 20% below normal fees. PPOs are often formed as a competitive reaction to Health Maintenance Organizations (HMOs) by physicians who contract out with insurance companies, employers, or third-party administrators. A patient can use a physician outside of the PPO providers, but he or she will have to pay a greater portion of the fee.

Preferred Providers—Physicians, hospitals, and other healthcare providers who contract to provide health services to persons covered by a particular health plan.

Preferred Therapeutic Class—A specific drug class or classes selected as the most appropriate for treatment of a particular disease or condition as determined by a Pharmacy and Therapeutics (P & T) Committee or similar entity using the best available scientific evidence.

There is usually a reduced copayment if the patient uses a specific drug from such a class of drugs. For example, the P & T Committee may determine that H2-blocking agents rather than Proton Pump Inhibitors are the most appropriate first-line therapy for Gastro-Esophageal Reflux Disease (GERD).

Premium—The amount paid to a carrier for providing coverage under a contract. Premiums are typically set in coverage classifications such as individual, two-party, and family; employee and dependent unit; employee only, employee and spouse, employee and child, and employee, spouse, and child.

Preventive Care—Health care with an emphasis on prevention, early detection, and early treatment of conditions, generally including routine physical examination, immunization, and wellness care.

Primary Care Physician/Provider (PCP)—Sometimes referred to as a "gatekeeper," the primary care physician is usually the first doctor a patient sees for an illness. This physician then treats the patient directly, refers the patient to a specialist (secondary care), or admits the patient to a hospital when necessary. Often, the primary care physician is a family physician or internist.

Prior Authorization—The process of obtaining certification or authorization from the health plan or pharmacy benefit manager for specified medications or specified quantities of medications. Often involves appropriateness review against pre-established criteria. Failure to obtain prior authorization often results in a financial penalty to the subscriber.

Private-Sector Healthcare Programs—Signifies healthcare companies not directly affiliated with any federal, state, or local government. Normally, they are enterprises that perform services for a profit.

PRO—*See Professional Review Organization.*

Professional Review Organization (PRO)—An organization that reviews the activities and records of a healthcare provider, institution, or group. The reviewer is generally a physician if a physician is the subject of the review; a group of administrators, physicians, and allied healthcare personnel if a hospital is the subject of the review; etc. The PRO can be state sponsored or independent. May also be referred to as a Peer Review Organization.

Prospective Payment—A prospective payment is a payment that is received before care is actually needed. It gives the provider organization a financial incentive to use fewer resources, because they get to keep the difference between what is prepaid and what is actually used.

Provider—Any supplier of services (i.e., physician, pharmacist, case management firm, etc.).

PSAO—*See Pharmacy Services Administrative Organization.*

Pure Community Rating—*See Rating, Standard Community Rating.*

Q

QA—*See Quality Assurance.*

QALY—*See Quality-Adjusted Life-Year.*

QI—*See Quality Improvement.*

QOL—*See Quality of Life.*

Quality-Adjusted Life-Year (QALY)—This unit of measure is one way to quantify health outcomes resulting from some type of intervention. The number of quality-adjusted life-years is the number of years at full health that would be valued equivalently to the number of years of life experienced in a less desirable health state.

Quality Assurance (QA)—Quality assurance or quality assessment is the activity that monitors the level of care being provided by physicians, medical institutions, or any health care vendor in order to ensure that health plan enrollees are receiving the best possible care. The level of care is measured against pre-established standards, some of which are mandated by law.

Quality Improvement (QI)—A continuous process that identifies problems in health care delivery, examines solutions to those problems, and regularly monitors the solutions for improvement.

Quality of Life (QOL)—A patient's perceptions of how they deal with their disease or with their everyday life when suffering from a particular condition. It is subjective because information cannot be measured objectively; however, it has been in the health care literature for at least 20 years.

Quality of Life Measures—An assessment of the patient's perceptions of how they deal with their disease or with their everyday life when suffering from a particular condition. It is subjective in the sense that the kinds of information cannot be measured objectively; however, it has been in the healthcare literature for at least 20 years. It has been used in the area of pharmaceuticals most recently in the last five or six years. Through statistical means, the indices that have been developed to measure various aspects of quality of life have been validated over time, and we know that these measures are reliable and reproducible.

R

Rating—The method that is used to determine the cost of premiums to the members of a managed healthcare or indemnity insurance plan.

> **Adjusted Community Rating**—A rating method under which a health plan or MCO divides its members into classes or groups based on demographic factors such

as geography, family composition, and age, and then charges all members of a class or group the same premium. The plan cannot consider the experience of a class, group, or tier in developing premium rates. Also known as modified community rating.

Blended Rating—For groups with limited recorded claim experience, a method of forecasting a group's cost of benefits based partly on an MCO's manual rates and partly on the group's experience.

Community Rating—A rating method that sets premiums for financing medical care according to the health plan's expected costs of providing medical benefits to the community as a whole rather than to any sub-group within the community. Both low-risk and high-risk classes are factored into community rating, which spreads the expected medical care costs across the entire community.

Experience Rating—A rating method under which an MCO analyzes a group's recorded healthcare costs by type and calculates the group's premium partly or completely according to the group's experience.

Manual Rating—A rating method under which a health plan uses the plan's average experience with all groups—and sometimes the experience of other health plans—rather than a particular group's experience to calculate the group's premium. An MCO often lists manual rates in an underwriting or rating manual.

Modified Community Rating—*See Rating, Adjusted Community Rating.*

Pure Community Rating—*See Rating, Standard Community Rating.*

Standard Community Rating—A type of community rating in which an MCO considers only community-wide data and establishes the same financial performance goals for all risk classes. Also known as pure community rating.

Rebate—A monetary amount that is returned to a payer from a prescription drug manufacturer based on use by a covered person or purchases by a provider.

Referral—The request for additional care, usually of a specialty nature as requested by a primary care physician or another specialist needing additional medical information on behalf of the patient.

Reinsurance—An insurance arrangement whereby the managed care organization or provider is reimbursed by a third-party for costs exceeding a pre-set limit, usually an annual maximum. *See also Stop-Loss Insurance.*

Risk—The change or possibility of loss. For example, physicians may be held at risk if hospitalization rates exceed agreed upon thresholds. The sharing of risk is often employed as a utilization control mechanism within the HMO setting. Risk is also defined in insurance terms as the possibility of loss associated with a given population.

Risk Adjustment—A system of adjusting rates paid to managed care providers to account for the differences in beneficiary demographics, such as age, gender, race, ethnicity, medical condition, geographic location, etc.

Risk Contract—Also known as a Medicare risk contract. A contract between a Health Maintenance Organization (HMO) or competitive medical plan (CMP) and the Centers for Medicare & Medicaid Services (CMS) to provide services to Medicare beneficiaries under which the health plan receives a fixed monthly payment for enrolled Medicare members and then must provide all services on an at-risk basis. This type of contract may be between physicians and an HMO, placing the physician at risk for costs of services provided.

Risk Pool—A defined account (e.g., defined by size, geographic location, claim dollars that exceed a certain level per individual) to which revenue and expenses are posted. A risk pool attempts to define expected claim liabilities of a given defined account as well as required funding to support the claim liability.

S

Screening—The method by which managed care organizations limit access to health care for unnecessary reasons. In most Health Maintenance Organizations (HMOs), a phone call to the physician or his or her medical office staff is required before an office visit can be arranged. "Gatekeepers" and concurrent review are other methods of screening patients.

Self-Funded/Self-Insured—Clients that obtain benefits on a self-funded basis. The company assumes all of the financial risk and liability that would normally be covered by an insurance company.

Shared Risk—An arrangement where any two entities, such as a health plan and a provider, agree to share in the risk to some contracted percentage of hospital or other medical costs that may come in over budget, but also allows the sharing of profits for care provided under budget.

Skilled Nursing Facility (SNF)—Typically an institution for convalescence or a nursing home, the skilled nursing facility provides a high level of specialized care for long-term or acute illnesses. The SNF is an alternative to extended hospital stays or difficult home care.

SNF—*See Skilled Nursing Facility.*

Staff Model HMO—*See Health Maintenance Organization, Staff Model.*

Standard Benefit Package—A set of specific health benefits that are offered by delivery systems.

Standard Community Rating—*See Rating, Standard Community Rating.*

Standard of Care—A diagnostic and treatment process that a clinician should follow for a certain type of patient, illness, or clinical circumstance.

Standards of Quality—Authoritative statement of minimum levels of acceptable performance, excellent levels of performance, or the range of acceptable performance.

Stop-Loss Insurance—A type of insurance coverage that enables provider organizations or self-funded groups to place a dollar limit on their liability for paying claims and requires the insurer issuing the insurance to reimburse the insured organization for claims paid in excess of a specified yearly maximum.

Surgicenter—A separate, free-standing medical facility specializing in outpatient or same-day surgical procedures. Surgicenters drastically reduce the costs associated with hospitalizations for routine surgical procedures because extended inpatient care is not required for specific disorders.

T

Technology Assessment—To evaluate new or existing diagnostic and therapeutic devices and procedures. Technology assessment evaluates the effect of a medical procedure, diagnostic tool, medical device, or pharmaceutical product. In the past, technology assessment meant primarily evaluating new equipment and focused on the clinical safety and efficacy of an intervention. However, in today's health care world, it includes both a broader view of clinical outcome, such as the effect on a patient's quality of life, and the effect on society, such as cost-benefit analysis.

Telemedicine—The ability to use centralized medical expertise to provide care to patients of rural areas, and for centralized physicians to speak and share images with rural doctors through two-way visual and audio networks that allow an electronic house call; telemedicine, such as teleradiology, precludes the rural patient's need for transportation to an urban area to receive care, and reduces other staff or equipment costs in rural areas, servicing nearly a third of today's rural hospitals.

Tertiary Care—Tertiary care is administered at a highly specialized medical center. It is associated with the utilization of high-cost technology resources.

Therapeutic Substitution—Involves the dispensing of a chemically different drug, considered therapeutically equivalent (i.e., will achieve the same outcome) in place of a drug originally prescribed by a physician. The drugs are not generically equivalent. Therapeutic substitutions are done in accordance with procedures and protocols set up and approved by physicians in advance. Therefore, the pharmacist would not have to seek the prescribing physician's approval for each interchange.

Third-Party Administrator (TPA)—Clients who handle the administration of the program for a group or insurance company. The TPA is considered the plan sponsor and is therefore financially responsible.

Third-Party Payer—A public or private organization that pays for or underwrites coverage for healthcare expenses for another entity, usually an employer, such as Blue Cross and Blue Shield, Medicare, Medicaid, or commercial insurers. The individual enrollee generally pays a premium for coverage in all private and some public programs, then the organization pays bills on the patient's behalf, which are called third-party payments; also called third-party carrier.

Tiered Copayment Benefits—A pharmacy benefit design that financially rewards patients for using generic and formulary drugs by requiring the patient to pay progressively higher copayments for brand-name and non-formulary drugs. For example, in a three-tiered benefit structure, copayments may be $5.00 for a generic, $10.00 for a formulary brand product, and $25.00 for a non-formulary brand product.

TPA—*See Third-Party Administrator.*

Triage—The evaluation of patient conditions for urgency and seriousness, and establishment of a priority list for multiple patients. In the setting of managed care, triage is often performed after office hours on the telephone by a nurse or other health professional to screen patients for emergency treatment.

Triple Option—A type of health plan in which employees may choose from a Health Maintenance Organization (HMO), a Preferred Provider Organization (PPO), and an indemnity plan.

U

U&C —*See Usual and Customary Price.*

UCR—*See Usual, Customary and Reasonable.*

UM—*See Utilization Management.*

Underwriter—A reviewer of prospective and renewing cases for appropriate pricing, risk assessment, and administrative feasibility.

Unique Physician Identification Number (UPIN)—A unique identification number assigned to a physician that is used to identify the prescriber on prescription drug claims.

UPIN—*See Unique Physician Identification Number.*

UR—*See Utilization Review.*

Urgent Care Center—A medical facility where ambulatory patients can be treated on a walk-in basis, without an appointment, and receive immediate, non-emergent care. The urgent care center may be open 24 hours a day; patients calling an Health Maintenance Organization (HMO) after hours with urgent, but not emergent, clinical problems are often referred to these facilities.

Usual and Customary (U&C) Price—The amount that a pharmacist would charge a cash-paying customer for a prescription.

Usual, Customary and Reasonable (UCR)—The amount commonly charged for a particular medical service by physicians within a particular geographic region. UCR fees are used by traditional health insurance companies as the basis for physician reimbursement.

Utilization Guidelines—A utilization review resource that indicates accepted approaches to care for common, uncomplicated healthcare services.

Utilization Management (UM)—Managing the use of medical services to ensure that a patient receives necessary, appropriate, high-quality care in a cost-effective manner.

Utilization Review (UR)—Performed by the Health Maintenance Organization (HMO) to discover if a particular physician-provider or other provider (e.g., pharmacy) is spending as much of the HMO's money on treatment or any specific portion thereof (e.g., specialty referral, drug prescribing, hospitalization, radiologic or laboratory services) as his or her peers.

V

VA National Formulary—A drug formulary implemented in 1997 by the Veterans Health Administration (VHA) intended to help control costs and improve quality of prescribing in the VHA's hospitals, ambulatory facilities, nursing homes, and other health care facilities.

Validity—Relationship between the recommended care and the substance and quality of evidence.

Variances—The differences obtained from subtracting actual results from expected or budgeted results.

Vertical Integration—The connecting of dissimilar or other than strictly horizontal entities such as an Health Maintenance Organization (HMO), hospitals, physician practices, Preferred Provider Organization (PPO), or Physician-Hospital Organization (PHO) into one care system from parts that use to exist as a supplier-customer relationship; linked to enhance coordination and value to patient care and support, while aiding proper utilization by the system; may be formed through joint ventures, mergers or acquisitions, new service development, or meaningful affiliations; also called full-service integration. *See also Horizontal Integration.*

W

Wellness Programs—*See Health Promotion Programs.*

Withhold Fund—The portion of the monthly payment to physicians withheld by the HMO until the end of the year or other time period to create an incentive for efficient care. If the physician exceeds utilization norms in comparison with other members of his group or geographic region, he or she loses a percentage of the withhold. The principle of the withhold fund may be applied to hospital services, specialty referrals, laboratory usage, etc.

Workup—The total patient evaluation, which may include laboratory assessments, radiologic series, medical history, and diagnostic procedures.

Workers' Compensation—A state-governed system that addresses work-related injuries. Under this system, employers assume the cost of medical treatment and wage losses stemming from a worker's job-related injury. In return, employees give up the right to sue employers.

SOURCES

1. Modified from *Medical Interface-Managed Care A-Z Managed Care Terms.* Published by Medicom International, Inc., Bronxville, NY.
2. Modified from *Managed Care Pharmacy Practice.* RP Navarro and AMCP. Published by Aspen Publishers, Inc., Gaithersburg, Maryland.
3. Modified from *Managed Care at a Glance: Common Terms,* Boston: Tufts Managed Care Institute, 1996.
4. Modified from *Negotiating Successful Managed Care Contracts,* Bruce W. Clark, *Healthcare Financial Management* (August 1995). Copyright 1995 by the Healthcare Financial Management Association.
5. Other public sources

INDEX